Timeline for Application/Admission

This should be considered a general guide for applicants. It is important that an app[...]
medical school consult with his or her pre-health advisor to devise a schedule that w[...]

COLLEGE YEAR 1	• **Fall semester** o Meet pre-health advisor and investigate pre-health advisory program[...] o As applicable, ensure that pre-health advisor receives course directors' evaluations o Successfully complete first-semester required premedical coursework and other degree requirements • **Spring semester** o Visit "Considering a Career in Medicine" Web site at *www.aamc.org/students* o Identify summer employment/volunteer medically related opportunities o Successfully complete second-semester required premedical coursework and other degree requirements o Ensure that pre-health advisor receives course directors' evaluations
SUMMER 1	• Complete summer employment/volunteer medically related experience • Attend summer school, if desired or necessary
COLLEGE YEAR 2	• **Fall semester** o Check in with pre-health advisor and participate in pre-health activities o Investigate available volunteer/paid medically related clinical or research activities o Successfully complete first-semester required premedical coursework and other degree requirements o Ensure that pre-health advisor receives course directors' evaluations • **Spring semester** o Check in with pre-health advisor and participate in pre-health activities o Participate in volunteer/paid medically related clinical or research activities o Identify summer employment/volunteer medically related opportunities o Successfully complete second-semester required premedical coursework and other degree requirements o Ensure that pre-health advisor receives course directors' evaluations
SUMMER 2	• Complete summer employment/volunteer medically related experience • Participate in a summer health careers program, if available • Attend summer school, if desired or necessary

COLLEGE YEAR 3	• **Fall semester**
	o Check in with pre-health advisor and participate in pre-health activities
	o Continue participation in volunteer/paid medically related activities
	o Investigate:
	  • Medical education options in MSAR and *www.aamc.org/members/listings/msalphaae.htm*
	  • Medical College Admission Test (MCAT®) Web site *www.aamc.org/mcat*
	  • Information about the Medical College Admission Test (MCAT®) and American Medical College Application Service (AMCAS) fee assistance on the AAMC Fee Assistance Program Web site *www.aamc.org/fap*, as appropriate
	  • AAMC's "Applying to Medical School" Web site *www.aamc.org/students/applying/start.htm*
	  • As applicable, information for students from groups underrepresented in medicine on the AAMC Minorities in Medicine Web site *www.aamc.org/students/minorities/start.htm*
	o Begin preparation and register for desired MCAT® administration; visit MCAT® web site *www.aamc.org/mcat* for available test date options
	o Successfully complete first-semester required premedical coursework and other degree requirements
	o Ensure that pre-health advisor receives course directors' evaluations
	• **Spring semester**
	o Consult regularly with pre-health advisor regarding:
	  • Schedule for completion of school-specific requirements for advisor/committee evaluation
	  • Advice about medical education options
	o Continue participation in volunteer/paid medically related activities
	o Prepare for and take desired MCAT® administration; visit MCAT® web site *www.aamc.org/mcat* for available test date options

continued...

continued from page one

COLLEGE YEAR 3	o Continue review of medical education options
	o Take desired MCAT® administration. Registration opens for summer MCAT® administrations
	o Investigate information about medical school application services:
	  • the American Medical College Application Service (AMCAS) on the AMCAS Web site *www.aamc.org/amcas*
	  • the Texas Medical and Dental Schools Application Service (TMDSAS) on the TMDSAS Web site *www.utsystem.edu/tmdsas/*
	  • the Ontario Medical School Application Service (OMSAS) on the OMSAS Web site *www.ouac.on.ca/*
	  • the American Association of Colleges of Osteopathic Medicine Application Service (AACOMAS) on the AACOMAS Web site *https://aacomas.aacom.org/*
	o Investigate as applicable, the AAMC Curriculum Directory Web site *http://services.aamc.org/currdir* for information about medical school curricula and joint, dual, and combined-degree programs
	o Successfully complete second-semester required premedical coursework and other degree requirements
	o Ensure that pre-health advisor receives course directors' evaluations

SUMMER 3	• Participate in a summer health careers program, if available
	• Complete AMCAS application
	• Take desired MCAT® administration
	• Attend summer school, if desired or necessary
	• Become familiar with:
	  o AAMC Recommendations for Medical School Applicants document *www.aamc.org/students/applying/policies*
	  o AAMC Recommendations for Medical School Admission Officers document *www.aamc.org/students/applying/policies*

COLLEGE YEAR 4	• **Fall semester**
	  o Complete supplementary application materials for schools applied to
	  o Consult regularly with pre-health advisor regarding:
	    • Completion of school-specific requirements for advisor/committee evaluation
	    • Status of application/admission process at medical schools applied to
	  o Continue participation in volunteer/paid medically related activities
	  o Interview at medical schools
	  o Continue review of medical education options
	  o Investigate:
	    ■ Financial aid planning process process
	    ■ Financial aid forms required by school of interest with the AAMC *Financial Aid Forms Required by Medical Schools* searchable database *http://services.aamc.org/msar_reports/*
	  o Successfully complete first-semester elective science and non-science coursework and other degree requirements
	  o Ensure that pre-health advisor receives course directors' evaluations
	• **Spring semester**
	  o Make interim and final decisions about medical school choice
	  o Immediately notify medical schools which you will not be attending
	  o Ensure that all IRS forms are submitted as early as possible for financial aid consideration
	  o Successfully complete second-semester elective science and non-science coursework and other degree requirements
	  o Graduate

SUMMER 4	o Prepare for medical school enrollment: purchase books and equipment and make appropriate living arrangements o Relax and prepare for medical school o Attend orientation programs and matriculate at medical school

AAMC
Tomorrow's Doctors, Tomorrow's Cures®

Medical School Admission Requirements (MSAR™)

The Most Authoritative Guide to U.S. and Canadian Medical Schools

2010–2011

Includes Newly-Accredited Medical Schools:

- The Commonwealth Medical College
- Florida International University College of Medicine
- San Juan Bautista School of Medicine
- Texas Tech El Paso Foster School of Medicine
- University of Central Florida College of Medicine

Association of
American Medical Colleges

Medical School Admission Requirements, 2010–2011, United States and Canada

AAMC Staff

MSAR Guide Program Staff

Tami Levin,
Senior Web and Technology Specialist
Academic Affairs

Kim Reed,
Web and MSAR Content Specialist
Academic Affairs

Content Specialist
Henry M. Sondheimer, M.D.,
Senior Director,
Student Affairs and Programs
Academic Affairs

Consultants
Stephen Fitzpatrick,
Program Director, AMCAS
Mission Support

Susan Gaillard,
Database Specialist
Mission Support

Gwen Garrison, Ph.D.,
Director, Student and Applicant Studies
Mission Support

Lily May Johnson,
Manager, Constituent Diversity Services
Office of the Executive Vice President

Jack Krakower,
Senior Director, Med School Financial
and Administrative Affairs
Mission Support

H. Collins Mikesell,
Senior Research Analyst
Mission Support

Karen Mitchell,
Senior Director,
Admissions Testing Services
Mission Support

Nancy-Pat Weaver,
Senior Education Debt Management
Specialist
Academic Affairs

Shelley Yerman,
Senior Specialist, Student Financial Aid
Academic Affairs

To order additional copies of this publication, please contact:
Association of American
Medical Colleges
Publications Department
2450 N Street, NW
Washington, DC 20037
Phone: 202-828-0416
Fax: 202-828-1123
E-mail: *publications@aamc.org*
Web site: *www.aamc.org/publications*

Price: $25.00, plus $8 shipping
(single copy)
Copyright 2009 by the Association of American Medical Colleges.

ISBN 978-1-57754-077-9

Printed in the United States of America

Revised annually; new edition available in early spring.

Group on Student Affairs (GSA) Steering Committee, 2009–2010

Chair
Molly Osborne, M.D., Ph.D.
Associate Dean for Student Affairs
Oregon Health & Science University
School of Medicine

Chair Elect
Michael G. Kavan, Ph.D.
Associate Dean for Student Affairs
Creighton University School of Medicine

Vice Chair
Maureen J. Garrity, Ph.D.
Associate Dean for Student Affairs
University of Colorado School of Medicine

Immediate Past Chair
Georgette Dent, M.D.
University of North Carolina
School of Medicine

Chair, GSA-Minority Affairs Section
Cynthia E. Boyd, M.D.
Associate Vice President and Director,
Medical Staff Operations
Rush Medical College of Rush
University Medical Center

Chair, Central Region
Linda Bissell
Director of Financial Services
University of Iowa
Roy J. and Lucille A. Carver
College of Medicine

Chair, Western Region
Neil H. Parker, M.D.
Senior Associate Dean for Education
and Student Affairs, and GME
University of California Los Angeles
David Geffen School of Medicine

Chair, Southern Region
Marc J. Kahn, M.D.
Senior Associate Dean for Admissions
and Student Affairs
Tulane University School of Medicine

Chair, Northeast Region
Lori Alvord, M.D.
Associate Dean, Student
and Minority Affairs
Dartmouth Medical School

Chair, Committee on Admissions
Robert Witzburg, M.D.
Associate Dean and Director of
Admissions
Boston University School of Medicine

Chair, Committee on Student Affairs
Samuel K. Parrish, M.D.
Associate Dean for Student Affairs
Drexel University School of Medicine

Chair, Committee on Student Financial Assistance
Carrie Steere-Salazar
Director, Student Financial Services
University of California, San Francisco
School of Medicine

Chair, Committee on Student Records
Karen Lewis
Assistant Vice President for Enrollment
Management Student Services and
Registrar
Meharry Medical College

Council of Deans Liaison
Jay Perman, M.D.
Dean, College of Medicine
Vice President for Clinical Affairs
University of Kentucky
School of Medicine

Chair, Organization of Student Representatives
Matthew Rudy
Medical College of Georgia

National Association of Advisors for the Health Professions
Jeremiah L. Putnam, Ph.D.
Chief Health Professions Advisor
Davidson College

Association of American Medical Colleges

The Association of American Medical Colleges (AAMC) has as its purpose the advancement of medical education and the nation's health. In pursuing this purpose, the Association works with many national and international organizations, institutions, and individuals interested in strengthening the quality of medical education at all levels, searching for biomedical knowledge, and applying these tools to providing effective health care.

As an educational association representing members with similar purposes, the primary role of the AAMC is to assist those members by providing services at the national level that will facilitate the accomplishment of their missions. Such activities include collecting data and conducting studies on issues of major concern, evaluating the quality of educational programs through the accreditation process, providing consultation and technical assistance to institutions as needs are identified, synthesizing the opinions of an informed membership for consideration at the national level, and improving communication among those concerned with medical education and the nation's health. Other activities of the Association reflect the expressed concerns and priorities of the officers and governing bodies.

The Association of American Medical Colleges is a not-for-profit association representing all 130 accredited U.S. and 17 accredited Canadian medical schools; nearly 400 major teaching hospitals and health systems, including 68 Department of Veterans Affairs medical centers; and nearly 90 academic and scientific societies. Through these institutions and organizations, the AAMC represents 125,000 faculty members, 70,000 medical students, and 104,000 resident physicians.

In addition to the activities listed above, the AAMC is responsible for the Medical College Admission Test (MCAT®) and the American Medical College Application Service (AMCAS®) and provides detailed admissions information to the medical schools and to undergraduate premedical advisors.

Important Notice

The information in this book is based on the most recent data provided by member medical schools prior to publication at the request of the Association of American Medical Colleges (AAMC).

This material has been edited and in some instances condensed to meet space limitations. In compiling this edition, the AAMC made every reasonable effort to assure the accuracy and timeliness of the information, and, except where noted, the information was updated as of January 2009. All information contained herein, however, especially figures on tuition and expenses, is subject to change and is non-binding for medical schools listed or the AAMC. All medical schools listed in this edition, as with other educational institutions, are also subject to federal and state laws prohibiting discrimination on the basis of race, color, religion, sex, age, handicap, or national origin. Such laws include Title VI of the Civil Rights Act of 1964, Title IX of the Education Amendments of 1972, Section 504 of the Rehabilitation Act of 1973, the Americans with Disabilities Act, and the Age Discrimination Act of 1975, as amended. For the most current and complete information regarding costs, official policies, procedures, and other matters, individual schools should be contacted.

In applying to U.S. or Canadian medical schools, applicants need not go through any commercial agencies. The AAMC does not endorse any organization or entity that purports to assist applicants to achieve admission to medical school other than undergraduate pre-medical advisors and medical school admissions officers.

All URLs in this book can be found at *www.aamc.org/msar.*

AAMC Commitment to Diversity

Diversity within medical education and the physician workforce is essential to the health of the nation. The benefits of diversity in medicine will continue to increase as the nation ages, becomes more diverse along many dimensions, and experiences inequities in health care. The AAMC's commitment to diversity in medicine and biomedical research spans more than three decades and is demonstrated by ongoing leadership and engagement in activities that promote diversity through programs, advocacy, and research. This commitment has been reaffirmed in the publication, Learn, Serve, Lead: The Mission, Vision, and Strategic Priorities of the AAMC, which states that the AAMC's mission is to serve and lead the academic medicine community to improve the health of all. To support its mission, AAMC's vision and that of its members is, in part, to establish "…a healthy nation and world in which… [t]he nation's medical students, biomedical graduate students, residents, fellows, faculty, and the health care workforce are diverse and culturally competent…." As a result, leading efforts to increase diversity in medicine is among the AAMC's nine strategic priorities.

To achieve this end, the AAMC works with its members to:

- advance diversity in academic medicine and biomedical research that fully embraces the diversity of the nation;

- generate and coordinate research, collect evidence, and disseminate studies pertinent to diversity in academic medicine and biomedical research;

- lead policy and advocacy efforts for diversity in academic medicine and biomedical research;

- direct pipeline programs and services across the education continuum to increase diversity in academic medicine and biomedical research;

- communicate the relationship of diversity in medicine and biomedical research to ameliorating disparities in health and health access outcomes; and

- supply resources and guidance to educators seeking to maximize the benefits of diversity across the medical education continuum.

Contents

List of Tables and Charts

Alphabetical Listing of Medical Schools

Geographical Listing of Medical Schools

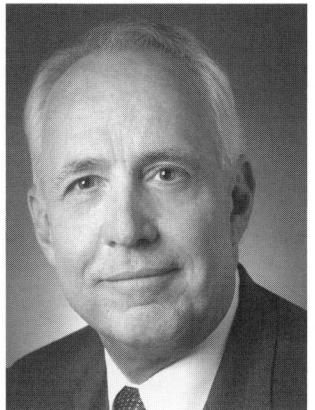

Maybe it was the great feeling you had from volunteering, or the profound concern stirred by a family member's illness that made you think about becoming a doctor. Or, perhaps it was the thrill you experienced in solving a complex research problem that inspired you to dream about finding the next "big cure." Whatever reason led you to consider a career in medicine, you have come to the right place: the Medical School Admissions Requirements (MSAR™).

Published annually by the Association of American Medical Colleges (AAMC)—the national association representing all 130 accredited U.S. and 17 accredited Canadian medical schools—the MSAR is the only medical school application guide authorized by the schools themselves. As you page through it, you will learn about each school's focus, mission, and curriculum, as well as its entrance requirements and selection factors.

You also will find details about financial aid and costs, and see the degree of diversity represented by 2008–09 matriculants. And, in what I think is one of the MSAR Guide's best features, you will see that diversity reflected in the number of accepted applicants at each school who took certain premed courses, performed community service, or worked in research or other medically related positions. In other words, you will read about students who, only a few years ago, went through the same decision-making process you are undertaking now.

Should you decide to apply to medical school, I think you will find it is an extraordinary time to be a doctor. You will be entering medicine at a time when the country needs your services most, given predicted physician shortages in coming years, and when national attention is sharply focused on the need of all Americans for access to high-quality, affordable care. It is also a time when our profession is undergoing an exciting period of transformative change, with clinical care becoming increasingly patient-centered and team-based, biomedical research more technically sophisticated and collaborative, and medical education itself evolving into a continuum of lifelong learning.

Whatever career you decide to pursue, please accept my best wishes for success. And, if being a doctor is the path you choose, please know that the AAMC stands ready to help you. It would be a special pleasure for me if—during your education and training—our paths should cross and we have the opportunity to meet.

Darrell G. Kirch

Darrell G. Kirch, M.D.
President and CEO
Association of American Medical Colleges

Organization of Student Representatives 2009–2010

A philosopher once said, "A journey of a thousand miles begins with a single step." Undoubtedly, you have already taken many steps along the road to medical school. As you take this next step toward a career in medicine, this book will serve as a trustworthy roadmap and guide. Medical School Admission Requirements (MSAR™) will provide you with current information of interest for each U.S. and Canadian medical school.

As Chair of the AAMC Organization of Student Representatives (OSR), which is charged with expressing the voice and perspective of 70,000 medical students enrolled in 130 Liaison Committee on Medical Education (LCME)-accredited medical schools in the United States, I would like to congratulate you on the steps that you have already taken and welcome you on the road toward an exciting and rewarding career in medicine.

The mission of the medical education system is to serve the public by educating and training a diverse physician workforce to be engaged in a variety of healthcare functions: clinical medicine, public health, biomedical and health services research, and medical education. In addition, there is a need for physicians who can contribute to the fields of public policy, law, ethics, business, and journalism. We are training in a time of great change, not only in our technical and scientific capabilities but also in the system in which we practice. Opportunities abound within the medical field and are limited only by your imagination and ideals as a medical professional. As the future of medicine unfolds before our eyes, the field is in need of dedicated innovators to lead health care into the next generation. Now is the perfect time to begin considering what your ideals for the future of this profession are and how you would like to play a role in shaping it.

The medical school application process is a challenge in its own right. The demands of time, attention, and finances should not deter you from your ultimate goals, nor should the opinions of others who say it cannot be done. Many resources are available to help with any challenges you might face, such as support for those in need of financial assistance and counseling for those in need of direction. I cannot overemphasize the fact that a career in medicine is available to applicants from all types of backgrounds with all sorts of goals.

As you prepare to apply to medical school, consider your choices broadly and carefully, as each medical school will provide you with unique learning and life experiences. Consult many resources, including your mentors, advisors, and peers, as well as medical school faculty and medical students. Most importantly, do not underestimate the support and encouragement offered by family and friends. Utilize your medical school interviews to explore the academic and extracurricular opportunities offered at each prospective institution; these are experiences that will enrich your life for years to come.

You have chosen to pursue a fulfilling and important career dedicated to relieving human suffering and improving humanity's health and well-being. I wish you great success on your journey and congratulate you on these first steps toward becoming a doctor.

Matthew Paul Rudy
Medical Student
Medical College of Georgia
2008–2009 Chair, AAMC Organization of Student Representatives

Chapter 1

Medicine as a Career

For those interested in a career in medicine, the choices are almost limitless.

From clinical practice to medical administration, to public health, to military medicine, to medical education, to community health, to biomedical research — medicine is an inclusive profession that offers incredibly varied opportunities to its physician ranks. Ideally, all physicians aspire to be:

- altruistic, compassionate, trustworthy, and truthful in their relationships with patients, patients' family members, and professional colleagues. They understand the history of medicine, medicine's compact with society, their ethical responsibilities as physicians, and their obligations under the law. They act with integrity and honesty; they respect patients' privacy and dignity. They seek to understand the meaning of patients' stories in the context of patients' beliefs and family and cultural values. They avoid being judgmental when patients' beliefs and values conflict with their own. They continue to care for dying patients even when disease-specific therapy is no longer available or desired.

- knowledgeable about the scientific basis of medicine and the normal and abnormal functioning of the body. They have sufficient knowledge of the structure and function of the body, its major organ systems, and the molecular, cellular, and biochemical mechanisms that maintain the body's homeostasis in order to comprehend disease and incorporate modern diagnostic and therapeutic modalities in their practices. They engage in lifelong learning to remain current in their understanding of the scientific bases of medicine.

- skillful in communicating with and providing care to their patients. They obtain from patients an accurate medical history that includes all relevant information, and they perform skillfully a physical examination and those diagnostic procedures warranted by their patients' conditions. They obtain, interpret properly, and manage information from those studies relating to the patients' conditions, and they seek consultation from other physicians and health professionals, when indicated. They understand the etiology, pathogenesis, and various manifestations of the diseases and conditions they are likely to confront in the practice of their specialty. They understand the scientific basis and evidence of effectiveness for each of the therapeutic options available for patients at different times in the course of their conditions, and discuss those options with patients in an honest and objective fashion. They communicate with patients and their families about their concerns regarding the patients' health and well-being. They are sufficiently knowledgeable about both traditional and non-traditional modes of care to provide intelligent guidance to their patients.

- dutiful in working with other physicians and health care professionals to promote the health of individual patients and all community members. They are well-informed about risk factors for disease and injury; they understand disease and injury prevention practices. They promote healthy behaviors through counseling individual patients and their families and public education and action; they actively support traditional public health practices in their communities. They advocate for improving access to care for everyone, especially members of traditionally underserved populations. They understand the economic, psychological, occupational, social, and cultural factors contributing to the development and/or perpetuation of conditions that impair health. They apply principles of evidence-based medicine and cost-effectiveness in making decisions about the utilization of limited medical resources. They collaborate with other physicians, other health care professionals, and individuals representing a wide variety of community agencies. As members of a team addressing individual or population-based health care issues, they lead, when appropriate, and defer to the leadership of others, when indicated. They acknowledge and respect the roles of other health professionals in providing needed services to individual patients, populations, or communities.

Which Path Is Right for You?

Men and women bring to the profession of medicine a broad range of personal interests, educational backgrounds, and occupational histories, as well as unique sets of skills, abilities, experiences, and philosophies. Aspiring physicians seek to achieve lofty, but attainable professional goals in a variety of specialties and clinical settings:

- The satisfaction of enduring patient relationships is one attraction of family medicine or internal medicine, where the "art" of medicine flourishes in each encounter with every patient. Others with a commitment to social justice and the well-being of a community, and an interest in fulfilling the health care needs of the underserved and disadvantaged, can meet these challenges in urban and rural clinics, in community medicine and public health, or as medical missionaries.

- An interest in scientific investigation and the desire to expand the boundaries of medical knowledge are traits of those in the nation's private and public laboratories and research institutions. Physicians interested in communicating their colleagues' laboratory-derived discoveries and interpreting their impact on society

enjoy their roles as medical editors, journalists, or experts in medical ethics.

- Careers in general surgery often suit those physicians with a desire for direct feedback about the results of their interventions. Plastic and reconstructive surgery draws others with artistic skills, excellent eye-hand coordination, and aesthetic interests.

- Those interested in mind-body interactions and the emotional lives of their patients might find a home in neurology or psychiatry. Others interested in national defense or the challenges inherent in emergency situations use their skills as flight surgeons or in aerospace or military medicine.

- The economic and public policy aspects of health care guide some physicians to lead think tanks and health-related associations and organizations, as well as to serve in the legislative and executive branches of government. The more visceral aspects of medicine draw some to work with crime and accident victims as emergency medicine physicians or trauma surgeons; others work in orthopedic surgery with patients who have bone, joint, or other musculoskeletal problems.

- For those fascinated by the issues facing groups of patients with age-defined illnesses and problems — from the risks of infancy and early childhood to the challenges of later life — fulfillment can come as pediatricians and geriatricians. Others prefer to pursue detailed knowledge about the intricacies of a single body organ or system, such as that required of ophthalmologists, dermatologists, or neurosurgeons.

- Assisting patients in overcoming complex fertility and gestational problems is the hallmark of the specialties of reproductive endocrinology and obstetrics and gynecology. Those with a long-range interest in reducing the incidence of birth defects and inherited syndromes might find their calling in the field of medical genetics.

- The detection, prevention, and eradication of injury and disease in groups and populations, both in this country and abroad, draw people to preventive medicine and epidemiology at such organizations as the Centers for Disease Control and Prevention or the World Health Organization. Those same interests at the local level can be fulfilled in forensic pathology, coroners' and medical examiners' offices, and state or county health departments.

The possibilities in medicine are almost endless. No matter what your personal interests, skills, or needs may be, medicine encourages and permits you to find your individual niche. Should your interests, abilities, or needs change with time and experience, medicine — because of its emphasis on lifelong learning and its periodic requirements for demonstrating competence — affords ongoing opportunities for refining your skills and reorienting your practice.

Career Guidance and Decision-Making

Medical schools recognize the critical role they play in helping medical students to assess their personal values and interests, identify career options, determine their personal "fit" with those options, and make well-informed decisions about specialty choice. This recognition is reflected in the Careers in Medicine™ program, created by the AAMC in collaboration with its 130 member medical schools. The four-phase career decision-making format used in this program is similar to that used by premedical students in deciding on medicine as a career, and in deciding which medical schools would be an appropriate match.

In Phase 1 of Careers in Medicine, Understanding Yourself, medical students explore who they are, what activities they enjoy, the values that underlie their lives and work, and the nature of their relationships with other people. During Phase 2, Exploring Options, tools are provided for exploring specialties and other career options. Phase 3, Choosing a Specialty, focuses on comparing the personal information obtained in Phase 1 with the specialty and career options garnered in Phase 2. Finally, in Phase 4, Getting into Residency, plans are laid for application to residency training programs and related activities, such as completing personal statements and interviews.

The process of career-planning and decision-making is dynamic and ongoing. Consider familiarizing yourself with the Careers in Medicine program at *www.aamc.org/careersinmedicine* as you work on plans for application to medical school and a medical education.

Combined, Dual, and Joint Degree Programs

The U.S. medical education system is designed to support the process of identifying and attaining your place in medicine. During both the four years of medical school — known as undergraduate medical education — and in the residency and fellowship training that follows (graduate medical education), opportunities abound for specialized education and training. At medical schools and residency training programs across the country, students and residents are enrolled in combined, dual, and joint degree programs that prepare them well for future careers. Federally funded Medical Scientist Training Programs (MSTPs) assist students in obtaining both the M.D. and Ph.D. degrees in areas related to medical research, and in working with mentors to prepare for careers as academic physicians and physician-scientists (see Chapter 11).

Medical schools on university campuses provide dual M.D./graduate and professional degree programs in a variety of academic disciplines, including the basic sciences, business administration, computer science, education, law, and public health. Graduates of such programs may pursue careers as National Institutes of Health scientists, medical

school faculty members, hospital administrators, health care entrepreneurs, medical informatics and diagnostic experts, or forensic scientists and medical examiners; they also become authorities in epidemiology, public health, and community and preventive medicine.

Information about combined college/M.D. programs for high school students can be found in Chapter 10 and on the AAMC Curriculum Directory Web site at *http://services.aamc.org/currdir*. Information about combined, dual, and joint M.D./graduate and professional degree programs (e.g., M.Ed., M.P.H., J.D., M.B.A., and various Ph.D. specializations) can be found in a database that is searchable by school and program type, also accessible at the AAMC Curriculum Directory Web site. The information in the Curriculum Directory is provided, and periodically updated, by medical school personnel through the AAMC Curriculum Management and Information Tool (CurrMIT).

Characteristics of U.S. and Canadian Medical Schools

The missions of the 130 accredited U.S. and 17 accredited Canadian allopathic medical schools vary as widely as the motivations of individual medical students. (Allopathic medical schools grant the M.D. degree, while osteopathic medical schools grant the D.O. degree.) Each U.S. medical school is periodically required to document that it has met strict accreditation standards set by the Liaison Committee on Medical Education (LCME, *www.lcme.org*), the joint accrediting body of the American Medical Association (AMA, *www.ama-assn.org*), located in Chicago, and the AAMC (*www.aamc.org*), located in Washington, D.C. Canadian medical schools are jointly accredited by the LCME and the Committee on Accreditation of Canadian Medical Schools of the Association of Faculties of Medicine of Canada (*www.afmc.ca*).

Fundamental elements of medical education are shared by all schools: acquisition of basic science knowledge and elementary clinical skills during the first component of the curriculum, and acquisition of more advanced clinical skills under the supervision of attending physician faculty members during the second component of the curriculum. Medical schools also vary on many important characteristics, including institutional mission, curricular emphasis and structure, class size and applicant pool, cost, ownership, and clinical affiliations.

What Kind of School for You?

As an applicant embarks on the path toward a medical career, consideration of the type of medical school is important. Some medical school curricula emphasize the education and training of primary care physicians, typically meaning general pediatricians, general internists, and family physicians (although obstetrician/gynecologists and others who are the first point of contact for patients are also sometimes included). Some medical schools emphasize the education and training of physicians who will serve the needs of rural patients. Still other schools emphasize the acquisition of research skills and provide opportunities for investigative activities on the part of medical students, with their graduates going on to careers in academic medicine and basic and clinical research. Some schools were founded by state legislatures with a curricular emphasis on the needs of a particular patient population, such as older patients.

Many medical schools provide educational opportunities at multiple branch and regional campuses. At some schools, students complete their first two years in classrooms and laboratories on a central campus, then disperse to separate clinical campuses to complete core and elective clinical experiences in their final two years. At other institutions, the opposite occurs.

In 2008, the entering class sizes at U.S. medical schools ranged from 50 to 308 students. Applicant pools at U.S. schools also vary greatly. Some public medical schools in smaller states have small pools, with first-year classes selected primarily from state residents. Other private schools select new entrants from national pools of several thousand applicants, with little regard to each applicants' state of legal residence.

In June 2006, the AAMC issued a call for LCME-accredited medical schools to increase their enrollments by 30 percent by 2015, with expansion accomplished by both increasing enrollments in existing schools and establishing new medical schools. This recommendation was based on data suggesting that current medical school enrollments would result in a physician shortage in the United States within the next several decades unless fundamental changes occur in the demand and need for health care and/or the way health care is provided. This recommendation was further supported by data from a growing number of specialty and state-specific studies concluding that shortages exist or will soon exist in particular specialties or states. Additional information about physician workforce projections and the need for more physicians can be found on the AAMC Web site at *www.aamc.org/workforce/*.

Public or Private?

Medical schools generally fall into two categories as a function of their funding sources: public and private. Public medical schools usually receive some of their operating revenue from state or federal governments, while private schools usually generate revenue from other sources, including endowments and tuition. Determining the "real"

annual expense associated with attendance at a state-supported or private medical school can be complex. Tuition and fees at public schools are often less than those at private schools, especially for state residents, because educational costs are underwritten with tax revenues. However, this tuition differential usually disappears for students who are not state residents, and tuition at public medical schools for non-residents often equals that of private institutions. On the other hand, some private medical schools with large endowments are able to provide substantial scholarship aid to qualifying students, thus lowering the "effective tuition" rate significantly and permitting those students to graduate with less educational debt than they would have accumulated if they had attended a public medical school in their state of residence.

Some medical schools, both public and private, own and manage their own hospitals, outpatient facilities, and health care systems. Others, sometimes referred to as community-based schools, establish ongoing affiliations with existing inpatient and ambulatory care facilities in their surrounding communities, where students complete the clinical components of their education under the supervision of faculty members.

While all medical schools were established to educate future physicians, they can differ substantially in their educational programs. This and other information about U.S. and Canadian medical schools is presented in greater detail in the school profile pages that begin on page 112. Complete information can also be found on each school's Web site, links to which can be found on the AAMC Web site at *www.aamc.org/medicalschools*, as well as in institutional academic bulletins, brochures, and related publications.

Chapter 2

The Process of Medical Education

The path to medical practice consists of five phases:

- undergraduate premedical education (college)

- undergraduate medical education (medical school)

- graduate medical education (residency and fellowship training)

- licensure and certification

- continuing medical education

While each of these educational elements is separate and distinct from the others, the successful completion of each component is a building block, laying a strong, broad foundation for the eventual independent practice of medicine.

Undergraduate Premedical Education

For future physicians, college affords opportunities for excelling in the natural sciences, the social sciences, and the humanities; for fostering inquiry and problem-solving abilities; for honing communication and interpersonal skills; and for developing intellectual discipline and time-management skills. College begins to prepare students for the academic and personal rigors of a medical education. There they learn to appreciate the continuum of human experience and to learn from the experiences of others — to recognize the impact of culture and family dynamics on human development and thus to value the uniqueness of the doctor-patient relationship.

Medicine is practiced in a social context. Physicians must be able to communicate effectively with people from a variety of backgrounds and life experiences. Medical school admission committees seek to enroll students who bring diverse talents and interests to medicine; their goal is to identify students whose personal and career aspirations are compatible with society's health care needs, whether coping with the international AIDS epidemic, responding to bioterrorism, natural disasters, or other crises, or caring for persons who are medically underserved or economically disadvantaged.

Undergraduate Medical Education

Curricula at U.S. and Canadian medical schools have common elements, although they vary in educational approaches. All medical schools share the goals of preparing students in the art and science of medicine, and providing them with the background necessary to enter a three- to seven-year-long period of graduate medical education following receipt of the M.D. degree. A significant amount of periodically updated information about medical school curricula and institutional characteristics can be found in the AAMC databases at *http://services.aamc.org/currdir*.

Each medical school's faculty establishes standards for students' academic performance, personal and professional conduct, clinical proficiency, and promotion and graduation. Many schools have developed comprehensive learning objectives for their educational programs, along with detailed descriptions of the means by which students will be assessed at various stages along the educational continuum. Faculty members determine whether students have met curricular learning objectives by requiring them to demonstrate mastery of both course content and clinical skills — through written tests, oral examinations, and laboratory exercises — and by observing and assessing their clinical acumen. Many schools require students to complete local and national standardized examinations before they can progress to further clinical training. The frequency and methods of evaluation vary from school to school. In recent years medical schools have continued to revise their educational programs, moving from more passive approaches to learning to more active ones and from an emphasis on large-group to small-group learning activities. As possible, lecture formats have been systematically replaced with learning opportunities that promote self-assessment, problem-solving, integration of the basic and clinical sciences, and collaboration with faculty and peers. Increasingly, schools are also requiring students to complete year-end and overall comprehensive examinations prior to promotion and graduation.

Grading procedures at medical schools vary. Many schools have pass/fail or honors/pass/fail grading systems, while others use letter grades. Whatever the assessment structure, students' knowledge and skills are carefully scrutinized on a periodic basis by members of the faculty. Increasingly, schools are differentiating the assessment of students' academic achievement from that of their personal and professional behavior, with complementary evaluations during each classroom and clinical experience. In the clinical environment, one-on-one relationships between faculty members and students permit close and ongoing observation and feedback.

At three percent, the rate of attrition at U.S. medical schools is remarkably low. Students who are deficient in certain areas often have opportunities for remediation and assistance. Nevertheless, all medical school faculties reserve the right to dismiss any student whose academic or personal characteristics are incompatible with a physician's professional responsibilities.

The first two years. Initially, students learn those basic sciences essential to the practice of medicine. The normal structure and function of human systems are taught through gross and microscopic anatomy, biochemistry, behavioral science, physiology, and neuroscience.

Subsequently, the educational focus shifts to abnormalities of structure and function, disease, and general therapeutic principles through exposure to microbiology, immunology, pathology, and pharmacology.

Throughout the first two years, the clinical significance of basic science material is continuously stressed.

In addition to the core scientific work, students are exposed to a wide variety of topics:

• nutrition

• medical ethics

• genetics

• laboratory medicine

• health care delivery systems

• substance abuse

• human values

• research

• preventive medicine

• community health

• geriatrics

• human sexuality

Lecture-style teaching no longer dominates the classroom. Small-group learning, multi-disciplinary clinical conferences, peer-to-peer learning, and case-based and problem-based approaches all have a place in the first two years. These experiences can be with actual patients and with people trained to simulate pathological conditions, known as standardized patients. In addition, interdepartmentally inte-

grated courses are being developed at many schools as an alternative to previous discipline or department-based courses.

By the end of these two years, students have learned the scientific underpinnings of medicine. They also have learned the basics of interviewing and obtaining historical data from patients, as well as of conducting physical examinations, interpreting laboratory findings, and considering diagnostic and treatment alternatives. Students are now prepared to make the transition to the clinical environment on a full-time basis.

The second two years. The second period of undergraduate medical education consists of a series of required clinical rotations, or clerkships, usually lasting from 4 to 12 weeks each, during which medical students work with patients and their families in various inpatient and outpatient settings. Here, they function under the supervision of physician faculty members — known as attending physicians — and residents, and collaborate with other members of the clinical team, including nurses, social workers, psychologists, pharmacists, and technical staff. The pattern, length, and number of rotations differ from school to school, but core clinical training usually includes clerkships in internal medicine, obstetrics/gynecology, pediatrics, psychiatry, and surgery. Depending on the school, required clerkships can also include family medicine, primary care, neurology, a community or rural medicine preceptorship, or an acting internship.

During clinical clerkships, students are assigned to an outpatient clinic or inpatient hospital unit where they assume responsibility for "working-up" a number of patients each week; that is, collecting relevant data and information from them and presenting pertinent findings to a faculty member for diagnosis and treatment planning. Students also participate in the ongoing clinical care of patients assigned to the medical team. Ideally, students follow their patients over time, either during hospitalizations or through the course of outpatient treatment. When appropriate, students also relate to patients' family members — providing information, answering questions, and preparing them for the outcome of patients' care.

During these clinical education experiences, students learn to apply their basic science knowledge and clinical skills in diagnosing and treating patients' illnesses and injuries. They learn clinical decision-making and patient management skills. They interact daily with faculty members, whether at the bedside, during inpatient team discussions ("rounds"), on patient visits, or in case-based lectures and small-group discussions.

Electives. Most medical schools provide curricular opportunities to assist students in pursuing special interests through supplemental educational experiences known as electives, which are offered in the basic, behavioral, and clinical sciences, as well as in basic and clinical research. While electives are typically available during the final year of medical school, they may also be available at other times in the curriculum. Students can complete electives on their own campuses, at other medical schools, through federal and state agencies (such as the Institute of Medicine, *www.iom.edu*; the Indian Health Service, *www.ihs.gov*; and the Centers for Disease Control and Prevention, *www.cdc.gov*), in international settings, and through external non-academic service organizations.

Clinical electives include opportunities in the entire range of medical and surgical specialties and subspecialties. Students seek these experiences for several reasons: to acquaint themselves with additional career options, to broaden and enrich their educational experience, and to expose themselves to areas of specialization that are one-time opportunities.

Residency or specialty. During the fourth year of medical school, students choose a medical specialty and apply to graduate medical education programs (residencies) through such services as the Electronic Residency Application Service (ERAS, *www.aamc.org/eras*) and the National Resident Matching Program (NRMP, *www.nrmp.org*). ERAS is an application service that transmits residency applications, letters of recommendation, transcripts, and other supporting credentials from applicants and medical schools to internship, residency, and fellowship programs using the Internet. The NRMP is a Web-based program that matches applicants' preferences for specific residency programs with program directors' preferences for specific applicants.

Graduate Medical Education

The third phase of medical training prepares physicians for independent practice in an area of specialization. Residency programs focus on the acquisition of detailed factual knowledge and the development of clinical skills and professional competencies in a particular specialty. These programs are based in hospitals or other health care institutions and, in most specialties, utilize both inpatient and outpatient settings for teaching purposes. Residency programs are accredited by the Accreditation Council for Graduate Medical Education (ACGME, *www.acgme.org*) and its associated Residency Review Committees. Residents, also known as house officers or house staff, typically complete educational requirements for certification through a specialty board recognized by the American Board of Medical Specialties (ABMS, *www.abms.org*). Information about medical specialties and subspecialties can also be found on the Careers in Medicine Web site at *www.aamc.org/careersinmedicine*.

For medical students who decide to practice in a medical or surgical specialty, the requirements of that specialty's certifying board will influence the choice of the first-postgraduate-year (PGY1) program. Family medicine,

internal medicine, pediatrics, and general surgery encourage students to enter PGY1 programs in that specialty directly, and to continue in these programs until they have completed all specialty board requirements.

Satisfactory completion of three years of training in family practice, internal medicine, or pediatrics or five years of training in general surgery generally qualifies an individual to take the board certification examinations in each of those specialties.

Students seeking careers in other medical or surgical specialties (e.g., dermatology, physical medicine and rehabilitation, radiology) are first exposed to a broad range of clinical experiences during their PGY1 year. Usually these students complete this first residency training clinical year in internal medicine or general surgery or in a diversified "transitional year" program, with the expectation that they will enter a program in the specialty of their choice in the second postgraduate year (PGY2). In some cases, the year of broad clinical exposure may be in the same institution where subsequent subspecialty training occurs. In other instances, specialty training must be completed elsewhere. Education and training in a medical or surgical subspecialty (e.g., cardiology, pulmonology, geriatrics, hematology/ oncology, cardiothoracic surgery) take place for varying periods of time after completion of the appropriate preparatory residency training. These trainees in a medical or surgical subspecialty are sometimes referred to as "fellows."

Licensure and Certification

The fourth phase of medical training involves licensure to practice medicine and certification in a specialty. Medical practice is regulated by each individual state or jurisdiction. Each state has a statute, known as a medical practice act, that describes the practice of medicine and identifies the public agency in the state that has responsibility for licensing physicians and regulating medical practice. These agencies protect the public from potentially unprofessional or incompetent physicians.

All states require applicants for a medical license to document that they have both completed appropriate educational and training programs and achieved passing scores on licensure examinations approved by the relevant state agency or board. In 1990, the Federation of State Medical Boards (FSMB, *www.fsmb.org*) and the National Board of Medical Examiners (NBME, *www.nbme.org*) established the United States Medical Licensing Examination, (USMLE, *www.usmle.org*), a single, three-step licensing examination utilized by all U.S. licensing jurisdictions.

USMLE Step 1 assesses whether the examinee can understand and apply important concepts of the sciences basic to the practice of medicine, with special emphasis on principles and mechanisms underlying health, disease, and modes of therapy. Step 1 ensures mastery of the sciences that provide a foundation for the safe and competent practice of medicine in the present, and the scientific principles required for the maintenance of competence through lifelong learning.

USMLE Step 2 consists of two components: Clinical Knowledge (CK) and Clinical Skills (CS). USMLE Step 2 assesses the examinee's ability to apply medical knowledge, skills, and understanding of clinical science essential for the provision of patient care under supervision, and includes emphasis on health promotion and disease prevention. Step 2 ensures that due attention is devoted to principles of clinical sciences and basic patient-centered skills that provide the foundation for the safe and competent practice of medicine.

USMLE Step 3 assesses whether the examinee can apply medical knowledge and understanding of biomedical and clinical science essential for the unsupervised practice of medicine, with an emphasis on patient management in ambulatory settings. Step 3 provides a final assessment of a physician's ability to assume independent responsibility for delivering general medical care.

In addition to receiving a license from a state medical board, physicians are strongly encouraged to apply voluntarily for certification in a medical or surgical specialty from one of the 24 approved boards of the American Board of Medical Specialties (ABMS, *www.abms.org*). Through comprehensive examinations, these specialty boards determine if candidates have been appropriately prepared in accordance with established educational standards. Those who have satisfied all board requirements are certified and are known as "diplomates" of the specialty board; periodic recertification is offered at intervals of 7 to 10 years. More than 85 percent of licensed physicians in the U.S. have been certified by at least one ABMS member board.

Continuing Medical Education

The fifth and final phase of medical training is continuing medical education, or CME. Physicians continue the educational process in the specific medical specialty in which they completed residency training; CME reflects the commitment to lifelong learning that is a hallmark of the medical profession. By attending CME programs regularly, practicing physicians maintain their clinical competence over time and enhance their knowledge and skills. The Accreditation Council for Continuing Medical Education (ACCME, *www.accme.org*) provides a system of voluntary accreditation for providers of continuing medical education programs.

Chapter 3

Undergraduate Premedical Preparation

During college, the successful premedical student completes several important tasks, including:

- the selection of a personally challenging and appealing major

- the timely completion of all required premedical courses

- the pursuit of advanced coursework in areas of special interest

- the establishment of an ongoing relationship with an informed premedical advisor

- participation in a variety of extra-curricular activities and experiences

- the mastery of both course content and academic skills

- the balancing of intellectual development and social and interpersonal growth

Academic Preparation

Choice of major. Medical schools recognize the importance of a strong foundation in the natural sciences — biology, chemistry, physics, and mathematics — and most schools have established minimum course requirements for admission. These courses usually represent about one-third of the credit hours needed for degree completion. This approach deliberately leaves room for applicants from a broad spectrum of college majors, including those in the humanities and social sciences. No medical school requires a specific major of its applicants or matriculants. Admission committee members are aware that medical students can develop the essential skills of acquiring, synthesizing, applying, and communicating information through a wide variety of academic disciplines.

Nevertheless, many premedical students choose to major in a scientific discipline. Ideally, they do so because they are fascinated by science and perceive that such a major can be the foundation for a variety of career options. Choosing science primarily to enhance one's chances for admission to medical school is not in a student's long-term best interest. Medical school admission committees seek students whose intellectual curiosity leads them to a variety of disciplines and whose intellectual maturity assures that their efforts are persistent and disciplined.

Science preparation. The study and practice of medicine are based on modern concepts in biology, chemistry, and physics, and on an appreciation of the scientific method. Hence, mastery of these basic scientific principles is expected of all entering medical students. Medical schools typically require successful completion of one academic year (two semesters or three quarters) of biology and physics and one academic year each of general chemistry and organic chemistry. Each of these courses should be academically rigorous and acceptable for students majoring in those areas.

All science courses should include adequate laboratory experiences.

Although only a few medical schools require applicants to complete a specific course in mathematics, all schools appreciate mathematical competence as a strong foundation for understanding the basic sciences. In addition, a working knowledge of statistics helps both medical students and physicians to become critical evaluators of the medical literature. Familiarity with computers is helpful during the educational experience, as well as in medical practice. Thus, many medical schools recommend coursework in mathematics, statistics, and computer science.

Upper-level science coursework is not typically required by medical schools. Students may choose to take advanced science courses because of their own interests or undergraduate major requirements. Taking additional science courses that duplicate the basic science content of the first two years of medical school is not recommended. In fact, practicing physicians often recommend that premedical students, during their college years, take advantage of what might be their final opportunity for study in non-science areas (e.g., music, art, history, and literature) that might become the basis for avocational interests later in life. Table 3-A gives an overview of the most common courses required by medical schools.

AP and CLEP credit. Premedical students intending to apply college credit earned through Advanced Placement (AP) and College Level Examination Placement (CLEP) to meet premedical requirements should be aware that some medical schools restrict the use of such credit. In most cases, the restrictions involve the official reporting of AP and CLEP credit on the college transcript, establishing an upper limit of such credit toward courses required for admission, or requiring additional upper-level courses in the science areas where AP or CLEP credit was received. Premedical students should carefully review Chapter 7 and pertinent medical

school Web sites and publications for additional and current information.

Advanced work. Medical schools encourage honors, independent study, and research work by premedical students. These activities demonstrate in-depth, sustained scholarly exploration and the presence of lifelong learning skills that are essential to a career in the medical profession.

Development of Personal Attributes

Academic or scientific accomplishments alone are not sufficient for entry into medical school and the medical profession. Intellectual capacity is obviously important, but it is not sufficient; the most critical aspect of practicing medicine is the physician-patient relationship.

In a publication that outlines learning objectives for all medical students, the AAMC reported that, while physicians are certainly expected to be knowledgeable and skillful, they are also expected to be altruistic and dutiful. The required knowledge and skills are developed in part through the college and medical school educational processes. Dedication to duty, altruism, and the other essential attributes of medical professionals are nurtured through experience — with family, with friends, and with people in need.

In the Medical School Objectives Program: *Learning Objectives for Medical Student Education: Guidelines for Medical Schools* report (*www.aamc.org/meded/msop*):

Dutifulness is defined as:

- an appreciation of the complex non-biological determinants of poor health

- an awareness of community and public health issues

- the ability to identify risk factors for disease

- a commitment to the early identification and treatment of disease

- an acceptance of the responsibility for making scientifically based medical decisions and for advocating for the care of the underserved

- an understanding of basic issues in health care financing and delivery

Altruism is defined as involving:

- ethical decision-making

- compassion, respect, honesty, and integrity

- collaborative work with other team members

- advocacy on behalf of one's patients

- sensitivity to potential conflicts of interest

- the capacity to recognize one's limits

- the commitment to continuously improve one's knowledge and abilities

These basic elements of the "art" of medicine, along with other important characteristics such as motivation, persistence, and communication and interpersonal skills, evolve over time. Experience in a healthcare setting, caring for an ill or elderly family member, participating in basic or clinical science research efforts, working as an emergency medical technician, "shadowing"

TABLE 3-A

Subjects Required by 10 or More U.S. Medical Schools, 2010–2011 Entering Class

Required Subject	No. of Schools (n=130)	Required Subject	No. of Schools (n=130)
Biochemistry	13	Humanities	16
Biology or Biology/Zoology	128	Inorganic (General) Chemistry	122
Calculus	18	Organic Chemistry	123
College Mathematics	33	Physics	121
English	85	Social Sciences	10

NOTE: Figures based on data provided fall 2008.

---

a physician, or providing emotional support to people in a rape crisis center, emergency room, or social service agency — these types of service activities are recommended to those considering medicine as a career.

By participating in such activities, premedical students learn both about the medical profession and about themselves. They learn about their tolerance for stress, their ability to communicate and empathize with people from different backgrounds and cultures, their problem-solving skills, and their willingness to put others' needs before their own. They also come to better understand the nature of medical practice and the daily demands placed upon physicians and their family members. After learning these important lessons, they can decide whether medicine is an appropriate career choice for them.

Finally, premedical students should know how these experiences are assessed by medical school admission committees. At least three criteria are used: length of time invested, depth of the experience, and lessons learned. Short-term experiences such as day-long blood drives or one-time-only shadowing experiences are less enlightening than semester or year-long commitments. Passive activities such as observation are less instructive than those requiring active participation. Most important, admission committees want to know what students derived from these experiences. Applicants should be prepared to answer these kinds of questions about their community, clinical, or research experiences.

For the enrolled medical student, the satisfaction derived from these experiences is often the motivational factor that helps them to "pull through" the challenging demands of medical school, which affect even the best students.

Premedical Advising

Students investigating a career in medicine — no matter where they might be in the process — can get extremely valuable advice from their campus pre-health advisor. Depending on the individual school, pre-health advisors function on either a full- or part-time basis. They may be a faculty member (often in a science department), a staff member in the office of an academic dean or the career center, the director of an advising office for pre-professional students, or a physician in part-time practice. Ideally, pre-health advisors are knowledgeable and supportive, as well as well-informed about medical education programs, both locally and nationally. Advisors belong to organizations such as the National Association of Advisors for the Health Professions (NAAHP, *www.naahp.org*) that assist them in their work. They are able to provide information, guidance, and support to interested students and, at times, even challenge students to consider new options or reconsider their decisions.

Pre-health advisors assist premedical students to:

- identify college courses that satisfy premedical requirements

- determine an appropriate sequence for completing those courses

- find tutorial assistance, if needed

- plan academic schedules to accommodate both premedical coursework and other educational objectives, including a study program abroad, a dual major, or a senior honors thesis

- locate volunteer or paid clinical and research experiences

- strengthen the medical school application

- prepare for interviews and standardized tests

- arrange for letters of evaluation and recommendation

- determine the most appropriate career paths based on individual assets, liabilities, values, and life goals

Premedical students usually meet with pre-health advisors when they:

- enter into a premedical curriculum

- join a pre-health student society

- change majors or courses of study

- need information about medical school admission requirements

- prepare to apply to medical school

- get ready for medical school interviews

- seek community, clinical, or research experiences

- require advice about resolving academic problems

- want to discuss future career paths

- plan a postbaccalaureate premedical program or coursework

- prepare for health profession school admission tests

- need letters of evaluation or recommendation

Services provided by a pre-health advisor. Advisors' services typically vary according to the advisor's employment status, the number of premedical students to be served, and the philosophy and organizational structure of the institution. Students should contact their school's advisor to determine what services are available; they generally fall into five categories:

- Academics. Advisors are well informed about premedical coursework on their campuses and about developing suitable academic programs for pre-health students. They collaborate with campus academic staff in designing study, reading skill, and test preparation workshops, and in offering tutoring programs. Advisors publicize regional and national programs of interest to their students.

- Clinical and research experiences. Advisors often work with advisory groups composed of college and medical school teaching and research faculty and community clinicians. These groups help identify part-time jobs, volunteer positions, and opportunities for independent study credit in local laboratories and offices.

- Assistance to student organizations. Advisors often coordinate the activities of the local and national organizations and academic societies that serve pre-health students. These groups plan programs, identify funding sources, and arrange for campus visits from admissions and financial aid personnel, as well as medical school alumni and practicing physicians.

- Advising and support. Advisors help students to pursue realistic individual goals and maximize their potential. They meet with students individually, and they provide group opportunities for students to meet each other and community representatives from various health professions. Advisors establish peer advising and mentoring programs. They are sensitive to the needs of students, including their financial needs, their being a member of a group currently underrepresented in medicine, or their being first in their family to attend college.

- Sharing resources. Pre-health advisors disseminate information and publications from relevant organizations, including the AAMC and the National Association of Advisors for the Health Professions. They provide computer access to Web-based health careers programs and those on educational financing. They distribute information about local, regional, national, and international research and service opportunities. They stock a library of publications related to medical school and medical education, including Medical School Admission Requirements (MSAR™).

The pre-health committee letter of recommendation. One important service provided by the advisor to pre-health students, and frequently also to alumni, is the pre-health committee letter of recommendation. This is usually a composite letter written on behalf of a medical school applicant by the college or university's pre-health committee. The pre-health advisor may be a committee member or the committee chair, and is usually the liaison between students and the committee, facilitating letter-writing and the distribution of letters to schools.

This letter presents an overview of the student's academic strengths, exposure to health care and medical research environments, contributions to the campus and community, and personal attributes such as maturity and altruism. The letter may also address any extenuating circumstances that may have resulted in deficits in the student's performance during a course or semester, or provide perspective on challenges and problems the student may have encountered. The letter can also explain school-specific courses and programs in which the student has participated.

Some undergraduate institutions do not provide composite letters of recommendation. Instead, they collect individual letters of recommendation and evaluation during the student's enrollment and distribute them at the appropriate time to the medical schools where the student has applied. Students should inquire about the specific services that their institution's pre-health advisor provides.

Finding a pre-health advisor.
Students who have difficulty identifying an advisor on their own campus should contact the National Association of Advisors for the Health Professions (NAAHP, *www.naahp.org*). If a student's school does not have a pre-health advisor, volunteer advisors at other institutions may be identified. The NAAHP also offers publications to help students prepare for medical school. You can contact the NAAHP at:

National Association of Advisors
for the Health Professions
P.O. Box 1518
Champaign, IL 61824-1518
T (217) 355-0063 F (217) 355-1287
naahpja@aol.com

Special Programs

The majority of medical school applicants are seniors in college. However, numerous schools offer special programs to accommodate "non-traditional" pre-medical and medical students:

Combined college/medical school programs. These programs begin after high school and combine undergraduate and medical school curricula. About five percent of medical students begin their medical education in these programs, which vary by school. Most include the typical eight years of pre-medical and medical study, although a small number permit students to complete both college and medical school in six to seven years. Several programs limit participation to state residents, and many require prospective medical students to be enrolled at specific affiliated undergraduate institutions. Additional information can be found in Chapter 10.

Deferred entry. Many medical schools consider requests from accepted applicants who wish to defer matriculation, usually for a year, to take advantage of a special opportunity or for other personal reasons. Most schools require a written application and review requests on an individual basis. Some schools require deferred applicants to sign an agreement to attend that school the following year; others will hold a place in the next entering class until a mutually agreed upon date, even if the applicant decides to seek admission to other schools for the next year. Interested applicants are advised to obtain additional information about specific school requirements regarding deferred entry from individual medical schools as they differ from school to school and sometimes change on a year-to-year basis; the school-specific pages in Chapters 12 and 13 also provide relevant information.

Postbaccalaureate premedical programs. Not all medical school applicants are college seniors; some have already completed college. Some embarked on other careers after college, but then decided to apply to medical school. If these graduates were not previously science majors, they must complete required premedical coursework through postbaccalaureate premedical programs, which exist at colleges and universities across the country, both public and private. The programs range from formal, one- and two-year programs for full-time students to more informal part-time ones. Some specialize in applicants who are planning to change careers, while others focus on those attempting to enhance their prior academic performance. A searchable database of postbaccalaureate premedical programs can be found on the AAMC Web site at *http://services.aamc.org/postbac*.

Chapter 4

The Application Process

The annual medical school application process begins each spring, as applicants use one of three different processes for applying to U.S. medical schools:

- the American Medical College Application Service (AMCAS™) for the 129 U.S. schools and programs (including the M.D./Ph.D. programs of the Texas A&M University System Health Science Center College of Medicine, the University of Texas Southwestern Medical School at Dallas, the University of Texas Medical School at Houston, and the University of Texas Medical Branch at Galveston) that participated in AMCAS for the 2009 entering class (*www.aamc.org/amcas*)

- the Texas Medical and Dental Schools Application Service (TMDSAS™) for the seven public allopathic medical schools in Texas (*www.utsystem.edu/tmdsas*)

- school-specific application forms for two medical schools with their own individual application processes. Individual schools often supplement AMCAS and TMDSAS application materials with their own forms and materials, known as "supplemental" or "secondary" application materials.

Application Procedures

AMCAS, TMDSAS, and individual schools manage their application processes and the procedures by which applicant information is made available to medical school admission committee members. The authority and responsibility for selecting individuals who will be admitted to a medical school rest with each school's faculty. Acting through its standing admission committee, the faculty develops and approves criteria for admission. The administrative responsibility for receiving and processing applications rests with admissions officers and members of the admissions office staff. The responsibility for reviewing applicant information, interviewing candidates, and making decisions about admitting candidates rests with admission committee members.

Composition of the admission committee. Medical school admission committees typically include faculty representatives from both basic science and clinical departments. In addition, membership also frequently includes faculty from other colleges and schools in the university, community physicians, other community members, and medical students.

Application processing. Applications are screened and categorized by admissions office staff according to criteria established by the admission committee. Depending on the school, supplemental application materials (including letters of recommendation, an essay, legal residency and other school forms, and a fee) may be requested from all or some applicants, or only from those who meet specific criteria.

As applications are completed, applicants who are of greatest interest to schools are contacted by admissions office staff, and arrangements are made for campus visits and interviews with admission committee members. At some institutions, meetings with off-campus interviewers, including practicing physicians located near an applicant's home or school, may be required. As the process continues, other applicants may also be contacted and interviewed.

Applicants are typically interviewed by more than one committee member, either individually or in a group. After completion of the interview process, interviewers' evaluations are correlated with all other application materials and presented to the admission committee for discussion. Final decisions about admission are usually made by the committee acting as a whole.

All applicants, whether or not they are interviewed, are informed of the admission committee's decision according to the school's individual schedule. Committee decisions can range from an offer of immediate acceptance, to placement of the applicant in a "hold" category or on an alternate list, to non-acceptance. As the admission cycle continues, acceptances are offered until the required number of matriculants have been identified for that year's entering class.

Early Decision Program or regular application? One of an applicant's first decisions is whether to apply to a medical school through the Early Decision Program (EDP) or the regular application process. The fact that candidates applying through the EDP are informed about the outcome of their application at a participating school by October 1 affords them sufficient time to apply to other schools through the regular process if they are not accepted through the EDP.

The decision to apply through the EDP should be made carefully. While criteria for accepting EDP applicants vary among schools, a frequent criterion is that applicants show extraordinary credentials for admission. Applicants considering an EDP application should contact the medical school admissions office for more specific information.

EDP applicants must agree:

- not to apply through the EDP if they have already submitted an initial or secondary (AMCAS or non-AMCAS) application to the M.D. degree program at another U.S. allopathic medical school for the current entering class

- to apply to only one AMCAS medical school through the EDP

- not to submit additional (AMCAS or non-AMCAS) applications until they have received notification of non-acceptance through the EDP, or they have been formally released from the EDP commitment, or the October 1 EDP notification deadline has passed

- to attend the school if offered an EDP acceptance

All EDP applicants accepted by a medical school must adhere to the tenets of the program; any violation will result in an investigation by AMCAS. With regard to the EDP, medical schools agree to:

- notify each EDP applicant of the admission decision by October 1

- defer each EDP applicant to the regular applicant pool in those instances when an EDP non-acceptance decision is made

Timing of the application process. Each medical school establishes annual deadline dates for receipt of both primary and secondary application materials at the school. These dates are published in medical school bulletins and application materials, on school Web sites, and in Chapters 12 and 13. (Deadline dates range from mid-October to mid-December for receipt of primary application materials at AMCAS-participating schools and November 1 for TMDSAS-participating schools, with varying dates for school-specific applications.) Deadlines for receipt of all secondary application materials at medical schools also vary. Applicants should be aware of all deadline dates for all schools to which they are applying.

The deadline for receipt by AMCAS of the application, fee, and official transcripts for EDP applicants is August 1. (Contact the admissions office or see Chapters 12 and 13 for early decision application deadlines at schools that do not participate in AMCAS.) All secondary application materials must be received at the EDP school by the

school's deadline date. EDP candidates may be interviewed by admission committees in late August or September so that final decisions can be made and communicated to EDP candidates by October 1.

Admission committees generally interview candidates for regular admission during the fall, winter, and spring months. Most regular admission offers are made during the winter months. Medical schools collectively agree to issue, by March 30 of the matriculation year, a number of acceptances at least equal to the size of the first-year entering class. Applicants are therefore encouraged to submit their applications as early in the application process as possible. They are also responsible for ensuring that all required materials are received by the relevant application service and the individual medical school in a timely fashion. Medical schools are not responsible for notifying applicants if parts of their application file are missing.

Notification of acceptance. For the past four decades, AAMC-member medical schools, regardless of the type of application system used, have agreed to observe a set of acceptance procedures for first-year entering students, commonly referred to as the admission "traffic rules." Observing these recommendations (see Page 50 or *www.aamc.org/students/ applying/policies*) ensures that applicants and schools know, usually by June, who will be matriculating at each school in the fall. The deadline for notifying EDP applicants of EDP admission decisions is October 1. The earliest and latest dates for notifying regular applicants of acceptance, and the time allowed for applicants to respond to acceptance offers, are indicated in each school's entry in Chapters 12 and 13. The "traffic rules" also recommend that school deposits required of accepted applicants not exceed $100, and that they be refundable until May 15. The deposit amount and refund policy for each school are also indicated in Chapters 12 and 13.

Applicant responsibilities. Just as medical schools agree to a set of "traffic rules" in the application and admission process, applicants are also expected to observe a set of procedures (see Page 52 or *www.aamc.org/students/ applying/policies*), thus ensuring an orderly and timely selection process for other applicants and for schools.

Schools' and applicants' observance of these procedures helps to ensure that all applicants are afforded timely notification of the outcome of their medical school applications and timely access to available first-year positions and that schools are protected from having unfilled positions in their first-year entering classes.

Falsifications, omissions, or discrepancies in application materials or irregular behavior during administration of the MCAT® examination will be investigated in accordance with AAMC investigation policies.

The Medical College Admission Test

The Medical College Admission Test (MCAT®) is a standardized examination designed to assist medical school admission committees in assessing applicants' academic preparation, achievement in science, verbal reasoning skills, and written communication skills, and in predicting which applicants will perform adequately in the rigorous medical school curriculum. The MCAT examination consists of multiple-choice questions and a writing assessment administered as a computerized examination in most parts of the U.S. and Canada and in international locations. Current information about registration, scheduling, testing dates, and testing locations for the computerized MCAT can be accessed on the MCAT Web site at *www.aamc.org/mcat*.

The MCAT provides admission committees with standardized measures of performance for all examinees. The test content outline was developed with input from medical school admissions officers, premedical faculty members, medical educators, practicing physicians, residents, medical students, AAMC staff, and a group of testing experts under contract to the AAMC. The MCAT examination is also designed to encourage those interested in a medical career to pursue broad undergraduate study in the natural and social sciences and in the humanities. It assesses facility with scientific problem-solving, critical thinking skills, and writing ability, as well as the understanding of scientific concepts and principles identified as required for the study of medicine.

The four sections of the MCAT examination are Physical Sciences, Verbal Reasoning, Biological Sciences, and Writing Sample:

• Physical Sciences and Biological Sciences. These sections are constructed to assess material covered in introductory undergraduate courses in biology; chemistry, including inorganic chemistry and organic chemistry; and general, non-calculus physics. Both sections consist entirely of science problems and may include data presented in graphs, tables, and charts. Both sections are designed to evaluate knowledge of basic concepts, facility with scientific problem-solving, and the ability to interpret data presented in a tabular or graphic format.

• Verbal Reasoning. This section is designed to assess applicants' abilities to comprehend, reason, and think critically. It draws upon material from the humanities, social sciences, and natural sciences. Subject-matter knowledge is not evaluated; the content information necessary to answer test questions is presented in each passage. In preparation for this section, examinees are encouraged to familiarize themselves with the practice of critical thinking and the use of reasoning skills in these disciplines.

• Writing Sample. The essay topics that constitute this section are designed to provide examinees with an opportunity to demonstrate writing and analytic skills. Examinees are allotted 30 minutes to write an essay on a first assigned topic, then another 30 minutes to write an essay on a second assigned topic; each requires an expository response. Essay topics do not pertain to the technical content of biology, chemistry, physics, or mathematics; the medical school application process; reasons for desiring a career in medicine; social or cultural issues not part of the general experience of MCAT examinees; religious issues; or emotionally-charged subjects.

MCAT scoring. A total of five MCAT scores are reported, one for each MCAT section and a total score. Scores for the Physical Sciences, Verbal Reasoning, and Biological Sciences sections are presented on a numerical scale, ranging from a low of 1 to a high of 15. Scores for the Writing Sample section are presented on an alphabetical scale, ranging from a low of J to a high of T. A total score is also reported, which is the sum of the Physical Sciences, Verbal Reasoning, and Biological Sciences sections, along with the Writing Sample score: for example, 45T.

The MCAT is administered and scored by the MCAT Program Office at the direction of the AAMC. Information about the specific content of the examination, its organization, and the scoring system appears on the MCAT Web site at *www.aamc.org/mcat*.

Test dates. The MCAT will be administered on 24 days in 2009. On four of these days, the MCAT will be administered twice, once in the morning and once in the afternoon, for a total of 28 administrations throughout the year. The other 20 days will have either a morning or an afternoon administration.

The first administrations of the year will be in January 2009. In 2009, the MCAT will also be administered in each month from March to September (for specific dates, see the MCAT test administration calendar on the MCAT Web site at *www.aamc.org/mcat*). Most medical schools will utilize MCAT scores from as late as September 2009 MCAT administrations only for applications to their 2010 entering class. Applicants should check with individual schools to determine their policies regarding utilization of 2010 MCAT scores for applications to the 2010 entering class. Relevant information can also be found on the school-specific pages in Chapters 12 and 13.

Potential medical school applicants are advised to take the MCAT about 12–18 months prior to their expected entry into medical school. Many medical schools prefer that applicants take the MCAT early in the year because of the short time between the availability of late summer and September scores and school application deadlines. Taking the MCAT early in the calendar year also allows time for students to retake the test later, if necessary. For applicants enrolled in summer courses, a late-summer MCAT administration may be preferable. Scores will be returned to examinees and available to medical schools approximately 30 days after the test administration. This enables applicants to take the test as late as September and still have their scores available before school application deadlines.

Only those persons who intend to apply to a school of allopathic, osteopathic, podiatric, or veterinary medicine are permitted to take the MCAT; any other potential examinees must receive special permission prior to taking the examination.

Fees and registration. The examination fee is $225 for each of the 2009 MCAT administrations. Registration for the 2009 MCAT is available only online at *www.aamc.org/mcat*. Prior to regis-

tering for the MCAT, potential examinees must familiarize themselves with the information in the publication 2009 MCAT Essentials, which is available on the MCAT Web site.

Testing with accommodations. Potential examinees with appropriately documented disabilities that meet the definition of a disability under the Americans with Disabilities Act (ADA) may request testing accommodations. Examinees with chronic medical conditions or short-term disabilities that are not covered by the ADA and who have special testing needs should consult with the MCAT program about accommodations. Information about the documentation that is needed to request testing accommodations and application deadline dates is available at *www.aamc.org/mcat*.

Preparation for the MCAT. The MCAT is a "high stakes" admissions test; scores are carefully evaluated by medical school admission committees. Examinees should prepare for the MCAT by completing premedical introductory biology, general and organic chemistry, and physics coursework (see Chapter 3) prior to taking the MCAT examination for the first time. If some time has elapsed since the completion of premedical courses, review of course material prior to taking the MCAT is highly recommended. Potential examinees with ongoing challenges in reading speed or comprehension are advised to address and resolve those issues prior to taking the examination. Campus academic advising or academic skills staff are often well informed about these and related issues.

The MCAT should not be taken "cold" or for "diagnostic" reasons; the MCAT Practice Tests can be used for preparation. A variety of MCAT preparation materials are described at the end of the section.

Retaking the MCAT. Applicants who are not satisfied with their MCAT scores should confer with their pre-

health advisor about the advisability of retaking the test. Legitimate reasons for retaking the MCAT can include:

- a significant discrepancy between college grades and MCAT scores

- having taken the examination prematurely (i.e., without adequate preparation or prior to completion of all relevant premedical coursework)

- serious illness at the time of the examination

- a recommendation from a medical school admissions officer or admission committee member that the MCAT be retaken

Registration procedures for retaking the examination are identical to those for initial testing. The MCAT may be taken a maximum of three times during each calendar year; there are no exceptions to this policy.

Score reporting. Payment of the MCAT examination fee includes the reporting of test scores to AMCAS, other application services, and individual medical schools. MCAT scores are available approximately 30 days after the examination date. Examinees can view MCAT scores from 1991 to present through the MCAT Testing History (THx) System (*www.aamc.org/mcat*). Examinees who have tested in 2003 or later and have applied via AMCAS will automatically have their scores released to those institutions designated within the AMCAS application. Scores from tests taken prior to 2003 or any that are to be released to non-AMCAS institutions (regardless of year taken) must be released using the THx System. Once scores are released to AMCAS, they may not be withdrawn from current or future applications. To request MCAT scores prior to 1991, examinees must print and complete the request form available on the MCAT Web site (*www.aamc.org/mcat*). A fee is required for score reports older than 1991.

MCAT examinees are encouraged to request, at the time of registration or through the AMCAS application, that their scores be sent directly to their pre-medical advisors. This is a free service.

MCAT publications. The AAMC publishes a variety of practice materials, including a series of official practice tests. MCAT Practice Online provides previously administered tests. The practice materials feature automated scoring, integrated solutions, diagnostic reports, customized item selection, daily test-taking tips, and discussion boards. Free access to a single full-length MCAT with all the features of MCAT Practice Online is available at *www.e-mcat.com*.

Also available to students preparing for the MCAT is the new Official Guide to the MCAT Exam (2009). The guide includes test questions from real MCAT exams along with detailed descriptions of their solutions (written by the test developers). Also included is additional advice about retesting — for students who are unhappy with their scores — advice about applying to medical school, and data that show your probability of getting accepted.

MCAT publications are available for purchase online through the MCAT Web site (*www.aamc.org/mcat*).The MCAT Web site also contains detailed information about the format and content of the examination and outlines of the science, problem-solving, critical thinking, and communication skills tested by the MCAT.

American Medical College Application Service (AMCAS)

The American Medical College Application Service (AMCAS) is a non-profit, centralized application processing service for applicants to the first-year entering classes at participating U.S. medical schools. AMCAS policies and procedures are developed in consultation with representatives of participating medical schools. AMCAS bene-fits both schools and applicants by collecting, verifying, and processing application data and MCAT scores on behalf of participating medical schools and transmitting those data to them.

AMCAS also assists admission committees by providing rosters and statistical reports regarding the national and individual medical school applicant pools, as well as aggregate data about accepted applicants at medical schools across the nation. AMCAS data are used by the AAMC in various research efforts regarding the medical school applicant and matriculant pools.

AMCAS does not render admission decisions or advise applicants as to the medical schools to which they should apply. Each medical school, through its admission committee and admissions officer, is completely autonomous in its admission decisions.

For the 2009 entering class, 129 U.S. medical schools and programs (including the M.D./Ph.D. program of the Texas A&M University System Health Science Center College of Medicine, the University of Texas Southwestern Medical School at Dallas, the University of Texas Medical School at Houston, and the University of Texas Medical Branch at Galveston) will participate in AMCAS. The nine U.S. medical schools that will not participate in AMCAS for the 2009 entering class are:

- University of Missouri–Kansas City School of Medicine
- University of North Dakota School of Medicine and Health Sciences
- Texas A&M University System Health Science Center College of Medicine*
- Texas Tech University Health Sciences Center School of Medicine
- Texas Tech University Health Sciences Center, El Paso, Paul L. Foster School of Medicine
- University of Texas Southwestern Medical Center at Dallas* Southwestern Medical School*
- University of Texas Medical School at Galveston*
- University of Texas Medical School at Houston*
- University of Texas School of Medicine at San Antonio

The most current listing of participating schools and programs is available at *www.aamc.org/students/amcas/participatingschools.htm*.

The AMCAS application. The AMCAS application is available via the AMCAS Web site at *www.aamc.org/amcas*. On the AMCAS Web site, applicants will find links to key steps in starting an application, an application worksheet that previews the application content, an application timeline, important FAQs, and other resources to assist them with the application, such as an instruction booklet in PDF format.

The AMCAS application permits applicants to complete, certify, and submit their AMCAS application via the AMCAS Web site. The AMCAS application is accessible 24 hours a day, beginning on or about May 1, 2009, for the 2010 entering class.

* The M.D. Programs of the Texas A&M University System Health Science Center College of Medicine, the University of Texas Southwestern Medical School in Dallas, the University of Texas Medical School at Houston, and the University of Texas Medical Branch at Galveston participate in the Texas Medical and Dental School Application Service for the 2010 entering class, but their M.D.-Ph.D. programs participate in the American Medical College Application Service (AMCAS) for the 2010 entering class. Please refer to Chapter 12 for more information.

AAMC registration. The AAMC has a global registration system. Applicants who have previously registered for the MCAT THx System, the Fee Assistance Program, AMCAS, or other AAMC services have already selected an AAMC username and password and have been assigned an AAMC ID; they should use the same access information to enter the AMCAS application. Those who have not recently registered for AAMC services must complete the AMCAS registration form, select a username and password, and be assigned an AAMC ID. The AAMC secure username, login, and password sequence ensures the confidentiality of their application information.

Transcript requirements and deadlines. Applicants must request that an official transcript be forwarded to AMCAS by the registrar of every postsecondary school at which they have ever been registered.

AMCAS provides a "transcript request form" that expedites the cataloguing and processing of transcripts. To generate a transcript request form, the applicant must complete the "Identifying Information" and "Schools Attended" sections of the AMCAS application and follow the directions for printing the transcript request form. Prior to submitting this form to the registrar's office, the form should be carefully reviewed to ensure that the information is accurate and that the registrar's address is current. Simultaneously, applicants are encouraged to request personal copies of each transcript prior to completing the "Academic Record" section of the AMCAS application.

Transcripts are required from every junior college, community college, trade school, or professional school within the United States, Canada, or U.S. territories, regardless of whether or not credit was earned. This requirement applies also to college courses taken while in high school. Transcripts submitted to AMCAS for prior years' applications cannot be used to verify

coursework and grades for an application to the 2010 entering class.

Application materials and official transcripts for the Early Decision Program (EDP) must be received by AMCAS by August 1, 2009. For regular applicants, all official transcripts must be received no later than two weeks following the deadline date for application materials. Refer to the AMCAS online instruction booklet or help text for detailed information about official transcript requirements and deadlines; this information is available at *www.aamc.org/amcas*. AMCAS begins accepting official transcripts on or about May 1, 2009.

Completing the AMCAS application. The application is divided into different sections, which may be completed during multiple sittings. Extensive on-screen instructions and help text are provided. Payment is also received online.

Applicants are encouraged to print their application after submitting it to AMCAS. To ensure that the submission process was successfully completed, applicants should check the "Date Submitted" field in the upper left-hand corner of the first page of the application. The "Date Submitted" field should have been modified from "N/A" to the current date.

Applicant monitoring responsibilities. AMCAS provides a dynamic welcome page that details the status of each application. Applicants are responsible for checking this page and addressing identified errors and omissions. Applicants are also expected to thoroughly review changes made by AMCAS during the verification process and alert AMCAS to any issues regarding these changes.

Applicants may change certain information on their application and apply to additional medical schools, using their username, login, and password sequence, after their initial application has been submitted; each add/change requires that the applicant recertify and resubmit the application.

Processing of applications. Regardless of the number of AMCAS-participating schools to which an individual applies, only one application should be submitted to AMCAS. After receipt of the service fee and an official transcript from each postsecondary school at which the applicant has been registered, AMCAS verifies the accuracy of the academic record, as entered by the applicant, by comparing it with the official transcript(s) received in support of the application. Each year, AMCAS surveys postsecondary school registrars for grading system updates, and uses this registrar-provided information to assign AMCAS grades and calculate a normalized GPA for each applicant. Once processing of an application has been completed by AMCAS, AMCAS makes the application available to all designated medical schools. AMCAS also distributes MCAT scores, provided that the applicant has released those scores to AMCAS. All 2003 and later MCAT scores are automatically included in an applicant's AMCAS application. Scores from MCAT administrations in years prior to 2003 are provided to AMCAS only if the applicant has released those scores to AMCAS.

AAMC Fee Assistance Program (FAP)

The AAMC believes that the cost of applying to medical school should not be a financial barrier to individuals who are interested in becoming physicians. The AAMC Fee Assistance Program (FAP) assists MCAT examinees and AMCAS applicants who, without financial assistance, would be unable to take the MCAT or apply to these medical schools that use the AMCAS application.

Applicants who are approved for fee assistance receive the following benefits from the AAMC:

- Reduction of the MCAT registration fee from $225 to $85 for test administrations in 2009

- Waiver of the application fee of $490 for submitting the completed AMCAS application to up to 13 AMCAS-participating medical schools. Applicants pay $30 for each school beyond the 13 free applications.

- One free copy of The Official Guide to the MCAT Exam (2009)

In addition, most AMCAS-participating medical schools waive their supplemental application fees for applicants who have been granted fee assistance by the AAMC.

Eligibility

Eligibility decisions are now tied directly to the U.S. Department of Health and Human Services poverty level guidelines. For the 2009 calendar year, applicants whose annual family income is 300% or less of the federal poverty level for their family size will be approved for fee assistance.

How FAP works

Applying for fee assistance is simple. Upon submission of the FAP application online, the FAP program will immediately determine whether or not an applicant meets FAP eligibility requirements. If tentatively approved, the applicant will be asked to submit documentation in support of the application. If the applicant is determined to be ineligible, submission of documentation is not necessary.

Timeline

The FAP application is available online from January through December of each calendar year. However, applicants should note that the FAP application and all required supporting documentation should be received at least three weeks prior to the desired MCAT registration date and/or AMCAS application deadline.

Additional information about the FAP, including instructions, the application, and information about relevant deadline dates, is available at *www.aamc.org/fap*.

Chapter 5

Applicant and Accepted Applicant Data

In 2007–2008, 42,231 persons applied to the 2008 entering class at the 126* allopathic medical schools in the United States. By the fall of 2008, 19,135 applicants had been offered an acceptance to at least one medical school, and 18,036 accepted applicants had matriculated. These accepted applicants possessed a broad range of MCAT® scores and undergraduate grade point averages, as well as a wide variety of personal characteristics and life experiences. Both male and female applicants were distributed across numerous racial and ethnic groups. A small number applied through the Early Decision Program, but the majority used the regular application process.

This chapter contains graphic representations of relevant data for the entire applicant pool, as well as for accepted and non-accepted applicants, for the 2008 entering class. All data presented in this chapter are accurate as of October 10, 2008 [Source: AAMC Data Warehouse; Applicant Matriculant File]. In the following charts:

- "All Applicants" refers to all applicants to the 2008 entering class

- "Accepted Applicants" refers to those applicants accepted to at least one medical school

- "Not Accepted" applicants refers to those applicants not accepted to any medical school

A small number of accepted applicants chose not to matriculate in 2008.

By familiarizing themselves with this information, reviewing the school-specific data in Chapter 12, and comparing themselves with applicants to the 2008 entering class, potential applicants can determine their relative standing on a variety of admission-related factors and can, with their advisors' help, make decisions that are appropriate for them. Extensive information about medical school applicants and matriculants can also be found online at *www.aamc.org/data/facts*.

Chart 5-A

MCAT Verbal Reasoning Score Distribution, Year 2008 Applicants

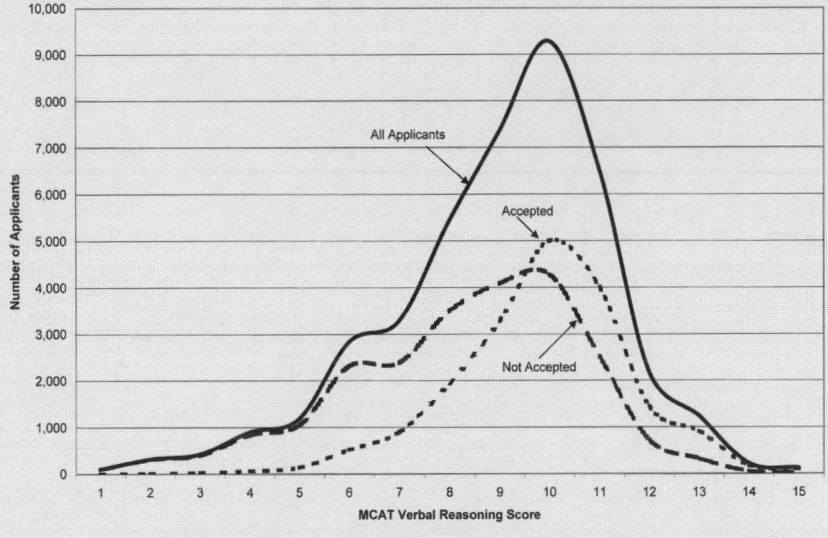

Source: AAMC Data Warehouse: Applicant Matriculant File   As of October 10, 2008

*The four medical schools accredited in 2008 will enroll their first matriculants in 2009.

Performance on the MCAT

Charts 5-A – 5-E present information about the performance of applicants on the MCAT:

- Chart 5-A shows that applicants achieved Verbal Reasoning (VR) scores at each score from 1 to 15; the largest number achieved a VR score of 10. Accepted applicants' scores ranged from 1 to 15, although very few had VR scores below 5 (just under 100). At a VR score of 10, the number of accepted applicants exceeded the number not accepted.

Chart 5-B

Physical Sciences Score Distribution, Year 2008 Applicants

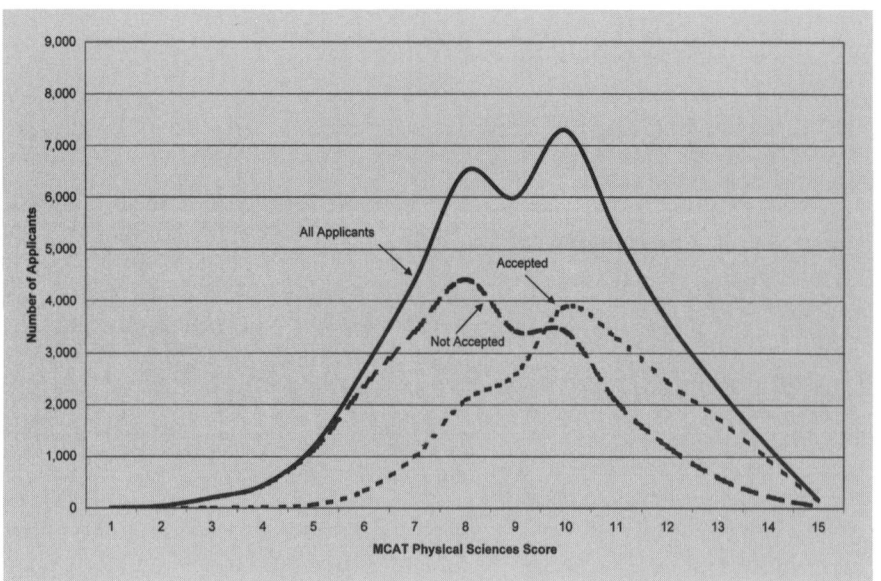

Source: AAMC Data Warehouse: Applicant Matriculant File   As of October 10, 2008

- Chart 5-B shows that applicants achieved Physical Sciences (PS) scores at each score from 1 to 15; the largest number achieved a PS score of 10. Accepted applicants' scores ranged from 1 to 15; fewer than 90 accepted applicants achieved a score of 5 or below. Accepted applicants exceeded not accepted applicants at a PS score of 10.

- Chart 5-C shows that applicants achieved Writing Sample (WS) scores at each score from J to T; the largest number achieved a WS score of Q. Accepted applicants' scores ranged from J to T; the number with scores of K and below was about 170. Accepted applicants exceeded not accepted applicants at a score of Q.

Chart 5-C

MCAT Writing Sample Score Distribution, Year 2008 Applicants

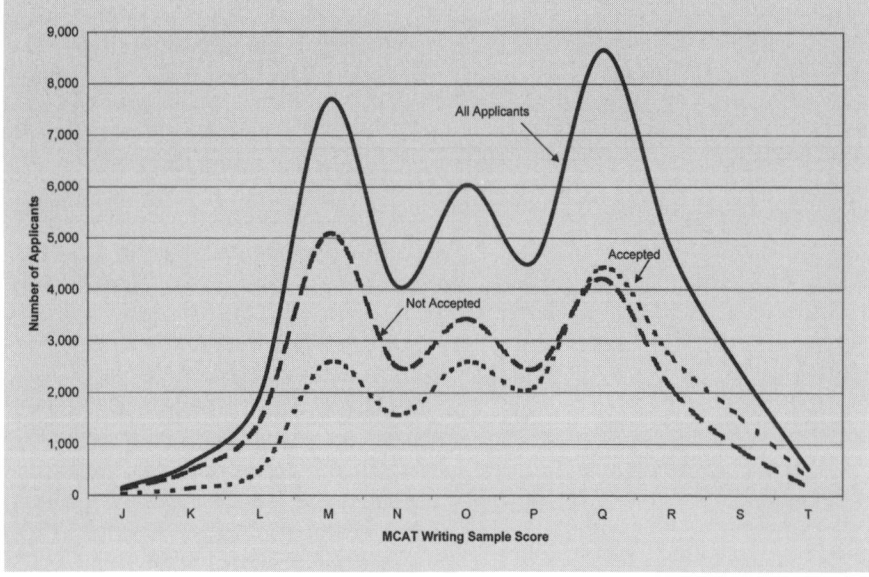

Source: AAMC Data Warehouse: Applicant Matriculant File   As of October 10, 2008

- Chart 5-D shows that applicants achieved Biological Sciences (BS) scores at each score from 1 to 15; the largest number achieved a BS score of 10. Accepted applicants' scores ranged from 1 to 15; about 45 scored 5 or below. Accepted applicants exceeded not accepted applicants at a score of 11.

- Chart 5-E — which shows total scores on the numerically scored sections of Verbal Reasoning, Physical Sciences, and Biological Sciences — reveals that applicants achieved total scores from 3 to 45; the largest number achieved a total score of 30. Accepted applicants achieved total scores from 7 to 45; the number of accepted applicants with total scores of 17 and below (an average of almost 6 on each section) was about 40. Accepted applicants exceeded not accepted applicants at a total score of 30.

No score on a single MCAT section and no total MCAT score "guarantees" admission to medical school. Charts 5-A, 5-B, and 5-D reveal that, while applicants with VR, PS, and BS scores of 10 and above had a higher probability of being accepted to medical school, a significant number of applicants with such scores were not accepted. The same holds true for the Writing Sample section; a score of Q and above is a likely, though not definite, barometer for acceptance. Finally, Chart 5-E shows that a substantial number of applicants with total MCAT scores of 29 and above were not accepted. These findings reveal the importance of factors other than MCAT performance — including undergraduate academic performance and a variety of personal characteristics and experiential variables — in the medical student selection process.

Chart 5-D
MCAT Biological Sciences Score Distribution, Year 2008 Applicants

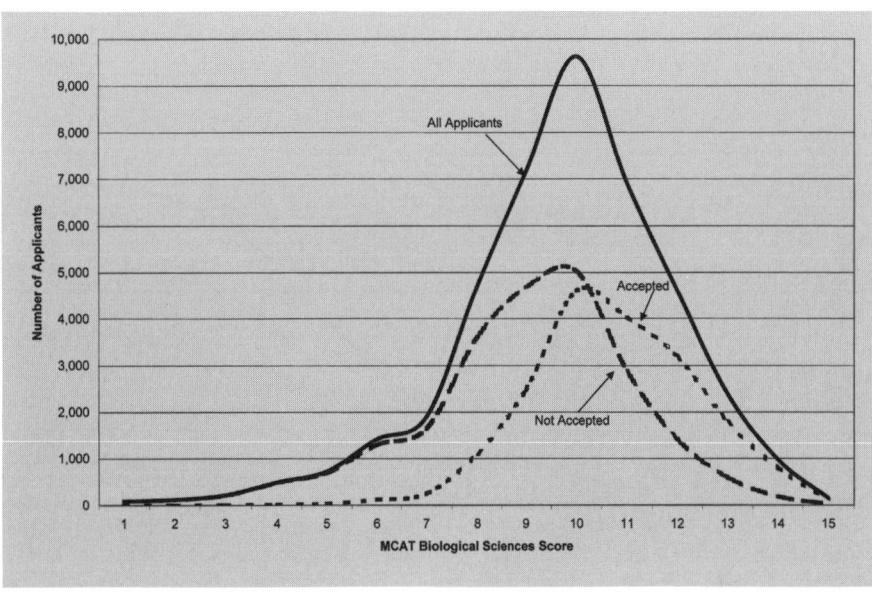

Source: AAMC Data Warehouse: Applicant Matriculant File   As of October 10, 2008

Chart 5-E
MCAT Total Numeric Score Distribution, Year 2008 Applicants

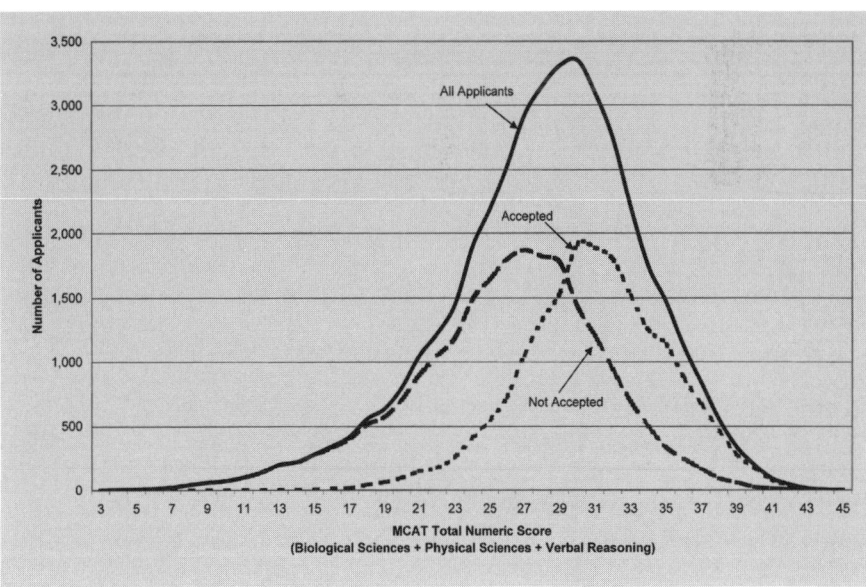

Source: AAMC Data Warehouse: Applicant Matriculant File   As of October 10, 2008

Chart 5-F

Science GPA Distribution, Year 2008 Applicants

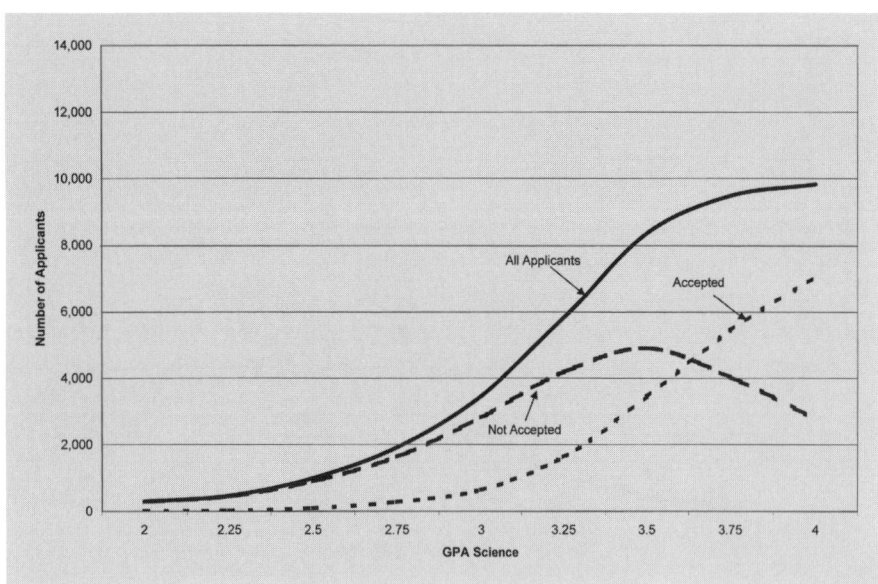

Source: AAMC Data Warehouse: Applicant Matriculant File

As of October 10, 2008

Chart 5-G

Non-Science GPA Distribution, Year 2008 Applicants

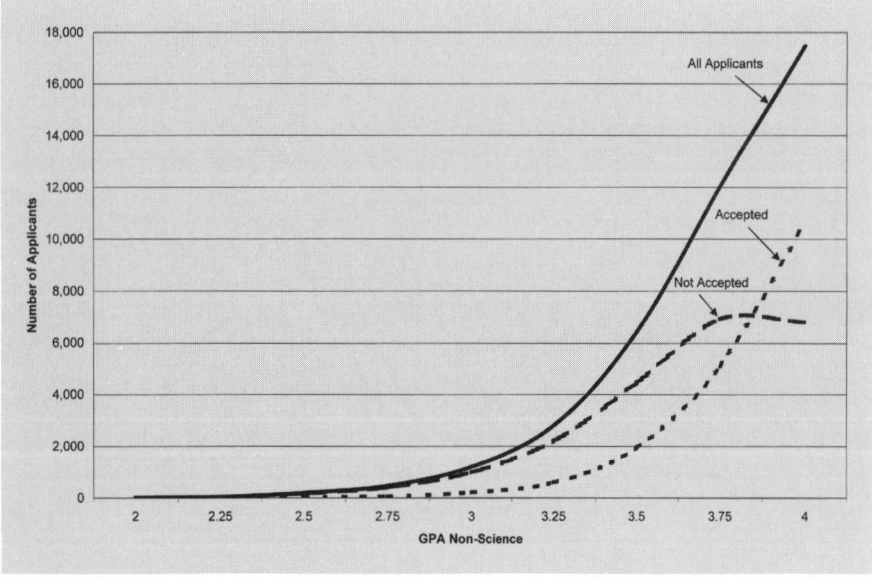

Source: AAMC Data Warehouse: Applicant Matriculant File

As of October 10, 2008

Undergraduate Grade Point Average (GPA)

Charts 5-F – 5-H present information about the undergraduate academic performance of applicants:

- Chart 5-F: undergraduate science GPA (Biology, Chemistry, Physics, and Mathematics)

- Chart 5-G: undergraduate non-science GPA

- Chart 5-H: undergraduate total GPA

Chart 5-F shows that the undergraduate science GPAs of all applicants were on a continuum from 2.0 to 4.0, on a 4.0 scale; most were between 3.75 and 4.0. Accepted applicants also had undergraduate science GPAs across the entire range, but few had GPAs of 2.50 or below (just under 120). The undergraduate science GPA at which accepted applicants exceeded those not accepted was between 3.50 and 3.75.

Chart 5-G shows applicants' undergraduate non-science GPAs along the continuum from 2.0 to 4.0, with most between 3.75 and 4.0. Accepted applicants' undergraduate non-science GPAs also ranged from 2.0 to 4.0, but only about 90 had a GPA of 2.75 or below.

At 3.75 to 4.0, accepted applicants exceeded not accepted applicants.

As shown in Chart 5-H, all applicants had total undergraduate GPAs from 2.0 to 4.0, and most were in the range of 3.50 to 3.75. Accepted applicants' total undergraduate GPAs also ranged from 2.0 to 4.0, but only about 100 possessed undergraduate total GPAs of 2.75 or below. Accepted applicants exceeded not accepted applicants at an undergraduate total GPA of between 3.50 and 3.75.

As is the case with MCAT data, GPA data in Charts 5-F – 5-H show that no undergraduate GPA assures admission to medical school. While applicants with undergraduate science, non-science, and total GPAs in the range of 3.50 to 3.75, 3.75 to 4.0, and 3.50 to 3.75, respectively, were more likely to be accepted to medical school, a significant number of such applicants were not accepted. Again, these findings underscore the importance of a wide variety of personal characteristics and experiential variables in the medical student selection process.

MCAT and Undergraduate GPA

Chart 5-I combines MCAT scores and undergraduate GPA for all applicants to medical school from 2005 to 2007. The data may not reflect your particular circumstances. As a result, we recommend that you go to *www.aamc.org/data/facts/* to see acceptance rates for particular demographic groups. Note that these results are presented without regard to any of the other selection factors.

Chart 5-H
Total GPA Distribution, Year 2008 Applicants

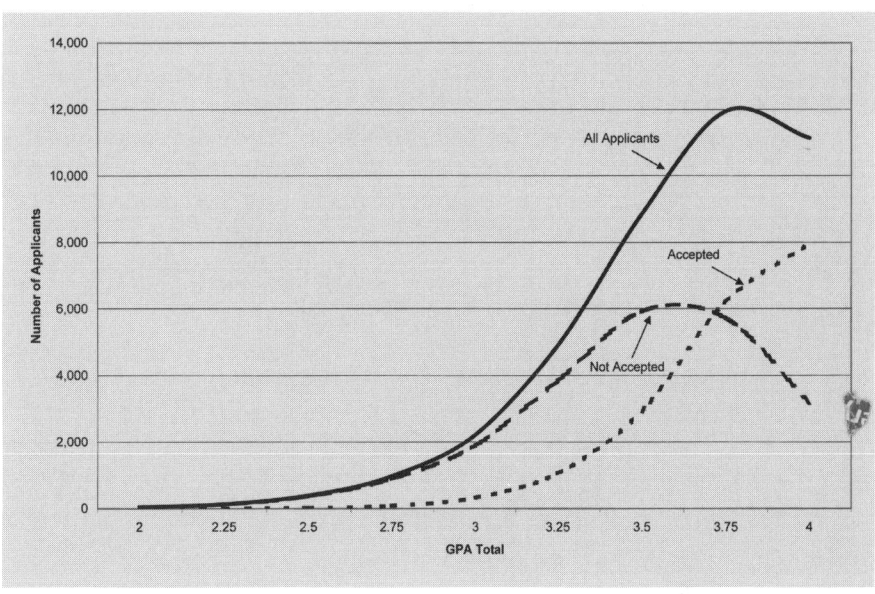

Source: AAMC Data Warehouse: Applicant Matriculant File

As of October 10, 2008

Chart 5-I
MCAT and Undergraduate GPA Combined

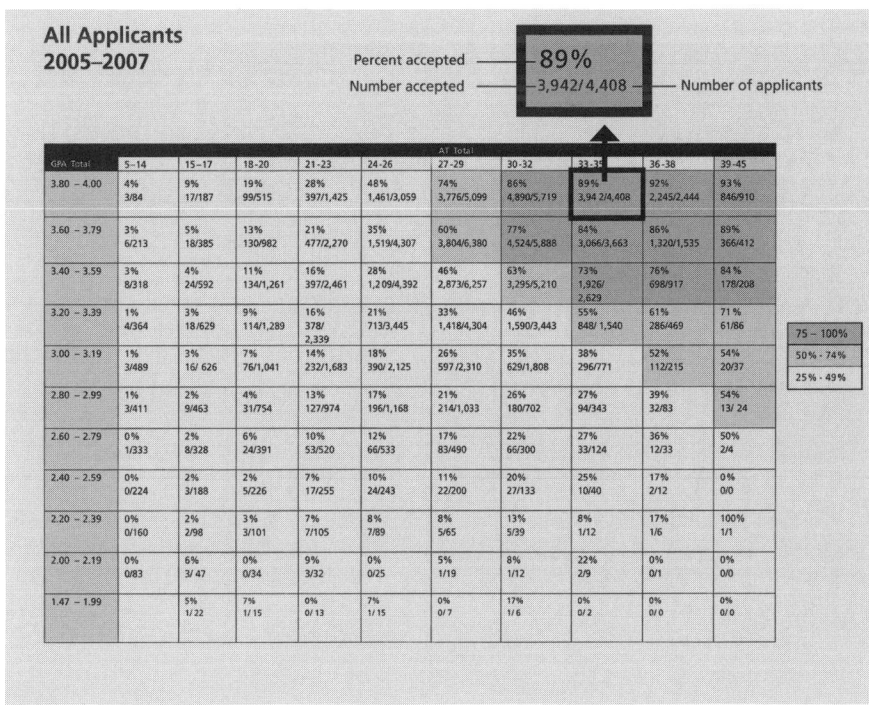

All Applicants 2005–2007

Percent accepted — **89%**
Number accepted — 3,942/4,408 — Number of applicants

GPA Total	5–14	15–17	18–20	21–23	24–26	27–29	30–32	33–35	36–38	39–45
3.80 – 4.00	4% 3/84	9% 17/187	19% 99/515	28% 397/1,425	48% 1,461/3,059	74% 3,776/5,099	86% 4,890/5,719	89% 3,942/4,408	92% 2,245/2,444	93% 846/910
3.60 – 3.79	3% 6/213	5% 18/385	13% 130/982	21% 477/2,270	35% 1,519/4,307	60% 3,804/6,380	77% 4,524/5,888	84% 3,066/3,663	86% 1,320/1,535	89% 366/412
3.40 – 3.59	3% 8/318	4% 24/592	11% 134/1,261	16% 397/2,461	28% 1,209/4,392	46% 2,873/6,257	63% 3,295/5,210	73% 1,926/2,629	76% 698/917	84% 178/208
3.20 – 3.39	1% 4/364	3% 18/629	9% 114/1,289	16% 378/2,339	21% 713/3,445	33% 1,418/4,304	46% 1,590/3,443	55% 848/1,540	61% 286/469	71% 61/86
3.00 – 3.19	1% 3/489	3% 16/626	7% 76/1,041	14% 232/1,683	18% 390/2,125	26% 597/2,310	35% 629/1,808	38% 296/771	52% 112/215	54% 20/37
2.80 – 2.99	1% 3/411	2% 9/463	4% 31/754	13% 127/974	17% 196/1,168	21% 214/1,033	26% 180/702	27% 94/343	39% 32/83	54% 13/24
2.60 – 2.79	0% 1/333	2% 8/328	6% 24/391	10% 53/520	12% 66/533	17% 83/490	22% 66/300	27% 33/124	36% 12/33	50% 2/4
2.40 – 2.59	0% 0/224	2% 3/188	2% 5/226	7% 17/255	10% 24/243	11% 22/200	20% 27/133	25% 10/40	17% 2/12	0% 0/0
2.20 – 2.39	0% 0/160	2% 2/98	3% 3/101	7% 7/105	8% 7/89	8% 5/65	13% 5/39	8% 1/12	17% 1/6	100% 1/1
2.00 – 2.19	0% 0/83	6% 3/47	0% 0/34	9% 3/32	0% 0/25	5% 1/19	8% 1/12	22% 2/9	0% 0/1	0% 0/0
1.47 – 1.99		5% 1/22	7% 1/15	0% 0/13	7% 1/15	0% 0/7	17% 1/6	0% 0/2	0% 0/0	0% 0/0

75 – 100%
50% – 74%
25% – 49%

Source: AAMC Data Warehouse: Applicant Matriculant File

As of February 27, 2008

Chart 5-J

Undergraduate Major Distribution, All Applicants, 1992–2008

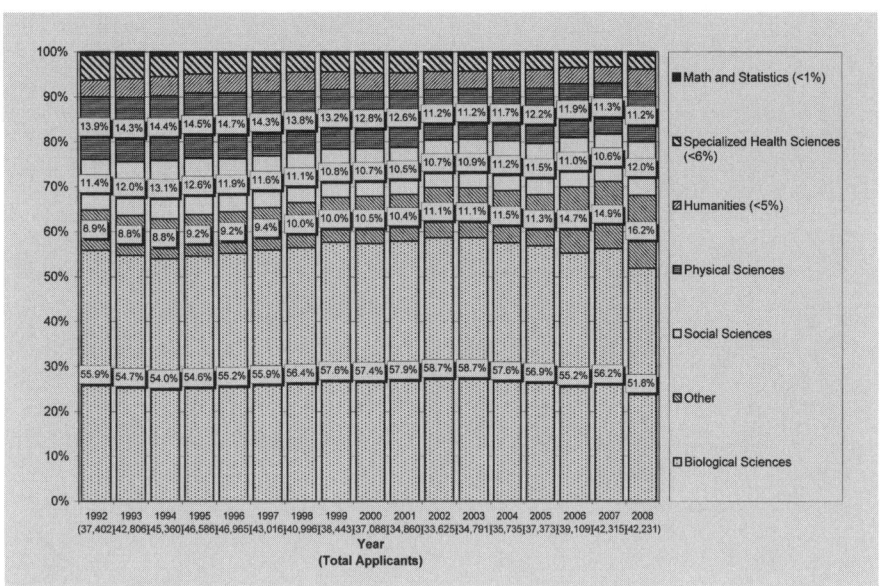

Source: AAMC Data Warehouse: Applicant Matriculant File

As of October 10, 2008

Chart 5-K

Undergraduate Major Distribution, Accepted Applicants, 1992–2008

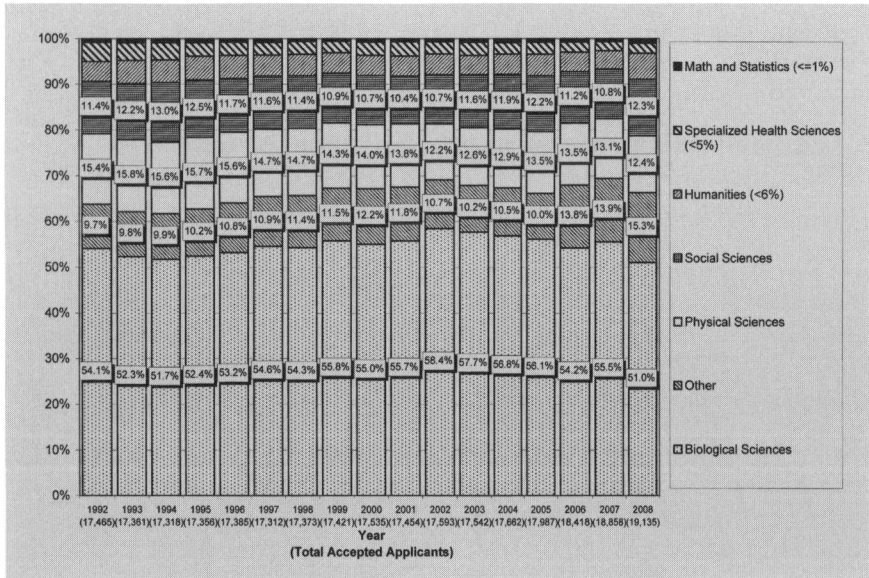

Source: AAMC Data Warehouse: Applicant Matriculant File

As of October 10, 2008

Undergraduate Major

Chart 5-J presents information about the undergraduate majors of all medical school applicants to the 1992–2008 entering classes. Over the past decade, approximately three-fifths of applicants reported undergraduate biological science majors, while the remainder reported a variety of majors, including the humanities, mathematics and statistics, physical sciences, social sciences, other health sciences, and a broad "other" category. The proportion of these majors has remained relatively constant over time, despite annual fluctuations in the applicant pool.

Chart 5-K presents similar information about the undergraduate majors of applicants accepted to the 1992–2008 entering classes. Comparisons of the majors of the total applicant pool with those of accepted applicants reveal acceptance rates, for various science-related majors, ranging from 33.9 percent for applicants with specialized health science majors, to 44.6 percent for biological science majors, to 50.0 percent for physical science majors, the highest rate of acceptance for science-related majors.

Gender

Chart 5-L presents information about the number and gender of the entire applicant pool and of accepted applicants for the 1992–2008 entering classes. The largest annual applicant pool during the past decade was for the 1996 entering class; since that year, the pool gradually declined until 2003, when there was a slight increase (3.5 percent) in applicants. The applicant pool increased again by 2.7 percent in 2004, by 4.6 percent in 2005, by another 4.6 percent in 2006, and by 8.2 percent in 2007. In 2008, the applicant pool held relatively steady, with a slight decrease of 0.2 percent. The number of male applicants to the 2008 entering class increased by about 290 from the number of male applicants to the previous year's entering class, but that number was still smaller than it had been for any other entering class from 1993 through 1998. The number of female applicants to the 2008 class decreased by about 375 over the number of female applicants to the previous year's entering class, the largest number of female applicants on record. While the number of accepted applicants remained fairly constant for 10 years, it has started to increase in recent years, from a low of 17,312 in 1997 to a high of 19,135 in 2008. The number of accepted male applicants has fluctuated from a high of 10,208 in 1992 to a low of 8,810 in 2003. The number of accepted female applicants has increased, with small fluctuations, from a low of 7,255 in the 1994 entering class to a high of 9,181 in 2008. The significant gaps between male and female applicants for the 1992 entering class (6,166) and the 1993 entering class (6,892) have disappeared; 553 and 301 more women than men applied to the 2003 and 2004 entering classes, respectively. In 2005, only 121 more men than women applied. In 2008, 1,510 more men than women applied to medical school. During the same time span, the gaps between accepted male and female applicants also dropped. Accepted male applicants outnumbered accepted female applicants by 2,951 for the 1992 entering class, but only by 773 for the 2008 entering class. The national ratio of male to female applicants was 49.2 : 50.8 percent for the 2003 entering class, the first time that the number of female applicants was greater than the number of male applicants to medical school. For the 2004 entering class, this trend continued, with a ratio of male to female applicants of 49.6 : 50.4. For the 2005 entering class, there were once again more male than female applicants, with a ratio of male to female applicants of 50.2 : 49.8. This trend continued in 2008, with a ratio of male to female applicants of 51.8 : 48.2.

Age

Chart 5-M shows that the age distribution for all applicants to the 2008 entering class was broad, with 16 applicants under the age of 19 at the

Chart 5-L
Applicants by Gender and Acceptance Status, 1992–2008

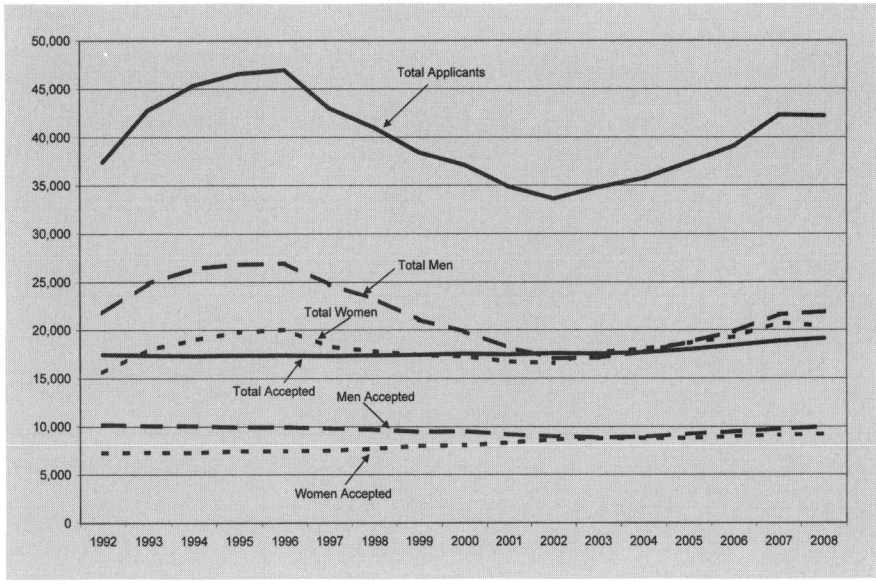

Source: AAMC Data Warehouse: Applicant Matriculant File   As of October 10, 2008

Chart 5-M
Age Distribution, Year 2008 Applicants

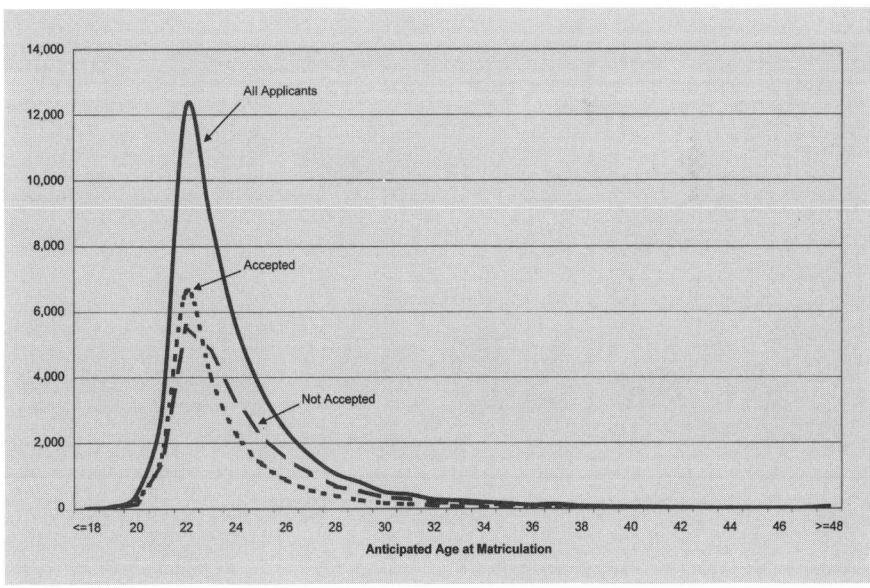

Source: AAMC Data Warehouse: Applicant Matriculant File   As of October 10, 2008

Chart 5-N

Total Applicants by Early Decision Program (EDP)
and Acceptance Status, 2008

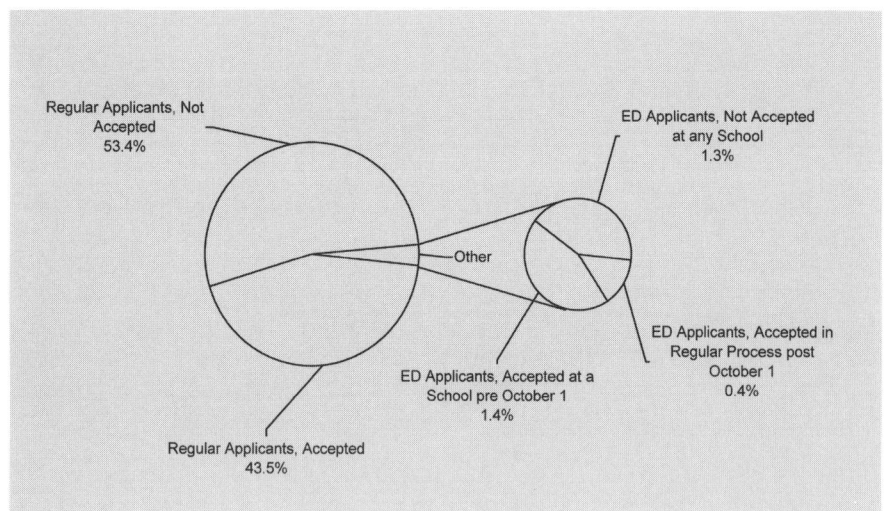

Source: AAMC Data Warehouse: Applicant Matriculant File

As of October 10, 2008

Chart 5-O

Distribution of Self-Reported Ethnicity and Race: All Applicants, 2002–2008

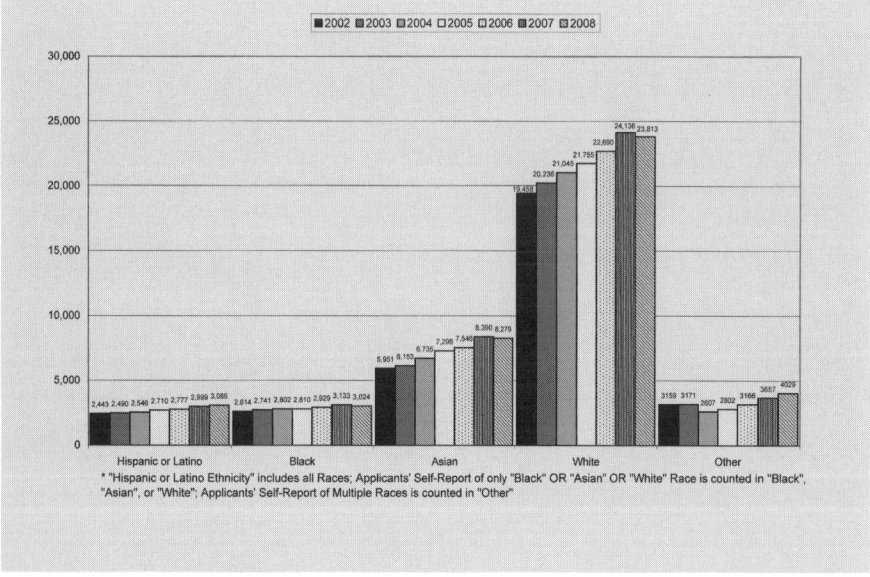

Source: AAMC Data Warehouse: Applicant Matriculant File

As of October 10, 2008

time of anticipated matriculation, and 71 applicants aged 48 and over. The largest contingent of applicants, 38,290, was between 21 and 28 at the time of anticipated matriculation; the rest of the applicant pool were either under 21 (529) or over 28 (3,412) at the time of anticipated matriculation. Chart 5-M illustrates a similar finding for accepted applicants. Accepted applicants for the 2008 entering class were between 17 and 55 years of age at the time of expected matriculation.

Type of Application

Chart 5-N presents information about application outcomes for Early Decision Program (EDP) and regular applicants to the 2008 entering class: 96.9 percent were regular applicants and 3.1 percent were EDP applicants. Of all applicants, 43.5 percent were accepted to at least one medical school through the regular application process; 1.4 percent were accepted to one medical school through EDP prior to October 1; and 0.4 percent were accepted to at least one medical school after not having been accepted through EDP before October 1. Conversely, 53.4 percent of regular applicants and 41.5 percent of the 3.1 percent of applicants who applied through EDP were not accepted to any medical school for 2008.

Race and Ethnicity

In accordance with the requirements of the U.S. Office of Management and Budget Directive 15, data about race and ethnicity were collected differently by AMCAS for applicants to the 2002 through 2008 entering classes than they were for applicants to prior years' entering classes. For that reason, this section presents applicant race and ethnicity data beginning with 2002 only. Additional applicant data regarding race and ethnicity for prior years are presented on the AAMC Web site at *www.aamc.org/data/facts*.

Chart 5-O shows applicant self-reported race and ethnicity data for all applicants to the 2002 through 2008 entering classes. Chart 5-P shows applicant self-reported race and ethnicity data for all accepted applicants to the 2002 through 2008 entering classes. The following changes occurred in the self-reported racial and ethnic make-up of the applicant pool from 2007 to 2008:

- The number of self-described white applicants in 2007 was 24,136; the number of white applicants in 2008 was 23,813, a decrease of 1.3 percent.

- The number of self-described Asian applicants in 2007 was 8,390; the number of Asian applicants in 2008 was 8,279, a decrease of 1.3 percent.

- The number of self-described black applicants in 2007 was 3,133; the number of black applicants in 2008 was 3,024, a decrease of 3.5 percent.

- The number of self-described Hispanic applicants in 2007 was 2,999; the number of Hispanic applicants in 2008 was 3,086, an increase of 2.9 percent.

- The number of applicants in 2007 whose self-description of their race or ethnicity was in some other category was 3,657; the number of applicants in this cohort in 2008 was 4,029, an increase of 10.2 percent from 2007.

Simultaneously, the following changes occurred among those applicants accepted to the 2007 and 2008 entering classes:

- The number of self-described white accepted applicants in 2007 was 11,284; the number of white accepted applicants in 2008 was

Chart 5-P

Distribution of Self-Reported Ethnicity and Race:
All Accepted Applicants, 2002–2008*

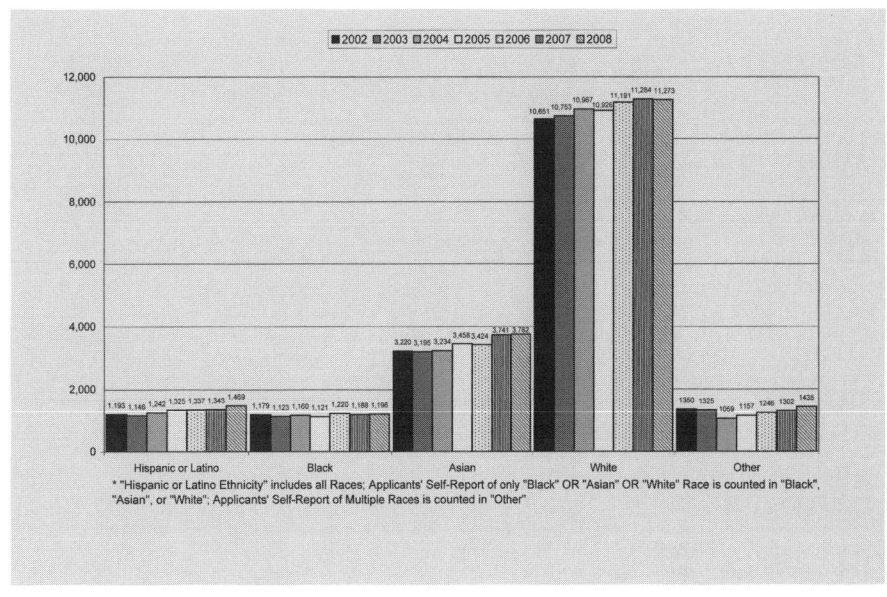

Source: AAMC Data Warehouse: Applicant Matriculant File

As of October 10, 2008

11,273, a decrease of 0.1 percent.

- The number of self-described Asian accepted applicants in 2007 was 3,741; the number of accepted Asian applicants in 2008 was 3,762, an increase of 0.5 percent.

- The number of self-described black accepted applicants in 2007 was 1,188; the number of accepted black applicants in 2008 was 1,196, an increase of 0.7 percent.

- The number of self-described Hispanic accepted applicants in 2007 was 1343; the number of Hispanic

accepted applicants in 2008 was 1,469, an increase of 9.4 percent.

- The number of accepted applicants in 2007 whose self-description of their race or ethnicity was in some other category was 1,302; the number of accepted applicants in this cohort in 2008 was 1,435, an increase of 10.3 percent from 2007.

Additional information of interest to applicants from groups under-represented in medicine is available in Chapter 6.

Chapter 6

Increasing Diversity in Medical School

The Association of American Medical Colleges (AAMC) believes that both medical education and health care delivery benefit from diversity among medical students, faculty, physicians, researchers, and administrators. The AAMC recognizes that diversity is a broad concept that can encompass a variety of factors, including, among others, race and ethnicity, gender, socioeconomic status, sexual orientation, life experiences, and personal characteristics. Individual medical schools determine how best to embrace diversity on their campuses so that their students can obtain the educational benefits that flow from a diverse student body and from diversity among faculty and administrators.

Within this general context, the AAMC has paid particular attention for more than three decades to medical students who are from racial and ethnic populations that are underrepresented in the medical profession. (For more information about the AAMC's definition of "underrepresented in medicine," see *www.aamc.org/meded/urm*.) In particular, the AAMC's Diversity Policy and Programs has been, and continues to be, engaged in a number of programs designed to increase diversity in academic medicine. These programs, while open to all students, are sensitive to the challenges and needs of individuals from racial and ethnic groups underrepresented in medicine, as well as of those persons from disadvantaged backgrounds. Examples of programs that may be useful in exploring medicine as a career are described below.

Enrichment programs. Medical schools nationwide provide programs and resources specifically designed to assist in preparing and recruiting students for medical education. Some of these programs are held during the school year, while others take place during the sum-

mer. Some are designed for high school students, others for college students, and still others for postbaccalaureate students. The AAMC is affiliated with two such programs:

- The annual Minority Student Medical Career Awareness Workshops and Recruitment Fair for high school and college students and their family members, which is held each fall during the AAMC's annual meeting. Representatives from all 130 AAMC-member medical schools are invited, and students have the opportunity to talk with them about preparing for medical school, enrichment programs, admission policies and procedures, financial aid, and more. Workshops are also sponsored for family members, guidance counselors, and health professions advisors. The dates and locations of upcoming AAMC fairs can be found at *www.aamc.org/careerfair*.

- The Summer Medical and Dental Education Program (SMDEP) is a free, six-week, academic enrichment program for freshman and sophomore college students interested in a career in medicine or dentistry. Program activities include science and mathematics-based courses, learning and study skills seminars, career development activities, clinical experiences, and a financial planning workshop. SMDEP is funded by The Robert Wood Johnson Foundation and is offered at 12 U.S. medical and dental schools across the nation. The AAMC's Diversity Policy and Programs, in conjunction with the American Dental Education Association, functions as the national program office. For additional information, visit *www.smdep.org*, or call the toll-free number at 866-56SMDEP.

AspiringDocs.org®. The AAMC sponsors a campaign designed to interest undergraduate students from groups underrepresented

Table 6-A Matriculants by Medical School and Race and Ethnicity 2008*

School State	School Name	Mexican American	Cuban	Puerto Rican	Other Hispanic or Latino	Total Hispanic or Latino	Chinese	Asian Indian	Pakistani	Filipino	Japanese	Korean	Vietnamese	Other Asian	Total Asian	Native American (incl AK)	Black	Native Hawaiian/OPI	White	Total Matriculants
AL	Alabama	1	0	0	0	1	6	13	1	1	0	3	0	0	24	1	14	1	138	176
	South Alabama	0	0	0	0	0	1	4	2	0	0	1	0	0	8	1	5	0	62	74
AR	Arkansas	2	0	1	2	5	1	6	1	1	0	0	2	1	13	0	14	1	124	154
AZ	Arizona	10	0	2	5	16	9	14	1	1	1	4	3	5	36	1	4	1	112	158
CA	Loma Linda	2	1	2	13	17	16	6	1	7	1	13	4	2	45	1	10	1	100	165
	Southern Cal-Keck	20	1	1	6	26	24	10	1	0	8	3	4	3	48	4	9	1	88	159
	Stanford	6	3	0	4	13	8	8	1	0	2	3	2	6	30	3	2	0	46	86
	UC Berkeley/SF Joint Prog	1	0	0	0	3	2	8	1	0	0	1	0	0	4	0	0	0	10	15
	UC Davis	8	0	1	1	10	14	8	3	2	1	3	7	5	40	2	5	1	57	103
	UC Irvine	6	0	0	6	13	14	9	0	1	1	5	5	3	38	0	4	2	58	104
	UC San Diego	9	0	2	2	14	28	12	0	0	2	2	9	5	55	2	1	0	68	134
	UC San Francisco	16	0	0	10	26	23	6	1	6	3	5	4	6	50	4	15	2	81	152
	UCLA Drew	9	0	0	3	12	0	0	0	1	0	1	0	0	3	0	8	0	4	24
	UCLA-Geffen	17	1	0	3	21	17	14	0	4	5	2	8	6	57	4	11	0	78	163
CO	Colorado	5	2	0	3	9	0	2	0	0	2	6	5	2	17	4	5	0	126	156
CT	Connecticut	4	0	0	5	8	2	6	0	0	0	1	0	3	11	0	7	0	61	85
	Yale	4	0	0	5	8	13	6	0	0	1	3	0	3	29	1	10	0	53	100
DC	George Washington	0	1	0	4	4	5	34	1	3	0	3	2	3	50	1	26	0	88	177
	Georgetown	2	2	2	5	11	15	15	3	2	1	5	5	4	49	0	13	1	125	194
	Howard	3	1	3	4	11	1	12	1	1	0	1	1	1	19	2	80	2	8	114
FL	Florida	0	1	0	8	14	5	10	1	3	0	1	1	3	22	0	8	0	103	132
	Florida State	1	10	1	9	19	5	15	1	3	0	1	3	1	24	0	9	0	81	118
	Miami-Miller	0	24	1	5	28	6	12	3	5	0	4	5	5	34	0	14	0	143	194
	South Florida	1	2	4	1	7	3	15	3	0	2	2	1	1	25	2	10	1	84	120
GA	Emory	1	1	0	1	2	3	6	1	0	1	5	0	4	17	0	13	0	90	128
	MC Georgia	1	2	0	1	4	7	25	1	0	1	6	1	4	45	0	15	0	128	190
	Mercer	0	0	0	1	1	2	2	2	1	0	2	1	3	10	2	1	0	79	90
	Morehouse	0	0	0	0	0	3	3	2	1	0	3	0	2	11	0	42	6	3	56
HI	Hawaii-Burns	0	0	0	0	0	18	1	0	6	27	4	0	2	45	0	0	6	17	62
IA	Iowa-Carver	9	0	0	1	10	4	10	0	0	1	3	3	1	21	1	6	1	112	148
IL	Chicago Med-Franklin	2	0	0	2	3	10	26	6	2	1	12	3	4	61	0	13	0	104	187
	Chicago-Pritzker	5	0	0	0	5	10	6	0	0	1	5	3	0	26	0	11	0	60	100
	Illinois	23	3	4	23	51	17	34	5	6	1	15	2	13	91	3	28	2	162	308
	Loyola-Stritch	3	1	1	2	6	3	6	5	2	2	4	0	0	19	0	10	2	111	145
	Northwestern-Feinberg	2	2	1	7	10	25	28	2	1	1	9	0	3	69	0	1	2	84	169
	Rush	3	0	0	7	10	8	16	3	2	1	3	1	3	36	0	4	0	89	130
	Southern Illinois	0	1	0	1	2	0	2	0	3	0	2	0	1	8	0	11	0	54	72
IN	Indiana	3	0	0	7	10	14	17	3	1	2	5	3	4	44	3	16	0	237	308
KS	Kansas	7	0	0	1	8	4	10	0	1	0	0	5	4	21	4	11	0	138	175
KY	Kentucky	2	0	0	0	2	2	2	0	0	0	2	1	1	7	0	4	1	95	113
	Louisville	2	1	0	1	4	4	9	0	3	0	0	0	1	19	0	13	0	118	155
LA	LSU New Orleans	2	1	0	8	10	5	6	0	6	0	0	4	2	17	1	10	2	146	179
	LSU Shreveport	0	1	0	2	2	3	1	0	3	1	0	1	1	8	2	3	0	103	116
	Tulane	0	1	0	2	3	9	10	2	1	2	3	0	4	34	1	2	0	141	178
MA	Boston	8	2	1	8	18	21	20	0	2	1	4	4	4	56	0	16	0	96	178
	Harvard	5	1	2	6	14	24	16	1	3	2	3	1	8	57	3	16	0	81	165
	Massachusetts	1	1	2	1	5	1	4	0	0	0	2	0	3	10	0	6	0	99	114
	Tufts	5	2	0	4	11	22	12	3	0	0	5	0	1	43	1	10	1	124	178
MD	Johns Hopkins	1	1	1	2	5	14	10	1	2	0	3	2	1	31	0	7	1	70	118
	Maryland	1	1	1	2	4	10	12	1	2	0	4	1	5	35	0	17	0	102	160
	Uniformed Services-Hebert	2	2	3	6	13	7	1	0	6	1	6	2	5	22	2	4	2	144	171
MI	Michigan	0	0	0	6	9	13	12	3	3	0	6	1	5	44	2	5	1	110	169
	Michigan State	2	0	1	5	8	3	14	6	3	0	2	4	5	23	2	8	0	114	156
	Wayne State	1	1	0	1	3	9	36	6	3	0	5	1	6	64	4	14	1	184	290
MN	Mayo	2	0	0	1	2	5	4	1	1	0	0	0	2	13	0	1	3	32	50
	Minnesota	4	0	3	1	7	9	5	1	1	2	2	0	3	24	2	9	1	130	170
	Minnesota Duluth	0	0	0	0	0	0	0	0	0	0	0	0	1	1	6	0	0	54	60
MO	Missouri Columbia	0	0	0	2	2	2	5	3	0	0	0	0	1	12	4	6	1	75	95
	Missouri Kansas City	1	0	0	1	2	1	17	1	2	0	0	5	38	40	0	2	0	39	86
	St Louis	6	1	1	2	5	11	17	2	6	3	7	3	5	54	0	10	1	111	176
	Washington U St Louis	0	1	0	2	7	16	9	0	0	0	4	0	1	31	1	8	0	70	122
MS	Mississippi	0	1	0	1	3	1	3	0	1	0	1	1	2	9	1	10	0	91	110
NC	Duke	0	3	0	0	3	12	8	0	2	0	2	0	3	25	0	18	0	49	100
	East Carolina-Brody	0	0	0	0	0	1	2	4	0	0	0	1	2	10	2	11	0	49	76
	North Carolina	1	1	0	2	3	7	5	2	1	0	0	1	2	15	0	23	0	123	160
	Wake Forest	1	0	0	1	2	3	9	0	1	0	2	1	2	17	2	9	0	92	120
ND	North Dakota	1	0	0	0	5	0	0	1	1	0	0	0	0	2	8	0	0	50	62
NE	Creighton	3	2	0	0	5	2	5	0	1	3	3	0	0	15	0	4	1	103	126
	Nebraska	3	0	0	0	3	0	0	1	1	0	3	1	1	5	2	4	0	114	124

Table 6-A Matriculants by Medical School and Race and Ethnicity 2008*

	Matriculants 2008	Mexican American	Cuban	Puerto Rican	Other Hispanic or Latino	Total Hispanic or Latino	Chinese	Asian Indian	Pakistani	Filipino	Japanese	Korean	Vietnamese	Other Asian	Total Asian	Native American (incl AK)	Black	Native Hawaiian/OPI	White	Total Matriculants
NH	Dartmouth	1	0	0	4	5	5	2	1	2	0	0	1	0	11	0	1	1	47	78
NJ	UMDNJ New Jersey	0	3	5	12	20	18	33	4	5	0	15	1	2	73	0	17	0	94	194
	UMDNJ-RW Johnson	2	2	2	5	10	11	21	3	2	2	7	0	1	46	0	15	0	97	166
NM	New Mexico	17	1	0	9	25	4	2	1	1	1	0	0	1	5	5	1	0	60	75
NV	Nevada	0	1	0	0	1	2	7	1	2	1	1	0	1	15	5	1	0	44	62
NY	Albany	2	2	1	1	4	12	25	2	1	2	3	4	3	49	2	2	0	86	143
	Buffalo	1	0	0	0	1	14	9	2	2	0	4	2	2	33	2	4	0	98	136
	Columbia	3	0	1	3	7	14	5	0	1	0	5	2	4	26	2	25	0	88	153
	Cornell-Weill	3	0	4	9	12	8	3	1	1	2	10	2	4	15	1	8	0	72	101
	Einstein	2	1	4	9	14	15	7	1	3	1	5	1	4	45	2	11	0	113	182
	Mount Sinai	2	5	2	7	16	22	9	2	0	0	8	4	4	34	0	10	2	82	140
	New York Medical	1	3	2	2	9	22	15	1	5	3	7	4	4	57	0	10	0	110	187
	New York University	1	3	2	3	8	9	11	1	0	2	3	1	4	52	1	5	0	100	165
	Rochester	2	0	2	6	10	9	11	7	4	4	11	2	0	17	0	12	0	69	104
	SUNY Downstate	0	0	1	8	8	24	9	7	2	4	2	0	6	64	1	16	0	93	183
	SUNY Upstate	1	0	1	1	3	6	11	2	2	1	5	1	1	24	1	20	0	106	160
	Stony Brook	0	6	1	2	8	11	11	2	2	1	6	0	6	36	1	12	0	72	124
OH	Case Western	2	1	0	4	7	11	12	1	2	0	5	1	6	61	2	9	0	104	194
	Cincinnati	3	0	1	1	5	4	22	2	2	0	5	3	4	35	1	11	0	106	159
	Northeastern Ohio	1	0	0	3	4	16	24	4	0	1	5	3	3	34	0	3	0	73	114
	Ohio State	6	4	1	1	12	7	20	2	3	1	2	1	3	55	2	10	0	141	211
	Toledo	0	0	0	2	4	4	9	0	0	1	3	1	3	38	1	10	0	127	176
	Wright State-Boonshoft	2	0	1	0	2	4	4	0	1	0	4	6	3	19	1	8	0	74	100
OK	Oklahoma	2	0	0	3	5	4	5	0	2	0	3	4	3	21	9	1	0	138	166
OR	Oregon	3	0	1	1	4	4	4	1	6	4	1	7	7	27	1	1	1	84	115
PA	Drexel	4	2	0	10	16	18	67	5	6	2	7	7	2	105	3	21	1	129	256
	Jefferson	3	6	2	6	16	14	23	0	2	3	9	0	2	57	3	3	0	172	255
	Penn State	2	1	1	3	7	9	10	2	1	0	3	0	3	27	0	7	0	99	143
	Pennsylvania	3	1	1	13	17	14	10	1	2	2	0	1	3	31	2	13	0	106	154
	Pittsburgh	3	1	0	6	9	16	12	0	0	0	2	2	3	35	2	16	0	86	147
	Temple	2	4	2	10	15	16	16	2	3	0	0	0	4	40	2	10	1	126	182
PR	Caribe	0	4	49	4	56	0	0	2	1	0	0	0	1	3	0	4	0	40	65
	Ponce	1	3	55	2	60	1	0	0	0	0	0	0	0	2	0	6	0	46	65
	Puerto Rico	0	3	106	0	106	0	0	0	0	0	0	0	0	0	0	5	0	71	108
	San Juan Bautista	1	3	41	6	49	1	0	1	1	0	1	0	2	5	0	8	2	46	60
RI	Brown-Alpert	7	3	0	2	9	12	13	2	2	3	3	0	3	35	3	10	1	38	94
SC	MU South Carolina	1	0	0	0	1	10	7	1	1	1	1	0	1	13	2	21	1	128	165
	South Carolina	0	0	0	1	1	3	6	0	0	0	0	3	1	12	0	6	0	66	83
SD	South Dakota-Sanford	0	0	0	0	0	2	0	0	0	0	0	1	0	2	0	0	0	51	54
TN	East Tennessee-Quillen	0	0	0	1	1	0	5	0	0	0	0	1	1	7	0	1	0	51	60
	Meharry	2	0	2	2	5	0	3	2	0	0	0	3	0	8	0	82	0	6	100
	Tennessee	1	0	0	0	3	3	18	2	2	1	2	0	3	25	0	11	0	114	150
	Vanderbilt	3	0	1	2	6	24	10	0	4	1	2	3	1	16	1	12	1	70	105
TX	Baylor	15	3	1	5	23	10	36	3	2	2	1	4	6	74	6	9	1	86	176
	Texas A & M	12	0	0	3	16	10	20	1	5	2	2	4	5	45	2	8	0	80	139
	Texas Tech	6	1	0	3	10	10	12	1	1	0	3	3	17	39	2	2	0	90	140
	UT Galveston	30	0	3	7	39	12	9	0	1	0	2	5	9	37	2	24	0	142	230
	UT Houston	24	1	3	17	45	28	6	1	1	0	3	4	8	29	2	10	0	170	230
	UT San Antonio	28	1	0	11	38	12	7	3	1	1	3	13	16	39	0	11	0	152	221
	UT Southwestern	19	0	1	4	24	28	24	3	2	0	5	3	16	86	0	8	0	115	221
UT	Utah	5	0	0	5	8	3	4	1	4	3	2	3	3	20	3	1	4	82	102
VA	Eastern Virginia	2	0	0	1	4	5	4	2	1	5	2	3	5	22	1	3	0	78	115
	Virginia	2	2	3	9	16	8	8	1	2	1	2	2	3	25	1	9	0	107	145
	Virginia Commonwealth	0	2	1	0	3	11	26	1	2	1	7	7	6	56	1	8	2	122	192
VT	Vermont	0	0	1	7	8	5	2	0	2	2	3	7	3	14	0	2	0	92	111
WA	U Washington	8	0	0	4	12	9	8	1	3	5	5	3	5	45	4	4	0	175	216
WI	MC Wisconsin	9	1	0	0	10	18	14	0	0	3	4	3	2	44	3	10	1	153	212
	Wisconsin	5	1	1	5	11	9	11	0	5	4	2	2	4	30	0	8	0	129	163
WV	Marshall-Edwards	0	0	0	1	1	0	1	0	1	0	0	1	2	14	0	1	0	61	78
	West Virginia	0	0	0	0	0	7	2	2	1	2	0	2	2	16	0	0	0	93	109
	Totals	**492**	**161**	**358**	**471**	**1416**	**1125**	**1378**	**167**	**190**	**146**	**408**	**252**	**450**	**3940**	**172**	**1293**	**62**	**11925**	**18036**

Source: AAMC Data Warehouse: Applicant Matriculant File as of 10/10/2008. *Hispanic Ethnicities are alone or in combination with some other Hispanic Ethnicity and include any Race. Ethnicity Counts include U.S. Citizens and Permanent Residents only. Race Counts include U.S. Citizens and Permanent Residents only, are alone or in combination with some other Race, and include both Hispanic and Non-Hispanic Ethnicity. The total represents an unduplicated count and also includes matriculants for whom we have no race data or who are foreign.

in medicine by providing information and support. The centerpiece of the campaign, a free and comprehensive Web site at *www.AspiringDocs.org*, engages, encourages, and educates visitors to the site through a variety of online features, such as Ask the Experts, Ask the Experts podcasts, Hot Topics, and Inspiring Stories. The site provides clear information about applying to medical school, financing a medical education, and navigating the medical school application process. AspiringDocs.org includes testimonials from, and question-and-answer opportunities with, practicing physicians, medical students, medical school admissions officers, minority affairs officers, and other real-world experts about what it really takes to get into and succeed in medicine.

Other AAMC resources. The AAMC offers a wide variety of information and hyperlinks in the "Minorities in Medicine" section of the AAMC's Web site at *www.aamc.org/students/minorities/*, as well as on the AAMC's Diversity Web site at *www.aamc.org/diversity*. Some programs are highlighted below.

- *Minority Student Opportunities in United States Medical Schools (MSOUSMS).* Diversity Policy and Programs produces a biennial publication that contains information supplied by individual medical schools about student recruitment and admission, as well as other topics related to enhancing diversity in the academic environment. Information about enrichment programs offered by medical schools is also listed on a school-by-school basis. *MSOUSMS* is designed to be used in conjunction with Medical School Admission Requirements (MSAR). Details about the content of *MSOUSMS* and data tables on Applicants and Graduates are available at *www.aamc.org/msousms*.

- **Enrichment programs online.** Diversity Policy and Programs supports

the Web site for "Enrichment Programs on the Web." This site includes a database resource to help undergraduate students locate summer enrichment programs on medical school campuses. Information is available at *http://services.aamc.org/summerprograms/*.

- **Medical School Career Fairs and Events Calendar.** The calendar allows the AAMC and its constituents, such as the Group on Student Affairs-Minority Affairs Section (GSA-MAS), to coordinate the scheduling of recruitment and other events pertinent to students and constituents to reduce overlap and allow for maximum attendance. For example, students can easily search for recruitment events at schools in their state or in a specific date range. Information is available at *www.aamc.org/calendar/careerfairs*.

- **Fee Assistance Program (FAP).** The AAMC's FAP helps students with extreme financial limitations whose inability to pay the full Medical College Admissions Test (MCAT®) registration fee or the American Medical College Application Service (AMCAS) fee would prevent them from taking the MCAT or applying to medical school. Details about the FAP can be found at *www.aamc.org/fap* and in Chapter 4.

- **Medical Minority Applicant Registry (Med-MAR).** Students applying to medical school who self-identify as members of groups that are underrepresented in medicine or who are economically or educationally disadvantaged are given the opportunity to register for Med-MAR at the time they take the MCAT. The Med-MAR program then circulates basic biographical information about the examinee and the examinee's MCAT scores to all U.S. medical schools. Details about the registry can

be found at *www.aamc.org/students/minorities/resources/medmar.htm*.

- **Data about race and ethnicity in medicine.** The AAMC has a great deal of information about medical education, including detailed data about medical students from an array of racial and ethnic groups.

  - AAMC information about recent matriculant data for each medical school is presented in this publication in Table 6-A, Matriculants by Medical School and Race and Ethnicity, 2008.

  - Chapter 5 of this publication includes a section on the self-reported racial and ethnic identification of medical school applicants and accepted applicants for the 2008 entering class.

  - Additional data about medical school applicants, matriculants, and graduates are available on the AAMC Web site at *www.aamc.org/data/facts*.

  - Data on medical school faculty—including information on faculty by race and ethnicity—can be found at *www.aamc.org/data/facultyroster/reports.htm*.

  - The AAMC publication entitled *Diversity in Medical Education, Facts & Figures 2008* provides race and ethnicity data on medical school applicants, accepted applicants, matriculants, enrollment, graduates, and faculty, along with detailed tables. The full text of *Facts & Figures* can be accessed without charge at *www.aamc.org/publications*.

School-based resources. Students should also take advantage of resources that exist at undergraduate and medical schools. Several examples are listed below.

- **Medical school Web sites.** The AAMC maintains a list of both U.S. and Canadian M.D.-granting medical schools at *www.aamc.org/medical schools.htm*. This list includes links to each school's Web site.

- **Premedical school programs at undergraduate colleges.** Pre-health advisors at undergraduate colleges provide pertinent information on application and admission to medical school or refer students to appropriate contacts. Pre-health advisors also are knowledgeable about programs and resources that students from underrepresented groups and disadvantaged backgrounds are likely to find useful.

- **Medical school minority affairs officers.** Each medical school has a designated minority affairs officer. These individuals are dedicated to increasing diversity among medical students at their schools, and they are an excellent source of information for potential applicants and applicants. To get in touch with a minority affairs officer, students should contact a medical school in their local area or the medical schools in which they have a potential interest.

Directory of Minority Affairs Administrators. The Directory of Minority Affairs Administrators is a searchable database of the Group on Student Affairs-Minority Affairs Section (GSA-MAS) institutional representatives at U.S. medical schools. Students can use this directory to obtain the name of the minority affairs contacts at any of the 130 U.S. medical schools. The directory is searchable by name, location, and institution and is available at *http://services.aamc.org/minorityaffairs directory/*.

Financial assistance for medical school. Any individual with an interest in a medical career should not rule out medical school solely because of financial circumstances. Public and private medical schools work hard to offer a variety of financial aid plans to both accepted applicants and already enrolled students. Applicants to medical schools should discuss possibilities for financial assistance with the financial aid officer at the medical schools that interest them, as well as discuss how best to plan effectively for the financing of their medical education. More than four-fifths of medical students nationally receive some type of financial aid to assist them in paying for their medical education. General information about financing a medical education also can be found in Chapter 9 of this publication and at *www.aamc.org/students/minorities/ scholarships.htm*.

Programs at medical schools. Once students enroll in medical school, academic and personal support programs are available to them. These programs assist students from various backgrounds to successfully complete their medical studies, with the ultimate goal of increasing racial and ethnic diversity among physicians entering careers in patient care, teaching, and research, and of eliminating racial and ethnic disparities in health care and health status. The staff members at each medical school who are primarily responsible for these programs are identified in the school-by-school entries in Chapters 12 and 13 of this publication.

Selection

Decisions about the acceptance and admission of applicants to medical school are based upon multiple criteria that are developed by the faculty of each medical school and are consistent with the school's specific mission and goals. In general, all schools admit applicants who, on the basis of materials presented during the application process, have documented that they possess the personal characteristics desired in future physicians, the ability to successfully complete the academically rigorous curriculum, and the potential to fulfill the institution's mission and goals.

Personal Characteristics

Candidates' personal attributes and experiences are very important factors in selection decisions. All admission committees seek information about the following qualities in an applicant's personal statement, in evaluations and letters of recommendation from premedical advisors and others who know the applicant well, and in personal interviews:

- psychological maturity

- character and integrity

- self-discipline

- altruism

- judgment

- compassion and empathy

- communication skills

- concern for helping others

- intellectual curiosity and enthusiasm

- motivation and persistence

- reliability and dependability

- resilience and adaptability

- accountability

- experience with, and knowledge of, medicine

- leadership skills

- experience in overcoming hardship or disadvantage

Some medical schools supplement these with other characteristics, such as research experience and potential, commitment to caring for the underserved and disadvantaged, volunteer and community service experience, knowledge about health care delivery systems, and potential for enhancing diversity in the educational environment. "Diversity" is meant to account for the contributions that students with different backgrounds, cultures, perspectives, races, ethnicities, characteristics, and personal experiences can make to the educational experience of all students and to the school's cultural, social, and learning milieu.

Letters of Evaluation and Recommendation

Medical schools usually ask applicants to indicate the names of those persons who will be submitting letters of evaluation and recommendation on their behalf. Schools typically require at least one letter from the premedical advisor or committee at the undergraduate school where the applicant completed required premedical coursework. Additional letters are usually sought from college faculty members and other advisors who have both personal knowledge of the applicant's accomplishments and the ability to objectively assess the applicant's abilities, interests, and plans. Admission committee members give less weight to subjective recommendations from personal friends, family members, and political figures. If an applicant had significant employment or military experience during or after college, letters from employers, supervisors, and commanding officers are also appropriate.

Personal and Professional Conduct

An applicant's personal and professional conduct is a crucial factor in admission decisions. Information regarding personal and professional conduct is typically made available to medical schools in three ways:

- **Self-disclosure.** Applicants are expected to disclose any disciplinary action taken against them by an institution of higher learning for violation of institutional regulations or codes of conduct. Applicants are also expected to report any legal action taken against them for violating the law and to submit a straightforward explanation of the circumstances and penalties. Applicants should discuss, as appropriate, the lessons learned and the implications of these incidents for their personal growth.

AMCAS requires an applicant to disclose on the AMCAS application any felony and misdemeanor convictions, any history of dishonorable or general discharge from the Armed Forces of the United States, and any history of institutional action. Those medical schools that do not participate in AMCAS typically require such disclosures, as well.

Failure to disclose or falsification of any official college or legal action is taken very seriously by both the AAMC and medical schools, and can prompt an official AAMC investigation that may result in the withdrawal of an admission offer.

- **Letters of Evaluation and Recommendation.** Information regarding personal and professional history is also often reported in the premedical advisor's or premedical committee's letter. Applicants should be aware that any discrepancies

between self-disclosure and disclosure within a letter of evaluation or recommendation will be carefully scrutinized by medical schools.

- **Criminal Background Checks.** In July 2005, the AAMC recommended that a criminal background check be completed on all applicants accepted annually to medical school entering classes. This recommendation resulted from a desire to bolster the public's continuing trust in the medical profession, to ensure the safety and well-being of patients, to ascertain the ability of accepted applicants and enrolled medical students to eventually become licensed physicians, and to minimize the liability of medical schools and their affiliated clinical facilities. The AAMC worked with a group of representative medical schools to develop an AAMC-administered national, centralized process for completing and reporting on criminal background checks to AAMC-member medical schools. It is reasonable to expect that a large proportion of medical schools will choose to participate in this ongoing test for the 2010 entering class. Additional information will be made available to applicants and their premedical advisors as this testing process continues and decisions are made about implementation of policies and procedures for all interested schools.

Academic Ability

Admission committees seek to enroll students who have acquired the academic skills and knowledge necessary to progress successfully through the medical curriculum and who can be active learners throughout their medical careers. Committee members rely on an applicant's academic record and MCAT® scores in evaluating academic ability.

The former measures an applicant's academic competitiveness over time; the

latter provides objective information about the applicant's knowledge base compared with others in the national applicant pool.

Academic history. Given the challenges inherent in a medical education, an applicant's academic history allows admission committee members to determine whether the applicant's study skills, persistence, course of study, and grades predict success in medical school. The "Academic Record" on the AMCAS application, containing verified and standardized grades from college transcripts, is carefully reviewed by committee members to determine the:

- grades earned in each course and laboratory

- number of credit hours carried in each academic period

- distribution of coursework among the biological, physical, and social sciences and the humanities

- need for remediation of unsatisfactory academic work

- frequency of incomplete grades and course withdrawals

- number of years taken to complete the degree program

Although each medical school establishes its own admission criteria, schools usually prefer applicants who have completed their college degrees in a timely manner, carried respectable course loads, balanced science and humanities coursework, and consistently earned 3.0–4.0 grades (on a 4.0 scale). Chapter 5 contains information about the range of science, non-science, and total grade point averages of all applicants for the 2009 entering class.

In assessing an applicant's academic work, admission committees also consider the characteristics of the undergraduate academic institution.

Coursework at colleges known for rigorous academic standards frequently get greater weight. Because medical schools vary on accepting high school AP and CLEP credits, the admission policies of individual schools in Chapters 12 and Chapter 13 should be carefully reviewed. Additional information can be achieved on a school's Web site, in its academic bulletin, or from discussions with admissions office personnel.

An applicant who has earned less-than-competitive grades in a given course or academic period should not simply decide to forgo a career in medicine. With the help of a premedical advisor and with additional academic work completed more competitively, an applicant with prior academic problems may still be able to generate a successful application. Just as in medical care and practice, the ability to persist successfully in the face of initial adversity may be perceived as an important attribute in the application and admission process.

MCAT scores. Scores on the MCAT can provide supplementary information about a candidate's academic ability and potential. Each medical school decides how MCAT scores are factored into determining an applicant's ability to accomplish the academic work in the medical curriculum. Some schools average multiple MCAT scores, some accept the highest score in each section from multiple MCAT administrations, and others emphasize the most recent set of MCAT scores. Chapters 12 and 13 present school-specific policies about the oldest and most recent MCAT scores considered for admission. In addition, the data in Chapters 12 and 13 indicate that the range of MCAT scores deemed acceptable for admission varies among schools.

MCAT scores may receive greater attention from admission committees when a candidate's academic record is marginal or when committee members are not familiar with the candidate's undergraduate institution. In addition, a

comparison of grades with MCAT scores can provide committee members with more information than either provides on its own.

Since an applicant's academic ability is a critical selection factor for medical schools, assessing it typically includes a review of both grades and scores on the four sections of the MCAT. Evaluating the academic preparation and ability of applicants who are not recent college graduates usually includes, in addition to the overall college record, a review of achievement in postbaccalaureate courses. Similarly, the academic abilities of candidates from groups underrepresented in medicine and from educationally and socioeconomically disadvantaged groups require special attention; additional information can be found in Chapter 6 and in the AAMC publication, Minority Student Opportunities in U.S. Medical Schools (*www.aamc.org/msousms*).

Interviews

Medical school policies for granting and scheduling admission committee interviews vary. A few public schools in smaller states grant an interview to all candidates who are state residents, while the majority of schools invite candidates only after an extensive screening and prioritizing process. In some instances, the interview is a final step in the assessment process for applicants already deemed to be highly attractive candidates. In other instances, the interview process occurs before any preliminary decision-making by the admission committee. Almost always, an interview is required before a final admission decision is made.

Information about a school's interview policies and procedures is usually provided to applicants in the initial stages of the selection process. Questions and requests for clarification should be directed to staff in the school's admissions office.

Applicant interviews are typically held on the medical school campus. Sometimes an applicant will be asked to interview with a graduate of the school or with a physician in the applicant's area. Some schools have designated interviewers in different geographic regions to minimize time and expense for applicants, but many schools do not offer these off-campus opportunities.

At some schools, interviews are held with individual admission committee members; at others, group interviews are the norm. Some interviewers have prior access to the applicant's information, including grades, MCAT scores, and letters of evaluation, but other interviewers do not, and they focus instead on the candidate's experiential attributes. The interview can be an excellent opportunity for applicants to visit a campus; view the basic science and clinical facilities; meet faculty, staff, and students; and have their questions answered by members of the faculty and staff who are knowledgeable about the school and its educational and clinical programs.

The interview provides candidates with opportunities to discuss their personal histories and motivation for a medical career, as well as any aspects of their application that merit emphasis or explanation. Candidates should be prepared to discuss all aspects of their application, including their interest in the specific institution. Applicants should be forthright, open, and informative in their meetings with interviewers. Since most admission committee members are experienced interviewers who want to learn about the "real" person, applicants should not try to "game" the interview or paint a picture they believe the interviewer wants to see. For those applicants who are apprehensive about the process, practice interviews with a trusted advisor or friend can help them to present themselves in the best possible light.

AAMC Policies and Procedures for Investigating Reported Violations of Admission and Enrollment Standards

Purpose

Two significant responsibilities of the Association of American Medical Colleges (AAMC) are to promote integrity in the processes associated with entry into medical school or a graduate medical education program, and to encourage high standards during the course of enrollment. These policies and procedures have been developed to advance these purposes by addressing cases that arise in the following areas, while ensuring the rights of all concerned parties.

Policies

The AAMC requires applicants to present accurate and current information at the time application materials are submitted and during all phases of the admission process for entry into medical school or a graduate medical education program.

It is the policy of the AAMC to investigate discrepancies in credentials, attempts to subvert the admission process, and any other irregular matter that occurs in connection with application activities.

Testing Cases

The AAMC requires candidates for the MCAT examination to present accurate and current information at the time registration materials are submitted and to adhere to all Test Center Regulations and Procedures as outlined in the MCAT Essentials. It is the policy of the AAMC to investigate discrepancies, attempts to subvert eligibility requirements, violations of Test Center Regulations, and irregular behavior exhibited during the administration of the MCAT or other tests affiliated with the AAMC.

This investigation is distinct from a Score Validity Inquiry conducted by the MCAT Program, which pertains to the legitimacy of test scores as accurate representations of the individual's performance.

Other Cases

The AAMC may investigate and/or facilitate the reporting of certain cases that occur subsequent to an individual's enrollment in medical school. Such cases include, but are not limited to, academic and ethical violations and criminal activities. In addition, reports documenting cases submitted by other educational agencies may be disseminated by the AAMC to legitimately interested parties after notice and opportunity to comment are afforded the subject of the reports.

Reporting of Cases

The AAMC will prepare and issue a report documenting the nature of a confirmed case and any attachments provided by the individual in accordance with the procedures outlined below. With the issuance of a report, the AAMC makes no judgment as to the culpability of any person with respect to matters reported and does not assess the suitability of an individual to study or practice medicine. Rather, the AAMC strives to communicate complete and accurate information to legitimately interested parties. Evaluation of this information is the responsibility of the recipient of the report.

Procedures

Investigation Proceedings
The subject of any case is informed of the existence of the investigation and is offered an opportunity to respond to the allegations. The individual is also provided with the opportunity to review a draft of any report proposed for distribution prior to issuance. Unless otherwise requested, the final report will include any explanation or justification provided by the individual during the course of the investigation.

A pending investigation may interrupt the processing of application, registration, or testing materials of questionable validity. Such action by the AAMC, however, does not relieve the individual of the responsibility for the payment of normal processing fees.

Arbitration
The AAMC offers the option and reserves the right to request arbitration should the individual conclude that a draft report inaccurately characterizes the matter under investigation or when an agreement between parties on the content and language of the report cannot be reached. Such arbitration must be requested prior to the conclusion of an investigation and the issuance of a final report.

Arbitration is conducted by a neutral arbitrator selected by the Washington, D.C., office of the American Arbitration Association. The arbitrator acts solely on the basis of a written record submitted by both parties and no hearing or oral arguments are held. The arbitrator will have final authority to conclude whether: (1) the report should be distributed as written or (2) the report should be modified in accordance with the arbitrator's directions before distribution or (3) no report should be distributed. In addition, the arbitrator determines which party is responsible for the arbitration fee. All other costs associated with arbitration are borne by the party incurring them.

Report Recipients
The report in final form will be issued to all medical schools or residency programs to which the individual has applied or matriculated during the current cycle and medical schools and residency programs to which the applicant applies or matriculates in the future. If, at the time of the investigation, the individual is enrolled in a medical school or graduate medical education program, the report will be forwarded to the current institution of attendance and will be distributed in response to all future application or matriculation activity.

In addition to its members, the AAMC provides services to other educational institutions. For example, the MCAT examination is used by a variety of health profession and graduate programs in addition to medicine. The report in final form is therefore subject to issuance in response to application or matriculation at such institutions of which the AAMC has knowledge.

Reports may contain information relevant to academic or disciplinary proceedings, criminal investigations, and decisions relative to entry into graduate medical education programs and professional licensure. It is the position of the AAMC to cooperate with duly constituted agencies by responding to official requests for such reports.

Chapter 8

Acceptance

Medical schools make admission offers to applicants on a continuous basis during the months before the medical school fall semester — as early as September of the year prior to matriculation for Early Decision Program (EDP) applicants, and as late as the first day of class for regular applicants. This process can sometimes become complex, especially when an applicant is admitted to more than one school. Both schools and applicants have rights and responsibilities in this process.

All 130 AAMC-member medical schools agree to observe a set of recommendations on medical school acceptance procedures for first-year entering students (see Page 50 or *www.aamc.org/ students/applying/policies*). These are commonly referred to as the admission "traffic rules." Applicants should be familiar with them, as they ensure that application and acceptance processes are timely and fair for all concerned. These recommendations:

- contain important dates all applicants should know

- reserve the right of applicants to hold places at multiple schools without losing an acceptance deposit, usually until May 15

- indicate policies for schools to follow after May 15 regarding applicants who continue to hold multiple places

- set forth prohibitions about a medical school's offering admission to applicants who have already enrolled in, or begun orientation programs at, another medical school. Individual schools' acceptance policies are presented in Chapters 12 and 13, although applicants are encouraged to contact the schools that are of interest to them, as well.

Applicants also have responsibilities (*www.aamc.org/students/applying/policies*). During the application process for the 2008 entering class, 8,044 applicants were accepted to two or more medical schools. Although multiple family, personal, and financial factors can affect applicants' ultimate decisions about which school to attend, they are strongly encouraged to hold only one medical school acceptance at a time. Once applicants make a final decision, they should withdraw their applications promptly from other schools. When possible, applicants holding multiple acceptances should accept their first-choice offer and withdraw from other schools that have made an offer of admission. If a subsequent and more highly preferred admission offer is received, applicants can accept the new offer and withdraw from the school at which they were originally accepted. Immediately upon matriculating at a medical school or participating in an orientation program associated with the beginning of the first-year curriculum, applicants must withdraw their applications to all other medical schools at which they remain under consideration.

Citizenship and Residency

Citizenship. The 2008 entering class at U.S. medical schools included 289 students who were not U.S. citizens or who were not permitted to reside permanently in this country by U.S. Citizenship and Immigration Services, a bureau of the Department of Homeland Security. This relatively small number of international matriculants results from several factors:

- Many public medical schools limit enrollment to state residents.

- State residency statutes require that applicants be either U.S. citizens or permitted to reside permanently or indefinitely in the U.S.

- Many private medical schools require international applicants to document their ability to independently finance a medical education.

- Many countries impose severe restrictions on the exportation of currency.

- Federal financial aid sources generally require students to be either U.S. citizens or permitted to reside permanently or indefinitely in the U.S.

- Many medical schools require completion of premedical coursework at a U.S. college or university.

- Medical schools require documentation of English language proficiency, either from an American undergraduate college or the official agency in the applicant's home country. Information about the Test of English as a Foreign Language (TOEFL) can be found at *www.toefl.org*.

Private medical schools are more likely to accept international students than public schools. However, they frequently require international matriculants to show evidence of a U.S. bank account containing sufficient resources to cover tuition and expenses for one or more years of medical education. International applicants should be aware of these issues and be prepared to meet all special requirements.

State residency. State-supported medical schools generally give preference for admission and transfer to state residents. Some states have additional requirements regarding county or regional residence. Requirements are established by state legislatures and are usually available from school officials or on the school's or state's Web site. For students who are financially independent of their parents, documentation of state residency typically involves:

- payment of state resident income taxes

- voter registration in the state

- physical residence in the state for a prescribed period of time

- possession of a state driver's license

- motor vehicle registration in the state

For students who are financial dependents, the state of residence is usually the same as that of their parents. A school's state residency definition for the purpose of in-state tuition and fee eligibility may differ from definitions for other purposes, such as voting. An applicant can usually have official state residency in only one state at a time. Because of the relationship between state of residence and probability of admission, applicants are strongly encouraged to clarify their official residency status with preferred schools before initiating a formal application.

State residents enrolled in public schools customarily pay lower tuition than nonresidents. Some private schools also show preference for state residents for at least some of their places because the school receives state government support. Some states without a public medical school participate in special interstate and regional agreements to provide their residents with access to a medical education. Registrars and residency officers, located either on the medical school or parent institution's campus, can assist applicants with state residency issues.

The individual school entries in Chapter 12 present data about resident and non-resident applicants and matriculants. Nationally, 61.8 percent of 2008 matriculants attended schools in their home states; 79.5 percent of students in public schools and 34.1 percent in private schools were state residents. Public schools are unlikely to admit nonresidents unless they have exceptionally strong credentials or strong ties to the state through prior residency, employment, education, or family members.

Special Regional Opportunities for Applicants

Six interstate agreements provide special opportunities for residents of certain states:

1. The Delaware Institute of Medical Education and Research provides payment to Jefferson Medical College of Thomas Jefferson University to reserve at least 20 admissions each year for Delaware residents. To be eligible, applicants must be Delaware residents, meet the premedical academic requirements of Jefferson Medical College, and apply through the American Medical College Application Service (AMCAS). Applicants' undergraduate degrees can be from any accredited U.S. college or university. Additional information is available at *http:// dhcc.delaware.gov/information/ dimer.shtml*, or from:

   Delaware Institute of Medical Education and Research
   The Delaware Higher Education Commission
   Carvel State Office Building
   820 North French Street
   Wilmington, DE 19801
   (302) 577-5240
   (800) 292-7935

2. The Finance Authority of Maine's (FAME) Maine Access to Medical Education Program — through relationships with participating medical schools, including Dartmouth Medical School and the University of Vermont College of Medicine — ensures preference each year for 20 first-year places for Maine residents certified as eligible by the state. FAME seeks applicants who are most likely to practice primary care in underserved areas of the state. The program pays the school a fee for each student. Although students' tuition and fees are not reduced, they do receive priority for need-based forgivable loans of $5,000 to $25,000 annually.

Students must commit to completing at least two primary care clinical rotations in Maine following completion of the medical school's core curriculum. Applicants should know that the state of Maine will encourage them to select primary care specialties and to practice in the state following completion of their training. Maine's Advisory Committee on Medical Education reviews all applications, but individual medical schools make final admission decisions. Additional information can be found at *www.famemaine.com*, or from:

Maine Access to
Medical Education Program
Finance Authority of Maine
P.O. Box 949
Augusta, ME 04332-0949
(800) 228-3734

3. University of Utah School of Medicine Idaho Contract-The State of Idaho has contracted to provide access for eight Idaho students each year to attend the University of Utah School of Medicine. Students must be certified through Idaho State University as residents of Idaho prior to applying. Accepted students attend the University of Utah School of Medicine and pay the equivalent of Utah resident tuition. Students also pay a surcharge to a fund administered by the Idaho State Board of Education that is designed to encourage participants to return to a primary care practice in a rural or underserved area in Idaho.

Information about this program is available at *http://medicine.utah.edu/admissions/begin/residency.htm* or by calling (208) 282-2475.

University of Utah School of Medicine
Office of Admissions
30 North 1900 East Room 1C029
Salt Lake City, Utah 84132-2101
801.581.7498
deans.admissions@hsc.utah.edu

4. Under the auspices of the Southern Regional Education Board (SREB), some students from Alabama, North Carolina, and Tennessee, who have been accepted at Meharry Medical College, can pay reduced tuition at that school. For more information, see the SREB Web site at *www.sreb.org*, or contact the SREB at:

Southern Regional Education Board
592 10th St. N.W.
Atlanta, GA 30318
(404) 875-9211
acm-rcp@sreb.org

5. The Western Interstate Commission for Higher Education (WICHE) supports the Professional Student Exchange Program, enabling students from Montana and Wyoming, after certification by their states and contingent on the availability of funding, to attend a participating medical school and to pay in-state tuition at a public school or reduced tuition at a private school. The student's home state pays a fee to the admitting medical school to help cover costs. Additional information can be obtained from the certifying office in the student's home state; contact information for each state's certifying office can be found on the WICHE Web site at *www.wiche.edu/SEP/PSEP/cert-off.asp*. A student must apply though the home state certifying office by October 15th for priority consideration.

6. The WWAMI (Washington, Wyoming, Alaska, Montana, and Idaho) program of decentralized medical education, begun in 1972, provides access to a publicly supported medical education to students from the five participating states. WWAMI students complete their first year at participating institutions in their home states and their second year at the University of Washington School of Medicine in Seattle. Clerkship options are available for third- and fourth-year

students in community settings throughout the five-state region. Additional information is available at *www.uwmedicine.org/education/wwami*, or from:

Office of Admissions
School of Medicine
University of Washington
A-300 Health Sciences Building
Box 356340
Seattle, WA 98195-6340
(206) 543-7212
askuwsom@u.washington.edu

Deferring Entry into Medical School

An accepted applicant may encounter a special, one-time opportunity that is too attractive to pass up, or be invited to spend an additional year in an ongoing research project, or want to live abroad for a period of time. In recent years, most medical schools have developed delayed matriculation programs that allow applicants to pursue these opportunities without giving up their medical school places.

These deferred-entry programs usually require that the applicant submit a written request, and some schools may also ask for a report at the end of the deferral period. Delays of matriculation are usually granted for one year, although some schools may defer for longer periods of time. Some schools require delayed matriculants to sign an agreement to not apply to other medical schools in the interim, while others permit delayed matriculants to apply to other schools. Deferred matriculants will receive instructions from the school granting the deferral about requirements for another application for the year of actual matriculation. The number of deferrals may be limited, and there may be a deadline date for such applications. Interested applicants should seek specific information from schools that interest them, and schools are encouraged to define their expectations of the deferred applicant in a written document that is signed by both an appropriate school official and the applicant. The school-specific pages in Chapters 12 and 13 also contain information about deferred entrance.

Multiple Acceptances and Final Decisions

Applicants fortunate enough to receive multiple admission offers should not delay their fellow applicants' receipt of an acceptance offer by holding those acceptances for an extended time. Decisions should be made and schools notified as promptly as possible. In the spring, AMCAS shares acceptance information with all medical schools. By mid-May, the AAMC expects that all medical schools will have notified accepted applicants of their financial aid awards and that accepted applicants will have sufficient information to determine which school to attend. May 15 is the deadline for acceptance deposit refunds and for applicants' final decisions about medical schools; after May 15, schools can require applicants to choose the one school that they will attend from among those schools that have offered an acceptance. Under no circumstances should applicants be required to withdraw from other schools' waiting lists as a condition of accepting a medical school place. Ultimately, decisions about where to attend belong to applicants, not schools.

Orientation Programs

Most medical schools hold orientation programs for entering students just prior to the start of the first term. These programs familiarize students with their new environment; provide opportunities to meet fellow students, staff, and faculty; facilitate book and equipment purchases; and start to acculturate students to medicine's professional codes and responsibilities.

Once these orientation periods have begun, students can no longer accept admission offers from other schools, and they should withdraw their names from all waiting lists at other schools.

AAMC Recommendations for Medical School Admission Officers

The following recommendations are promulgated by the Association of American Medical Colleges (AAMC) to ensure that M.D. and M.D.–Ph.D. applicants are afforded timely notification of the outcome of their applications and timely access to available first-year positions and that schools and programs are protected from having unfilled positions in their entering classes. These recommendations are being distributed for the information of prospective M.D. and M.D.–Ph.D. students, their advisors, and personnel at the medical schools and programs to which they have applied.

The AAMC recommends that:

1. Each school:

   a. Publish annually, amend publicly, and adhere to its application, acceptance, and admission procedures.

   b. Utilizing an application service abide by all conditions of its participation agreement with that application service.

2. Each school:

   a. Between August 1 and March 15, notify the AAMC Section for Medical School Application Services of all admission actions within four weeks of those actions being taken.

   b. Between March 16 and the first day of class, notify the AAMC Section for Medical School Application Services of all admission actions within seven days of those actions being taken.

3. Each school notify all applicants — other than combined college/M.D., Early Decision Program (EDP), and deferred matriculation applicants — of acceptance to medical school only after October 15 of each admission cycle. It may be appropriate to communicate notifications of decisions other than acceptance to medical school to applicants prior to October 15.

4. By March 30 of the matriculation year, March 15 for M.D.–Ph.D. programs, each school have issued a number of offers of acceptance at least equal to the expected number of students in its first-year entering class and have reported those acceptance actions to the AAMC Section for Medical School Application Services.

5. Prior to May 15 of the matriculation year (April 15 for schools whose first day of class is on or before July 30), April 30 for M.D.–Ph.D. programs, each school or program permit ALL applicants (except for EDP applicants) — including those to whom merit or other special scholarships have been awarded:

   a. A minimum two-week time period for their response to the acceptance offer.

   b. To hold acceptance offers from any other schools or programs without penalty.

AAMC Recommendations for Medical School Admission Officers
continued

6. After May 15 of the matriculation year (April 15 for schools whose first day of class is on or before July 30), April 30 for M.D.–Ph.D. programs, each school or program implement school-specific procedures for accepted applicants who, without adequate explanation, continue to hold one or more places at other schools or programs. These procedures:

   a. May require applicants to:

      i. Respond to acceptance offers in less than two weeks.

      ii. Submit a statement of intent, a deposit, or both.

   b. Should recognize the problems of applicants with multiple acceptance offers, applicants who have not yet received an acceptance offer, and applicants who have not yet been informed about financial aid opportunities at those schools to which they have been accepted.

   c. Should permit accepted applicants to remain on other schools' waiting lists and to withdraw if they later receive an acceptance offer from a preferred school or program.

7. Each school's acceptance deposit not exceed $100 (except for EDP applicants) and be refundable until May 15, April 30 for M.D.–Ph.D. applicants. If the applicant enrolls at the school, the school is encouraged to credit the deposit toward tuition.

8. After June 1, May 15 for M.D.–Ph.D. programs, any school that plans to make an acceptance offer to an applicant already known to have been accepted by another school or program for that entering class ensure that the other school is advised of this offer at the time that the offer is made. This notification should be made immediately by telephone and promptly thereafter by written correspondence delivered by regular or electronic methods. Schools and programs should communicate fully with each other with respect to anticipated late roster changes in order to minimize interschool miscommunication and misunderstanding, as well as the possibility of unintended vacant positions in a school's first-year entering class.

9. No school make an acceptance offer, either verbal or written, to any individual who has enrolled in, or begun an orientation program immediately prior to enrollment at, a U.S. or Canadian school. Enrollment is defined as being officially matriculated as a member of the school's first-year entering class.

10. Each school treat all letters of recommendation submitted in support of an application as confidential, except in those states with applicable laws to the contrary. The contents of a letter of recommendation should not be revealed to an applicant at any time.

Approved: AAMC Council of Deans Administrative Board, February 17, 2009

AAMC Recommendations for Medical School and M.D.–Ph.D. Applicants

The following recommendations are promulgated by the Association of American Medical Colleges (AAMC) to ensure that M.D. and M.D.–Ph.D. applicants are afforded timely notification of the outcome of their applications and timely access to available first-year positions and that schools and programs are protected from having unfilled positions in their entering classes. These recommendations are being distributed for the information of prospective M.D. and M.D.–Ph.D. students, their advisors, and personnel at the medical schools and programs to which they have applied.

The AAMC recommends that:

1. Each applicant be familiar with, understand, and comply with the application, acceptance, and admission procedures at each school or program to which the applicant has applied, as well with as these recommendations.

2. Each applicant provide accurate and truthful information in all aspects of the application, acceptance, and admission processes for each school or program to which the applicant has applied.

3. Each applicant submit all application documents (e.g., primary and secondary application forms, transcript[s], letters of evaluation/recommendation, fees) to each school in a timely manner and no later than the school's or program's published deadline date.

4. Each applicant promptly notify all relevant medical school application services and all medical schools or programs with independent application processes of any change, permanent or temporary, in contact information (e.g., mailing address, telephone number, e-mail address).

5. Any applicant who will be unavailable for an extended period of time (e.g., during foreign travel, vacation, holidays) during the application/admission process:

    a. Provide instructions regarding his or her application and the authority to respond to offers of acceptance to a parent or other responsible individual in the applicant's absence.

    b. Inform all schools or programs at which the applicant remains under consideration of this individual's name and contact information.

6. Each applicant respond promptly to a school's or program's invitation for interview. Any applicant who cannot appear for a previously scheduled interview should notify the school or program **immediately** of the cancellation of the appointment in the manner requested by the school or program.

7. Each applicant in need of financial aid initiate, as early as possible, the steps necessary to determine eligibility, including the early filing of appropriate need-analysis forms and the encouragement of parents, when necessary, to file required income tax forms.

8. In fairness to other applicants, when an applicant has made a decision, prior to May 15, April 30 for M.D.–Ph.D. applicants, not to attend a medical school or program that has made an offer of acceptance, the applicant **promptly** withdraw his or her application from that (those) other school(s) or program(s) by written correspondence delivered by regular or electronic methods.

9. By May 15 of the matriculation year (April 15 for schools whose first day of class is on or before July 30), April 30 for M.D.–Ph.D. programs, each applicant who has received an offer of acceptance from more than one school choose the specific school at which the applicant prefers to enroll and withdraw his or her application, by written correspondence delivered by regular or electronic methods, from all other schools or programs from which acceptance offers have been received.

10. Immediately upon enrollment in, or initiation of an orientation program immediately prior to enrollment at, a U.S. or Canadian school or program, each applicant withdraw his or her application from consideration at all other schools or programs at which he or she remains under consideration.

Approved: AAMC Council of Deans Administrative Board, February 17, 2009

Chapter 9

Financing a Medical Education

After being accepted to medical school, a prospective student must finalize an individual plan for covering the significant costs of a medical education, including, among other typical expenses, tuition, fees, books, equipment, living expenses, medical and disability insurance, and transportation. Two major skills are involved: the ability to develop realistic and proactive financing plans and the ability to manage educational debt. There are several factors that a student should consider in making financial decisions:

- Students are typically able to cover the cost of their medical educations with student loans.

- Medical school tuition and fees have increased significantly over the past decade.

- Student educational loans are the most common form of financial assistance.

- Primary financial responsibility for medical school rests with students and their families.

- Most medical students are unable to supplement their income with employment.

- Students with a history of credit problems may not qualify for the private loans that, in some cases, supplement federal borrowing.

- Credit card and other consumer debt obligations cannot be met with student financial aid.

- Available non-loan financial assistance, such as scholarships and grants, is finite, especially for living expenses.

- Criteria for awarding institutional financial aid differ from school to school.

- Funding and eligibility requirements for federal financial aid programs are determined by federal regulations, which can change periodically.

Information about the financial aid forms required by each medical school can be found in the searchable database on the AAMC Web site at *http://services.aamc.org/msar_reports*.

FIRST *for Medical Education* is an AAMC program that provides a wide range of services, resources and tools for medical school applicants and students, among others. The FIRST Web site (*www.aamc.org/first*) offers students information and tools to help them make smart decisions about student loans, effectively manage their education debt, and expand their financial literacy. Several resources for applicants and students are available to help provide a better understanding of financial aid, such as the library of FIRST Fact Sheets (*www.aamc.org/programs/first/students/factsheets.htm*) — short, informational sheets on a variety of financial aid related topics, and interactive Budget Worksheet (*www.aamc.org/programs/first/facts/budget_worksheet.pdf*).

TABLE 9-A

Tuition, Fees and Health Insurance for 2008–2009 First-Year Students in U.S. Medical Schools (in Dollars)

Categories of Students	Private Schools		
	Range	Median	Average
Resident	$15,278 – $51,968	$43,480	$41,225
Nonresident	$23,242 – $52,236	$43,896	$42,519

Categories of Students	Public Schools		
	Range	Median	Average
Resident	$10,234 – $36,773	$24,809	$23,581
Nonresident	$18,709 – $74,748	$43,543	$43,587

Figures based on data provided summer 2008. Three schools do not accept nonresident students and therefore do not report nonresident data: University of Arizona, University of Massachusetts, and Mercer University. This table excludes the Uniformed Services University of the Health Sciences, a public institution that does not charge tuition or student fees.

TABLE 9-B

Federal Loan Programs for Students

Characteristic	Primary Care Loan	Federal Perkins	Federal Subsidized/ Unsubsidized Stafford	Graduate PLUS Loan
Lender	Medical school financial aid office on behalf of the Department of Health and Human Services	Medical school financial aid office on behalf of the federal government	Bank or other lending institution, the federal government or an eligible institution	Bank or other lending institution, the federal government or an eligible institution
Based on need	Note[1]	Yes	Subsidized: Yes Unsubsidized: No	No
Citizenship requirement	U.S. citizen, U.S. national, U.S. permanent resident, or asylum status	U.S. citizen, U.S. national, U.S. permanent resident, or asylum status	U.S. citizen, U.S. national, U.S. permanent resident, or asylum status	U.S. citizen, U.S. national, U.S. permanent resident, or asylum status
Borrowing limits	Up to cost of attendance (Third- and fourth-year students may receive additional funds to repay previous educational loans received while attending medical school)	$6,000/year $40,000 aggregate undergraduate and graduate	$47,167 less subsidized Stafford $8,500 annual maximum; $224,000 less subsidized Stafford $65,500 maximum premed and medical borrowing[2]	Annual cost of attendance minus other financial aid
Interest rate	Note[3]	5%	For loans first disbursed since July 1, 2006, 6.8% for the life of the loan	For loans first disbursed since July 1, 2006, 8.5% for the life of the loan
Borrower is responsible for interest during school:	No	No	Subsidized: No Unsubsidized: Yes	Yes

1. Yes; in addition, borrower must agree upon signing loan agreement to enter and complete a primary care residency and practice in a primary care field until the loan is repaid in full. Family resource information is required for consideration.
2. Both annual and cumulative maximum are subject to change, pending congressional action.
3. Five percent; however, rate is recomputed at 18% from the date of noncompliance should borrower fail to meet primary care requirements (for primary care loans made on or after November 13, 1998).

(MD)[2]: Monetary Decisions for Medical Doctors

(MD)[2]: Monetary Decisions for Medical Doctors is a comprehensive, Web-based program (*www.aamc.org/md2*) developed by the AAMC to assist premedical and medical students in their financial planning. Divided into three sections — The Premedical School Years, The Medical School Years, and The Residency and Early Practice Years — (MD)[2] provides information that is tailored to the specific needs of students during the different phases of their education. Information covered includes types of financial aid, the financial aid application process, and credit and consumer debt, along with relevant reference materials.

Planning for the Financing of a Medical Education

In 2008, those medical students who graduated with educational debt reported an average educational debt of $155,000. Tuition and other expenses vary from school to school; entries in Chapter 12 provide information about individual schools' tuition and fee schedules, as well as about cost of attendance (minus tuition and fees) and average educational indebtedness for 2008 graduates.

Since most students rely on loans to pay for medical school, they should be aware of two general borrowing concepts:

• Borrowing encumbers future income. When taking an educational loan, the student is obligating future income to pay that loan off, which means that future income may be limited for opening a practice, purchasing a home, buying a car, or starting a family. Some financial analysts estimate that three dollars of future income are needed to pay off every dollar of current borrowing. Medical students should be aware of the implications of borrowing.

• The borrower must decide whether the value of a medical degree is approximately equal to the future income necessary to satisfy

TABLE 9-B (continued)

Federal Loan Programs for Students

Characteristic	Primary Care Loan	Federal Perkins	Federal Subsidized/ Unsubsidized Stafford	Graduate PLUS Loan
Deferments	No	No	Subsidized: No Unsubsidized: Yes	Yes
Grace period	No	No	Subsidized: No Unsubsidized: Yes	N/A
Grace period	1 year after graduation	9 months after graduation	6 months after graduation	None
Deferments*	During school and primary care residency; check your promissory note or ask your financial aid officer.	During school. Check your promissory note or ask your financial aid officer.	During school. Check your promissory note or ask your financial aid officer.	During school. Check your promissory note or ask your financial aid officer.

* See Deferment Chart — pg. 13 of the Education Debt Manager at *www.aamc.org/programs/first/debtmanager.pdf*

Characteristic	Primary Care Loan	Federal Perkins	Federal Subsidized/ Unsubsidized Stafford	Graduate PLUS Loan
Repayment requirements	Minimum: $40/month; 10 to 25 years to repay; not eligible for loan consolidation	Minimum: $40/month including interest; maximum 10 years to repay; eligible for loan consolidation	Minimum: $50/month; level, graduated, income sensitive, and extended repayment options available; eligible for loan consolidation	Minimum: $50/month; level, graduated, income sensitive and extended repayment options available; eligible for loan consolidation
Prepayment penalties	None	None	None	None
Allowable cancellations	Death or total and permanent disability	Death or total and permanent disability	Death or total and permanent disability	Death or total and permanent disability

educational loans. While borrowing for educational purposes is a good investment in one's future, it has an impact on personal and professional lifestyle choices. Only the individual borrower can assess whether the potential return is worth the initial investment.

Debt Management

Learning to manage money takes constant practice, and formulating and living within a budget are essential elements. Thoughtful spending choices can result in less borrowing now and more disposable income later. Several practices are key to good budgeting:

- Have a spending plan. Prepare a strategy for allocating resources and anticipating periodic expenses, such as car insurance premiums, and unexpected emergencies, such as medical bills.

- Use credit prudently. Possessing one low-interest, no-fee credit card and paying the full balance monthly are highly recommended. Timely payments enhance personal credit ratings and prevent late fees.

- Use financial windfalls wisely. Use the "rule of thirds" for unexpected gifts or tax refunds: one-third to savings, one-third to pay down debt, and one-third to spending.

- Calculate ownership costs. Owning a house or car involves insurance and maintenance costs in addition to mortgage and loan payments.

- Plug spending leaks. Even minor expenditures such as restaurant meals, if they are incurred daily or weekly, add up over time.

- Limit careless shopping. Impulse buying can ruin even the best financial plan. Shop with a list and buy only when specific items are needed.

- Save whenever possible. Saving even a small amount each week can quickly add up.

- Practice delayed gratification. Answering these questions can pare down spending: Is this a "want" or a "need"? Must I have it now? Can I pay less elsewhere? Can I borrow or rent it instead?

- Live on less. Even the essential expenses of housing, transportation, and food can be reduced by living with a roommate, carpooling, using public transportation, or preparing meals at home.

In addition to good budgeting, debt management also requires good recordkeeping. The borrower is responsible for maintaining records on monies owed, terms and conditions of each loan, the agencies that service loans, deadline dates, and deferment policies. Copies of application forms and promissory notes should be kept in a safe place. Many loan programs and financial institutions help in this process by providing access to information on their Web sites. Carefully tracking due dates and deadlines is also very beneficial.

Borrowers are also responsible for keeping loan providers and servicers notified of changes in name, contact information, and enrollment status. Borrowers who fail to maintain contact with lenders risk becoming delinquent in their loan payments or defaulting on their loans. Either of these situations can cause serious long-term consequences to the borrower's credit rating and can endanger future borrowing.

Financial Aid Philosophy

Financial aid provides assistance for postsecondary education and opportunities for students to attend schools of their choice. The philosophy of financial aid is that a student's family bears primary responsibility, to the extent possible, for paying educational expenses. From undergraduate to graduate and professional education, there is a decided shift in expectations about who bears the main responsibility for paying educational expenses, as

explained below. Eligibility for financial aid is generally determined by answering three questions:

1. **How much does it cost?** The answer varies by school and by year in school. Cost is composed of three components: tuition and fees; books, supplies, and equipment; and living expenses. These are frequently referred to as the "cost of attendance" or the "student financial aid budget." Cost of attendance figures by school year should be available from each medical school's financial aid officer.

2. **What are the student's resources?** The amount that a student's family can contribute to a medical education is called the "expected family contribution." It is determined through a need-analysis formula at the time of the financial aid application, which ensures that all students are treated equitably. Unlike most undergraduate students, graduate and professional students are considered financially independent in determining the expected family contribution for most types of federal financial aid; both income and assets are taken into account. However, eligibility for some types of federal aid requires reporting of family financial information, even though the student is technically considered to be independent. This is also the case at some institutions in determining eligibility for institutional grants, scholarships, and school-based loans. In theory, this approach ensures that certain types of aid are awarded to those students with the greatest need. When school officials request financial information of parents or family members, they are assessing ability, rather than willingness, to pay. In applying for aid, applicants and students should work closely with their medical school financial aid officers.

3. **What additional resources are needed?** The financial aid officer compares the student's expected family contribution and other resources with the institution's total cost of attendance to determine how much assistance is needed for the academic year. The student then receives an award letter that describes the actual package of financial aid from all available sources.

General Eligibility Criteria

Financial aid programs usually require that the applicant or student is:

- a U.S. citizen, a permanent resident, or permitted to reside indefinitely in the United States by U.S. Citizenship and Immigration Services, a bureau of the Department of Homeland Security.

- making satisfactory academic progress

- in compliance with Selective Service registration requirements

- not in default on other loans

An applicant or student who has defaulted on prior loans will not qualify for most federal programs and may thus be prevented from attending medical school, as the federal government is the most substantial source of financial aid. Some educational financing programs may also require a service commitment, following completion of training, as a condition of assistance.

Types of Financial Aid

In general, there are two types of financial assistance available to medical students:

- **Grants and scholarships.** The type and amount of this support vary by school and may include state and institutional funds. Grants and scholarships do not have to be repaid, but their availability may be very limited. The medical school financial aid officer is the best source of information on which grants and scholarships are available to individual students and how to qualify.

- **Loans.** Most medical student funding is in the form of loans, and details on various loan programs are available from the financial aid officer and from (MD)[2]. There are two types of loans: subsidized and unsubsidized. Subsidized loans carry no interest cost to borrowers during the in-school period, grace period, and any deferment periods, and thus are the most desirable. Unsubsidized loans accrue interest from the date of disbursement. While borrowers are not required to pay interest on unsubsidized loans during school enrollment, grace, and any deferment periods, they will be responsible for the interest costs which will be capitalized (i.e., added back to the loan principal). Private loans, used to supplement other types of aid including federal loans, are examples of unsubsidized loans. Borrowers should seek out private loans very carefully.

While medical students may also be able to work or receive funding through work-study programs offered by sponsoring colleges or universities, participation in these programs is not the norm for medical students.

Credit Issues

Students must not only show a cost of attendance that supports their borrowing from private loan programs, they must also be "credit ready," meaning that they have either a positive credit history or no credit history at all. Students with a history of late payments on consumer obligations are likely to find themselves excluded from private loans until they can resolve their credit problems.

Some medical schools require a credit history as a part of the financial aid application; applicants are advised to request their credit report prior to applying for aid. The applicant may be able to resolve any problems that may be identified before the financial aid application process gets underway. Alternately, the applicant may choose to defer matriculation until these problems can be resolved and expunged from the credit record. Many medical schools will grant a delay of matriculation to an accepted applicant who must address credit problems. Even prospective students with excellent credit histories, but with significant consumer debt, may encounter difficulty in financing medical school.

In all instances, applicants are strongly advised to make early contact with the financial aid officers at medical schools of interest to them to discuss financial aid eligibility and, if necessary, resolve any outstanding credit problems.

Service Commitment Programs

Service commitment programs — awards available through the U.S. Army, Navy, and Air Force, federal agencies, and some state agencies — provide financial assistance to enrolled medical students or residents in return for physician services after completion of medical training. While these programs are not need or cost-based or, strictly speaking, a form of financial aid, they may be of assistance in financing a medical education or in repaying student loans borrowed for medical school expenses.

- **Armed Forces Health Professions Scholarship Program (HPSP) and Financial Assistance Programs (FAP).** The Department of Defense is implementing significant enhancements to the benefits offered in the Armed Forces Health Professions Scholarship Program (HPSP) and Financial Assistance Programs (FAP).

  The HPSP provides payment for educational expenses for students enrolled in a course of study leading to a degree in medicine. Educational expenses include tuition, books, equipment, fees and laboratory expenses, as well as a monthly stipend, in exchange for an active duty military service commitment. The monthly stipend for all program participants is more than $1,900 per month. Additionally, the Army and Navy are presently offering a $20,000 sign on bonus.

  The FAP offers monetary benefits to health care professionals in postgraduate specialty training, also in exchange for an active duty service commitment. FAP participants receive the same monthly stipend provided to Health Professions Scholarship Program participants in addition to an annual monetary grant. The current annual grant amount for FAP participants is $28,454, subject to annual adjustments.

  Persons participating in the HPSP program are commissioned as officers in the Individual Ready Reserve (IRR). While pursuing their course of medical study, they serve for 45 days of active duty at the rank of second lieutenant/ensign with full pay and allowances during each year they are in the program. FAP members pursuing specialized training serve on active duty in a grade commensurate with their educational level for 14 days during each year of participation. Active duty service begins after completion of training. For HPSP participants, there is a year-for-year obliga-

TABLE 9-C

Armed Forces Health Professions Scholarship Programs (HPSP)

Characteristic			
Provider	Navy	Air Force	Army
	Navy Recruiting Command 5722 Integrity Drive, Bldg 784, Millington, TN 38054 *www.navy.com/ healthcare opportunities/* 800-USA-NAVY	USAF Recruiting Service Headquarters 550 D Street, Suite 1 Randolph AFB, TX 78150-4527 *www.airforce.com/ opportunities/ healthcare/ education/* 800-558-5260	Recruiting Command Attn: RCRO-HS-MC, 1307 Third Avenue, Fort Knox, KY 40121-2726 *www.goarmy. com/amedd/* 800-955-6966
Based on need	No	No	No
Citizenship requirement	U.S. citizen only	U.S. citizen only	U.S. citizen only
Service commitment	Yes	Yes	Yes

Each branch of the Armed Services has a variety of programs. For specific details please see their Web sites or call the above-reference telephone numbers.

tion, with a minimum of three years on active duty. For FAP, active duty obligation consists of the length of the FAP benefit plus one year.

Applications are handled by local area military recruiters with contact information listed in telephone books or on the Internet. Prospective applicants also may want to speak with current military physicians who can provide a comprehensive perspective on the practice of military medicine. Applicants for the HPSP/FAP undergo a competitive screening process. Interested medical students are highly encouraged to apply for HPSP since the Armed Forces have not awarded all available scholarships over the past several years. Additional information is provided in Table 9-C.

• **The National Health Service Corps (NHSC).** The NHSC is a part of the federal Health Resources and Services Administration's (HRSA) Bureau of Health Professions. The NHSC's mission is to improve the health of the nation's underserved populations by assisting communities to recruit and retain community-responsive, culturally competent primary care clinicians. The NHSC offers a variety of programs to dedicated students and clinicians interested in pursuing careers in primary care for the underserved, including the NHSC's Scholarship Program and Loan Repayment Program. Both programs offer financial support in exchange for the opportunity to practice in communities of greatest need throughout the nation. The NHSC Scholarship Program is available to qualifying students upon matriculation. Information on NHSC Scholarship and Loan Repayment opportunities, as well as on all NHSC opportunities to serve the underserved, can be found at *http://nhsc.bhpr.hrsa.gov* or obtained by calling 1-800-221-9393; in the AAMC's State and Other Loan Repayment/Forgiveness and Scholarship Programs database, available online at *www.aamc.org/stloan*; from school financial aid officers; and from on-campus faculty NHSC "Ambassadors" in health professions schools across the country. A list of Ambassadors can be found on the NHSC Web site or obtained by calling 1-800-221-9393.

• **State loan forgiveness or repayment programs.** State programs are frequently available to students and graduates in return for a commitment to serve in the state's areas of need. Most often available to residents and practicing physicians, these programs are sometimes open to enrolled medical students, as well. Information can be found in the searchable database on the AAMC Web site at *www.aamc.org/stloan*, and from school financial aid officers.

Chapter 10

Information on Combined Undergraduate/M.D. Programs

About one quarter of U.S. medical schools offer combined college/M.D. programs for high school students. These programs range in length from six to nine years. The first two to four years of the curriculum consist of undergraduate courses, including required premedical courses; the remaining years are devoted to the medical school curriculum. Graduates receive both a bachelor's degree from the undergraduate institution and an M.D. degree from the medical school.

The purposes of these programs vary by institution:

• to permit highly qualified students to plan and complete a broad liberal arts education before initiating their medical studies

• to attract highly capable students to the sponsoring medical school

• to enhance diversity in the educational environment

• to reduce the total number of years required to complete the M.D. degree

• to educate physicians likely to practice in particular geographic areas or to work with medically underserved populations

• to reduce the costs of a medical education

• to prepare physician-scientists and future leaders in health policy

Potential applicants should familiarize themselves with the mission and goals statement of each combined degree program in which they have an interest in order to ensure a match between their educational and professional goals and those of the program.

These programs typically represent relationships between a medical school and one or more undergraduate colleges located in the same geographic region. They are sometimes part of the same university system, or they can be independent institutions.

Admission is open to highly qualified, mature high school students who are committed to a future career in medicine. State-supported schools generally admit few out-of-state applicants to their combined college/M.D. programs; private schools tend to have greater flexibility regarding state of residency.

While academic requirements vary among the schools sponsoring these programs, they typically include biology, chemistry, physics, English, mathematics, and social science courses. Calculus and foreign-language courses are also frequently required; a computer science course is sometimes recommended. Admission to the medical curriculum may occur immediately or after a student completes a prescribed number of semesters with a minimum grade point average (GPA). In some programs, students are not required to take the MCAT®; in other programs, a minimum MCAT score must be attained for progression through the program.

Progressing through the program from the undergraduate to the medical curriculum is usually contingent on a student's achieving specific criteria in terms of standardized test scores and GPAs and meeting the school's expectations regarding personal and professional behavior.

High school students interested in a combined college/M.D. program should consult their high school guidance counselor to ensure that they are enrolled in a challenging college preparatory curriculum, one which incorporates the specific courses required for admission to the program. The program descriptions that follow were compiled from responses to a survey sent to all medical schools sponsoring programs of interest to high school students. For additional information, contact each school directly.

The following abbreviations are used in the school entries in this chapter:

ACT
American College Testing Program

AP
Advanced Placement

BCPM
Biology, Chemistry, Physics, and Mathematics

CEEB
College Entrance Examination Board

FAFSA
Free Application for Federal Student Aid

GPA
Grade Point Average

MCAT
Medical College Admission Test

SAT
Scholastic Aptitude Test

USMLE
United States Medical Licensing Examination

List of Medical Schools Offering Combined Undergraduate/M.D. Programs, 2010–2011

Alabama
University of Alabama School of Medicine

University of South Alabama College of Medicine

California
University of California, San Diego School of Medicine

University of Southern California College of Letters, Arts, and Sciences and Keck School of Medicine

Connecticut
University of Connecticut

District of Columbia
The George Washington University School of Medicine and Health Sciences and The Columbian School of Arts and Sciences

Howard University

Florida
University of Florida College of Medicine

University of Miami

Illinois
Northwestern University Feinberg School of Medicine

University of Illinois at Chicago College of Medicine

Massachusetts
Boston University

Michigan
Wayne State University School of Medicine

Missouri
Saint Louis University School of Medicine

University of Missouri—Kansas City School of Medicine

New Jersey
University of Medicine and Dentistry of New Jersey— New Jersey Medical School

Rutgers University and UMDNJ— Robert Wood Johnson Medical School

New York
Brooklyn College and SUNY Downstate Medical Center

Hobart and William Smith Colleges/SUNY Upstate Medical University

Rensselaer Polytechnic Institute and Albany Medical College

St. Bonaventure University/The George Washington University School of Medicine and Health Sciences

Siena College and Albany Medical College

Sophie Davis School of Biomedical Education at the City University of New York

Stony Brook University and Stony Brook University School of Medicine

Union College and Albany Medical College

University of Rochester School of Medicine and Dentistry

Ohio
Case Western Reserve University
School of Medicine

Northeastern Ohio Universities
College of Medicine

The Ohio State University
College of Medicine

University of Cincinnati
College of Medicine

Pennsylvania
Drexel University and Drexel
University College of Medicine

Lehigh University and Drexel
University College of Medicine

Pennsylvania State University
and Jefferson Medical College

Temple University School of Medicine

Villanova University and Drexel
University College of Medicine

Wilkes University/SUNY-Upstate
Medical University

Rhode Island
Warren Alpert Medical School
of Brown University

Tennessee
Fisk University and Meharry
Medical College

Texas
Rice University and Baylor
College of Medicine

University of Texas School of
Medicine at San Antonio

Virginia
Eastern Virginia Medical School

Virginia Commonwealth University
School of Medicine

**List of Medical Schools Offering
Combined Undergraduate/M.D.
Programs, 2010–2011**

6 Years
University of Missouri—Kansas City
School of Medicine

6-7 Years
University of Miami

Northeastern Ohio Universities
College of Medicine

Pennsylvania State University and
Jefferson Medical College

7 Years
The George Washington University
School of Medicine and Health
Sciences and The Columbian
School of Arts and Sciences

University of Florida
College of Medicine

Northwestern University
Feinberg School of Medicine

University of Illinois at Chicago
College of Medicine

Boston University
(8-year option available)

University of Medicine and Dentistry
of New Jersey—New Jersey
Medical School

Rensselaer Polytechnic Institute
and Albany Medical College

Sophie Davis School of Biomedical Education/City University of New York

The Ohio State University College of Medicine

Drexel University and Drexel University College of Medicine

Lehigh University and Drexel University College of Medicine

Villanova University and Drexel University College of Medicine

Fisk University and Meharry Medical College

University of Texas School of Medicine at San Antonio

8 Years
University of Alabama School of Medicine

University of South Alabama College of Medicine

University of California, San Diego School of Medicine

University of Southern California College of Letters, Arts, and Sciences and Keck School of Medicine

University of Connecticut and University of Connecticut School of Medicine

Howard University

Michigan State University College of Human Medicine

Wayne State University School of Medicine

Saint Louis University School of Medicine

Rutgers University and University of Medicine and Dentistry of New Jersey—Robert Wood Johnson Medical School

Brooklyn College and SUNY Downstate Medical Center

Hobart and William Smith Colleges/SUNY Upstate Medical University

St. Bonaventure University/The George Washington University School of Medicine and Health Sciences

Siena College and Albany Medical College

Stony Brook and Stony Brook University School of Medicine

Union College and Albany Medical College

University of Rochester School of Medicine and Dentistry

Case Western Reserve University School of Medicine

University of Cincinnati College of Medicine

Temple University School of Medicine

Wilkes University/SUNY-Upstate Medical University

Brown Medical School

Rice University and Baylor College of Medicine

Eastern Virginia Medical School

Virginia Commonwealth University School of Medicine

9 Years
University of Cincinnati College of Medicine (College of Engineering—undergraduate)

University of Alabama
School of Medicine

Birmingham, Alabama

Address Inquiries To:
Amelia Johnson
Program Administrator
UAB Honors Academy, HUC 531
University of Alabama at Birmingham
1530 3rd Avenue, South, Birmingham, Alabama 35294-1150
T (205) 996-9842 **F** (205) 996-9838
honorsacademy@uab.edu
www.uab.edu/emsap

Purpose

The UAB Early Medical School Acceptance Program (EMSAP) is designed to give exceptional high school graduates an opportunity to take advantage of the best resources of the undergraduate and medical programs through a mentored relationship with medical school faculty. A medical school professor advises students from high school graduation until the second year of the medical program, establishing a unique relationship. This is not an accelerated program, rather a program to allow gifted students to explore a broad range of educational, research and community service opportunities beyond the typical premedical experiences.

Requirements for Entrance

Students are selected in their senior year of high school. Both residents and non-residents of Alabama are eligible to apply to the program. Applicants must submit the following documents: (1) a UAB application; (2) a completed EMSAP application; (3) two letters of recommendation from high school administrators, counselors, or teachers describing their suitability for a career in medicine; (4) a brief essay incorporating information about themselves and their career objectives and expectations for contributing to society; and (5) a resume listing their academic achievements, honors received, activities, employment, health-related experience, etc. Applicants must meet the requirements for freshman admission to the university and be admitted to the University by the EMSAP application deadline, December 15, 2009.

Selection Factors

Required high school courses include: four years of English, four years of mathematics, one year of chemistry or physics, and one year of biology. Minimum GPA: 3.5 overall GPA (on a 4.0 scale). Test scores: at least 30 ACT or a minimum 1320 SAT (critical reading + math). Selected applicants are invited for a required interview.

Curriculum

This eight-year program leads to a baccalaureate degree awarded by the University of Alabama at Birmingham (UAB), and to the M.D. degree granted by the University of Alabama School of Medicine. Students must meet the regular undergraduate course requirements for the University of Alabama at Birmingham, complete two required EMSAP (Early Medical School Acceptance Program) seminars and live on campus during their first two years. Applicants may apply to one of three other Honors programs in the Honors Academy. The deadline to apply for both programs is December 15. In order to matriculate to the medical school phase of the program, students must: (1) take the MCAT and receive a minimal total score of 28; (2) maintain an overall GPA of 3.6 and a math and science GPA of 3.5; (3) receive their baccalaureate degree; and (4) meet all requirements

and conditions to remain in good standing for their acceptance into the University of Alabama School of Medicine. After the second year of medical school, students must pass the USMLE Step 1 in order to be promoted and graduate. Passing the USMLE Step 2 Clinical Knowledge (CK) examination and sitting for the Step 2 Clinical Skills (CS) examination are required in order to graduate from the medical school. Passing an Observed Structured Clinical Examination (OSCE) is also required for graduation from medical school.

Expenses	Resident Tuition and Fees	Non-resident Tuition and Fees
Undergraduate	$4,715	$10,400
U.S. Medical School	$18,871	$49,379

Financial Aid

UAB awards comprehensive federal, state, institutional, and private financial aid on the basis of merit, financial need, or both. Each year, the university offers more than 1,500 scholarships, including approximately $1.5 million in merit-based awards. Applicants are automatically considered for all academic scholarships when accepted to the university. As academic scholarships are awarded on a first come-first served basis, applicants are encouraged to apply no later than December 1 (prior to EMSAP application deadline) of the senior year of high school.

Application and Acceptance Policies

Filing of application:
  Earliest date: September 1, 2009
  Latest date: December 15, 2009
Application fee: $30   Fee Waiver Available: Yes
Acceptance notice:
  Earliest date: Mid-February 2010
  Latest date: Late February 2010
Applicant's response to acceptance offer:
  Latest date: May 1, 2010
Deposit to hold place in class: None
Starting date: Mid-August 2010

Information on 2008–2009 Entering Class

Number of	In-State	Out-of-State	Total
Applicants	73	37	110
Applicants Interviewed	20	8	28
New Entrants	6	4	10
Total number of students enrolled in program: 34			

University of South Alabama College of Medicine

Mobile, Alabama

Address Inquiries To:
Donna Pigg, Assistant Director of Admissons
University of South Alabama Meisler Hall, Room 2500
Mobile, Alabama, 36688-0022
T (251) 460-6141 **F** (251) 460-7876
dpigg@usouthal.edu
www.southalabama.edu/com/

Purpose

Candidates selected for the program will receive early acceptance from the University of South Alabama and its College of Medicine. Students participating in the program are expected to enter the University of South Alabama College of Medicine in the fall after completion of the baccalaureate degree.

Requirements for Entrance

Students in the senior year of high school or recently graduated individuals who have not yet entered college are eligible to apply for the program. Both residents and non-residents of Alabama may apply.

Selection Factors

Candidates must have a minimum high school GPA of 3.5, as computed by the University of South Alabama, and must present a minimum enhanced composite ACT score of 30 (or comparable SAT score). Candidates must also have demonstrated evidence of leadership qualities, community service, communication skills, and motivation for the study of medicine.

Curriculum

The curriculum will include core requirements for the selected baccalaureate program and prerequisites for matriculation in medical school. Students in the program must maintain a minimum overall GPA of 3.5 and a minimum GPA of 3.4 in the sciences (biology, chemistry, physics) and mathematics. All required courses must be taken at the University of South Alabama unless otherwise approved in advance by the student's undergraduate program director and the Director of Admissions for the College of Medicine. Students will be required to participate in CP-200 (Career Planning; Clinical Observation) for a minimum of four quarters. Students will be given the opportunity to participate in a special summer premedical clerkship. These activities will be planned to give participants a broad exposure to medical education. Students will be required to take the MCAT for admission to the College of Medicine and will be required to achieve a composite score of 27. A formal assessment, including an interview, will be conducted after the student has completed 96 quarter hours of academic work. At this time, students' academic performance and continued interest in a medical career will be assessed.

Expenses

Expenses	Resident Tuition and Fees	Non-resident Tuition and Fees
Undergraduate	$6,500	$13,000
U.S. Medical School	$17,990	$33,088

Financial Aid

Information can be obtained from the Office of Financial Aid, Meisler Hall, Room 1200, University of South Alabama, Mobile, Alabama 36688-0002; by phone at (251) 460-6231; or on the school Web site at *www.finaid2.usouthal.edu*.

Application and Acceptance Policies

Filing of application:
Earliest date: December 15, 2009
Latest date: June 11, 2010
Application fee: $25   Fee Waiver Available: No
Acceptance notice:
Earliest date: March 1, 2010
Latest date: Until program is filled
Applicant's response to acceptance offer:
Maximum time: Two weeks
Deposit to hold place in class: None
Starting date: August 18, 2010

Information on 2008–2009 Entering Class

Number of	In-State	Out-of-State	Total
Applicants	100	45	145
Applicants Interviewed	31	14	45
New Entrants	12	3	15

Total number of students enrolled in program: 60

University of California, San Diego School of Medicine

La Jolla, California

Address Inquiries To:
Yvonne Coleman, Director of Medical Scholars Program
University of California, San Diego School of Medicine
Office of Admissions, 0621
9500 Gilman Drive, La Jolla, California 92093-0621
T (858) 534-3880 **F** (858) 534-5282
somadmissions@ucsd.edu
http://meded.ucsd.edu/groups/med-scholars/

Purpose

The Medical Scholars Program was established to encourage the recruitment of unusually talented high school students, who would then be attracted to both the University of California, San Diego, (UCSD) undergraduate and medical schools, and to promote the goal of increasing diversity on both campuses.

Requirements for Entrance

Students are selected for this program during their senior year of high school. The program is open to California residents only. Applicants must meet course requirements for UCSD undergraduate admission. They must take either the SAT or ACT and achieve a minimum score of 2250 on the SAT or 34 on the ACT.

Selection Factors

To be eligible for consideration, applicants must have a minimum high school GPA of 4.0 and 2250 on the SAT or 34 on the ACT. The average high school grade-point average for the 2008 entering class was 4.28. Applicants must also demonstrate strong extracurricular involvement, particularly in community service and leadership. Letters of recommendation and an essay are additional considerations. An interview is required. The MCAT is not required.

Curriculum

This program leads to a baccalaureate degree granted by the University of California, San Diego, and to the M.D. degree granted by the UCSD School of Medicine. It takes eight years to fulfill the requirements for both degrees. The specific course requirements for the baccalaureate degree include a minimum of 6 quarters in either humanities or social sciences and 15 quarters in the natural and physical sciences. Students must take Step 1 of the USMLE after the second year of medical school. Passing Steps 1 and 2 of the USMLE is required in order to be promoted and to graduate.

Expenses

	Resident Tuition and Fees	Non-resident Tuition and Fees
Undergraduate	$8,906	$29,813
U.S. Medical School	$23,031	$35,276

Financial Aid

Sources of financial aid include scholarships, grants, loans, and work-study. Additional information is available from the undergraduate financial aid office: Building 201, University Center, La Jolla, California 92093-0013, or at *www.ucsd.edu/finaid*.

Application and Acceptance Policies

Filing of application:
  Earliest date: February 15, 2010
  Latest date: March 15, 2010
Application fee: None   Fee Waiver Available: n/a
Acceptance notice:
  Earliest date: April 21, 2010
  Latest date: April 28, 2010
Applicant's response to acceptance offer:
  Maximum time: 1 week
Deposit to hold place in class: None
Starting date: September 2010

Information on 2008–2009 Entering Class

Number of	In-State	Out-of-State	Total
Applicants	209	n/a	209
Applicants Interviewed	24	n/a	24
New Entrants	10	n/a	10
Total number of students enrolled in program: 43			

University of Southern California
College of Letters, Arts, and Sciences
and Keck School of Medicine
Los Angeles, California

Address Inquiries To:
Karen Rowan-Badger, Director of Admission
College of Letters, Arts, and Sciences
University of Southern California
Los Angeles, California 90089-0152
T (213) 740-5930 **F** (213) 740-1338
admission@college.usc.edu
www.usc.edu/schools/college/admission/baccalaureatemd/

Purpose

The goal of this program is to encourage bright and motivated students to expand the breadth of their education through a diverse liberal arts education. Students accepted into this program have the opportunity to study a wide variety of disciplines beyond the course of the standard premedical curriculum. It is the hope of the university to graduate physicians who are educated in medical science, the arts, and the humanities.

Requirements for Entrance

Students are selected for this program in the senior year of high school. Both residents and non-residents of California and international students are eligible to apply. Although there are no specific high school course requirements, applicants are required to take either the SAT or ACT.

Selection Factors

Academic factors considered include grades and standardized test scores. Participation in extracurricular activities and demonstrated leadership and community service are valued. Students who enrolled in 2008 had a mean high school GPA of 4.34 (weighted) and a mean SAT score of 2190. An interview is required and is granted by invitation following careful evaluation of an applicant's file.

Curriculum

This program leads to a baccalaureate degree awarded by the University of Southern California, and to the M.D. degree granted by the University of Southern California Keck School of Medicine. This is not an accelerated program; all students must complete four years of undergraduate education and four years of medical school. Students must complete requirements for the bachelor's degree and may pursue any major offered in the university that is compatible with the requirements of the program. There are specific requirements for the bachelor's degree, which include the humanities and social, natural, and physical sciences. Advancement to the medical school phase of the program is based on acceptable academic performance and MCAT scores as defined by the program. The MCAT is required and must be taken by the spring of the junior year. Students must take USMLE Steps 1 and 2, and pass Step 1 of the USMLE in order to graduate from the School of Medicine.

Expenses

	Resident Tuition and Fees	Non-resident Tuition and Fees
Undergraduate	$37,096	$37,096
U.S. Medical School	$44,188	$44,188

Financial Aid

Sources of aid include scholarships, grants, work-study programs, and loans. For additional information, contact the Office of Financial Aid, University of Southern California, Los Angeles, California 90089-0912; call (213) 740-1111; or visit *www.usc.edu/admission/fa/*.

Application and Acceptance Policies

Filing of application:
  Earliest date: August 1, 2009
  Latest date: December 1, 2009
Application fee: $65   Fee Waiver Available: Yes
Acceptance notice:
  Earliest date: April 1, 2010
  Latest date: April 1, 2010
Applicant's response to acceptance offer:
  Maximum time: 1 month
Deposit to hold place in class: $300; nonrefundable
Starting date: August 2010

Information on 2008–2009 Entering Class

Number of	In-State	Out-of-State	Total
Applicants	295	222	517
Applicants Interviewed	60	38	98
New Entrants	23	8	31

Total number of students enrolled in program: 101

University of Connecticut
Storrs, Connecticut

Address Inquiries To:
Keat Sanford, Ph.D., Assistant Dean for Admissions
Office of Undergraduate Admissions
Special Programs in Medicine & Dental Medicine
University of Connecticut, 2131 Hillside Road, U-88
Storrs, Connecticut 06269-3088
T (860) 486-3137 **F** (860) 486-1476
http://medicine.uchc.edu/prospective/admissions/babs_md/index.html

Purpose
This program offers gifted and talented high school students, who are focused on a career in medicine, the opportunity to combine a broad-based liberal arts program with a medical education. This program links undergraduate preparation with four years of medical education, resulting in dual degrees: a B.A. or B.S. degree and the M.D. degree.

Requirements for Entrance
Students are selected for this program during the senior year of high school. Both residents and non-residents of Connecticut are eligible to apply. Applicants must take either the SAT I or ACT.

Selection Factors
To be considered for this program, the student should have the following: a high school class ranking in the top five percent; an overall high school grade-point average of 3.5 (4.0 scale); an SAT combined score of 1300 or an ACT composite score of 30; a completed regular undergraduate admission application and a supplemental application for the program in medicine by the January 1 postmark deadline; and, an interview at the School of Medicine. In addition, recommendations from teachers/advisors, as well as evidence maturity, extracurricular activities, and a commitment to the health profession, are considered. To matriculate in the School of Medicine upon completion of undergraduate preparation, the student must meet additional criteria that include: maintaining a college 3.5 cumulative grade-point average (4.0 scale); ordinarily obtaining an MCAT score of 30+ (with a minimum score of 28), with section scores of 7 or greater; participation in clinical, research, and community service activities; and favorable interviews during the senior undergraduate year. For more information on the medical school program, please contact Dr. Keat Sanford, Assistant Dean for Medical School Admissions, at (860) 679-3874 or sanford@nso1.uchc.edu.

Curriculum
Students must complete requirements for a baccalaureate degree from the University of Connecticut. Requirements include courses in the humanities and social sciences. The curriculum typically takes eight years to complete: Years 1 through 4 in the liberal arts and sciences and Years 5 through 8 in the School of Medicine. The MCAT is required for admission to the medical school phase of the program. Students are required to pass Step 1 of the USMLE for promotion and Step 2 of the USMLE in order to graduate.

Expenses

Expenses	Resident Tuition and Fees	Non-resident Tuition and Fees
Undergraduate	$7,200	$21,912
U.S. Medical School	$25,548	$48,195

Financial Aid
All enrolled candidates will be automatically considered for merit scholarships. A full range of financial aid options based on student financial need is available, as well. Candidates for need-based aid must submit the Free Application for Federal Student Aid (FAFSA) by March 1. For more information about student aid programs, contact the University of Connecticut's Office of Student Financial Aid Services at (860) 486-2819; write to U-4116, Storrs, Connecticut 06269; or visit the UConn homepage at *www.uconn.edu*.

Additional Information
Students are provided with enrichment experiences while completing the undergraduate program. Programming includes: courses offered at the main University campus by faculty from the School of Medicine (these have included Mini-Medical School and The Patient and the Healer.); a summer research fellowship opportunity at the School of Medicine; placements to obtain clinical experience; placements to obtain community service experience; and assigned advisory committees for each student including faculty from the School of Medicine.

Application and Acceptance Policies
Filing of application:
 Earliest date: September 1, 2009
 Latest date: January 1, 2010
Application fee: $70   Fee Waiver Available: Yes
Acceptance notice:
 Earliest date: March 1, 2010
 Latest date: Until full
Applicant's response to acceptance offer:
 Latest date: May 1, 2010
Deposit to hold place in class: $150; nonrefundable
Starting date: August 2010

Information on 2008–2009 Entering Class

Number of	In-State	Out-of-State	Total
Applicants	108	156	264
Applicants Interviewed	25	15	40
New Entrants	4	1	5

Total number of students enrolled in program: 44

The George Washington University School of Medicine and The Columbian College of Arts and Sciences

Washington, D.C.

Address Inquiries To:
Office of Undergraduate Admissions
The George Washington University
2121 I Street N.W., Suite 201
Washington, D.C. 20052
T (202) 994-6040
gwadm@gwu.edu
http://gwired.gwu.edu/adm/apply/honors.html

Purpose

A joint program of The George Washington (GW) University Columbian College of Arts and Sciences and the School of Medicine and Health Sciences, the seven-year B.A.–M.D. program is designed for the high school senior who exhibits academic excellence, leadership in activities, and community service and healthcare experience, and who has confirmed the goal to become a physician. The purpose of the program is to encourage a liberal arts focus in preparation for medical school. Students typically choose majors in a wide variety of fields ranging from economics and psychology to religion and biology. The new, state-of-the-art GW Hospital opened in 2002. Housed on the 6th floor of the new GW Hospital is the GW Clinical Skills Center. Dedicated to education and research, this floor of the hospital features cutting-edge technology in a setting that is among the most innovative in the nation. Through the use of the Surgical Simulation and Demonstration Area and the Standardized Patient Examining Area, medical students gain the comprehensive clinical exposure, feedback, and evaluation they need to become both technically adept and humane caregivers for their patients.

Requirements for Entrance

Students are selected in their senior year of high school. Applicants must be a U.S. citizen, U.S. permanent resident, or Canadian citizen in order to apply. Applicants are expected to complete the SAT or ACT, as well as the SAT Subject Tests in Mathematics, Science, and English. Competitive SAT scores for the program are (equivalent) 2100 and above.

Selection Factors

Academic factors considered in selecting applicants include the strength of the academic program, grades in high school, class rank, and standardized test scores. In addition to academic factors, extra-curricular and health-related activities, community service, essays, and letters of recommendation are reviewed. Competitive applicants are those who rank in the top ten percent of their high school class, have shown leadership ability through participation in extracurricular activities, have demonstrated interest in the medical field through experience, and have taken advantage of advanced course offerings. An interview is required and is by invitation only.

Curriculum

A special faculty committee reviews each student's progress throughout the program annually. To continue each year in the program, students must maintain a minimum of a "B" in courses required for admission to the medical school and an overall 3.6 average. Students do not take the MCAT. Students participate in seminars of interest and are involved in community service and health care experiences throughout the undergraduate portion of the curriculum. The review committee will make a final recommendation concerning promotion to the medical school curriculum at the end of the third year. In the fourth year,

students enroll in the School of Medicine and Health Sciences and begin their formal medical training. The baccalaureate degree is received before entrance to the M.D. program. The integration of clinical skills begins in the first and second years of medical school, as students spend time with physicians, learning the art and skill of patient interviewing and physical diagnosis. The sixth and seventh years are devoted to developing clinical expertise in a wide variety of hospitals in the D.C. metropolitan area. At the end of the seventh year, students are awarded the M.D. degree.

Expenses

Expenses	Resident Tuition and Fees	Non-resident Tuition and Fees
Undergraduate	$53,647	$53,647
U.S. Medical School	$46,267	$46,267

Financial Aid

Information may be obtained from The George Washington University, Office of Student Financial Assistance, 2121 "I" Street, N.W., #310, Washington, D.C. 20052. The Office of Student Financial Assistance may be reached by phone at 1-800-222-6242.

Additional Information

Students accepted to the 2010 seven-year B.A.–M.D. program recieve a $15,000 award yearly, resulting in combined tuition and fees of $38,647. Tuition and fees remain the same for each year of the seven-year program.

Application and Acceptance Policies

Filing of application:
  Earliest date: September 1, 2009
  Latest date: December 10, 2009
Application fee: $70   Fee Waiver Available: Yes
Acceptance notice:
  Earliest date: April 2010
  Latest date: April 2010
Applicant's response to acceptance offer:
  Maximum time: May 1, 2010
Deposit to hold place in class: $800; nonrefundable
Starting date: August 2010

Information on 2008–2009 Entering Class

Number of	In-State	Out-of-State	Total
Applicants	n/a	700	700
Applicants Interviewed	n/a	55	55
New Entrants	n/a	6	6
Total number of students enrolled in program: 105			

Howard University College of Medicine

Washington, D.C.

Address Inquiries To:
Julie Andrist, Assistant Coordinator/Counselor
Center for Preprofessional Education
College of Arts and Sciences, 2225 Georgia Avenue N.W., Room 518,
Howard University
Washington, D.C. 20059
T (202) 238-2363 **F** (202) 588-9820
preprofessional@howard.edu, www.howard.edu/library/preprof/

Purpose

The goal of this combined-degree program is to encourage talented undergraduate students to choose medicine as a career and to retain these excellent students in the Howard University College of Medicine.

Requirements for Entrance

Students can be selected for this program during the senior year of high school or during the first year of college. There are no state residence requirements. Applicants are expected to have completed the following courses by the time they graduate from high school: at least two years of a foreign language; at least one year each of biology, chemistry, and physics; two years of mathematics; and, four years of English, including literature. They must take either the SAT or the ACT Assessment.

Selection Factors

The academic factors considered in offering admission to an applicant are rank in high school class, GPA, and test scores. Applicants are expected to be in the top five percent of their high school class. In the 2008–2009 entering class, the average GPA was 3.7, and the average SAT combined score was 2000. ACT Assessment cumulative scores ranged from 26 to 30. Personal qualities considered are: superior writing skills, maturity, positive self-confidence, realistic self-appraisal, a realistic assessment of the medical profession, good leadership skills, and sustained demonstration of service to people who are less fortunate. An interview is required.

Curriculum

This program leads to a bachelor's degree awarded by the College of Arts and Sciences at Howard University and to the M.D. degree granted by the Howard University College of Medicine. Students must complete work for a baccalaureate degree. They are expected to complete at least 40 semester hours of humanities and social sciences courses to fulfill general education requirements and at least 46 semester hours of natural and physical sciences courses. Students meet with the director (the advisor) of the Center for Preprofessional Education to design a curriculum tailored to their individual needs. The specific course selection must have the advisor's approval. Students are encouraged to select a major of personal interest. The curricula for both degrees are completed in six years. In the first two years, the curriculum focuses on work toward the bachelor's degree and premedical requirements, and in the last four years the focus is on studies related to medicine. Students in this program must take the MCAT in April of the second year. The results of the MCAT, the GPA, the demonstration of a high level of maturity, and a strong commitment to service in

areas where there is a shortage of health professionals are factors in gaining admission to the medical school phase of the combined degree program. Students are also expected to take Steps 1 and 2 of the USMLE while at Howard University College of Medicine; they must pass these examinations prior to promotion and graduation.

Expenses

Expenses	Resident Tuition and Fees	Non-resident Tuition and Fees
Undergraduate	$15,010	$15,010
U.S. Medical School	$34,081	$34,081

Financial Aid

Information can be obtained from the Office of Financial Aid, Howard University, Johnson Administration Building, 2400 6th Street, N.W., Washington, D.C. 20059.

Application and Acceptance Policies

Filing of application:
 Earliest date: March 1, 2010
 Latest date: March 1, 2010
Application fee: $45   Fee Waiver Available: No
Acceptance notice:
 Earliest date: varies
 Latest date: varies
Applicant's response to acceptance offer:
 Maximum time: July 15, 2010
Deposit to hold place in class: $150; nonrefundable
Starting date: August 2010

Information on 2008–2009 Entering Class

Number of	In-State	Out-of-State	Total
Applicants	5	55	60
Applicants Interviewed	3	15	18
New Entrants	0	10	10
Total number of students enrolled in program: 10			

University of Florida
College of Medicine
Gainesville, Florida

Address Inquiries To:
Denise Chichester
Medical Selection Committee
University of Florida College of Medicine P.O. Box 100216
Gainesville, Florida 32610
T (352) 273-7990 **F** (352) 392-1307
http://jhmp.sites.medinfo.ufl.edu

Purpose

The Junior Honors Medical Program is for undergraduate students who have chosen a career in the medical profession and who have demonstrated superior scholastic ability and personal development during their first two academic years of college enrollment. Experience in health care, community service, and medically related research are extracurricular activities that are considered valuable for these applicants.

Requirements for Entrance

Students are selected for this program during the sophomore year of college enrollment. Admission is open to all possible candidates who are Florida residents. There are no specific high school course requirements. However, admission tests such as the SAT and/or ACT achievement tests are required. The minimum GPA required for application is 3.75 on college coursework; the minimum required SAT score is a 1200. The courses listed must be completed by the spring semester of the applicant's sophomore year: General Chemistry I & II (both with labs), Organic Chemistry I & II (both with labs), General Biology I & II (both with labs) and Calculus I & II. The following courses may be completed in the junior year: General Physics I & II (both with labs) and Biochemistry.

Selection Factors

The academic factors considered in offering admission to an applicant include sophomore standing (two years of college classroom enrollment), competitive SAT or ACT scores, competitive GPA, and completion of prerequisite courses. Involvement in medically related research prior to application is considered positively as well as consistent health care experience and community service. The MCAT is currently not required. Selected applicants are invited for a required interview held in March and April. Acceptance decisions are not made until grades for the Spring semester are posted and an official transcript is received in the UF COM Admissions Office, usually in May.

Curriculum

The most frequent major for the baccalaureate degree is the B.S. in interdisciplinary biological and medical sciences through the College of Liberal Arts and Sciences. Some students choose nutrition as a major through the College of Agricultural and Life Sciences; this option requires approval. The junior year in the program includes undergraduate college required courses and seminars with College of Medicine faculty. During the junior year, JHMP students must complete an Honors Thesis prior to entering medical school. Completion of the thesis earns the designation of honors or high honors in research at graduation for the MD degree. The bachelor's degree is awarded after the fourth year of college enroll-ment, which is concurrently the first year of medical school. The University of Florida College of Medicine awards the Doctor of Medicine degree. It takes seven years to complete requirements for both degrees. All courses in the first two years are liberal arts courses. In Year 3, half of the curriculum is in the liberal arts and half in medicine. In Years 4 through 7, all courses are in medicine.

Expenses	Resident Tuition and Fees	Non-resident Tuition and Fees
Undergraduate	$1,888	$10,311
U.S. Medical School	$26,514	$55,754

Financial Aid

Several sources of financial aid are available to students, including college scholarships and loans, federal Stafford loans, and state National Merit and Robert Byrd Scholarships, if eligible. For more information, contact Eileen Parris, UF COM Office of Financial Aid, P.O. Box 100216 HSC, Gainesville, Florida 32610, (352) 273-7939; or E-mail eparris@ufl.edu.

Additional Information

For the research requirement, the Junior Honors student is assigned a faculty member in a department of interest to the student. The faculty member supervising the research is a mentor to the student. Continued interest in the research area can be achieved during the medical school years either through the Medical Sciences Research Program or the M.D./Ph.D. Program.

Application and Acceptance Policies

Filing of application:
    Earliest date: N/A
    Latest date: January 30, 2010
Application fee: None   Fee Waiver Available: n/a
Acceptance notice:
    Earliest date: May 15, 2010
    Latest date: August 15, 2010
Applicant's response to acceptance offer:
    Maximum time: 2 weeks
Deposit to hold place in class: None
Starting date: August 2010

Information on 2008–2009 Entering Class

Number of	In-State	Out-of-State	Total
Applicants	63	0	63
Applicants Interviewed	23	0	23
New Entrants	12	0	12
Total number of students enrolled in program: 59			

University of Miami

Coral Gables, Florida

Address Inquiries To:
Yamilet Medina-Lopez, Admissions Officer
Office of Admissions, University of Miami
P.O. Box 248025
Coral Gables, Florida 33124
T (305) 284-4323
webrequest.admission@miami.edu
http://www6.miami.edu/UMH/CDA/UMH_Main/0,1770,2613-1;14415-3,00.html

Purpose

The Honors Program in Medicine (HPM) offers exceptionally motivated and talented high school students, who have reached a mature and independent decision to study medicine, an opportunity to earn the B.S. and M.D. degrees in seven or eight years.

Requirements for Entrance

Applicants must be U.S. citizens or permanent residents. Both residents and non-residents of Florida are considered for admission. Applicants must be in their last year of high school at the time of application. Applicants must have a minimum combined score of 1400 on the SAT or a composite score of 32 on the ACT, an unweighted GPA of at least 3.75, and take the SAT II Subject Tests in Mathematics, and one science (a minimum score of 600 is required in each). All applicants must have completed eight semesters of mathematics and English and two semesters each of biology and chemistry by the time of graduation from high school.

Selection Factors

Academic factors taken into account include scores on standardized tests, the quality of the high school curriculum (including the number and nature of Advanced Placement courses and/or International Baccalaureate coursework), and the amount of university-level work already completed. Of equal importance to academic achievements are personal factors such as maturity of thought and action, common sense, empathy, interpersonal skills, appropriate freedom from parental influence, and social cognizance. Most important, the applicant must have made a practical decision to study medicine based on self-initiated patient-contact experiences.

Curriculum

The first three years are spent on the Coral Gables campus taking required science and humanities courses and focusing almost exclusively on work related to the bachelor's degree. The undergraduate portion of the curriculum may be extended to four years if the student is in good academic standing and has established a clear plan of academic and personal growth. All HPM students must have a 3.7 science GPA and a 3.7 cumulative GPA and an MCAT composite score of 28 to be promoted to the School of Medicine after three years. Students can be promoted at the end of four years with a cumulative and science GPA of at least 3.5 and a minimum MCAT score of 28. All students must develop a continuous history of involvement at the undergraduate level in a variety of experiences that must include patient contact, and some combination of research, campus or community service, study abroad, or employment, consistent with a sincere desire to study and practice medicine. HPM students may attend either the parent medical campus in Miami or the regional medical campus located in Boca Raton, Florida, on the campus of Florida Atlantic University. The missions of the educational programs at both campuses are identical but the regional medical campus emphasizes continuity of care and community medicine. Students at the Miami campus receive their clinical training at Jackson Memorial Hospital and other hospitals affiliated with the Miller School of Medicine, while students at the regional campus will receive their clinical training at John F. Kennedy Community Hospital.

Expenses

	Resident Tuition and Fees	Non-resident Tuition and Fees
Undergraduate	$34,834	$34,834
U.S. Medical School	$30,048	$39,254

Financial Aid

Scholarships, work-study, loans, and state tuition grants are sources of financial assistance. Information on undergraduate financial aid is available from the Office of Admissions on the Coral Gables campus.

Application and Acceptance Policies

Filing of application:
    Earliest date: October 1, 2009
    Latest date: November 1, 2009
Application fee: $55   Fee Waiver Available: No
Acceptance notice:
    Earliest date: April 1, 2010
    Latest date: April 1, 2010
Applicant's response to acceptance offer:
    Maximum time: May 1, 2010
Deposit to hold place in class: $300; nonrefundable
Starting date: August 2010

Information on 2008–2009 Entering Class

Number of	In-State	Out-of-State	Total
Applicants	170	92	262
Applicants Interviewed	80	99	179
New Entrants	9	10	19
Total number of students enrolled in program: 63			

Northwestern University Feinberg School of Medicine

Evanston, Illinois

Address Inquiries To:
Dr. Marianne Green, Associate Dean for Medical Education
Office of Admission and Financial Aid Northwestern University
1801 Hinman Avenue
Evanston, Illinois 60204-3060
T (312) 503-8915 **F** (312) 503-0840
ug-ad@northwestern.edu
www.medschool.northwestern.edu/hpme

Purpose

The Honors Program in Medical Education (HPME), one of the oldest in the nation, offers a unique opportunity for gifted and highly motivated students who seek careers in medicine or medical science. The HPME provides a broad, flexible and challenging undergraduate education free from many of the pressures related to gaining acceptance to medical school.

Requirements for Entrance

Students are selected for this program during their senior year of high school. Both residents and non-residents of Illinois are eligible to apply. Applicants must meet the following high school course requirements: English, eight semesters; mathematics, including differential and integral calculus, eight semesters; chemistry, two semesters; physics, two semesters; biology, two semesters; and, foreign language, four semesters. They must take either the SAT Reasoning Test or the ACT Assessment with Writing, plus the SAT Subject Tests (in mathematics level 2 and chemistry).

Selection Factors

Academic factors considered in selecting applicants include class rank, grades in high school, and scores on college entrance tests. Average test scores of students in the 2008–2009 entering class were: SAT Critical Reading, 732; SAT Mathematics, 775; SAT Writing 750; CEEB Subject Tests – Chemistry, 764; Mathematics II, 788; ACT plus Writing, 34. Non-academic factors considered are motivation for a career in medicine, concern for others, maturity, team work, and leadership. An interview is required.

Curriculum

The degrees offered in the honors program are a baccalaureate degree (B.A., B.S. in medicine, B.S. in biomedical engineering, or B.S. in communication) and the M.D., all from Northwestern University. Students must complete requirements for a baccalaureate degree in addition to the required science courses (inorganic and organic chemistry, calculus-based physics, biological science sequence). The majority of students in the Feinberg College of Arts & Science major in biological sciences but have many other options within the college. Students in the McCormick School of Engineering & Applied Sciences major in biomedical engineering and take the basic and advanced engineering courses, in addition to non-science courses. The program in the School of Communication includes special courses in communication sciences and disorders. The curriculum usually takes seven or eight years to complete, and students are encouraged to develop a unique curricular path. During the undergraduate years, the curriculum consists of courses in the liberal arts and sciences, engineering, or speech. After matriculation to Feinberg School of Medicine, the curriculum focuses on medicine. The MCAT is not required. Students must take Steps 1 and 2 of the USMLE and record passing grades in order to graduate from the medical school.

Expenses

Expenses	Resident Tuition and Fees	Non-resident Tuition and Fees
Undergraduate	$36,756	$36,756
U.S. Medical School	$41,926	$41,926

Financial Aid

Sources of aid include Northwestern University and federal, state, and private programs. Undergraduate applicants can receive more information from the Office of Admission and Financial Aid, 1801 Hinman Avenue, Evanston, Illinois 60204-3060; or phone (847) 491-7271. Information about medical school financial aid can be obtained from Financial Aid Professional Schools, Abbott Hall, 710 Superior Street, Chicago, Illinois 60611.

Additional Information

Students are encouraged to explore focused areas of concentration during their undergraduate years that may prepare them personally and professionally for their careers in medicine. Students spend their undergraduate years on the Evanston Northwestern Campus; the medical school curriculum is conducted at the Feinberg School of Medicine Chicago Campus. Tours of the Evanston Campus are given on a regular basis, however, tours are not generally offered for the Chicago Campus. For more detailed information about the program, please see our Web site: *www.medschool.northwestern.edu/hpme.*

Application and Acceptance Policies

Filing of application:
  Earliest date: n/a
  Latest date: January 1, 2010
Application fee: $65   Fee Waiver Available: Yes
Acceptance notice:
  Earliest date: April 1, 2010
  Latest date: n/a
Applicant's response to acceptance offer:
  Latest Date: May 1, 2010
Deposit to hold place in class: $400; nonrefundable
Starting date: September 15, 2010

Information on 2008–2009 Entering Class

Number of	In-State	Out-of-State	Total
Applicants	109	575	684
Applicants Interviewed	27	120	147
New Entrants	6	23	29

Total number of students enrolled in program: 88

University of Illinois at Chicago College of Medicine

Chicago, Illinois

Address Inquiries To:
Josephine Volpe, Assistant Director Academic Affairs/Special Scholarship Programs
University of Illinois at Chicago, 2506 University Hall, M/C 115
601 S. Morgan Street
Chicago, Illinois 60607
T (312) 355-2477 **F** (312) 355-1233
gppauic@uic.edu
www.uic.edu/depts/oaa/spec_prog/gppa/

Purpose

The Guaranteed Professional Program Admissions (GPPA) initiative is a combined effort of the University of Illinois at Chicago (UIC) Honors College on the undergraduate campus and the College of Medicine. This program is offered only to high school seniors from Illinois. The GPPA guarantees incoming freshmen a seat in the College of Medicine at one of the four locations provided they qualify upon completion of their undergraduate studies at UIC.

Requirements for Entrance

This program is limited to Illinois residents. Students are selected for this program during the senior year of high school. There are no specific high school course requirements.

Selection Factors

The academic factors considered are rank in high school class, grade-point average, and test scores. Applicants must be in the top 15 percent of their high school class. Applicants must have a minimum ACT composite score of 28, or its SAT equivalent score. In addition to academic factors, extracurricular health-related activities and letters of recommendations are required. All applicants are invited for a required interview. A selected number of applicants are invited to return for a second interview.

Curriculum

The GPPA-Medicine program is designed to be completed in four years of undergraduate education at the University of Illinois at Chicago. Students are free to choose any of UIC's majors in eight undergraduate colleges. Throughout their undergraduate education, students participate in a number of required seminars and courses that will introduce them to various aspects of the medical profession. The final course is the Independent Study Seminar, which is a "capstone" project and presentation. Students must maintain a 3.5/4.0 cumulative grade-point average throughout their undergraduate education. During the year proceeding expected entry into medical school, students must take the Medical College Admissions Test (MCAT). Students must earn a MCAT score of at least the mean of the matriculating students into the College of Medicine in the year prior to expected entry, with no score below 9 in any segment of the exam. Students successfully completing the GPPA requirements are guaranteed a seat in one of the four UIC College of Medicine campuses. However, students are not required to attend the UIC College of Medicine. Once enrolled in the College of Medicine, students in the program are bound by the policies in force at the time of their matriculation.

Expenses

Expenses	Resident Tuition and Fees	Non-resident Tuition and Fees
Undergraduate	$11,800	N/A
U.S. Medical School	$29,564	N/A

Additional Information

Interested students should consult the GPPA-Medicine Conditions of Acceptance for more detailed information. All students are assigned a faculty mentor from the College of Medicine for their undergraduate years. All undergraduate classes take place in Chicago. UIC College of Medicine has four campuses, Chicago, Urbana/Champaign, Peoria and Rockford.

Application and Acceptance Policies

Filing of application:
  Earliest date: September 15, 2009
  Latest date: December 15, 2009
Application fee: $0   Fee Waiver Available: n/a
Acceptance notice:
  Earliest date: March 15, 2010
  Latest date: April 1, 2010
Applicant's response to acceptance offer:
  Maximum time: May 1, 2010
Deposit to hold place in class: None
Starting date: August 2010

Information on 2008–2009 Entering Class

Number of	In-State	Out-of-State	Total
Applicants	352	n/a	352
Applicants Interviewed	90	n/a	90
New Entrants	29	n/a	29
Total number of students enrolled in program: 100			

Boston University
School of Medicine
Boston, Massachusetts

Address Inquiries To:
Anthony J. Orlando
Assistant Director of Undergraduate Admissions
Boston University
Office of Undergraduate Admissions, 121 Bay State Road
Boston, Massachusetts 02215
T (617) 353-2300 **F** (617) 353-9695
admissions@bu.edu; www.bu.edu/bulletins/und/item14.html

Purpose
This combined degree program, one of the oldest in the nation, provides an undergraduate premedical preparation that also emphasizes the humanities and social sciences and affords a quality medical education even though the overall period of study is shortened.

Requirements for Entrance
Students are selected for the program at Boston University during the senior year of high school (or after high school if they have not been enrolled in any other degree-granting program). There are no state residence requirements. Students who are completing their high school graduation requirements in three years in order to graduate early are not eligible for this program. Applicants are expected to have completed the following courses by the time they graduate from high school: four years each of English and mathematics (one year of calculus is required); three years each of social sciences and a foreign language; and one year each of biology, chemistry (AP chemistry is strongly recommended), and physics. Applicants must take the SAT or the ACT with Writing. They must take SAT Subject Tests in Mathematics Level 2 and Chemistry. An SAT Subject Test in a foreign language is recommended.

Selection Factors
The academic factors taken into account in offering admission to an applicant include the following: the high school GPA, the SAT or the ACT with Writing score, scores on the SAT Subject Tests, rank in high school class, and the nature of the applicant's high school curriculum. In the 2008–2009 entering class, the average high school GPA was an unweighted 3.9 on a 4.0 scale, and rank in class was in the top two percent. The average combined Critical Reading and Math SAT score was 1531. The average SAT Writing score was 746. SAT Subject Test scores in Chemistry averaged 754. SAT Subject Tests in Mathematics Level 2 averaged 776. Personal characteristics sought in applicants are motivation, maturity, integrity, and an understanding of a career in medicine. An interview with College of Arts and Sciences and School of Medicine faculty is required.

Curriculum
This program leads to a baccalaureate degree granted by the College of Arts and Sciences at Boston University and to the M.D. degree awarded by Boston University School of Medicine. Students must complete work for the baccalaureate degree in three years with a major in medical science and a minor concentration in a division of the College of Arts and Sciences. Students must also satisfy the course distribution and language requirements of the college. Requirements for this degree include nine one-semester courses in the natural and physical sciences and two one-semester courses in the humanities, mathematics and computer science, and social sciences. The program is seven years in length, with an eight-year option. Students must meet GPA and MCAT requirements of the program. They are also required to take Step 1 of the USMLE during the medical school portion of the program. Taking Step 2 of the USMLE is not a requirement for graduation, but is strongly recommended.

Expenses

	Resident Tuition and Fees	Non-resident Tuition and Fees
Undergraduate	$36,540	$36,540
U.S. Medical School	$45,286	$45,286

Financial Aid
The usual sources of financial aid are available to students during the undergraduate portion of this program. Once in the medical school, students can qualify for need-based, low-interest, and government-sponsored loans. More information about aid can be obtained from the Office of Financial Assistance, Boston University, 881 Commonwealth Avenue, Boston, Massachusetts 02215, or by phone (617) 353-2965.

Application and Acceptance Policies
Filing of application:
Earliest date: September 1, 2009
Latest date: December 1, 2009
Application fee: $75   Fee Waiver Available: Yes
Acceptance notice:
Earliest date: April 1, 2010
Latest date: April 15, 2010
Applicant's response to acceptance offer:
Maximum time: May 1, 2010
Deposit to hold place in class: $650; non-refundable
Starting date: September 2010

Information on 2008–2009 Entering Class

Number of	In-State	Out-of-State	Total
Applicants	61	481	542
Applicants Interviewed	13	86	99
New Entrants	4	19	23

Total number of students enrolled in program: 75

Wayne State University
School of Medicine

Detroit, Michigan

Address Inquiries To:
Nancy Galster, Program Coordinator,
Irvin D. Reid Honors College
Wayne State University
2100 Undergraduate Library
Detroit, Michigan 48202
T (313) 577-8523 **F** (313) 577-6425
honors@wayne.edu
www.honors.wayne.edu/medstart.php

Purpose
The MedStart Program is intended to train medical innovators and creative thinkers. As undergraduates, students are treated as part of the medical community, with an emphasis on mentoring and research.

Requirements for Entrance
Students are selected for this program during their senior year of high school. Applicants must be citizens or permanent residents of the United States or citizens of Canada. Although there are no specific high school course requirements, applicants are required to take the ACT.

Selection Factors
To be considered for this program, applicants must have a minimum ACT score of 25 and a high school GPA of at least 3.5. Community service, team activities, leadership, extracurricular activities, and experience in health care are among the personal attributes and experiential factors sought in applicants. An interview is also required. Once admitted into the program, students are expected to maintain an overall GPA of 3.3 in the freshman year and a 3.50 GPA in the sciences and overall in subsequent years of their undergraduate studies. For subsequent admission to Wayne State University School of Medicine, students in this program must complete all prerequisite courses, take the MCAT (with a minimum total score of 27 and no less than an eight in any individual section), and submit an AMCAS application.

Curriculum
The program, eight years in duration, allows students to obtain a baccalaureate degree from Wayne State University and the M.D. degree from Wayne State University School of Medicine. During the four years of their undergraduate studies, 100 percent of their coursework will be related to the bachelor's degree. The coursework in the four years of medical school will be spent in achieving the medical degree. Students must meet university requirements for the Irvin D. Reid Honors College and degree completion. Throughout the eight-year baccalaureate-medical program, monthly seminars are held which are relevant to medical fields and topics in medicine. Students may apply for a ten-week paid clinical research experience in the summer following the junior undergraduate year.

Expenses

Expenses	Resident Tuition and Fees	Non-resident Tuition and Fees
Undergraduate	$7,592	$16,244
U.S. Medical School	$28,425	$57,515

Financial Aid
Information about financial aid can be obtained from the Office of Scholarships and Financial Aid, Welcome Center, P.O. Box 4230, Detroit, MI 48202; by telephone (313) 577-3378; or visit *www.financialaid.wayne.edu*.

Application and Acceptance Policies

Filing of application:
    Earliest date: November 1, 2009
    Latest date: January 15, 2010
Application fee: $30   Fee Waiver Available: No
Acceptance notice:
    Earliest date: April 1, 2010
    Latest date: varies
Applicant's response to acceptance offer:
    Maximum time: May 1, 2010
Deposit to hold place in class: None
Starting date: September 2010

Information on 2008–2009 Entering Class

Number of	In-State	Out-of-State	Total
Applicants	182	68	250
Applicants Interviewed	22	8	30
New Entrants	12	3	15
Total number of students enrolled in program: 55			

Saint Louis University School of Medicine

St Louis, Missouri

Address Inquiries To:
Alexa Barnoski Serfis, Ph.D., Director, Preprofessional Health Studies
Preprofessional Health Studies, Verhaegen Hall Room 314
3634 Lindell Blvd.
St. Louis, Missouri 63108-3302
T (314) 977-2840 **F** (314) 977-3660
prehealth@slu.edu
www.slu.edu/colleges/AS/phs/medScholars.html

Purpose

This combined-degree program awards special recognition to exceptional first-year (freshmen) premedical students. It is intended to enhance the educational experience and reduce the stress associated with premedical-medical education.

Requirements for Entrance

Students apply to this program when they apply to Saint Louis University for undergraduate admission. Both residents and non-residents of Missouri are eligible to apply to the program. Applicants are required to complete the following courses prior to graduation from high school: one year of biology, one year of chemistry, and three years of mathematics. In addition to meeting these requirements, applicants must take either the ACT (minimum score of 30) or SAT (minimum score of 1320).

Selection Factors

Outstanding academic achievement in high school is a favorable factor in qualifying for the combined-degree program at Saint Louis University. Selected applicants usually rank in the top ten percent of their high school class. It is required that all candidates achieve a minimum ACT score of 30 or SAT score of 1320. An interview is not required. Students are required to take the MCAT in April of the junior year (no minimum score required). MCAT scores are not a factor for promotion or admission to the medical school phase of the program.

Curriculum

This eight-year program leads to a baccalaureate degree awarded by Saint Louis University and to the M.D. degree granted by the Saint Louis University School of Medicine. Students have much flexibility in choosing a major and are encouraged to study in an area of their choice. During the first four years of the curriculum, students will spend 100 percent of their time in coursework related to the bachelor's degree, which includes 42 to 46 semester hours of natural and physical science, 3 to 4 semester hours of mathematics, and 12 semester hours of humanities. There are strict GPA requirements to remain in the program. The remaining four years focus on achieving the M.D. degree.

Expenses	Resident Tuition and Fees	Non-resident Tuition and Fees
Undergraduate	$30,330	$30,330
U.S. Medical School	$44,435	$44,435

Financial Aid

Information can be obtained from the Office of Financial Aid/Scholarships, DuBourg Hall 121, Saint Louis University, 221 North Grand Boulevard, St. Louis, MO 63103.

Application and Acceptance Policies

Filing of application:
    Earliest date: October 1, 2009
    Latest date: December 1, 2009
Application fee: None   Fee Waiver Available: n/a
Acceptance notice:
    Earliest date: March 1, 2010
    Latest date: n/a
Applicant's response to acceptance offer:
    Maximum time: May 1, 2010
Deposit to hold place in class: $200; non-refundable
Starting date: Mid-August 2010

Information on 2008–2009 Entering Class

Number of	In-State	Out-of-State	Total
Applicants	141	347	488
Applicants Interviewed	0	0	0
New Entrants	40	70	110

Total number of students enrolled in program: 263

University of Missouri-Kansas City School of Medicine

Kansas City, Missouri

Mary Anne Morgenegg, Admissions Coordinator
Council on Selection
University of Missouri – Kansas City School of Medicine
2411 Holmes, Kansas City, Missouri 64108-2792
T (816) 235-1870 **F** (816) 235-6579
medicine@umkc.edu
www.med.umkc.edu

Purpose

This combined baccalaureate–M.D. degree program integrates the humanities, social sciences, basic sciences, and clinical medicine throughout the curriculum so that graduates will have the background for lifelong learning in order to meet the needs of their patients, families, and communities.

Requirements for Entrance

The program is primarily designed for high school graduates who are entering college. Residents and non-residents of Missouri are eligible to apply. An applicant's high school curriculum must include, at a minimum, the following: eight semesters of English; eight semesters of mathematics; six semesters of science, including two semesters of biology and two semesters of chemistry; six semesters of social studies; two semesters of fine arts; and four semesters of a foreign language. Applicants must meet a minimum academic screen based on the ACT composite score and rank in high school class.

Selection Factors

Applicants' academic potential is judged by the quality of high school courses, rank in high school class, and scores on the ACT. In the 2008–2009 entering class, the average test score for MO residents was in the 92nd percentile, and the average rank in class was in the 93rd percentile. For residents of other states, the average test score was at the 97th percentile, and the average rank was at the 94th percentile. Personal qualities include maturity, leadership, reliability, motivation for medicine, range of interests, interpersonal skills, compassion, and job experience. Qualified applicants are invited for a required interview.

Curriculum

The six-year curriculum leads to a baccalaureate degree granted by the University of Missouri, Kansas City (UMKC) College of Arts and Sciences or the UMKC School of Biological Sciences and the doctor of medicine degree granted by the School of Medicine. Students must complete requirements for the bachelor's degree. Students have a choice of majors, but most select liberal arts or psychology. Course requirements for the bachelor's degree in liberal arts include 21 semester hours of humanities, 21 semester hours of social sciences, and 50 semester hours of natural and physical sciences. The curriculum typically takes six years to complete. During the first two years of the curriculum, students spend 75 percent of their time in coursework related to the bachelor's degree. Conversely, in the last four years, students spend 75 percent of their time in courses, clerkships, and electives related to the M.D. degree. Thus, the study of liberal arts, basic sciences, and clinical

medicine is integrated throughout the entire curriculum. Students are assigned a faculty advisor (docent), and younger students are paired with older students. During the last four years of the curriculum, students attend a general medicine outpatient clinic for a half-day each week. Students in this program do not take the MCAT. They must pass Steps 1 and 2 of the USMLE for graduation. An alternate path is available for extended study.

Expenses

	Resident Tuition and Fees	Non-resident Tuition and Fees
Undergraduate	N/A	N/A
U.S. Medical School	$28,810	$56,279

Financial Aid

Contact the UMKC Financial Aid Office at the Administrative Center, 5115 Oak, Kansas City, Missouri 64110, (816) 235-1154.

Application and Acceptance Policies

Filing of application:
   Earliest date: August 1, 2009
   Latest date: November 1, 2009
Application fee: $35   Fee Waiver Available: No
Acceptance notice:
   Earliest date: April 1, 2010
   Latest date: n/a
Applicant's response to acceptance offer:
   Latest date: May 1, 2010
Deposit to hold place in class: $100; refundable by May 14, 2010
Starting date: August 2010

Information on 2008–2009 Entering Class

Number of	In-State	Out-of-State	Total
Applicants	332	474	806
Applicants Interviewed	141	142	283
New Entrants	53	47	100
Total number of students enrolled in program: 623			

Chapter 10: Information on Combined Undergraduate/M.D. Programs   77

University of Medicine and Dentistry of New Jersey-New Jersey Medical School

Newark, New Jersey

Address Inquiries To:
Lisa Houston, Admissions Coordinator
Office of Admissions
UMDNJ – New Jersey Medical School
P.O. Box 1709
Newark, New Jersey 07101-1709
T (973) 972-4631 **F** (973) 973-7986
njmsadmiss@umdnj.edu
http://njms.umdnj.edu/education/admissions/seven_year_ba_md.cfm

Purpose

The New Jersey Medical School (NJMS) currently has baccalaureate/M.D. degree programs in collaboration with nine undergraduate institutions. The goal of these programs is to give highly qualified students the best opportunity to broaden their premedical preparation, while establishing their career path.

Requirements for Entrance

Applicants must be high school seniors who are in the top ten percent of their class and have a combined SAT Critical Reading and Math test score of 1400. Please note that we only consider the Critical Reading and Math sections and not the Essay section of the SAT. Applicants must be either U.S. citizens or permanent residents of the U.S. The most qualified and dedicated applicants will receive the highest consideration.

Selection Factors

Applicants are screened on the basis of academic credentials, letters of recommendation, and an essay. Those meeting the criteria are invited for an interview at the undergraduate school. The undergraduate schools then forward credentials of qualified applicants to NJMS for review and selection for a NJMS interview. The application deadline to the undergraduate institution is January 4, 2010.

Curriculum

The program consists of three years at an undergraduate school followed by a four-year medical program. Although not used to determine admission, the MCAT must be taken prior to medical school matriculation. Promotion to the medical school is contingent upon achieving grades of "B" or better in all premedical courses and maintaining an overall grade point average of at least 3.5 each semester. The baccalaureate degree is awarded by the undergraduate institution upon completion of the first year of medical school. The M.D. degree is awarded by NJMS upon successful completion of all NJMS degree requirements. Students are required to pass Step 1 of the USMLE for promotion to the third year. Passing Step 2 of the USMLE is required for graduation. Nine programs are currently available: Boston University provides an emphasis in liberal arts or humanities and the program is for NJ residents only. For more information contact: admissions@bu.edu. Caldwell College provides a well-rounded program that incorporates course work in the humanities, liberal arts and social behavioral sciences, as well as the premedical sciences. For additional information contact: schoi@caldwell.edu. Drew University offers premedical preparation in all sciences and liberal arts subjects. For more information contact: ksmall@drew.edu. Montclair State University offers premedical preparation in biology, chemistry, biochemistry, molecular biology, computer science, mathematics, psychology, and anthropology. For more information contact: shillcockj@mail.montclair.edu. New Jersey Institute of Technology offers undergraduate study in the Honors Premedical Curriculum within the Engineering Science Program. For more information contact: honors@njit.edu. Rutgers University-Newark Campus offers premedical preparation in the sciences. For more information contact: nyeste@ugadm.rutgers.edu. Stevens Institute of Technology offers premedical preparation in chemical biology. For more information contact: mhadidi@stevens.edu. The College of New Jersey offers preparation in biology, chemistry, history, philosophy, and psychology. For more information contact: shevlin@tcnj.edu. The Richard Stockton College of New Jersey offers preparation in chemistry, biology, physics, and liberal arts. For more information contact: admissions@stockton.edu. NJMS also offers Articulated Programs, which allow students in their second year of college to apply to matriculate at NJMS after completion of their third year of college through programs with: St. Peter's College (contact lsciorra@spc.edu), Rutgers University-Newark (contact jmaiello@andromeda.rutgers.edu) and Rutgers University – New Brunswick (contact hpo@biology.rutgers.edu).

Expenses

Expenses	Resident Tuition and Fees	Non-resident Tuition and Fees
Undergraduate	$25,218	$39,461
U.S. Medical School	$26,113	$40,356

Financial Aid

Financial aid packages for the undergraduate years are determined by the undergraduate schools.

Application and Acceptance Policies

Filing of application:
    Earliest date: Varies by school
    Latest date: January 5, 2010
Application fee: Varies   Fee Waiver Available: n/a
Acceptance notice:
    Earliest date: Varies by school
    Latest date: April 14, 2010
Applicant's response to acceptance offer:
    Maximum time: Varies by undergraduate school.
Deposit to hold place in class: No
Starting date: Varies

Information on 2008–2009 Entering Class

Number of	In-State	Out-of-State	Total
Applicants	213	n/a	213
Applicants Interviewed	111	n/a	111
New Entrants	30	n/a	30
Total number of students enrolled in program: 151			

Rutgers University and UMDNJ Robert Wood Johnson Medical School

Piscataway, New Jersey

Address Inquiries To:
Betsi Platt, Administrative Assistant
Rutgers, The State University of New Jersey Bachelor/Medical
Degree Program Nelson Biological Laboratory, Room A207, 604
Allison Road Piscataway, New Jersey 08854-8082
T (732) 445-5667 **F** (732) 445-6341
hpo@biology.rutgers.edu
http://lifesci.rutgers.edu/~hpo/BAMD.htm

Purpose

The program permits the early identification and admission of quality medical students. It also integrates medical studies with liberal arts study.

Requirements for Entrance

This program is open to all students enrolled at Rutgers University who are citizens or permanent residents of the United States. Students are selected for this program at the end of their sophomore year. Students must have a 3.50 overall GPA by the end of their third semester and sustain this GPA through the fourth semester at Rutgers University. Residents and non-residents of New Jersey are considered.

Selection Factors

An applicant's high school and college transcripts and faculty recommendations are taken into account in offering admission. In the 2008–2009 entering class, matriculants had achieved an average GPA of 3.9 at the end of the first two years of college. They had average scores of 660 on the Critical Reading section, 730 on the Mathematics section, and 710 on the Writing section. Maturity, motivation, and broad interests are personal characteristics sought in applicants. An interview is required. The MCAT is not used.

Curriculum

This program leads to the baccalaureate degree awarded by Rutgers University and to the M.D. degree granted by the University of Medicine and Dentistry of New Jersey–Robert Wood Johnson Medical School. Students must complete requirements for a baccalaureate degree. The most frequent majors for that degree are biological sciences, followed by biochemistry. The program is eight years in duration. The basic sciences and the liberal arts are studied together during a four-year period. While in medical school, students must take and pass Steps 1 and 2 of the USMLE.

Expenses	Resident Tuition and Fees	Non-resident Tuition and Fees
Undergraduate	$11,562	$21,776
U.S. Medical School	$26,462	$40,695

Financial Aid

Undergraduates should contact the Office of Financial Aid, Rutgers University, 620 George Street, New Brunswick, New Jersey 08901-1175; call (732) 932-7057; or visit the Web site at *http://studentaid.rutgers.edu.*

Application and Acceptance Policies

Filing of application:
  Earliest date: April 1, 2010
  Latest date: May 25, 2010
Application fee: None   Fee Waiver Available: n/a
Acceptance notice:
  Earliest date: July 1, 2010
  Latest date: n/a
Applicant's response to acceptance offer:
  Maximum time: 2 weeks
Deposit to hold place in class: None
Starting date: August 1, 2010

Information on 2008–2009 Entering Class

Number of	In-State	Out-of-State	Total
Applicants	33	0	33
Applicants Interviewed	23	0	23
New Entrants	10	0	10
Total number of students enrolled in program: 19			

Brooklyn College and SUNY Downstate Medical Center

Brooklyn, New York

Address Inquiries To:
Dr. Steven B. Silbering, Director, B.A.–M.D. Program
2231 Boylan Hall, Brooklyn College
2900 Bedford Avenue
Brooklyn, New York 11210-2889
T (718) 951-5471 F (718) 951-4559
silbering@brooklyn.cuny.edu
http://bamd.brooklyn.cuny.edu/bamdmain.html

Purpose

The aims of this program are to produce physicians who are humanists and who are concerned with the caring, as well as curing, dimensions of medicine and to offer an economically affordable baccalaureate and medical school education.

Requirements for Entrance

Students are selected in their senior year of high school. Admission is limited to residents of the states of New York, New Jersey, and Connecticut, with preference given to New York State residents. Applicants are recommended to have at least a 90 percent CAA (College Admission Average, academic subjects only) and a combined score of at least 1200 on the Mathematics and Critical Reading sections of the SAT Reasoning Test.

Selection Factors

The academic factors taken into account in offering admission to applicants include the high school GPA, SAT scores, New York State Regents Examination scores, and scores on Advanced Placement tests. In the 2008 entering class, most students had a high school average above 90, and the sum of the SAT Mathematics and Critical Reading scores was between 1300 and 1450. Non-academic factors include community service, participation in scientific research projects and other extracurricular activities. Maturity and motivation are qualities highly sought after among the applicants. An interview is required.

Curriculum

This program leads to a baccalaureate degree from Brooklyn College and an M.D. degree from SUNY Downstate Medical Center College of Medicine. Students in the baccalaureate portion of the B.A.–M.D. program are encouraged to choose a non-science major; however, if a science major is chosen, the student must have a non-science minor. While in Brooklyn College, B.A.–M.D. students fulfill not only the requirements for the major and minor, but also must complete a liberal arts (Core) requirement. Three core courses must be honors sections. In addition, students must complete the pre-med requirement, which includes various biology, chemistry and physics courses. No student is permitted to remain in the undergraduate portion of the B.A.–M.D. program if either the overall or science GPA's fall below 3.5 in any semester after the freshman year. The MCAT examination must be taken no later than the summer following the junior year. If a score on any of the three sections of the MCAT examination is less than 9, the MCAT must be repeated. Students are permitted to take the MCAT three times in order to achieve a 9 on each section on the same examination. Aside from the academic requirements of the undergraduate

B.A.–M.D. students, there is a clinical internship requirement of 320 hours that must be fulfilled during any of the summers except the one following the senior year. Also, during every semester after the freshman year, B.A.-M.D. students must perform 60 hours of non-clinical community service. After four years, the students graduate from Brooklyn College and matriculate into the four-year medical school program at SUNY Downstate.

Expenses

Expenses	Resident Tuition and Fees	Non-resident Tuition and Fees
Undergraduate	$4,000	$5,400
U.S. Medical School	$19,370	$34,070

Financial Aid

All students admitted to the B.A.–M.D. program are provided with full-tuition Presidential scholarships. If any student receives TAP financial aid, the Presidential scholarship will cover the remainder of the tuition.

Application and Acceptance Policies

Filing of application:
 Earliest date: September 14, 2009
 Latest date: December 31, 2009
Application fee: None   Fee Waiver Available: No
Acceptance notice:
 Earliest date: April 1, 2010
 Latest date: April 1, 2010
Applicant's response to acceptance offer:
 Latest date: April 21, 2010
Deposit to hold place in class: None
Starting date: August 27, 2010

Information on 2008–2009 Entering Class

Number of	In-State	Out-of-State	Total
Applicants	281	8	289
Applicants Interviewed	90	0	90
New Entrants	15	0	15
Total number of students enrolled in program: 60			

Hobart and William Smith Colleges/ SUNY Upstate Medical University

Geneva, New York

Address Inquiries To:
Renee Nearpass, Pre-Health Advisor
Elizabeth Blackwell Medical Scholars Program
Hobart & William Smith Colleges
Office of Admissions, 629 South Main Street
Geneva, New York 14456
T (800) 852-2256 **F** (315) 781-3914
admissions@hws.edu; www.hws.edu/admissions/adm_apply/firstyear.asp

Purpose

The Elizabeth Blackwell Medical Scholars program is designed for exceptional high school seniors who wish to attend medical school. Applicants to this program must be from a rural community, a group underrepresented in medicine, or be a first generation college student.

Requirements for Entrance

Students apply to the program in their senior year of high school. They must have a minimum SAT I score of 1250 (Mathematics and Critical Reading only) or a 28 ACT score and a high school grade point average of 90 or higher, as well as have demonstrated a commitment to a career in medicine. Students accepted into this program will complete their undergraduate degree at Hobart and William Smith Colleges and are guaranteed admission to Upstate Medical University's College of Medicine, pending all program standards are met.

Selection Factors

This program is for high school students who are from rural areas, from groups underrepresented in medicine, or who are among the first generation in their families to attend college. The following factors are taken into consideration in assessing applicants for admission into this program: grades, rank in class, SAT (ACT) scores, and extracurricular activities. Selected applicants are invited for a required interview.

Curriculum

This eight-year program leads to a baccalaureate degree awarded by Hobart and William Smith Colleges, and to the medical degree awarded by SUNY Upstate Medical University. Students in this program are not required to take the MCAT for promotion or for admission to the medical school.

Expenses

Expenses	Resident Tuition and Fees	Non-resident Tuition and Fees
Undergraduate	$38,860	$38,860
U.S. Medical School	$19,956	$34,656

Financial Aid

Blackwell Scholars are awarded a full-tuition scholarship to attend Hobart and William Smith Colleges. To retain the full-tuition scholarship, awardees must maintain a GPA of at least 3.0 during each semester while at Hobart and William Smith Colleges. More information about financial aid at Hobart and William Smith Colleges can be found at: *www.hws.edu/admissions/fin_edu.aspx* or *www.upstate.edu/prospective/tuition.php*.

Application and Acceptance Policies

Filing of application:
    Earliest date: August 2009
    Latest date: January 15, 2010
Application fee: $45   Fee Waiver Available: Yes
Acceptance notice:
    Earliest date: Within two weeks of interview
    Latest date: n/a
Applicant's response to acceptance offer:
    Maximum time: 2 weeks after offer is sent
Deposit to hold place in class: $100;
refundable by May 15 of year of entry
Starting date: The fall following graduation from Hobart and William Smith Colleges

Information on 2008–2009 Entering Class

Number of	In-State	Out-of-State	Total
Applicants	33	10	43
Applicants Interviewed	4	1	5
New Entrants	3	0	3
Total number of students enrolled in program: 10			

Rensselaer Polytechnic Institute and Albany Medical College

Troy, New York

Address Inquiries To:
Dean of Undergraduate Admissions
Rensselaer Polytechnic Institute
110 Eighth Street
Troy, New York 12180-3590
T (518) 276-6216 **F** (518) 276-4072
admissions@rpi.edu
www.rpi.edu/dept/admissions/resources/Physician-ScientistProgramAccelerated.pdf

Purpose

The Accelerated Physician-Scientist Program offers qualified individuals the opportunity to become physicians who are intensively trained in medical research. This innovative approach provides a well-rounded perspective that prepares future practitioners and physician-scientists to perform with confidence and care in a technologically changing environment.

Requirements for Entrance

Students are selected for this program during the senior year of high school. Residents of New York, as well as non-residents of the state, are eligible to apply. Applicants are expected to have completed the following courses by the time they graduate from high school: four years of English; one year each of biology, chemistry, and physics; and four years of mathematics (through pre-calculus). They must take the SAT Reasoning Test and two SAT Subject Area Tests: one mathematics and one science. In lieu of these tests, American College Testing (ACT) Assessment program scores, including the Writing Test, may be submitted. All tests must be completed by the December testing date prior to the proposed September matriculation.

Selection Factors

Academic factors considered in offering admission to an applicant include the quality and nature of coursework in high school, performance in those courses, rank in high school class, and test scores. The 2008–2009 entering class had an average score of 689 on the SAT Critical Reading, 765 on the SAT Mathematics, and 728 on the SAT Writing. Personal qualities sought in applicants are motivation, maturity, and intellectual capacity necessary to pursue the accelerated course of study. An interview is required.

Curriculum

The program leads to a B.S. degree awarded by Rensselaer Polytechnic Institute and the M.D. degree granted by Albany Medical College (AMC). The curriculum for the B.S. and M.D. degrees usually requires seven years to complete. During the first three years of the program spent at Rensselaer, the curriculum involves 70 percent premedical science courses and 30 percent liberal arts courses. Students take 18 courses in the natural and physical sciences and 8 elective courses in the humanities and social sciences. The cornerstone of the program is a mentored research project. During the sixth semester, students split their time between Rensselaer and AMC and begin research that extends over the third and final year at Rensselaer and into the summer preceding the first year of medical school. The research continues throughout the freshman year at AMC and into the following summer. Training in making oral and written scientific presentations is also included. At the medical college, basic and clinical sciences are integrated into themes (primarily organ systems) stressing normal function in Year 1 and pathological processes in Year 2. There are also five longitudinal themes that are integrated throughout the curriculum: clinical skills, ethical and health systems issues, evidence-based medicine, nutrition and informatics. In every theme, student learning is focused on clinical resentations. Basic science seminars reinforce the importance of the basic sciences in Years 3 and 4. Emphasis is placed on primary care throughout the four years, with an increased emphasis on care in ambulatory settings in the clinical rotations of Year 3. Year 4 emphasizes specialty care in various required rotations. Additional electives are available in Year 4. Students admitted to the program are not required to take the MCAT for admission to Albany Medical College. Students are expected to pass Steps 1 and 2 of the USMLE while at Albany Medical College.

Expenses

Expenses	Resident Tuition and Fees	Non-resident Tuition and Fees
Undergraduate	$36,950	$36,950
U.S. Medical School	$44,623	$44,623

Financial Aid

Sources of financial aid are restricted and include endowed scholarships based on need, merit scholarships, work-study, and student loans through federal and institutional programs. Applicants can receive more information by contacting the Financial Aid Office of Rensselaer Polytechnic Institute at (518) 276-6813 or Albany Medical College at (518) 262-5435.

Application and Acceptance Policies

Filing of application:
   Earliest date: September 1, 2009
   Latest date: November 1, 2009
Application fee: $50   Fee Waiver Available: Yes
Acceptance notice:
   Earliest date: March 2010
   Latest date: Until class is filled
Applicant's response to acceptance offer:
   Latest date: May 1, 2010
Deposit to hold place in class: $300; nonrefundable
Starting date: August 2010

Information on 2008–2009 Entering Class

Number of	In-State	Out-of-State	Total
Applicants	128	207	335
Applicants Interviewed	20	25	45
New Entrants	3	4	7

Total number of students enrolled in program: 31

St. Bonaventure University/George Washington University School of Medicine Dual Degree (BSMD) Program

St. Bonaventure, New York

Address Inquiries To:
Dr. Allen Knowles, III, Director
Franciscan Health Care Professions Programs
Biology Department
De La Roche Hall, Room 219
St. Bonaventure, New York 14778
T (716) 375-2656
prehealth@sbu.edu; aknowles@sbu.edu
www.sbu.edu

Purpose

A joint program of St. Bonaventure University (SBU) and the George Washington University School of Medicine and Health Sciences in Washington, DC (GW), the eight-year B.S.–M.D. program is designed for the high school senior who exhibits academic excellence, leadership in activities, and community service and healthcare experience, all of which have resulted in a passion for a career as a physician. The goal is to prepare the student with a strong background in the natural sciences in preparation for the rigors of medical school. SBU opened its new science facilities that will coordinate with the educational processes at GW, utilizing the state-of-the-art GW hospital. The GW Clinical Skills Center is dedicated to education and research with cutting-edge technology. Through the Surgical Simulation and Demonstration Area, medical students gain comprehensive and clinical exposure and feedback and skill improvement to enable them to become technically adept and humane caregivers. More information on the GW M.D. program can be found at *http://www.gwumc.edu/smhs*.

Requirements for Entrance

Students are selected in their senior year of high school. Applicants must be U.S. or Canadian citizens or Permanent Residents of the U.S. Applicants must complete the SAT (Verbal/Mathematics of at least 1300) or ACT (minimal score of 29), as well as the SAT Subject Test in Biology (preferably M).

Selection Factors

Academic factors considered in selecting applicants include high school grades, class rank, and standardized test scores. In addition, extracurricular and health-related activities, community service, volunteerism, research, medical field exposure, personal essays, and letters of recommendation are reviewed. Rank must be in the top 10% of the class, with a GPA of greater than 90 percent. Qualities demonstrating leadership, interest in the medical field through experiences, and AP and Honors courses are considered. An interview is required at SBU and GW and is by invitation only.

Curriculum

The student's progress is reviewed on a regular basis. Students must maintain a minimum of a "B" in courses required for admission to the medical school and an overall 3.6 average. The recommended major is biology, with interests outside of the sciences being encouraged. Students do not take the MCAT. Students are required to remain active in community service, volunteer programs, research components, and internships established through SBU. Students attend presentations and interact with GW M.D. students on the Medical Center campus. At the end of four years, the student is granted the B.S.

degree from SBU. In the first and second years at GW, the integration of clinical skills begins, as students spend time with physicians, developing patient interviewing skills, conducting physical examinations, and assisting in diagnosis. The third and fourth years at GW are used to develop clinical expertise in a variety of hospitals in the greater D.C. metropolitan area. Upon completion of all requirements, the M.D. degree is awarded by GW.

Expenses

	Resident Tuition and Fees	Non-resident Tuition and Fees
Undergraduate	$23,920	$23,920
U.S. Medical School	$46,267	$46,267

Financial Aid

For information on financial aid, fees, and expenses, please refer to the Web sites for each institution (*www.sbu.edu* and *www.gwumc.edu*) or contact the Financial Aid Offices.

Application and Acceptance Policies

Filing of application:
    Earliest date: September 1, 2009
    Latest date: December 15, 2009
Application fee: $30   Fee Waiver Available: Yes
Acceptance notice:
    Earliest date: March 15, 2010
    Latest date: n/a
Applicant's response to acceptance offer:
    Latest date: May 1, 2010
Deposit to hold place in class: $500; nonrefundable
Starting date: Late August 2010

Information on 2008–2009 Entering Class

Number of	In-State	Out-of-State	Total
Applicants	n/c	77	77
Applicants Interviewed	n/c	42	42
New Entrants	n/c	17	17
Total number of students enrolled in program: 17			

Siena College and Albany Medical College

Loudonville, New York

Address Inquiries To:
Office of Admissions
Siena College
515 Loudon Road
Loudonville, New York 12211-1462
T (518) 783-2423
admit@siena.edu
www.siena.edu/amc

Purpose

The Science, Humanities, and Medicine Program offers an eight-year continuum of education that has a special emphasis on the humanities and on community service to the medically underserved, while providing a sound understanding of both the natural and social sciences.

Requirements for Entrance

Students are selected for this program during the senior year of high school. Both residents and non-residents of New York are eligible to apply. Candidates for admission to the Siena/Albany Medical College program must have completed: four years of laboratory science (including biology, chemistry, and physics) and four years of mathematics (including a minimum of pre-calculus [calculus preferred]). Typically, successful candidates will have enrolled in, or completed, advanced-level courses by the end of their senior year in high school. A well-rounded background and demonstrated leadership experience are also important. Of equal significance is the student's proven concern for others and for the community. Applicants must take either the SAT Reasoning Test or ACT Assessment, including the optional Writing test. Tests must be completed by the November testing date prior to the proposed September matriculation.

Selection Factors

Academic factors considered in offering admission to an applicant include: required and elective courses taken, grades earned, class standing, SAT Reasoning Test or ACT scores, including the Writing test, honors received, letters of recommendation, and unique academic experiences. Of great importance to the admission committee are such factors as extracurricular activities, evidence of intellectual curiosity, and interest in the humanities and in the sciences. Students generally rank among the top ten percent of their high school class. The 2008–2009 entering class had an average score of 660 on the SAT Critical Reading section and 706 on the SAT Mathematics section. An interview is required.

Curriculum

This program offers a coordinated eight-year curriculum of premedical and medical education. The undergraduate phase offers an equal distribution of science and non-science courses. Students graduate in four years with a bachelor of arts degree in biology with a minor in the humanities. The undergraduate phase of the program also includes a required summer of human service in a health-related agency, usually in an urban setting or developing nation. Passage from the undergraduate college to the medical school requires achievement of a 3.40 GPA and a continued interest in the human service dimension of the program. At the medical college, basic and clinical sciences are integrated into themes (primarily organ systems) stressing normal function in Year 1 and pathological processes in Year 2. There are also five longitudinal themes integrated throughout the curriculum: clinical skills, ethical and health systems issues, evidence-based medicine, nutrition, and informatics. In every theme, student learning is focused on clinical presentations. The summer between the sophomore and junior years is dedicated to medically related volunteer service, usually in a rural or inner city clinic. Seminars reinforce the importance of the basic sciences in Years 3 and 4. Emphasis is placed on primary care throughout the four years, with an increased emphasis on care in ambulatory settings in Year 3 clinical rotations. Year 4 emphasizes specialty care in various required rotations. Additional electives are available in Year 4. Students admitted to the program are not required to take the MCAT for admission to AMC. Students must pass Steps 1 and 2 of the USMLE while at AMC.

Expenses

	Resident Tuition and Fees	Non-resident Tuition and Fees
Undergraduate	$24,015	$24,015
U.S. Medical School	$44,623	$44,623

Financial Aid

Applicants can receive more information by contacting the Siena College Financial Aid Office at (518) 783-2427 or the Albany Medical College Financial Aid Office at (518) 262-5435.

Application and Acceptance Policies

Filing of application:
  Earliest date: September 1, 2009
  Latest date: December 1, 2009
Application fee: $50   Fee Waiver Available: Yes
Acceptance notice:
  Earliest date: March 2010
  Latest date: Until classes are filled
Applicant's response to acceptance offer:
  Latest date: May 1, 2010
Deposit to hold place in class: $200; nonrefundable
Starting date: September 2010

Information on 2008–2009 Entering Class

Number of	In-State	Out-of-State	Total
Applicants	242	134	376
Applicants Interviewed	32	11	43
New Entrants	11	1	12

Total number of students enrolled in program: 52

Sophie Davis School of Biomedical Education at the City College of New York

New York, New York

Address Inquiries To:
Chris Wanyonyi, Director of Admissions
Sophie Davis School of Biomedical Education at the City College of New York
Office of Admission, Harris Hall, 160 Convent Avenue
New York, New York 10031
T (212) 650-7718 F (212) 650-7708
cwanyonyi@med.cuny.edu
med.cuny.edu/admissions.html

Purpose

The purposes of this combined-degree program are to train primary care physicians who will work in medically underserved urban areas, to increase the number of physicians from groups underrepresented in medicine, to intervene in the disparity of access to high quality pre-college science education, and create a medical school pipeline.

Requirements for Entrance

Students are selected for this program in the senior year of high school. Only residents of New York State are eligible to apply. Applicants are expected to have completed the following courses by the time they graduate from high school: two semesters each of chemistry and biology and six to eight semesters of mathematics. They must take the ACT Assessment and SAT tests.

Selection Factors

Academic factors taken into account in offering admission to an applicant are: high school GPA, SAT I scores, ACT Assessment scores, and scores on the New York State Regents Examinations. In the 2008 entering class, high school grades averaged 94 and the subscore on the Mathematics ACT Assessment averaged 29. The SAT Mathematics average was 650, and the SAT Verbal average was 633. Personal qualities sought in applicants include interest in people, concern for others, initiative, and leadership. An interview is required.

Curriculum

This seven-year program leads to a baccalaureate degree granted by The City College of New York (CCNY) and to the M.D. degree awarded by one of six participating medical schools (Albany Medical College, Dartmouth Medical College, New York Medical College, New York University, SUNY Brooklyn, or SUNY Stony Brook University). During the first five years of the program, students fulfill all requirements for the B.S. degree and study the preclinical portion of the medical school curriculum. After successfully completing the five-year sequence and passing Step 1 of the USMLE, students transfer to one of the participating medical schools for their final two years of clinical training. Students are expected to pass Step 1 of the USMLE to proceed to Years 3 and 4 of medical school. Additionally, students are expected to pass Step 2 of the USMLE to graduate. Students complete the core liberal arts curriculum of CCNY during the first two years. At this time, they also take courses emphasizing the importance of understanding cultural differences for good medical practice and, through community medicine courses, do field work at various community agencies, including many family practice clinics. The final years of the five-year sequence at CCNY include courses necessary in the first two years of medical school, including basic science courses and several community medicine courses. Students also benefit from counseling and academic support services.

Expenses

	Resident Tuition and Fees	Non-resident Tuition and Fees
Undergraduate	$4,129	N/A
U.S. Medical School	Varies	Varies

Financial Aid

Pell grants, New York State Tuition Assistance Program Awards, and NYC Merit Awards are all sources of financial aid. The school generally awards several scholarships to incoming students, including The Lois Pope L.I.F.E. scholarships and the William R. Hearst Endowed Scholarship. Scholarships available later in the program include those from the Alan Seelig Memorial Fund, the Aranow Fund, and the Sophie and Leonard Davis Scholarships. Applicants can contact the Financial Aid Office at (212) 650-5819.

Application and Acceptance Policies

Filing of application:
  Earliest date: September 2009
  Latest date: January 8, 2010
Application fee: None   Fee Waiver Available: n/a
Acceptance notice:
  Earliest date: March 25, 2010
  Latest date: April 1, 2010
Applicant's response to acceptance offer:
  Maximum time: May 1, 2010
Deposit to hold place in class: None
Starting date: Late August 2010

Information on 2008–2009 Entering Class

Number of	In-State	Out-of-State	Total
Applicants	750	n/a	750
Applicants Interviewed	244	n/a	244
New Entrants	78	n/a	78
Total number of students enrolled in program: 351			

Stony Brook University and
Stony Brook University School of Medicine

Stony Brook, New York

Address Inquiries To:
Undergraduate Admissions, Honors Programs
118 Administration Building
Stony Brook University
Stony Brook, New York 11794-1901
T (631) 632-6868 **F** (631) 632-9898
www.stonybrook.edu/ugadmissions/programs/honors.shtml
Judith.Burke-Berhannan@stonybrook.edu

Purpose

The Scholars for Medicine Program offers conditional acceptance to the Stony Brook University School of Medicine to a select number of outstanding and highly motivated students through one of three programs: The Honors College, WISE (Women in Science and Engineering) and the Engineering Program of Stony Brook University. In addition to acquiring a solid background in the sciences, accepted students have access to a wide array of liberal arts courses through the university. Students also have access to medical school programs in research and a series of health-related seminars.

Requirements for Entrance

Students are selected for this program only during the senior year of high school. There are no state residency requirements. No specific courses are required. Applicants must take the SAT. For non-U.S. citizens, documentation of permanent residency status will be required of accepted students prior to matriculation.

Selection Factors

To be considered for this program, applicants must have a minimum SAT score of 1350 (Critical Reading and Mathematics) and an unweighted high school GPA of 95. The applicant's high school academic record, standardized test reports, essay, history of interests and activities, and required interview at the School of Medicine are factors taken into account in offering admission.

Curriculum

This eight-year program leads to the baccalaureate and M.D. degrees granted by Stony Brook University. Students are expected to complete the requirements for any of the baccalaureate degrees awarded by the university as well as the requirements for either the Honors College, WISE Program or Engineering Program. Undergraduate work taken must include courses required by the School of Medicine, including one year each of biology, physics, inorganic chemistry, organic chemistry (all with lab), and English. No specific major is required for the premedical undergraduate phase. The program provides a seminar series of health-related lectures given by nationally and internationally recognized individuals in health care delivery. In addition, students have an opportunity to engage in cutting-edge research. Admission to the School of Medicine is contingent upon maintaining a minimum specified GPA during the first three undergraduate years. All scholars are required to take the MCAT no later than spring of their junior year in college and must attain a specified minimum MCAT score. USMLE Steps 1 and 2 are required for promotion and graduation from the School of Medicine. USMLE Steps 1 and 2 are required for promotion and graduation from the School of Medicine.

Expenses	Resident Tuition and Fees	Non-resident Tuition and Fees
Undergraduate	$7,542	$15,442
U.S. Medical School	$22,595	$38,198

Financial Aid

Financial aid available to enrolled students includes federal Perkins loans, Equal Opportunity Program, federal work-study, federal Pell Grants, Federal Supplemental Educational Opportunity, NY State Tuition Assistance Program (TAP), and NY State Aid for Part-Time Students. Applicants can receive more information by contacting the Office of Financial Aid and Student Employment at Stony Brook University at (631) 632-6840 or visiting the Web site at *www.stonybrook.edu/ugadmissions/financial/*. Please contact the programs directly concerning scholarship opportunities.

Application and Acceptance Policies

Filing of application:
    Earliest date: November 1, 2009
    Latest date: December 31, 2009
Application fee: n/a   Fee Waiver Available: n/a
Acceptance notice:
    Earliest date: March 1, 2010
    Latest date: April 4, 2010
Applicant's response to acceptance offer:
    Latest date: May 1, 2010
Deposit to hold place in class: $100; refundable
Starting date: September 2010

Information on 2008–2009 Entering Class

Number of	In-State	Out-of-State	Total
Applicants	472	151	623
Applicants Interviewed	19	5	24
New Entrants	5	1	6
Total number of students enrolled in program: 25			

Union College and Albany Medical College

Schenectady, New York

Address Inquiries To:
Associate Dean of Admissions
Union College
Schenectady, New York 12308
T (518) 388-6112 **F** (518) 388-8034
admissions@union.edu
www.medicine.union.edu/LIM

Purpose

The Leadership in Medicine Program is specifically designed for students who want to prepare for the challenge of medical leadership by taking advantage of additional educational opportunities as part of their undergraduate education. In addition to offering the standard coursework required for attaining the degrees of B.S., M.S. or M.B.A., and M.D., the integrated program focuses on three areas essential for future leaders in medicine: the economic and financial problems facing medicine, including health policy and health management; the increasing complexity of biomedical ethics; and the need to maintain a global perspective.

Requirements for Entrance

Students are selected for this program during the senior year of high school. Residents of New York, as well as non-residents of the state, are eligible to apply. Applicants are expected to have completed a challenging curriculum in high school, which must include biology, chemistry, and physics. They must take either the ACT Assessment or the SAT Reasoning Test and two SAT Subject Area Tests (one mathematics and one science). Tests must be completed by the December testing date prior to the proposed September matriculation.

Selection Factors

Academic factors considered in offering admission to an applicant include the quality and nature of coursework in high school, performance in those courses, rank in high school class, and standardized test scores. In the 2008–2009 entering class, the average score was 687 for SAT Critical Reading, 712 for SAT Mathematics, and 709 for SAT Writing. Personal qualities sought in applicants include motivation, maturity, and personal development. Interviews at Union College and Albany Medical College are required.

Curriculum

This program leads to B.S. and M.S. or M.B.A. degrees awarded by Union College and the M.D. degree granted by Albany Medical College. At Union College, students take 30 courses (15 science and 15 non-science) and complete an interdepartmental major in the humanities or social sciences. A special bioethics program supplemented by a health services practicum, a term abroad, and a program in health care management at the Union College Graduate Management Institute are also integral parts of the educational experience. The curriculum for the B.S., M.S., or M.B.A. and M.D. degrees requires eight years to complete. At the medical college, basic and clinical sciences are integrated into themes (primarily organ systems) stressing normal function in Year 1 and pathological processes in Year 2. Five longitudinal themes are inte-

grated throughout the curriculum: clinical skills, ethical and health systems issues, evidence-based medicine, nutrition, and informatics. In every theme, student learning is focused on clinical presentations. Basic science seminars reinforce the importance of the basic sciences in Years 3 and 4. Emphasis is placed on primary care throughout the four years, with an increased emphasis on care in ambulatory settings in Year 3 clinical rotations. Year 4 emphasizes specialty care in various required rotations. Additional electives are available in Year 4. Students admitted to the program are not required to take the MCAT for admission to Albany Medical College. Students are expected to pass Steps 1 and 2 of the USMLE while at Albany Medical College.

Expenses

Expenses	Resident Tuition and Fees	Non-resident Tuition and Fees
Undergraduate	$48,552	$48,552
U.S. Medical School	$44,623	$44,623

Financial Aid

Sources of financial aid include various programs based on need, student loans through federal and state assistance, work-study, and merit scholarships. For more information, contact the Financial Aid Office of Union College at (518) 388-6123 or at Albany Medical College at (518) 262-5435.

Application and Acceptance Policies

Filing of application:
    Earliest date: September 1, 2009
    Latest date: December 1, 2009
Application fee: $50   Fee Waiver Available: Yes
Acceptance notice:
    Earliest date: March 2010
    Latest date: Until class is filled
Applicant's response to acceptance offer:
    Latest date: May 1, 2010
Deposit to hold place in class: $500; nonrefundable
Starting date: September 2010

Information on 2008–2009 Entering Class

Number of	In-State	Out-of-State	Total
Applicants	153	176	329
Applicants Interviewed	26	32	58
New Entrants	6	11	17
Total number of students enrolled in program: 61			

University of Rochester
School of Medicine and Dentistry

Rochester, New York

Address Inquiries To:
Rochester Early Medical Scholars Coordinator
University of Rochester
Undergraduate Admissions, Box 270251
Rochester, New York 14627-0251
T (585) 275-3221 **F** (585) 461-4595
http://enrollment.rochester.edu/admissions/
admit@admissions.rochester.edu

Purpose

The Rochester Early Medical Scholars Program (REMS) provides both acceptance to the University of Rochester College of Arts, Sciences, and Engineering and conditional acceptance to the School of Medicine and Dentistry to a group of exceptionally talented and motivated students. REMS allows undergraduates the utmost flexibility in degree programs, mentoring relationships with medical school staff, and early exposure to the medical school curriculum through a series of lectures and seminars.

Requirements for Entrance

Students are selected for this program during their senior year of high school from a large pool. A recommended high school curriculum includes at least three years of foreign language and social studies, four years each of English, mathematics, and science. A transcript that includes honors, AP and/or IB courses is strongly recommended. Applicants are expected to take the SAT or ACT Assessment. SAT Subject Tests are highly recommended, especially, Mathematics Level 1C or Mathematics Level 2C, and Biology or Chemistry.

Selection Factors

Outstanding achievement in a challenging high school curriculum, character, interests, maturity, experience in health care or research settings, and motivation necessary for a career in medicine are required for consideration for entry into the REMS program. Fifty finalists will be invited to interview for REMS, and those interviews are required. In the 2007–2008 entering class, REMS students had an average SAT Verbal (Critical Reading) score of 720 and an average Mathematics score of 721. In order to take their place in the first-year medical school class, REMS students must carry at least a 3.3 overall GPA and a 3.3 biology-chemistry-physics-math GPA by the end of the freshman year, a 3.4 for the sophomore year, and 3.5 thereafter by the time of undergraduate graduation. In order to matriculate into medical school, all students must have and overall GPA of 3.5 and a biology-chemistry-physics-math overall GPA of 3.5. REMS students do not have to take the MCAT examination.

Curriculum

The eight-year program leads to a baccalaureate degree and the M.D. degree, both granted by the University of Rochester. Students must complete the baccalaureate degree in order to matriculate into medical school. The most popular major is biology, followed by chemistry, and health and society. However, an undergraduate science major is not required to matriculate into medical school. Undergraduates are encouraged to pursue a variety of academic disciplines in addition to completing their premedical course requirements. The University of Rochester School of Medicine and Dentistry's Double-Helix Curriculum (DHC) is a major innovation in medical education, focusing on a fully integrated basic and clinical science curriculum across all four years of medical school. Students begin their clinical clerkships in January of their first year and learn in an environment that fosters critical thinking, problem-solving and active learning in small group Problem-Based Learning sessions, lectures, laboratories and clinical skills workshops. See *www.urmc.rochester.edu/education/md* for details. As home of the "biopsychosocial model," Rochester values the art and science of medicine as a continuum, and fosters an educational model that is humanistic and patient-centered. REMS students also may apply for any of our combined degree programs, including the M.D./Ph.D., M.D./M.P.H., M.D./M.B.A., and M.D./M.S. programs. A "Take 5" program, offering a tuition-free, fifth undergraduate year, is available to selected REMS students. Summer research programs and extensive international experiences are available at both the undergraduate and medical school levels.

Expenses

	Resident Tuition and Fees	Non-resident Tuition and Fees
Undergraduate	$37,250	$37,250
U.S. Medical School	$42,204	$42,204

Financial Aid

University of Rochester scholarships and loans, plus governmental loans, are available. For more information, write the Financial Aid Office, University of Rochester, Box 270261, Rochester, New York 14627-0261, or phone (585) 275-3226 or (800) 881-8234. Web site: *http://enrollment.rochester.edu/financial.*

Application and Acceptance Policies

Filing of application:
    Earliest date: May 15, 2009
    Latest date: December 1, 2009
Application fee: $30   Fee Waiver Available: Yes
Acceptance notice:
    Earliest date: March 1, 2010
    Latest date: April 1, 2010
Applicant's response to acceptance offer:
    Maximum time: May 1, 2010
Deposit to hold place in class: $600; nonrefundable
Starting date: Early September 2010

Information on 2008–2009 Entering Class

Number of	In-State	Out-of-State	Total
Applicants	292	507	799
Applicants Interviewed	14	38	52
New Entrants	3	9	12
Total number of students enrolled in program: 67			

Case Western Reserve University School of Medicine

Cleveland, Ohio

Address Inquiries To:
Christine DeSalvo Miller, Senior Assistant Director
Office of Undergraduate Admission
Wolstein Hall, Case Western Reserve University
10900 Euclid Avenue; Cleveland, Ohio 44106-7055
T (216) 368-4450 **F** (216) 368-5111
admission@case.edu
http://admission.case.edu

Purpose

This program is intended to provide college students with a greater sense of freedom and choice in the pursuit of a premedical baccalaureate degree.

Requirements for Entrance

Students are selected for this program during the senior year of high school. Both residents and non-residents of Ohio are considered for admission. Applicants are expected to have completed the following courses by the time they graduate from high school: one year each of biology, chemistry, and physics and four years of mathematics. They must take either the ACT Assessment with the Writing Test or the SAT Reasoning Test.

Selection Factors

The applicant's high school academic record, standardized test reports, history of interests and activities, and a required interview are factors taken into account in offering admission. Evidence of strong interpersonal and leadership skills is also sought. While there is no minimum requirement for standardized test scores, in the Fall 2008 entering class, SAT scores ranged from approximately 650–800 on the Critical Reading section and 670–800 on the Math section and 640–800 on the Writing section. The average composite ACT score ranged from 33–35.

Curriculum

This eight-year program leads to the baccalaureate and M.D. degrees granted by Case Western Reserve University. Students are expected to complete the requirements for any of the baccalaureate degrees awarded by the colleges of the university. They are expected to satisfy all requirements of, and earn a baccalaureate prior to matriculating in, the School of Medicine. The work taken for the baccalaureate must include the studies specifically required of applicants by the School of Medicine, including one year of biology, two years of chemistry (including organic chemistry), one year of physics, and first-year (freshman) seminar. No specific major concentration is required for the premedical undergraduate phase. To date, the majors most commonly taken have been biology and biochemistry. Psychology, anthropology, chemistry, and biomedical engineering are also popular majors. The first four years of the program are devoted to study for the baccalaureate and the last four years to the curriculum in medicine. Students in the medical phase are required to pass Step 1 of the USMLE for promotion within the program and to pass Step 2 of the USMLE in order to graduate.

Expenses

Expenses	Resident Tuition and Fees	Non-resident Tuition and Fees
Undergraduate	$34,450	$34,450
U.S. Medical School	$43,966	$43,966

Financial Aid

Sources of aid for the undergraduate phase include merit and need-based aid, college work-study, and university grants and scholarships. For information about aid, contact the Office of University Financial Aid at (216) 368-4530.

Additional Information

The PPSP is intended to include a four-year undergraduate program of study and is not designed as an accelerated program. Matriculation at the School of Medicine will occur no earlier than four years after matriculation into the bachelor's degree program at Case Western Reserve University. Students who complete degree requirements in fewer than four years are required to pursue other significant experiences intended to enhance their professional and/or personal development during the terms following the receipt of their bachelor's degree and until study at the School of Medicine begins. Examples of this experience may include, but are not limited to: research, study abroad, community service and/or additional undergraduate or graduate coursework. This interim experience must be approved in advance by the Case Western Reserve University School of Medicine Admissions Committee.

Application and Acceptance Policies

Filing of application:
   Earliest date: n/a
   Latest date: December 1, 2009
Application fee: $35   Fee Waiver Available: Yes
Acceptance notice:
   Earliest date: n/a
   Latest date: Mid-April 2010
Applicant's response to acceptance offer:
   Maximum date: May 1, 2010
Deposit to hold place in class: $500; nonrefundable
Starting date: August 23, 2010

Information on 2008–2009 Entering Class

Number of	In-State	Out-of-State	Total
Applicants	234	533	767
Applicants Interviewed	10	35	45
New Entrants	1	9	10
Total number of students enrolled in program: 40–50			

Northeastern Ohio Universities College of Medicine

Rootstown, Ohio

Address Inquiries To:
Michelle Cassetty Collins, M.S.Ed., Director, Admissions and Student Services
Northeastern Ohio Universities College of Medicine
4209 State Route 44, P.O. Box 95
Rootstown, Ohio 44272-0095
T (330) 325-6270 **F** (330) 325-8372
admission@neoucom.edu
www.neoucom.edu/audience/applicants

Purpose

The mission of the Northeastern Ohio Universities College of Medicine (NEOUCOM) is to graduate qualified physicians oriented to the practice of medicine at the community level, with an emphasis on primary care (family medicine, internal medicine, pediatrics, and obstetrics-gynecology). NEOUCOM strives to improve the quality of health care in northeast Ohio. All graduates, regardless of specialty, are provided with a strong background in community and public health.

Requirements for Entrance

Students are selected for the B.S./M.D. program during their senior year of high school. During high school, applicants are expected to pursue a solid college preparatory curriculum, including 4 years of math and science, take either the ACT or the SAT, and be citizens or permanent residents of the U.S. Strong preference given to in-state applicants.

Selection Factors

Factors considered in admission include standardized test scores, high school overall and science/math GPAs, extracurricular involvement, medical exposure, coursework, and interview outcome. In 2008–2009, the mean high school GPA of matriculants was 3.85; average ACT test score was 30; average SAT was 1320 (verbal and math only). An interview is required and is offered by invitation only.

Curriculum

Students accepted into the combined B.S./M.D. program pursue the baccalaureate degree at The University of Akron, Kent State University, or Youngstown State University. The accelerated B.S./M.D. program may be completed in six or seven years. The M.D. degree is granted by NEOUCOM. The integrated curriculum is offered in five steps during the four years of medical study. The four-year Doctoring course includes the biomedical, behavioral, social, population health, clinical sciences, and humanities. Step 1: Instruction begins wtih a course to address issues of professionalism, doctor-patient relationships, clinical skills, and population health. Other curriculum emphasizes human anatomy, biochemistry, molecular pathology, and genetics. Step 2: Curriculum emphasizes physiological concepts in the practice of internal medicine, anatomy, physiology, and chemistry of the nervous system with basic clinical concepts and pathologies. Step 3: Curriculum is centered on systems and application in clinical settings. Step 4: Core clerkships in family medicine, internal medicine, obstetrics/gynecology, pediatrics, psychiatry, and surgery, and a four-week exploratory experience. Step 5: Curriculum includes electives and courses focusing on professionalism, humanities, and social science disciplines, along with vital skills needed as residents and interns.

Students must pass USMLE Step 1 for promotion to the third year and USMLE Step 2 Clinical Knowledge (CK) to graduate. USMLE Step 2 Clinical Skills (CS) must be taken to graduate.

Expenses

	Resident Tuition and Fees	Non-resident Tuition and Fees
Undergraduate	Varies	Varies
U.S. Medical School	$29,847	$57,708

Financial Aid

Campus-based financial aid (grants and low interest loans) is awarded on the basis of need. Students apply for aid by completing the FAFSA, the NEOUCOM financial aid application, and submitting copies of federal tax returns. A limited number of need-based grants are available, as well as other limited scholarship funds for disadvantaged students and students from groups underrepresented in medicine. Federal educational loans are a major part of the aid program. About 80 percent of enrolled students receive some form of financial aid. Financial need is not a factor in admission considerations.

Additional Information

In Fall of 2007, the first class of PharmD students enrolled for study in an interdisciplinary curriculum with the NEOUCOM medical students.

Application and Acceptance Policies

Filing of application:
    Earliest date: August 1, 2009
    Latest date: December 15, 2009
Application fee: $175*   Fee Waiver Available: Yes
Acceptance notice:
    Earliest date: December 19, 2009
    Latest date: March 20, 2010
Applicant's response to acceptance offer:
May 1, 2010
Deposit to hold place in class: None
Starting date: June 2010

Information on 2008–2009 Entering Class

Number of	In-State	Out-of-State	Total
Applicants	395	224	619
Applicants Interviewed	209	20	229
New Entrants	110	5	115
Total number of students enrolled in program: 239			

*The one fee is for application to NEOUCOM, The University of Akron, Kent State University and Youngstown State University.

Ohio State University College of Medicine
Early Admission Pathway

Columbus, Ohio

Address Inquiries To:
Lorna Kenyon, Director, Admissions Office
College of Medicine, The Ohio State University
155D Meiling Hall, 370 West 9th Avenue
Columbus, Ohio 43210
T (614) 292-7137 **F** (614) 247-7959
medicine@osu.edu
www.medicine.osu.edu/futurestudents/admissions/

Purpose

The Early Admission Pathway provides conditional acceptance into the College of Medicine after four years of undergraduate study for a select group of National Merit Finalists, National Achievement Finalists, and National Hispanic Finalists, entering The Ohio State University in Autumn Quarter.

Requirements for Entrance

Students are selected in their senior year of high school. Both residents and non-residents of Ohio are eligible to apply to the program. In addition to meeting the requirements for freshman admission, applicants are required to submit the results of the ACT Assessment or the SAT I.

Selection Factors

The following factors are taken into consideration in assessing applicants for admission: approval for University Honors affiliation; selection as a National Merit, National Achievement, or National Hispanic finalist; grade-point average; high school activities; leadership roles; and extracurricular activities. In the 2008 entering class, the average high school GPA was 4.47. The average SAT score was 1615 and the average ACT Assessment score was 33.9.

Curriculum

This eight-year program leads to a baccalaureate degree awarded by The Ohio State University and to the M.D. degree granted by The Ohio State University College of Medicine. The most frequent major for the baccalaureate degree is biology. Regardless of major, students must complete the prerequisites including one year of: biological sciences, general chemistry, organic chemistry with lab, physics with lab. Eligible EAP participants have the option to petition for entry into the College of Medicine after three years of undergraduate coursework and will be able to earn a Bachelor of Science degree in absentia after successful completion of the first year of medical school. Students with a cumulative grade point average of 3.50 or above in all coursework and in all courses in biological sciences, chemistry, physical sciences, and mathematics (BCPM) are not required to take the MCAT. The MCAT is required for students who have not met the above requirements by the end of Spring Quarter of the third year. They must: complete the baccalaureate degree prior to entry into medical school; register for and take the MCAT by October 1 of the fourth year and present a composite MCAT score of at least 32, with no subscore less than 9 in order to continue in good standing; work with the EAP academic advisor to determine appropriate course work for the remainder of their undergraduate program; and regain undergraduate college Honors affiliation by the end of Spring Quarter of the third year and maintain it through the completion of their undergraduate degree program. Students who lose and do not regain college Honors affiliation are no longer eligible for conditional acceptance into the College of Medicine. Students are held to the College of Medicine's standards of honor and professional conduct.

Expenses	Resident Tuition and Fees	Non-resident Tuition and Fees
Undergraduate	$8,679	$21,918
U.S. Medical School	$28,563	$43,701

Financial Aid

The sources of financial aid available are National Merit/Achievement/Hispanic Distinguished Scholarships valued at the current undergraduate resident tuition rate, plus other merit and need-based aid. For more information, contact the Office of Student Financial Aid, The Ohio State University, 517 Lincoln Tower, 1800 Cannon Drive, Columbus, Ohio 43210; (614) 292-0300.

Additional Information

EAP students have unique opportunities to meet and talk with distinguished College of Medicine faculty and students engaged in clinical and graduate education and research. Faculty and staff meet with EAP students to discuss opportunities for practical experience and the development of desired non-cognitive traits. Mentoring and medical career counseling are also provided. EAP students are expected to take full advantage of the opportunities to gain clinical exposure, participate in research activities, become involved in community and volunteer service, leadership and extracurricular activities. They are also encouraged to participate in enrichment activities sponsored by Alpha Epsilon Delta (AED), the premedical honor society at The Ohio State University.

Application and Acceptance Policies

Filing of application:
  Earliest date: October 1, 2009
  Latest date: March 1, 2010
Application fee: $40   Fee Waiver Available: No
Acceptance notice:
  Earliest date: April 15, 2010
  Latest date: May 1, 2010
Applicant's response to acceptance offer:
  Latest date: May 1, 2010
Deposit to hold place in class: None
Starting date: September 2010

Information on 2008–2009 Entering Class

Number of	In-State	Out-of-State	Total
Applicants	51	29	80
Applicants Interviewed	32	6	38
New Entrants	11	2	13
Total number of students enrolled in program: 59			

University of Cincinnati College of Medicine

Cincinnati, Ohio

Address Inquiries To:
Nikki Bibler, M.Ed., Assistant Director of Dual Admissions
University of Cincinnati College of Medicine
P.O. Box 670668
Cincinnati, Ohio 45267-0668
T (513) 558-5581 **F** (513) 558-6259
DualAdmissionsProgram@uc.edu
www.med.uc.edu/HS2MD

Purpose

The University of Cincinnati College of Medicine's Dual Admissions Program accepts high school seniors into one of three undergraduate Ohio colleges and into the College of Medicine. The College of Medicine has established a partnership with the following Ohio institutions: the University of Dayton, Miami University, and the University of Cincinnati undergraduate campus. Each undergraduate program will invite selected students already accepted into the university to apply for this program. Once accepted to this special program, students will receive an outstanding education while preparing for medical school and developing the qualities and characteristics to become excellent physicians.

Requirements for Entrance

Students are selected in their senior year of high school. Both residents and non-residents of Ohio are eligible to apply. Priority will be given to Ohio residents. Each university determines its own academic requirements, but the ACT and/or SAT are required.

Selection Factors

In making admissions decisions, the College of Medicine in conjunction with each undergraduate institution considers an applicant's academic record, standardized test performance, examples of leadership, interpersonal skills, and interest in and motivation for medicine. Mature and independent-thinking students who have good decision-making and coping skills are very desirable. Students are strongly encouraged to investigate each of the College of Medicine's undergraduate partners before applying. Only students who have applied to and been accepted by one of the affiliated undergraduate schools will be seriously considered for the Dual Admissions Program. Thus, students are encouraged to apply first to the undergraduate institution and then complete the Dual Admissions Application.

Curriculum

The course of study consists of four years at the undergraduate school, followed by four years in the College of Medicine. University of Cincinnati College of Medicine dual-admissions students are required to satisfactorily fulfill graduation requirements at their undergraduate institution. Students are strongly urged to complete a baccalaureate degree. Students must earn a 3.4 cumulative GPA and a 3.45 BCPM GPA by the beginning of the senior undergraduate year. At this time, they must also earn a composite score of 27 on the MCAT, with no less than a 9 in Biological Sciences and no less than an 8 in Verbal Reasoning or Physical Sciences. The student must pass Steps 1 and 2 of the USMLE in order to graduate from the College of Medicine. The USMLE Step 1 is administered at the completion of Year 2.

Expenses

	Resident Tuition and Fees	Non-resident Tuition and Fees
Undergraduate	Varies	Varies
U.S. Medical School	$26,910	$46,077

Financial Aid

More information about undergraduate financial aid can be obtained from the undergraduate partners' Office of Admissions.

Application and Acceptance Policies

Filing of application:
 Earliest date: October 1, 2009
 Latest date: January 7, 2010
Application fee: $25 Fee Waiver Available: Yes
Acceptance notice:
 Earliest date: April 1, 2010
 Latest date: Varies for students on the alternate list.
Applicant's response to acceptance offer:
 Maximum time: May 1, 2010
Deposit to hold place in class: None
Starting date: Varies by undergraduate program

Information on 2008–2009 Entering Class

Number of	In-State	Out-of-State	Total
Applicants	102	70	172
Applicants Interviewed	33	15	48
New Entrants	19	3	22

Total number of students enrolled in program: 131

Drexel University and
Drexel University College of Medicine

Philadelphia, Pennsylvania

Address Inquiries To:
Catherine Campbell-Perna, Associate Director
Drexel University
3141 Chestnut Street
Philadelphia, Pennsylvania 19104
T (215) 895-2400 **F** (215) 895-5939
enroll@drexel.edu
www.drexel.edu/em/undergrad/academic-programs/accelerated-degrees/

Purpose

This combined-degree program provides outstanding high school seniors, who are highly motivated toward the medical profession, an opportunity to combine a strong liberal arts undergraduate program in a highly technological environment with a medical education in seven years.

Requirements for Entrance

Students are selected for this program during their senior year of high school. Both residents and non-residents of Pennsylvania are eligible to apply. Students must be U.S. citizens or permanent residents and graduate from a U.S. high school. Prior to graduating from high school, applicants are required to complete one semester of biology, one semester of chemistry, one semester of physics, four years of English, and four years of mathematics. They must take either the SAT or the ACT Assessment.

Selection Factors

The academic factors taken into consideration for admission into the combined-degree program include SAT/ACT scores, high school GPA, and AP and honors courses. The average high school GPA for the 2008–2009 entering class was 3.9, with a mean score of 1470 on the SAT and a 33 Composite on the ACT. Medically related volunteer activities, leadership qualities, and community service are among the personal attributes sought in applicants. An interview at the college of medicine is also required. Once admitted into the program, students are expected to maintain an overall GPA of 3.5 in undergraduate studies; achieve a total minimum MCAT score of 30, or a score of 9 or better on each section of the MCAT; apply through AMCAS in the second year; complete all prerequisite courses; and receive no grade less than a C in any course. Receive in a single examination a minimum MCAT score of "9" or better in the verbal section and "10s" or better in the physical or biological science section, or a total minimum score of 31 (with no individual subsection score less than an 8) and a letter score of "P" or higher in the MCAT written section. Apply through AMCAS in the second year. The MCAT is a factor in admittance and promotion to the medical school phase of the program.

Curriculum

This seven-year program leads to a baccalaureate degree awarded by Drexel University and to the M.D. degree granted by the Drexel University College of Medicine. The most frequent major is biology, followed by chemistry. Students may also choose from a variety of humanities majors. During the first three years of the undergraduate phase, students spend 100 percent of their time in coursework related to the bachelor's degree, which includes 3 semester hours of natural and physical science.

Expenses

Expenses	Resident Tuition and Fees	Non-resident Tuition and Fees
Undergraduate	$37,420	$37,420
U.S. Medical School	$43,800	$43,800

Financial Aid

All Students are automatically considered for academic scholarships when applying for admission. Students should complete the FAFSA form by March 1st to be considered for need based financial aid.

Application and Acceptance Policies

Filing of application:
 Earliest date: Rolling
 Latest date: November 15, 2009
Application fee: $75   Fee Waiver Available: Yes
Acceptance notice:
 Earliest date: March 31, 2010
 Latest date: April 15, 2010
Applicant's response to acceptance offer:
 Latest date: May 1, 2010
Deposit to hold place in class: $300; nonrefundable
Starting date: September 20, 2010

Information on 2008–2009 Entering Class

Number of	In-State	Out-of-State	Total
Applicants	228	757	985
Applicants Interviewed	23	95	118
New Entrants	7	12	19
Total number of students enrolled in program: 87			

Lehigh University and
Drexel University College of Medicine

Bethlehem, Pennsylvania

Address Inquiries To:
Majed Dergham, Assistant Director
Office of Admissions
Lehigh University
27 Memorial Drive West
Bethlehem, Pennsylvania 18015
T (610) 758-3100 **F** (610) 758-4361
http://cas.lehigh.edu/CASWeb/Content/default.aspx?pageid=129

Purpose

This program is designed to give gifted high school students, who are highly motivated for a career in medicine, the opportunity to combine a liberal arts program with a medical education. The baccalaureate degree is awarded after Year 4 (the first year of medical school).

Requirements for Entrance

Applicants are expected to take the SAT Reasoning Test. SAT Subject tests are highly recommended in Mathematics Level 1 or Mathematics Level 2 and Chemistry. Applicants must be U.S. citizens or permanent residents.

Selection Factors

Generally, a combined SAT score of 1360 (or minimum 31 ACT), a class rank in the top 5 percent of the high school class, and a strong motivation for science are necessary for entrance into this program. Most recent matriculants had a high school GPA of 3.7, an SAT Verbal score of 720, and an SAT Mathematics score of 780. Maturity, stability, scholarship, flexibility, independence, and service to others are personal characteristics sought among applicants. An interview is required. Once admitted to the program, students are expected to maintain an overall grade point average of 3.5 or better and a science and math GPA of 3.5 or better with no grade less than a "C" in any courses. All program requirements must be completed at Lehigh University. Candidates are required to take the MCAT. Scores of either 9 or better on the verbal section of the MCAT and 10 or better on the science sections or a total minimum score of 31 (with no individual section score less than 8) are required.

Curriculum

This program, seven years in duration, allows students to obtain a bachelor's degree from Lehigh University and the M.D. degree from Drexel University College of Medicine. The Lehigh bachelor's degree is awarded after completion of the first year of study at Drexel. Students have the flexibility to pursue additional coursework or study abroad during the undergraduate portion of the program. However, specific course requirements for the degree include two semesters of English, three semesters of mathematics, eight semesters of natural and physical sciences, three semesters each of humanities and social sciences, a first year seminar, a writing intensive, and four elective courses. All students must pass USMLE Steps 1 and 2 in order to graduate from the medical school.

Expenses

	Resident Tuition and Fees	Non-resident Tuition and Fees
Undergraduate	$47,320	$47,320
U.S. Medical School	$43,800	$43,800

Financial Aid

Institutional scholarships and loans are available, as well as federal loan programs and armed services scholarships. More financial aid information can be obtained from the Financial Aid Office, Lehigh University, 218 W. Packer Avenue, Bethlehem, Pennsylvania 18015.

Application and Acceptance Policies

Filing of application:
  Earliest date: September 1, 2009
  Latest date: November 15, 2009
Application fee: $70   Fee Waiver Available: No
Acceptance notice:
  Earliest date: April 1, 2010
  Latest date: n/a
Applicant's response to acceptance offer:
  Latest date: May 1, 2010
Deposit to hold place in class: $500; nonrefundable
Starting date: August 2010

Information on 2008–2009 Entering Class

Number of	In-State	Out-of-State	Total
Applicants	35	188	223
Applicants Interviewed	10	50	60
New Entrants	1	2	3
Total number of students enrolled in program: 24			

Pennsylvania State University and Jefferson Medical College

University Park, Pennsylvania

Address Inquiries To:
Director of Admissions
Undergraduate Admissions Office
Pennsylvania State University, 201 Shields Building
University Park, Pennsylvania 16802
T (814) 865-5471 **F** (814) 863-7590
www.science.psu.edu/premedmed

Purpose

This accelerated, B.S.–M.D. premedical-medical program, which began in 1963 and has graduated over 900 students, is a cooperative effort between Pennsylvania State University, University Park, and Jefferson Medical College of Thomas Jefferson University in Philadelphia. Accepted students can select either a six- or seven-year schedule, which gives them either two years (with summers) or three years at Penn State before proceeding to four years at Jefferson Medical College. All students selecting the six-year option must begin their studies at the University Park campus in the summer session. Students selecting the seven-year option begin their studies at the University Park campus in the fall semester.

Requirements for Entrance

Students are selected for this program only during the senior year of high school. Both residents and non-residents of Pennsylvania are considered for admission, but preference is given to qualified applicants from Pennsylvania. Applicants are expected to have completed the following courses by the time they graduate from high school: four units of English, 1 1/2 units of algebra, one unit of plane geometry, one-half unit of trigonometry, three units of science, and five units of social studies, humanities, and/or the arts.

Selection Factors

To be considered for this program, applicants must be in the top ten percent of their high school class and offer a minimum combined score of 2100 on the critical reading and mathematics section of the SAT I or ACT score of 32. In the 2008–2009 entering class, the average combined score on the SAT (previous version) was 1545. Motivation, compassion, integrity, dedication, and performance in nonacademic areas are among the personal characteristics sought in applicants. An interview is required. Special attention is given to the student's progress during each semester while at Pennsylvania State University. Students must take a full course load and maintain a minimum GPA of 3.5 in both science and non-science courses. For subsequent admission to Jefferson Medical College, students in this combined-degree program must achieve an average score of 9 (average) or better on each section of the MCAT prior to matriculation in medical school.

Curriculum

This six-year program leads to a baccalaureate degree granted by Pennsylvania State University and to the M.D. degree awarded by Jefferson Medical College. Students begin this program in June immediately after high school graduation. They spend two full years on the Pennsylvania State, University Park, campus; they then proceed to Jefferson Medical College for the regular four-year curriculum. The B.S. degree from Pennsylvania State University is awarded after successful completion of the second year at Jefferson Medical College, and the M.D. degree is awarded after successful completion of the senior year at Jefferson Medical College. Students in the seven-year schedule spend three years at Pennsylvania State, but do not attend summer sessions. Their B.S. degree is awarded after Year 1 at Jefferson Medical College.

Expenses

	Resident Tuition and Fees	Non-resident Tuition and Fees
Undergraduate	$13,014	$24,248
U.S. Medical School	$43,033	$43,033

Financial Aid

At Penn State, scholarships, loans, and grants are the sources of financial assistance available. For more information, write the Office of Student Financial Aid, Pennsylvania State University, University Park, Pennsylvania 16802; or call (814) 865-5471. At Jefferson Medical College, financial aid application materials are mailed in January of the year of medical school matriculation. Students are encouraged to contact the University Office of Student Financial Aid to discuss all financial aid matters.

Application and Acceptance Policies

Filing of application:
    Earliest date: August 1, 2009
    Latest date: November 30, 2009
Application fee: $50   Fee Waiver Available: Yes
Acceptance notice:
    Earliest date: March 15, 2010
    Latest date: March 30, 2010
Applicant's response to acceptance offer:
    Latest date: May 1, 2010
Deposit to hold place in class: $300; nonrefundable
Starting date: Late June 2010

Information on 2008–2009 Entering Class

Number of	In-State	Out-of-State	Total
Applicants	110	308	418
Applicants Interviewed	28	66	94
New Entrants	7	23	30
Total number of students enrolled in program: 60			

Temple University School of Medicine

Philadelphia, Pennsylvania

Address Inquiries To:
Office of Admissions
Temple University School of Medicine
3500 North Broad Street, Suite 124
Philadelphia, Pennsylvania 19140
T (215) 707-3656 **F** (215) 707-6932
medadmissions@temple.edu
www.temple.edu/medicine/admissions/special_admissions.htm

Purpose

The Medical Scholars Program, in conjunction with three undergraduate institutions in Pennsylvania, provides an opportunity for outstanding high school seniors to gain a provisional acceptance to Temple University School of Medicine at the same time that they are accepted into their undergraduate school.

Requirements for Entrance

Students are selected for this program during their senior year of high school. Both residents and non-residents of Pennsylvania are eligible to apply. Although there are no specific high school course requirements, applicants are expected to have a substantial background in science and mathematics. AP coursework is viewed favorably, and students are required to take the SAT or ACT.

Selection Factors

In conjunction with the School of Medicine, each undergraduate institution considers an applicant's GPA, standardized test performance, extracurricular activities (including leadership roles), and interpersonal skills in making admission decisions. Substantial maturity and strong motivation are among the important personal qualities considered by the Admission Committee. The minimum SAT score required is 1350 in the combined Critical Reading and Mathematics sections, with no individual section less than 600 (including the new Writing section). The minimum composite ACT score required is 31. Students are expected to be in the top one to five percent of their high school graduating class. Academic ability should be demonstrated across a wide variety of courses, including AP science coursework. Selected applicants are required to interview with a representative of the undergraduate institution and a medical school admissions officer. Contact the partnering undergraduate institutions directly to obtain additional information about the Medical Scholars Program: Duquesne University, (412) 396-6335; Washington and Jefferson College, tklitz@washjeff.edu; and Widener University, (610) 499-4030.

Curriculum

Students in this combined-degree program will complete their baccalaureate degree at one of the three partnering universities listed above. The medical degree is granted by Temple University School of Medicine. Students may choose to be a science major, but are free to explore all available options as long as they complete the premedical science requirements. Matriculation to Temple University School of Medicine is conditional upon successful completion of all GPA and MCAT requirements as outlined by each institution's agreement. Educational innovations are unique at each undergraduate institution. All students are required to complete the M.D. program without deviation from the standard curriculum, including passing USMLE Steps 1, 2CS (Clinical Skills), and 2CK (Clinical Knowledge).

Expenses

Expenses	Resident Tuition and Fees	Non-resident Tuition and Fees
Undergraduate	Varies	Varies
U.S. Medical School	$40,774	$49,778

Financial Aid

For information about financial aid, contact the Financial Aid Office of the specific partnering undergraduate institution listed above. Financial aid available to medical students includes grants, scholarships, and student loans. For additional information, visit the School of Medicine Web site at: *www.temple.edu/sfs/med/*.

Application and Acceptance Policies

Filing of application:
  Earliest date: Varies by program
  Latest date: n/a
Application fee: $0   Fee Waiver Available: n/a
Acceptance notice:
  Earliest date: March 15, 2010
  Latest date: April 15, 2010
Applicant's response to acceptance offer:
  Latest date: May 1, 2010
Deposit to hold place in class: None
Starting date: Varies by undergraduate program

Information on 2008–2009 Entering Class

Number of	In-State	Out-of-State	Total
Applicants	n/a	n/a	115
Applicants Interviewed	n/a	n/a	37
New Entrants	n/a	n/a	14
Total number of students enrolled in program: 30			

Villanova University and
Drexel University College of Medicine
Villanova, Pennsylvania

Address Inquiries To:
John D. Friede, Ph.D., Health Professions Advisor
Office of University Admission
Villanova University
800 Lancaster Avenue, Villanova, Pennsylvania 19085
T (610) 519-4833 **F** (610) 519-8042
admission@villanova.edu
www.healthprofessions.villanova.edu/

Purpose
This combined-degree program provides outstanding high school seniors, who are highly motivated toward the medical profession, an opportunity to combine a strong liberal arts undergraduate program with a medical education in seven years.

Requirements for Entrance
Students are selected for this program in their senior year of high school. Both residents and non-residents of Pennsylvania are eligible to apply to the program; applicants must be U.S. citizens or permanent residents. Applicants are required to complete the following courses prior to graduation from high school: one year of biology, one year of chemistry, one year of physics, four years of English, and four years of mathematics. In addition to meeting these academic requirements, applicants are also required to submit the results of the ACT or SAT. An ACT score of at least 31 or an SAT score of 1360 (Critical Reading and Mathematics) is required. SAT II scores are recommended.

Selection Factors
The academic factors taken into consideration for admission into the combined-degree program include: SAT scores, high school GPA and class rank, and letters of recommendation. The average high school GPA for the 2007–2008 entering class was 3.80, unweighted. Extracurricular activities and community service are among the personal attributes sought in applicants; exposure to medicine is expected. An interview is required. Once admitted into the program, students are expected to maintain an overall GPA of 3.50 and a science GPA of 3.50, and they are required to achieve scores of either a 9 on the Verbal Reasoning and a 10 on the Physical Sciences and Biological Sciences sections or a combined score of 31 or better (with no score less than 8 on any section of the MCAT). A "P" or greater on the Writing Sample is required.

Curriculum
Students are required to complete a baccalaureate degree within the first year of medical school. The most frequent major is biology, followed by comprehensive science. This seven-year program leads to a baccalaureate degree awarded by Villanova University and to the M.D. degree granted by the Drexel University College of Medicine. During the undergraduate phase of the program, students will spend 100 percent of their time in coursework related to the bachelor's degree, which includes 41 semester hours of natural and physical science, six semester hours of mathematics, and 51 semester hours of humanities.

Expenses

Expenses	Resident Tuition and Fees	Non-resident Tuition and Fees
Undergraduate	$37,530	$37,530
U.S. Medical School	$43,800	$43,800

Financial Aid
For information on financial aid, visit *www.finaid.villanova.edu* and *http://webcampus.drexelmed.edu/admissions/financialaid.asp*.

Application and Acceptance Policies
Filing of application:
    Earliest date: September 1, 2009
    Latest date: November 1, 2009
Application fee: $75   Fee Waiver Available: Yes
Acceptance notice:
    Earliest date: March 15, 2010
    Latest date: March 30, 2010
Applicant's response to acceptance offer:
    Maximum time: May 1, 2010
Deposit to hold place in class: $700; nonrefundable
Starting date: August 23, 2010

Information on 2008–2009 Entering Class

Number of	In-State	Out-of-State	Total
Applicants	36	144	180
Applicants Interviewed	10	36	46
New Entrants	0	3	3
Total number of students enrolled in program: 21			

Wilkes University/SUNY-Upstate Medical University

Wilkes-Barre, Pennsylvania

Address Inquiries To:
Eileen Sharp
Coordinator for Health Science Professional Programs
Wilkes University, 84 West South Street
Wilkes-Barre, Pennsylvania 18766
T (570) 408-7812 **F** (570) 408-7812
sharp@wilkes.edu
www.wilkes.edu/pages/102.asp

Purpose

This cooperative program is motivated by the need for physicians interested in serving in rural and semi-rural health care delivery systems, as well as the interest of each institution in attracting students of superior ability and accomplishment.

Requirements for Entrance

Students apply to the program in their senior year of high school; applicants must be New York State residents. Candidates for admission must have completed the following high school course requirements: four years each of mathematics, English, science, and social science. Applicants must take the ACT or SAT examination.

Selection Factors

The following factors are taken into consideration in assessing the applicant for admission: grades, rank in class, SAT (ACT) scores, and extracurricular activities. Selected applicants are invited for a required interview.

Curriculum

This eight-year program leads to a baccalaureate degree awarded by Wilkes University and to the M.D. degree granted by SUNY Upstate Medical University. The most frequent major for the baccalaureate degree is biology, followed by chemistry and biochemistry. The M.D. portion of the curriculum does not depart from the "traditional" design. Upstate accepts a special responsibility to provide physicians to New York's underserved rural communities. A student from a rural setting or one subsequently trained there is more likely to practice there. This B.S.–M.D. program attracts students from rural areas who are not likely to otherwise find their way to medical school. Upstate also provides many special opportunities during medical school (Rural Medicine Program, Clinical Campus) to train students in community and rural settings. Students in this program are not required to take the MCAT for promotion or admission to the medical school. The USMLE Step 1 is required; it must be passed, prior to beginning clinical rotations, to be promoted and in order to graduate. Students must record a score on USMLE Step 2, but passing USMLE Step 2 is not a factor in graduation from the medical school.

Financial Aid

The sources of available financial aid are grants, scholarships, and student loans. For more information about financial aid, visit www.wilkes.edu/pages/567.asp, or contact the Financial Aid Office at SUNY Upstate Medical University by emailing FinAid@upstate.edu.

Expenses	Resident Tuition and Fees	Non-resident Tuition and Fees
Undergraduate	$25,170	$25,170
U.S. Medical School	$19,956	$34,656

Application and Acceptance Policies

Filing of application:
  Earliest date: August 1, 2009
  Latest date: November 10, 2009
Application fee: $45   Fee Waiver Available: Yes
Acceptance notice:
  Earliest date: Within two weeks of medical school interview
  Latest date: Two weeks after medical school interview
Applicant's response to acceptance offer:
  Maximum time: Two weeks from receiving acceptance offer
Deposit to hold place in class: $100; refundable
Starting date: The Fall following graduation from Wilkes

Information on 2008–2009 Entering Class

Number of	In-State	Out-of-State	Total
Applicants	6	n/a	6
Applicants Interviewed	6	n/a	6
New Entrants	1	n/a	1
Total number of students enrolled in program: 8			

The Warren Alpert Medical School of Brown University

Providence, Rhode Island

Address Inquiries To:
College Admission Office
Brown University, Box 1876
Providence, Rhode Island 02912
T (401) 863-2378
Admissions@Brown.edu
http://med.brown.edu/plme

Purpose

The Program in Liberal Medical Education (PLME) seeks to graduate physicians who are broadly and liberally educated, and who will view medicine as a socially responsible human service profession. Designed as an eight-year program, the PLME combines liberal arts and professional education. Great flexibility is built into the program. Working with PLME advising deans who are physicians, each student develops an individualized educational plan consistent with his or her particular interests. The PLME is a primary route of admission to The Warren Alpert Medical School.

Requirements for Entrance

Students are selected for the PLME in the senior year of high school. The Brown Admission Office recommends that applicants should have completed the following courses: four years of English, with significant emphasis on writing; three years of college preparatory mathematics; three years of a foreign language; two years of laboratory science above the freshman level; two years of history, including American history; at least one year of coursework in the arts; and at least one year of elective academic subjects. Prospective science or engineering majors should have taken physics, chemistry, and advanced mathematics. Familiarity with computers is recommended for all applicants. Applicants must take the SAT Reasoning Test and any two SAT Subject Tests (except for the SAT II Writing Test), or the ACT. (PLME applicants are encouraged to include a science SAT Subject Test).

Selection Factors

Students are selected on the basis of scholastic accomplishment and promise, intellectual curiosity, emotional maturity, character, motivation, sensitivity, caring, and particularly the degree to which they seem adapted to the special features of the program. In the 2008–2009 entering class, students, on average, were in the top two percent of their high school class and had achieved, on average, a score of 725 Verbal, 738 Mathematics, and 723 Writing on the SAT Reasoning Test. An interview is not required.

Curriculum

The PLME leads to a baccalaureate degree and to the M.D. degree granted by The Warren Alpert Medical School. Students must complete a baccalaureate degree in the field of their choice. Each student's educational plan is highly individualized. The PLME combines the flexibility and opportunities of an undergraduate education at Brown University with effective preparation for participation in an equally innovative medical education program.

Expenses

Expenses	Resident Tuition and Fees	Non-resident Tuition and Fees
Undergraduate	$43,144	$37,514
U.S. Medical School	$40,510	$40,510

Financial Aid

For undergraduates in the first four years of the PLME, financial aid is awarded by the Financial Aid Office at Brown University as a package. Students are awarded monies via scholarships, work-study, and loans. During the last four years of the PLME, financial aid is administered by the The Warren Alpert Medical School Office of Admissions and Financial Aid. Both loans and scholarships are available, although loans are the most common form of assistance.

Application and Acceptance Policies

Filing of application:
  Earliest date: November 1, 2009
  Latest date: January 1, 2010
Application fee: $70   Fee Waiver Available: No
Acceptance notice:
  Earliest date: December 15, 2009
  Latest date: Early April 2010
Applicant's response to acceptance offer:
  Latest date: May 1, 2010
Deposit to hold place in class: None
Starting date: September 2010

Information on 2008–2009 Entering Class

Number of	In-State	Out-of-State	Total
Applicants	50	2053	2103
Applicants Interviewed	n/a	n/a	n/a
New Entrants	5	46	51
Total number of students enrolled in program: 199			

Fisk University and Meharry Medical College

Nashville, Tennessee

Address Inquiries To:
Office of Admissions
1000 17th Avenue North
Nashville, Tennessee 37208
T (615) 329-8666 **F** (615) 329-8774
Kchandler@fisk.edu
www.mmc.edu

Purpose

The Joint Program in Biomedical Sciences is designed to address America's need to train bright young students from groups under-represented in medicine who are dedicated to finding solutions to biomedical problems through research and who will be future health care providers.

Requirements for Entrance

Students are selected at the end of their first semester of under-graduate coursework on the Fisk University campus. There are no specific high school course requirements. Applicants must have competitive scores on the ACT and/or the SAT. They must have completed at least one semester at Fisk University. Participants must submit an application with a personal statement which details their career goals and letters of recommendation from two college science or mathematics professors to the Office of Admissions.

Selection Factors

The courses taken and grades earned at Fisk University, plus ACT and/or SAT scores, are considerations for eligibility for this program. Applicants must rank in the top 20 percent of their high school class. Students must take the MCAT prior to admission into the clinical phase of the Medical program, and a satisfactory score is required for medical school admission.

Curriculum

The Joint Program in Biomedical Sciences, seven years in duration, allows students to obtain a baccalaureate degree from Fisk University and the M.D. degree from Meharry Medical College. Course requirements for the baccalaureate degree include 8 semesters of natural and physical sciences and 12 semesters each in the humanities and social sciences. Students are required to spend two summers in a structured academic enrichment program. Students must take Steps 1 and 2 of the USMLE during the medical school portion of the program. Passing these examinations is a factor in promotion and graduation from medical school. The most frequent major chosen by students is biology, followed by chemistry.

Expenses	Resident Tuition and Fees	Non-resident Tuition and Fees
Undergraduate	N/A	N/A
U.S. Medical School	$32,508	$32,508

Financial Aid

Applicants and students can apply for institutional scholarships and grants, U.S. Department of Education Title IV Federal Student Aid (work-study and loans), U.S. Department of Health and Human Services Student Aid Programs (loans and scholarships), Southern Regional Education Board Grants, and Tennessee Black Conditional Grants. Meharry's Office of Student Financial Aid makes available most federal, regional, and state financial aid applications and brochures on numerous funding opportunities. Visit *www.mmc.edu/students/studentfinancialaid.html* for sources of financial aid. The Meharry Medical College Library and local public libraries have publications on most sources of student financial aid. Applicants can receive more information from the Office of Student Financial Aid, Meharry Medical College, 1005 D.B. Todd Boulevard, Nashville, Tennessee 37208.

Additional Information

All students who are selected for the program are on scholarship while enrolled at Fisk University.

Application and Acceptance Policies

Filing of application:
  Earliest date: September 15, 2009
  Latest date: February 1, 2010
Application fee: None   Fee Waiver Available: n/a
Acceptance notice:
  Earliest date: February 15, 2010
  Latest date: March 15, 2010
Applicant's response to acceptance offer:
  Maximum time: 1 week
Deposit to hold place in class: None
Starting date: Retroactive second semester, undergraduate year one

Information on 2008–2009 Entering Class

Number of	In-State	Out-of-State	Total
Applicants	2	6	8
Applicants Interviewed	2	2	4
New Entrants	0	2	2
Total number of students enrolled in program: 5			

100   *Medical School Admission Requirements, 2010–2011*

Rice University and Baylor College of Medicine

Houston, Texas

Address Inquiries To:
Rice University, Office of Admissions—MS-17
P.O. Box 1892
Houston, Texas 77251-1892
T (713) 348-RICE **F** (713) 348-5323
admi@rice.edu
www.bcm.edu/medschool/baccmd.htm

Purpose

To promote the education of future physicians who are scientifically competent, compassionate, and socially conscious in order to apply insight from the extensive study of liberal arts and other disciplines to the study of modern medical science.

Requirements for Entrance

Students are selected for this program during their senior year of high school. Both residents and non-residents of Texas are considered for admission. Applicants are expected to have had a varied and rigorous high school program with high academic achievement. They must take the SAT Reasoning Test or ACT, plus three SAT Subject tests.

Selection Factors

The high school academic record, standardized test scores, course selection, extracurricular activities, and letters of recommendation are some of the factors taken into account in offering admission to an applicant. In the 2008–2009 entering class, students averaged above the top five percent in their high school class.

Curriculum

This is not an accelerated program; all students are expected to complete four years of undergraduate education and four years of medical school. Students earn a baccalaureate degree from Rice University, and are awarded the M.D. degree by Baylor College of Medicine. Minimum course requirements for this program include at least two semesters each in the humanities and social sciences and eight semesters in the natural and physical sciences. The medical part of the curriculum devotes approximately 1 ½ years to the basic sciences with clinical experience, and 2 ½ years to clinical science with some basic science coursework. The MCAT is not required for promotion or admission to the medical school. Students are required to take Step 1 of the USMLE in their second or third years. They are also required to take Step 2 of the USMLE, but passing these examinations is not a graduation requirement.

Expenses

Expenses	Resident Tuition and Fees	Non-resident Tuition and Fees
Undergraduate	$28,900	$30,486
U.S. Medical School	$12,803	$25,903

Financial Aid

Sources of financial aid include academic, athletic, and need-based scholarships. Applicants can receive more information from the Rice University Admission Office, M.S. 17, 6100 Main Street, Houston, Texas 77035.

Application and Acceptance Policies

Filing of application:
  Earliest date: November 1, 2009
  Latest date: December 1, 2009
Application fee: $60   Fee Waiver Available: Yes
Acceptance notice:
  Earliest date: n/a
  Latest date: Mid-April 2010
Applicant's response to acceptance offer:
  Latest date: May 1, 2010
Deposit to hold place in class: $300; refundable by August 2010
Starting date: August 2010

Information on 2008–2009 Entering Class

Number of	In-State	Out-of-State	Total
Applicants	135	170	305
Applicants Interviewed	16	26	42
New Entrants	6	5	11
Total number of students enrolled in program: 53			

University of Texas
School of Medicine at San Antonio
San Antonio, Texas

University of Texas School of Medicine at San Antonio
7703 Floyd Curl Drive, Mail Code 7790
San Antonio, Texas 78229
T (210) 567-6080 **F** (210) 567-6962
medadmissions@uthscsa.edu
http://som.uthscsa.edu/admissions/index.asp

Purpose
In partnership with the University of Texas-Pan American this program offers the opportunity to achieve conditional acceptance to medical school as early as the junior year at UT Pan American. Participants are provided mentorship by medical school faculty and educational enrichment and clinical experiences in the Summer Premedical Academy. Frequent meetings with medical school faculty during the year provide encouragement and support toward matriculation into medical school. Acceptance to medical school after three years of undergraduate school is possible.

Requirements for Entrance
Students are selected during their senior year of high school. The program is only open to residents of Texas who are citizens or permanent residents of the United States. While there are no specific high school course requirements, applicants are required to take the SAT and/or ACT. Concurrent or AP coursework is encouraged.

Selection Factors
Academic factors considered in selecting applicants include SAT/ACT scores and strength in science and mathematics coursework. In addition to an impressive academic portfolio, applicants must also demonstrate a sincere interest in medicine and present letters of recommendation from their high school counselors or teachers. An interview by members of the School of Medicine Admissions Committee is also required. Students are admitted to medical school based on a sliding scale of the ratio of MCAT scores and science GPA, an interview with the Admissions Committee as well as a demonstrated continued commitment to study medicine.

Curriculum
Students must maintain a science and overall GPA of 3.25 or better and are required to complete all medical school prerequisite coursework with a grade of "C" or better. Students also participate in six-week Summer Premedical Academies for which scholarships are provided. During each summer starting after their freshman year, students come to the medical school campus in San Antonio to participate in academic enrichment programs, as well as twice weekly clinical preceptorships. The program is designed to increase the students' academic preparedness for the next year's coursework and for an MCAT review course during the summer between their junior and senior years. The clinical preceptorships are designed to increase students' awareness of issues in clinical medicine and to develop a clear understanding of performance expectations while in medical school.

Expenses

Expenses	Resident Tuition and Fees	Non-resident Tuition and Fees
Undergraduate	$11,898	$26,361
U.S. Medical School	$13,450	$28,637

Additional Information
The Summer Premedical Academy provides academic enrichment coursework along with clinical preceptorships. Students are also mentored by faculty and students of the medical school. There is also an opportunity to meet with education specialists to assist with learning disabilities.

Application and Acceptance Policies
Filing of application:
   Earliest date: December 1, 2009
   Latest date: February 1, 2010
Application fee: None   Fee Waiver Available: n/a
Acceptance notice:
   Earliest date: April 1, 2010
   Latest date: April 1, 2010
Applicant's response to acceptance offer:
   Maximum time: Two weeks
Deposit to hold place in class: None
Starting date: May 20, 2010

Information on 2008–2009 Entering Class

Number of	In-State	Out-of-State	Total
Applicants	40	n/a	40
Applicants Interviewed	20	n/a	20
New Entrants	5	n/a	5
Total number of students enrolled in program: 20			

102   *Medical School Admission Requirements, 2010–2011*

Eastern Virginia Medical School

Norfolk, Virginia

Address Inquiries To:
Office of Admissions, Mail Code 3
Eastern Virginia Medical School
700 W. Olney Road
Norfolk, Virginia 23507-1607
T (757) 446-5812 F (757) 446-5896
www.evms.edu/admissions

Purpose

Eastern Virginia Medical School currently has combined programs with ten colleges and universities: Christopher Newport University, The College of William and Mary, Old Dominion University, Hampton University, Norfolk State University, Hampden-Sydney College, Saint Paul's College, Virginia State University, Virginia Union University and Virginia Wesleyan College. The purpose of these programs is to enlist outstanding undergraduate students into a track that provides great freedom and choice in the pursuit of a baccalaureate degree.

Requirements for Entrance

Students are selected during their sophomore year of college. Both residents and non-residents of Virginia are eligible to apply. There are no specific high school course requirements, but students must take the SAT.

Selection Factors

Applicants will be evaluated on their academic performance during their freshman year of college and the first semester of their sophomore year of college. An emphasis is placed on leadership skills and extracurricular activities, including medical volunteering. Selected applicants are invited for an interview.

Curriculum

The eight-year curriculum leads to a baccalaureate degree awarded by Christopher Newport University, The College of William and Mary, Old Dominion University, Hampton University, Norfolk State University, Hampden-Sydney College, Saint Paul's College, Virginia State University, Virginia Union University or Virginia Wesleyan College. The M.D. degree is granted by Eastern Virginia Medical School. Course requirements for the baccalaureate degree vary at each undergraduate institution. The most frequent major is biology. This early assurance program does, however, permit the student the opportunity for academic diversity. Students selected who have combined SAT scores greater than 1250 (math and verbal) will not be required to take the MCAT. Step 1 of the USMLE must be taken at the completion of the second year of medical school. Students must pass Steps 1 and 2 of the USMLE to complete the program and receive the M.D. degree.

Expenses

Expenses	Resident Tuition and Fees	Non-resident Tuition and Fees
Undergraduate	Varies	Varies
U.S. Medical School	$25,196	$45,544

Financial Aid

For information about financial aid during the undergraduate phase, contact the Office of Financial Aid at the undergraduate institutions identified. Ten programs are available: Christopher Newport University, Harold Grau, Ph.D., (757) 594-7946; The College of William and Mary, Beverley T. Sher, Ph.D., (757) 221-2852; Old Dominion University, Terri Mathews, (757) 683-5201; Hampton University, Michael Druitt, (757) 728-6757; Norfolk State University, Alicia McClain, Ph.D., (757) 823-8991; Hampden-Sydney College, H.O. Thurman, Ph.D., (434) 223-6177; Saint Paul's College, Sunday Adesuyi, Ph.D., (434) 848-6484; Virginia State University, Pamela Leigh-Mack, Ph.D., (804) 524-5285, Virginia Union University, Phillip W. Archer, Ph.D., (804) 257-5692 and Virginia Wesleyan College, Victor Townsend, Ph.D., (757) 455-3392. For information about financial aid during the medical school phase, contact the Office of Financial Aid at Eastern Virginia Medical School at (757) 446-5804.

Application and Acceptance Policies

Filing of application:
　　Earliest date: Varies
　　Latest date: Varies
Application fee: $35　　　　　Fee Waiver Available: No
Acceptance notice:
　　Earliest date: Varies
　　Latest date: Varies
Applicant's response to acceptance offer:
　　Maximum time: Varies
Deposit to hold place in class: $100; refundable by May 15, 2010
Starting date: August 2010

Information on 2008–2009 Entering Class

Number of	In-State	Out-of-State	Total
Applicants	15	13	18
Applicants Interviewed	12	3	15
New Entrants	6	1	7
Total number of students enrolled in program: n/a			

Virginia Commonwealth University School of Medicine

Richmond, Virginia

Address Inquiries To:
Dr. Anne L. Chandler, Senior Associate Dean
The Honors College
Virginia Commonwealth University
P.O. Box 843010, Richmond, Virginia 23284-3010
T (804) 828-1803 **F** (804) 827-1669
achandle@vcu.edu
www.pubapps.vcu.edu/honors/guaranteed/medicine/index.aspx

Purpose

The Guaranteed Admission Program of the Honors College offers academically capable, highly focused students an opportunity to pursue diverse, intellectually challenging programs of study. Students who successfully complete the Guaranteed Admission Program will be able to enter the medical school without the pressure of further competition. Close contact with the School of Medicine throughout the undergraduate program aids students in testing their career choice and in preparing for a lifelong commitment to learning in the profession.

Requirements for Entrance

Students are selected during their senior year of high school, and there are no state residency restrictions. All candidates are considered. The specific minimum high school course requirements are as follows: four units in English; three units in mathematics (to include algebra I and either geometry or algebra II); two units in science (at least one a laboratory science); and three units of history or social sciences or government. Students are strongly encouraged to present at least two units in a modern or ancient foreign language. Also required are standardized test scores on the ACT or SAT. The ACT composite score must be at or above 29. The combined SAT1 score must be at or above 1910 and obtained in a single sitting, with no score below 530. An unweighted GPA of 3.5 (on a 4.0 scale) is also required.

Selection Factors

Factors considered in offering admission to an applicant include: GPA, letters of reference, test scores, well-rounded and rigorous academic preparation, health care-related experience, and written and oral communication skills. The average GPA for students accepted for the 2008–2009 class was 3.85 (unweighted scale of 4.0), and the average SAT score was 2130. Selected applicants are invited for a required interview.

Curriculum

Students are required to complete a baccalaureate degree. The most frequent major is biology; the next most frequent major is chemistry. The undergraduate degree is awarded by Virginia Commonwealth University. Specific course requirements vary, depending upon the major. During the medical school program, there is a longitudinal clinical experience (Foundations of Clinical Medicine) in a community primary care practice that meets weekly for both of the first two years. Students are required to take Step 1 of the USMLE at the end of their second year. They must also take USMLE Step 2, but passing these examinations is not a promotion or graduation requirement. The doctor of medicine degree is also awarded by Virginia Commonwealth University. It takes eight years to fulfill the requirements for both degrees.

Expenses	Resident Tuition and Fees	Non-resident Tuition and Fees
Undergraduate	$6,779	$19,724
U.S. Medical School	$27,720	$41,525

Financial Aid

There are several sources of financial aid available to students, including scholarships, loans, grants, and work-study. For more information, contact the Virginia Commonwealth University Financial Aid Office, P.O. Box 842506, Richmond, Virginia 23284-2506; (804) VCU-MONY.

Application and Acceptance Policies

Filing of application:
   Earliest date: September 1, 2009
   Latest date: November 15, 2009
Application fee: $40   Fee Waiver Available: Yes
Acceptance notice:
   Earliest date: April 1, 2010
   Latest date: n/a
Applicant's response to acceptance offer:
   Maximum time: May 1, 2010
Deposit to hold place in class: $100; nonrefundable
Starting date: August 2010

Information on 2008–2009 Entering Class

Number of	In-State	Out-of-State	Total
Applicants	65	111	176
Applicants Interviewed	21	38	59
New Entrants	9	14	23
Total number of students enrolled in program: 93			

Chapter 11

Training of Physician-Scientists: M.D.-Ph.D. Programs

While most medical students will ultimately decide to devote their medical careers primarily to the care and treatment of patients, a smaller group of students at each medical school will choose a different career goal — to become physician-scientists (also referred to as research physicians and physician-investigators). Physician-scientists use their research and clinical skills both in the laboratory and at the bedside. They engage in basic and clinical research to advance medical knowledge, promote health, solve medical problems, combat disease, and improve medical care. They also attempt to bridge the gap between laboratory research and clinical medicine. They frequently are faculty members at academic medical centers and other research institutions; they also play important roles in biotechnology and at pharmaceutical companies.

Educational and Training

One path to a career as a physician-scientist is enrollment in a combined M.D.-Ph.D. program for a total of seven to eight years. An M.D.-Ph.D. student can complete the Ph.D. degree in any of a variety of scientific specializations. These include, among others, biochemistry, cell biology, biomedical engineering, developmental biology, genetics, immunology, pathology, pharmacology, physiology, biophysics, bioinformatics, epidemiology, molecular biology, and neuroscience. However, not every medical school offers each area of specialization. Another route to a career in medical research is through completion of a Ph.D. degree or a research fellowship following receipt of the M.D. degree, either in lieu of, or after completing, a residency in a medical specialty. Participation in an integrated M.D.-Ph.D. Program offers the opportunity to complete both the M.D. and Ph.D. degrees in a shorter time period than it would take to complete both degree programs separately.

Such programs are frequently referred to as "joint," "combined," or "dual" degree programs. It is important to note that some schools also use these terms to describe other educational programs linked to the M.D. degree, including Master's degree programs (e.g., in education, public health, and business administration) and other doctoral-level programs (e.g., in law, computer science, and history).

A complete and up-to-date listing of M.D.-Ph.D. programs at AAMC-member medical schools, including information about available areas of specialization, can be found on the AAMC Curriculum Directory Web site at *http://services.aamc.org/currdir*. Currently, almost all U.S. and Canadian medical schools have organized M.D.-Ph.D. programs in one or more areas of specialization. Some are relatively small in size (1–2 new students per year, with a dozen total students), while others are much larger (up to 20 new students annually, with a total enrollment of 150 students).

The typical M.D.-Ph.D. program is completed in a total of seven to eight years and includes:

- completion of the first two years of combined medical and graduate school coursework, followed by

- three to five years of doctoral research, including the completion of a thesis project, and

- a return to medical school for core clinical training and electives during the final years of the medical curriculum.

At most schools, integrated approaches to graduate and medical education and training have been introduced. These integrated approaches involve, among other educational innovations, interdisciplinary and interdepartmental seminars, summer research opportunities, and planned interactions with teams composed of both basic science and clinical investigators. While the national trend involves a move toward more integrated curricula, there is currently an array of curricular choices available.

Following receipt of both the M.D. and Ph.D. degrees, the physician-scientist usually completes residency training in a medical specialty, often followed by additional clinical and/or research training in a fellowship program, prior to initiating a career as a physician-scientist.

Application and Admission

For most medical schools participating in AMCAS, M.D.-Ph.D. programs have adopted a common application procedure. Students indicate their desire to apply to a M.D.-Ph.D. program on the AMCAS application and provide essays describing their reasons for wanting to pursue M.D.-Ph.D. training as well as their significant research experience. As with M.D. applications (see Chapter 4), schools differ in secondary application materials and how admissions committees process application. Potential applicants should investigate the M.D.-Ph.D. program Web site at each medical school of interest to learn about school specific variations in the application pocesses. At some schools, the application may first be referred to the admission committee for the regular M.D. program for assessment and an acceptance decision, with the applications of accepted students only then referred for further consideration by Ph.D. program faculty members. Other schools have a separate admission committee for M.D.-Ph.D. applicants. Still other schools will consider applicants for the Ph.D. component of the program only after their successful completion of the first year (or more) of medical school.

Because M.D.-Ph.D. applicants plan to become both physicians and scientists, admission committee members will

review primary and secondary application materials for evidence of the usual attributes and experiences that are important for admission of students to the M.D.-only program (see Chapter 7). In addition, however, they will seek, in the applicants' statement of career goals as a physician-scientist and in letters of recommendation from faculty members or investigators with whom the applicant has previously worked, additional evidence of:

- relevant and substantive research interest and experience during or after college

- an appreciation for, and understanding of, the work of physician-scientists, and

- intellectual drive, research ability and acumen, and perseverance

Some medical schools will accept applications from M.D.-Ph.D. candidates only for both degree programs, and will not consider applicants whose credentials are not deemed sufficient for enrollment in either program. Other schools permit the applicant who is not accepted to the M.D.-Ph.D. combined degree program to continue to pursue admission to the M.D.-only curriculum. Since school policies differ on this matter, applicants are well advised to clarify relevant application and admission policies at each school of interest prior to making application. Generally, an applicant who is not accepted to a combined M.D.-Ph.D. program, but who wishes to attend the M.D.-only educational program should express his or her continuing interest in the M.D.-only program to admission office staff.

Financing M.D.-Ph.D. Program Enrollment

Funding for M.D.-Ph.D. students vary from school to school. Many schools offer full support for both the M.D. and Ph.D. components of their education, including a stipend, tuition waivers, and health insurance. At other institutions, varying degrees of partial support are available, sometimes only for the Ph.D. components of the combined degree program. Applicants should ascertain from program officials the nature of financial support for students enrolled in the M.D.-Ph.D. program prior to applying and accepting a position in the program.

Sources of funding to support M.D.–Ph.D. students include institutional funds, as well as individual and institutional training grants, most often from federal sources. Federal sources of M.D.-Ph.D. training funds include Medical Scientist Training Program (MSTP) grants, awarded by the National Institute of General Medical Sciences (NIGMS) at the National Institute of Health (NIH) to more than 40 M.D.–Ph.D. programs. A full listing of such programs is available at *www.nigms. nih.gov/Training/InstPredoc/PredocInst-MSTP.htm*. (There are approximately 75 other medical schools that do not have NIGMS MSTP training grants, but that also offer opportunities for M.D.-Ph.D. studies.)

Careers in Academic Medicine and Medical Research

Approximately four-fifths of M.D.-Ph.D. graduates are employed as faculty members in academic medical centers, where they engage in substantial research activity and compete for available research funding from governmental, foundation, and other sources. One quarter of these graduates are faculty members in basic science departments, while three quarters are faculty members in clinical departments. They are also employed in clinical medicine, government, and industry, as well as in basic, clinical, translational, and epidemiological research.

Many physician-scientists at academic medical centers devote the majority of their time to their research, with the remainder of their time devoted to the other responsibilities of academic faculty members: clinical service, teaching, committee membership, and administration.

Advantages and Disadvantages of M.D.-Ph.D. Programs

One advantage of enrollment in a combined M.D.-Ph.D. program is the time saved from completing both programs separately. M.D.-Ph.D. students also enjoy opportunities for excellent research experiences and superb faculty mentoring frequently unavailable to the M.D.-only student. By virtue of these experiences, M.D.-Ph.D. students can significantly enhance their understanding and mastery of the basic science background underlying patients' clinical problems, and use that information to generate improvements in clinical diagnosis and treatment. Funding for the M.D.-Ph.D. student from MSTP and other federal and non-federal sources can result in a reduction in educational debt at program completion, although the long duration of training means that this type of support should not be a determinant of the decision to pursue admission to a combined M.D.–Ph.D program.

One disadvantage of M.D.-Ph.D. training is the length of enrollment in the program, followed by required residency and fellowship training, resulting in delayed onset of a professional career relative to M.D.-only peers. On average, however, M.D.-Ph.D. graduates begin their independent careers at about the same age as M.D.-only faculty. Another potential disadvantage is the several-year interval between the basic science and clinical years of medical school, which may require some M.D.-Ph.D. students to refresh their basic clinical skills before starting clinical clerkships. However, most M.D.-Ph.D. programs provide mechanisms for reintegration into clinical work.

Additional Information

For additional information and advice about application to, and enrollment in, a combined M.D.-Ph.D. program and the work of physician-scientists, contact your pre-health advisor and the M.D.-Ph.D. program director at medical schools of interest. In addition, the M.D.-Ph.D. Section of the AAMC Group on Graduate Research, Education, and Training (GREAT Group) is developing a Web site that will provide perspectives about M.D.-Ph.D. careers, training, and applications from M.D.-Ph.D. program Directors and Administrators.

For additional information regarding M.D.-Ph.D. training and careers, visit *www.aamc.org/great* to download M.D.-Ph.D. Training and Careers: A Guide for Potential Applicants, Current Trainees, and Advisors.

Chapter 12

Information About U.S. Medical Schools
Accredited by the LCME

Information about individual U.S. medical schools is given in the following two-page entries for the 130 schools (126 in the fifty states, four in Puerto Rico) that will be considering applications for the summer 2010 entering class. The schools presented here are accredited as of February 2009 by the Liaison Committee on Medical Education (LCME), which is sponsored by the Association of American Medical Colleges (AAMC) and the American Medical Association (AMA).

Individual school entries are each two pages, one devoted to narrative information and the other devoted to data and tabular information:

Page one: Narrative Information

- **Contact Information** — Admissions office staff, mail and e-mail addresses, phone and fax numbers, and Web site addresses for the medical school, admissions office, and financial aid office.

- **General Information** — Background and basic information about the medical school and its program.

- **Curricular Highlights** — Information about the medical education curriculum and educational philosophy and methodologies.

- **USMLE Step 1 and Step 2 Clinical Knowledge (CK) and Clinical Skills (CS) Policies** — United States Medical Licensing Examination (USMLE) policies and requirements for promotion and/or graduation. For the most current policies, see the AAMC Curriculum Directory Web site at *http://services.aamc.org/currdir/section1*.

- **Selection Factors** — Basic information regarding coursework, personal characteristics and experiences, and general requirements for applicants to be considered for acceptance and matriculation.

- **Financial Aid** — General information about the financial aid programs provid-

ed by the school, as well as additional contact information.

- **Information about Diversity Programs** — Information about the school's diversity initiatives and programs for students from groups underrepresented in medicine, as well as additional contact information.

- **Campus Information** — Information about total enrollment figures, campus setting, housing, special features, and satellite and/or regional campuses.

Page two: Data and Tabular Information

- **Application Process and Requirements for 2010–2011**

  - Primary Application Service — Notation of which type of application the school utilizes for primary applications (the American Medical College Application Service [AMCAS], the Texas Medical and Dental School Application Service [TMDSAS], or a school-specific application) and about the earliest and latest filing dates for the primary application.

  - Secondary Application — This section notes if a secondary application is required, to whom the secondary application is submitted, required fees, the potential availability of a fee waiver, and the earliest and latest filing dates for secondary application materials.

  - Latest MCAT® Considered — The most recent MCAT administration from which an MCAT score can be submitted in support of an application.

  - Oldest MCAT® Considered — The earliest MCAT administration from which an MCAT score can be submitted in support of an application.

  - Early Decision Program — This section notes if the school participates in an

Early Decision Program (EDP), when EDP applicants are notified about acceptance decisions, and if the Early Decision Program is available only to state residents or to both state residents and non-residents.

- Regular Acceptance Notice — The earliest and latest dates on which acceptance notices are sent to applicants. These dates do not refer to those applicants who have applied to special programs.

- Applicant's Response to Acceptance Notice – Maximum Time — The maximum period of time applicants are provided to respond to the acceptance offer.

- Requests for Deferred Entrance Considered — Information about deferred entrance opportunities at the school.

- Deposit — Information on the amount of the deposit required to hold a place in the next entering class, when the deposit is due, if the deposit is applied to tuition, if the deposit is refundable, and final date for requesting a deposit refund.

- Estimated Number of New Entrants — The number of regular, EDP and special program applicants expected to matriculate in the next year's entering class.

- Start Month/Year — The anticipated starting date in 2010 for the program.

- Interview Format — General information on how interviews are conducted and about the availability of regional interviews.

• **Other Programs** — Information regarding the availability of postbaccalaureate premedical, summer, and combined degree programs. Web sites and contact information are provided, as available.

• **Premedical Coursework** — Coursework and laboratories that applicants are either required or

recommended to complete prior to matriculation.

• **MCAT® Information for Accepted Applicants** — This chart displays, for each section of the MCAT, the median total numeric score for all 2008 accepted applicants, the Median Total Numeric MCAT score for all 2008 accepted applicants to all U.S. medical schools (the number in the shaded circle), the individual school's median MCAT scores for all 2008 applicants accepted to the school (the number in the white circle), and the range of scores on each MCAT section for all 2008 applicants accepted to the school (the gradient line behind the circled numbers). Where applicable, schools have noted if it is their policy to average an applicant's MCAT scores from various MCAT administrations. Note: Chart 5-E (Chapter 5) presents information about the likelihood of acceptance for applicants whose scores on all MCAT sections are at the lower end of the score range. Additionally, schools have noted whether the MCAT is required for admission and the percentage of accepted applicants who took the MCAT. Note: Several schools have special programs that do not require applicants to provide MCAT scores. Therefore, although the MCAT may be required for admission to the regular M.D. program, the percentage of accepted applicants who took the MCAT may be less than 100%.

The national median scores for each MCAT section published in this chapter represent median scores for the entire pool of accepted applicants to all medical schools. Thus, based on the fact that each acceptance of an applicant reflects an independent decision by each medical school, when an applicant has been accepted by more than one medical school, that applicant's MCAT scores are included in the calculation of the national median more than once.

• **Overall GPA Median and Science GPA**

Median — These data are for all applicants accepted to the medical school's 2008–2009 entering class.

• **Selection Factors** — Proportion of Accepted Applicants with Relevant Experience – These percentages were derived from applicant self-reports on the 2008 AMCAS application. They represent the percentage of accepted applicants who reported experiences in the categories of Community Service/Volunteer Work, Medically-Related Work, and Research Experience. Data provided from schools that participate in the TMDSAS application or that use a school-specific primary application were calculated in the same manner as those derived from the AMCAS application.

• **Acceptance & Matriculation Data for 2008–2009** — Data in this chart reflect verified applications, not initiated applications. The top half of the chart notes the number of applicants (resident, non-resident, international, and total) who applied, were interviewed, and/or deferred entrance.

The lower portion of the chart displays information about the number of resident, non-resident, international, and total matriculants who were accepted through any Early Assurance Program (EAP), the Early Decision Program (EDP), and any college/M.D. or M.D./Ph.D. program, as well as the total number of matriculants from any application process in the school's 2008–2009 entering class. Information is also noted regarding the school's ability to accept applications from international applicants.

• **Matriculant Demographics** — Information about the number of men and women who matriculated in the 2008 first-year class for the first time.

• **Matriculants' Self-Reported Race/Ethnicity** — This information reflects data that were self-reported by applicants on their applications.

Note: The sum of the columns may not reflect the actual number of matriculants. Applicants are permitted to select, in their racial and ethnic self-descriptions, more than one race and/or ethnicity. Each selection is counted. Therefore, if a given matriculant selects three races and/or ethnicities, that matriculant will be counted in three different columns. The total number of matriculants is presented in the row labeled "unduplicated."

- **Matriculants who were Science and Math Majors** — In this calculation, "Science and Math Majors" include: Aerospace Engineering, Agriculture, Anatomy, Astronomy, Biochemistry, Biology, Biomathematics, Biomedical Engineering, Biomedical Science, Biophysics, Botany, Chemical Engineering, Chemistry, Chemistry and Biology, Civil Engineering, Computer Science, Double Major Science, Electrical Engineering, Engineering, Environmental Studies, Forestry, Genetics, Geology, Geophysics, Human Biology, Mathematics, Mechanical Engineering, Meteorology, Microbiology, Molecular Biology, Natural Science, Neuroscience, Oceanography, Pathology, Pharmacology, Physics, Physiology, Premedicine, Psychobiology, Science General, Science–Other, Biology, Science–Other Physics, Statistics, and Zoology. These definitions reflect applicants' self-report on their AMCAS application; assistance was also provided by members of the National Association of Advisors for the Health Professions (NAAHP).

- **Matriculants with Baccalaureate and/or Graduate Degrees** — Information about the percentage of matriculants with baccalaureate and/or graduate degrees at the time of matriculation.

- **Specialty Choice** — The information in

this chart was derived from program directors' reports to the National Graduate Medical Education (GME) Census in GME Track™ for 2004, 2005, and 2006 graduates of each medical school.

- **Financial Information** — Cost of Attendance, Tuition and Fees, Other Expenses and Health Insurance information is derived from the 2008–2009 AAMC Tuition and Student Fees Questionnaire. Regarding health insurance, "can be waived" means that this fee may be waived for any student with existing and comparable health insurance coverage (e.g., through a parent or a spouse).

Data about % of Enrolled Students Receiving Financial Aid and Average 2008 Graduate Indebtedness are derived from the 2007–2008 Liaison Committee on Medical Education (LCME) 1B Survey. Note: Scholarship and Grant amounts include funding from programs with a service commitment.

Abbreviations

Listed below are the abbreviations used in the school entries in this chapter.

AMCAS® — American Medical College Application Service

CACMS — Committee on Accreditation of Canadian Medical Schools

CLEP — College Level Examination Program

EAP — Early Assurance Program

EDP — Early Decision Program

FAF — Financial Aid Form

FAFSA — Free Application for Federal Student Aid

FAP — AAMC Fee Assistance Program

GPA — Grade Point Average

LCME — Liaison Committee on Medical Education

LCME 1B — Liaison Committee on Medical Education 1B Survey

MCAT — Medical College Admission Test

NA — Non-Applicable

NC — Not Collected

NR — Not Reported

REC — Recommended

REQ — Required

TMDSAS — Texas Medical and Dental School Application Service

TSF — Tuition and Student Fees Questionnaire

USMLE — United States Medical Licensing Examination

WICHE — Western Interstate Commission for Higher Education

WWAMI — WWAMI is an enduring partnership between the University of Washington School of Medicine and the states of Wyoming, Alaska, Montana, and Idaho. Its purpose is to provide access to publicly supported medical education across the five-state region. "WWAMI" is derived from the first letter of each of the five cooperating states.

University of Alabama School of Medicine

Birmingham, Alabama

Medical Student Services/Admissions
University of Alabama School of Medicine
VH 100, 1530 3rd Ave. S.
Birmingham, Alabama 35294-0019
T 205 934 2433   **F** 205 934 8740

Admissions http://medicine.uab.edu/admissions
Main http://medicine.uab.edu
Financial http://medicine.uab.edu/financialaid
E-mail medschool@uab.edu

Public Institution

Dr. Robert R. Rich, Dean

Dr. Nathan B. Smith, Assistant Dean for Admissions

Dr. Anjanetta L. Foster, Assistant Dean for Diversity and Multicultural Affairs

Ann Little, Financial Aid Specialist

General Information

The School of Medicine was founded in Mobile in 1859 and has been located in Birmingham since 1945. The main campus is in Birmingham, with branch campuses, created in 1969, in Huntsville and Tuscaloosa.

Mission Statement

The School of Medicine is dedicated to the education of physicians and scientists in all of the disciplines of medicine and biomedical investigation for careers in practice, teaching, and research. Necessary to this educational mission are the provision of outstanding medical care and services and the enhancement of new knowledge through clinical and basic biomedical research.

Curricular Highlights

Community Service Requirement: Optional.
Research/Thesis Requirement: Optional.

The four-year program emphasizes the fundamentals underlying clinical medical practice, with attention to the emotional, cultural, and social characteristics of patients and to the importance of adapting care to meet their needs. The Preclinical curriculum integrates basic and clinical sciences around organ system modules co-directed by basic scientists and clinicians. The objective of the curriculum is for students to learn basic sciences in a clinically relevant context, teaching them to think comprehensively about organ function and disease rather than to memorize mountains of facts. The first two years also provide training in medical professionalism, interviewing, and physical examination. The third and fourth years consist of required rotations and electives, with clinical experiences in both hospital and ambulatory settings. There are structured opportunities for research.

USMLE

Step 1: Required. Students must record a passing score for promotion.
Step 2: Clinical Skills (CS): Required. Students must only record a score.
Step 2: Clinical Knowledge (CK): Required. Students must record a passing total score to graduate.

Selection Factors

The Admissions Committee is committed to admitting those applicants who possess the intelligence, skills, attitudes, and other personal attributes to become excellent physicians and to meet the health care needs of the state of Alabama. Desirable attributes include: solid academic performance, effective communication and interpersonal skills, evidence of service to others, empathy, emotional maturity, personal resilience, honesty, leadership ability, sense of purpose, and experiences to promote an understanding of what it means to be a physician (shadowing). Commitment and ability to meet the healthcare needs of Alabama's underserved populations (urban and rural), to biomedical research/academic careers, and to primary care careers are desirable. There is a special acceptance program for state residents committed to rural practice in Alabama. AP or CLEP coursework appearing on the AMCAS application will be accepted to meet a premedical requirement, although further coursework in biology and chemistry are desirable and may be necessary to be a competitive applicant. Other requirements: minimal total MCAT of 24 on the most recent exam, minimum grade of "C" on all required coursework, and completion of 90 hours of undergraduate credit from an accredited US college or university. With rare exceptions, completion of an undergraduate degree is required; all work toward current degrees must be completed prior to matriculation to the medical school.

Financial Aid

There are financial resources to fund an entire medical education. Resources include scholarships and low and higher interest loans. State merit scholarships are available in limited numbers to Alabama residents with exceptional academic records. State residents committed to rural practice in Alabama may qualify for aid.

Information about Diversity Programs

With the Office for Diversity Programs, the Admissions Committee attempts to identify and provide career counseling to students from groups under-represented in medicine.

Campus Information

Setting

The Birmingham campus is part of the UAB Medical Center, a world-renowned academic medical center with more than 70 research centers across 82 city blocks. All students complete the Pre-Clerkship Phase in Birmingham. For required clinical rotations, students are assigned to Birmingham or one of two branch campuses.

Enrollment

For 2008, total enrollment was: 733

Special Features

Students are encouraged to participate in mentored research opportunities, ranging from one-month projects to degree programs (MPH and MS). Students are required to complete a three month Scholarly Activity in the third year.

Housing

Housing is available on campus. Most medical students live off-campus and find affordable housing within a 15-minute commute to the campus.

Satellite Campuses/Facilities

Both the Huntsville and Tuscaloosa campuses offer students opportunities for community-based education, as well as rotations in regional medical centers offering a full range of medical specialties. Both campuses have new clinical education facilities.

Application Process and Requirements 2010–2011

Primary Application Service: AMCAS
Earliest filing date: June 1, 2009
Latest filing date: November 1, 2009

Secondary Application Required?: Yes
Sent to: Screened applicants
URL: Provided to invited applicants
E-mail: medschool@uab.edu
Fee: Yes, $75
Fee waiver available: Yes
Earliest filing date: August 1, 2009
Latest filing date: November 15, 2009

MCAT® required?: Yes
Latest MCAT® considered: September 2009
Oldest MCAT® considered: 2007

Early Decision Program: School does have EDP
Applicants notified: October 1, 2009
EDP available for: Residents only

Regular Acceptance Notice
Earliest date: October 15, 2009
Latest date: Until class is full
Applicant's Response to Acceptance Offer – Maximum Time: Two weeks

Requests for Deferred Entrance Considered: Yes

Deposit to Hold Place in Class: Yes
Deposit (Resident): $50
Deposit (Non-resident): $100
Deposit due: With acceptance offer
Applied to tuition: Yes
Deposit refundable: Yes
Refundable by: May 15, 2010

Estimated number of new entrants: 176
EDP: 15, special program: 41

Start Month/Year: July 2010

Interview Format: Individual interviews are held only on Thursdays, September through March. Regional interviews are not available.

Other Programs

PREPARATORY PROGRAMS
Postbaccalaureate Program: No
Summer Program: Yes, www.uasom.uab.edu/shep
Rural Medicine Programs: Yes, www.uasom.uab.edu/secondaryapplication/RMSPHome.html
Summer Health Enrichment Program: Yes, www.uasom.uab.edu/shep

COMBINED DEGREE PROGRAMS
Baccalaureate/M.D.: Yes, www.uab.edu/emsap
M.D./M.P.H.: Yes, www.soph.uab.edu/prospective/academicprograms
M.D./M.B.A.: No
M.D./J.D.: No
M.D./Ph.D.: Yes, www.uab.edu/uasom/mstp/

Premedical Coursework

Course	Req.	Rec.	Lab.	Hrs.
Inorganic Chemistry	•		•	8
Behavioral Sciences				
Biochemistry		•		
Biology	•		•	8
Biology/Zoology				
Calculus				
College English	•			6
College Mathematics	•			6

Course	Req.	Rec.	Lab.	Hrs.
Computer Science				
Genetics				
Humanities				
Organic Chemistry	•		•	8
Physics	•		•	8
Psychology				
Social Sciences				
Other				

Selection Factors: 2008 Accepted Applicants

Proportion of Accepted Applicants with Relevant Experience (Data Self-Reported to AMCAS®)		
Community Service/Volunteer		78%
Medically-Related Work		74%
Research		66%

Shaded bar represents school's accepted scores ranging from the 10th percentile to the 90th percentile. School Median ● National Median ◐

Overall GPA 2.0 2.1 2.2 2.3 2.4 2.5 2.6 2.7 2.8 2.9 3.0 3.1 3.2 3.3 3.4 3.5 3.6 3.7 (3.8) 3.9 4.0
Science GPA 2.0 2.1 2.2 2.3 2.4 2.5 2.6 2.7 2.8 2.9 3.0 3.1 3.2 3.3 3.4 3.5 3.6 3.7 (3.8) 3.9 4.0

MCAT® Total Numeric Score 9 10 11 12 13 14 15 16 17 18 19 20 21 22 23 24 25 26 27 28 29 30 (31) 32 33 34 35 36 37 38 39 40 41 42 43

Writing Sample			J	K	L	M	N	O	(P)	(Q)	R	S	T
Verbal Reasoning	3	4	5	6	7	8	9	(10)	11	12	13	14	15
Biological Sciences	3	4	5	6	7	8	9	(10)	(11)	12	13	14	15
Physical Sciences	3	4	5	6	7	8	9	(10)	(11)	12	13	14	15

Acceptance & Matriculation Data for 2008–2009 First Year Class

	Resident	Non-resident	International	Total
Applications	432	1580	22	2034
Interviewed	298	133	0	431
Deferred	3	1	0	4
Matriculants				
Early Assurance Program	0	0	0	0
Early Decision Program	13	0	0	13
Baccalaureate/M.D.	7	0	0	7
M.D./Ph.D.	1	8	0	9
Matriculated	157	19	0	**176**

Applications accepted from International Applicants: No

Specialty Choice

2004, 2005, 2006 Graduates, Specialty Choice (As reported by program directors to GME Track™)	
Anesthesiology	7%
Emergency Medicine	5%
Family Practice	10%
Internal Medicine	17%
Obstetrics/Gynecology	6%
Orthopaedic Surgery	4%
Pediatrics	12%
Psychiatry	3%
Radiology	5%
Surgery	8%

Matriculant Demographics: 2008–2009 First Year Class

Men: 100   **Women:** 76

Matriculants' Self-Reported Race/Ethnicity

Mexican American	1	Korean	3
Cuban	0	Vietnamese	0
Puerto Rican	0	Other Asian	0
Other Hispanic	0	Total Asian	24
Total Hispanic	1	Native American	1
Chinese	6	Black	14
Asian Indian	13	Native Hawaiian	1
Pakistani	1	White	138
Filipino	1	Unduplicated Number	
Japanese	0	of Matriculants	176

Science and Math Majors: 74%
Matriculants with:
   Baccalaureate degree: 99%
   Graduate degree(s): 10%

Financial Information

Source: 2007–2008 LCME I-B survey and 2008–2009 AAMC TSF questionnaire

	Residents	Non-residents
Total Cost of Attendance	$38,863	$69,371
Tuition and Fees	$18,871	$49,379
Other (includes living expenses)	$18,400	$18,400
Health Insurance (can be waived)	$1,592	$1,592

Average 2008 Graduate Indebtedness: $93,706
% of Enrolled Students Receiving Aid: 78%

Criminal Background Check

This medical school requires a criminal background check prior to matriculation.

University of South Alabama College of Medicine
Mobile, Alabama

Office of Admissions, MSB 241
University of South Alabama
College of Medicine
Mobile, Alabama 36688-0002
T 251 460 7176   F 251 460 6278

Admissions www.southalabama.edu/
com/admissions.shtml
Main www.southalabama.edu/com/
Financial www.finaid2.usouthal.edu/
E-mail mscott@usouthal.edu

Public Institution

Dr. Samuel J. Strada, Dean

Mark Scott, Director for Admissions

Dr. Margaret O'Brien, Associate Dean, Student Affairs

Dr. Hattie M. Myles, Assistant Dean, Special Programs and Student Affairs

General Information

The College of Medicine of the University of South Alabama was approved by the Board of Trustees of the university in 1967; the Alabama state legislature passed a resolution authorizing the college on August 19, 1967. The college admitted a charter class in January 1973. The basic medical sciences are housed on the university campus. The University of South Alabama Medical Center, operating continuously since 1831, has provided clinical medical education for more than a century. It is the major physician-staffed emergency facility in South Alabama and has been named a Level I trauma center by the Alabama Committee on Trauma. Other clinical training facilities include the USA Children's and Women's Hospital and the USA Mitchell Cancer Institute.

Mission Statement

To prepare talented, highly qualified students to become physicians, providing them the opportunity to develop basic science and clinical skills that will carry them successfully through residency and their career in medicine.

Curricular Highlights

Community Service Requirement: Optional.
Research/Thesis Requirement: Optional.

The first year is devoted to the basic sciences of anatomy, physiology, biochemistry, neuroanatomy, and embryology. Early introduction to clinical problems is also offered in courses through Clinical Correlation Conferences and Medical Practice and Society. The second year includes pathology, physical diagnosis, microbiology-immunology, pharmacology, and behavioral science. Public health/epidemiology and medical genetics round out the second-year curriculum. The third year has six clinical clerkships: medicine,

surgery, pediatrics, psychiatry/neurology, obstetrics-gynecology, and family practice. The fourth year is composed of nine rotations of four weeks each. Students are required to select one rotation each in clinical neuroscience, surgical subspecialties, ambulatory care, primary care, subspecialty in medicine, pediatrics or obstetrics-gynecology, an acting internship, and an in-house elective. Three of the rotations may be used for approved extramural experiences. Letter grades are given until the fourth year, where a pass/fail/honors system is used.

USMLE

Step 1: Required. Students must record a passing score for promotion.
Step 2: Clinical Skills (CS): Required. Students must record a passing total score to graduate.
Step 2: Clinical Knowledge (CK): Required. Students must record a passing total score to graduate.

Selection Factors

The Committee on Admissions will consider all candidates whose undergraduate grades and scores on the MCAT indicate that they can handle the rigorous curriculum of the College of Medicine. However, admission is based on more than scholastic achievement. Applicants will be considered on their potential to become conscientious and capable physicians. The University of South Alabama provides equal educational opportunities and is open to all qualified students without regard to race, creed, national origin, sex, or handicap with respect to all of its programs and activities. Because the college is state-supported, preference is given to Alabama residents. However, highly qualified out-of-state applicants are seriously considered. Disadvantaged, rural, and minority residents are strongly encouraged to apply. Fee waivers, based solely on economic need, are granted, when documented.

Financial Aid

The Office of Financial Aid coordinates the programs of assistance available to medical students demonstrating financial need. Scholarships are also available for entering freshmen and medical students who have demonstrated academic excellence and/or financial need.

Information about Diversity Programs

The school is committed to the enrollment and education of individuals from all disadvantaged groups. For information, contact Dr. Hattie M. Myles, Assistant Dean of Special Programs and Student Affairs.

Campus Information

Setting

The medical school is located in a suburban setting with easy access to restaurants, shopping, and the city's largest park system, which has both affordable golf and tennis facilities. Gulf Shores and Dauphin Island are less than an hour away, where students can enjoy some of the finest beaches in the United States. The hospitals and clinics are located throughout Mobile County and serve the health care needs of the community. These facilities include the only Level I trauma center in the region, as well as the latest in cancer treatments offered through the USA Mitchell Cancer Institute.

Enrollment

For 2008, total enrollment was: 296

Special Features

With only 74 students in each class and a large research-based clinical system consisting of four hospitals, students are exposed to significant procedural opportunities.

Housing

Very few, if any, students choose to live on campus due to the many safe and affordable housing options within a 5-mile radius of the campus. With the relative low cost of home ownership in the Mobile area, many students have found buying a small house or condo more cost-effective than leasing.

Satellite Campuses/Facilities

Students do their hospital training in any one of four hospitals, depending on the rotation. The College of Medicine also has clinic-based training with preceptors in facilities located throughout Alabama.

Application Process and Requirements 2010–2011

Primary Application Service: AMCAS
Earliest filing date: June 1, 2009
Latest filing date: November 15, 2009

Secondary Application Required?: Yes
Sent to: Screened applicants
URL: www.usouthal.edu
Contact: D. Mark Scott, (251) 460-7176
mscott@usouthal.edu
Fee: Yes, $75
Fee waiver available: Yes
Earliest filing date: June 15, 2009
Latest filing date: December 31, 2009

MCAT® required?: Yes
Latest MCAT® considered: September 2009
Oldest MCAT® considered: 2006

Early Decision Program: School does have EDP
Applicants notified: October 1, 2009
EDP available for: Residents only

Regular Acceptance Notice
Earliest date: November 15, 2009
Latest date: Until class is full
**Applicant's Response to Acceptance
Offer – Maximum Time:** Two weeks

**Requests for Deferred
Entrance Considered:** Yes

Deposit to Hold Place in Class: Yes
Deposit (Resident): $50
Deposit (Non-resident): $50
Deposit due: With response to acceptance offer
Applied to tuition: Yes
Deposit refundable: Yes
Refundable by: May 15, 2010

Estimated number of new entrants: 74

EDP: 15, special program: 5

Start Month/Year: August 2010

Interview Format: Students meet
one-on-one with three interviewers.
Regional interviews are not available.

Other Programs

PREPARATORY PROGRAMS
Postbaccalaureate Program: Yes, Dr. Cindy
Stanfield, (251) 380-2686, cthursto@usouthal.edu
Summer Program: Yes,
Dr. Hattie Myles, (251) 460-7313,
hmyles@usouthal.edu

COMBINED DEGREE PROGRAMS
Baccalaureate/M.D.: Yes, www.usouthal.edu
Chris Lynch, (251) 460-6141, admiss@usouthal.edu
M.D./M.P.H.: No
M.D./M.B.A.: No
M.D./J.D.: No
M.D./Ph.D.: Yes,
www.southalabama.edu/com/programs.shtml,
D. Mark Scott, (251) 460-7176, mscott@usouthal.edu

Premedical Coursework

Course	Req.	Rec.	Lab.	Hrs.
Inorganic Chemistry	•		•	8
Behavioral Sciences				
Biochemistry		•		
Biology	•		•	8
Biology/Zoology				
Calculus		•		
College English	•			6
College Mathematics	•			6

Course	Req.	Rec.	Lab.	Hrs.
Computer Science				
Genetics				
Humanities	•			6
Organic Chemistry	•		•	8
Physics	•		•	8
Psychology				
Social Sciences				
Other				

Selection Factors: 2008 Accepted Applicants

Proportion of Accepted Applicants with Relevant Experience (Data Self-Reported to AMCAS®)		
Community Service/Volunteer	79%
Medically-Related Work	71%
Research	65%

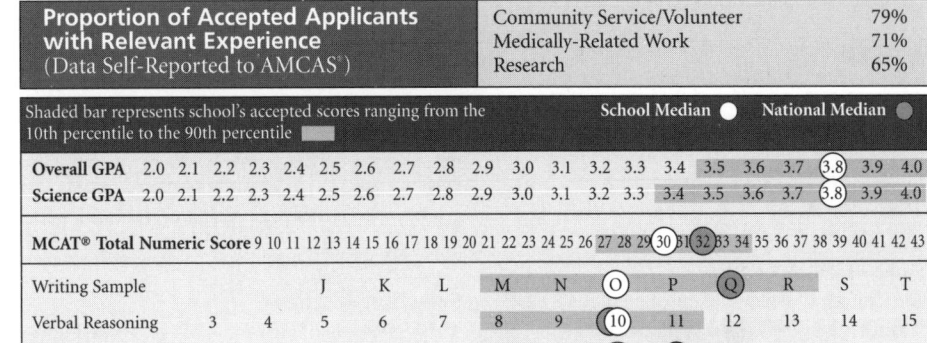

Shaded bar represents school's accepted scores ranging from the 10th percentile to the 90th percentile. School Median ● National Median ●

Overall GPA: 2.0 2.1 2.2 2.3 2.4 2.5 2.6 2.7 2.8 2.9 3.0 3.1 3.2 3.3 3.4 **3.5 3.6 3.7 (3.8)** 3.9 4.0
Science GPA: 2.0 2.1 2.2 2.3 2.4 2.5 2.6 2.7 2.8 2.9 3.0 3.1 3.2 3.3 **3.4 3.5 3.6 3.7 (3.8)** 3.9 4.0

MCAT® Total Numeric Score: 9 10 11 12 13 14 15 16 17 18 19 20 21 22 23 24 25 26 **27 28 29 (30) 31 32 33 34** 35 36 37 38 39 40 41 42 43

Writing Sample			J	K	L	M	N	(O)	P	(Q)	R	S	T
Verbal Reasoning	3	4	5	6	7	8	9	(10)	11	12	13	14	15
Biological Sciences	3	4	5	6	7	8	9	(10)	(11)	12	13	14	15
Physical Sciences	3	4	5	6	7	8	9	(10)	(11)	12	13	14	15

Acceptance & Matriculation Data for 2008–2009 First Year Class

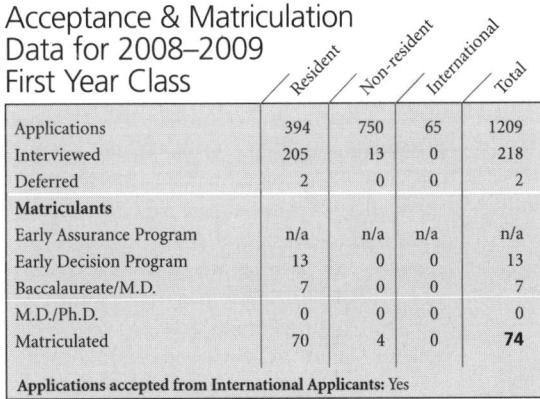

	Resident	Non-resident	International	Total
Applications	394	750	65	1209
Interviewed	205	13	0	218
Deferred	2	0	0	2
Matriculants				
Early Assurance Program	n/a	n/a	n/a	n/a
Early Decision Program	13	0	0	13
Baccalaureate/M.D.	7	0	0	7
M.D./Ph.D.	0	0	0	0
Matriculated	70	4	0	**74**

Applications accepted from International Applicants: Yes

Matriculant Demographics: 2008–2009 First Year Class

Men: 37 **Women:** 37

Matriculants' Self-Reported Race/Ethnicity

Mexican American	0	Korean	1
Cuban	0	Vietnamese	1
Puerto Rican	0	Other Asian	0
Other Hispanic	0	Total Asian	8
Total Hispanic	0	Native American	1
Chinese	1	Black	5
Asian Indian	4	Native Hawaiian	0
Pakistani	1	White	62
Filipino	0	Unduplicated Number	
Japanese	0	of Matriculants	74

Science and Math Majors: 81%
Matriculants with:
  Baccalaureate degree: 99%
  Graduate degree(s): 8%

Specialty Choice

2004, 2005, 2006 Graduates, Specialty Choice (As reported by program directors to GME Track™)	
Anesthesiology	3%
Emergency Medicine	4%
Family Practice	8%
Internal Medicine	25%
Obstetrics/Gynecology	8%
Orthopaedic Surgery	6%
Pediatrics	12%
Psychiatry	1%
Radiology	5%
Surgery	6%

Financial Information

Source: 2007–2008 LCME I-B survey
and 2008–2009 AAMC TSF questionnaire

	Residents	Non-residents
Total Cost of Attendance	$41,340	$56,438
Tuition and Fees	$17,990	$33,088
Other (includes living expenses)	$20,550	$20,550
Health Insurance (can be waived)	$2,800	$2,800

Average 2008 Graduate Indebtedness: $126,692
% of Enrolled Students Receiving Aid: 96%

Criminal Background Check

This medical school does not require a criminal
background check prior to matriculation.

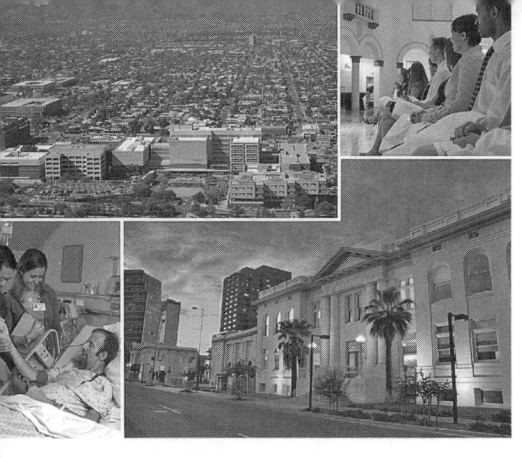

University of Arizona College of Medicine

Tucson, Arizona

Admissions Office, The University of Arizona
College of Medicine
P.O. Box 245075
Tucson, Arizona 85724-5075
T 520 626 6214(T), 602 827 2005(P)
F 520 626 3777(T), 602 827 2212(P)

Admissions www.admissions.medicine.arizona.edu
Main www.medicine.arizona.edu/
Financial www.medicine.arizona.edu/financial-aid
E-mail medapp@email.arizona.edu (T)
phxmed@email.arizona.edu (P)

Public Institution

Dr. Steven Goldschmid, Interim Dean - Tucson

Dr. Stuart D. Flynn, Dean - Phoenix

Dr. Ana Maria Lopez, Associate Dean, Office of Outreach & Multicultural Affairs

Maggie Gumble, Associate Director, Financial Aid

General Information

The College of Medicine enrolled its first class of students in 1967. As a professional and graduate college of The University of Arizona, its programs provide education and training for both the M.D. and Ph.D. degrees. The UACOM has two four-year campuses: the Tucson Campus, adjacent to the UA main campus, and the Phoenix Campus, located in downtown Phoenix.

Mission Statement

The Tucson and Phoenix campuses offer distinct, but related four-year educational programs leading to the M.D. degree. Both are designed for student achievement in the following six core competencies: (1) Medical Knowledge; (2) Patient Care; (3) Interpersonal and Communication skills; (4) Professionalism; (5) Practice-based Learning and Improvement; and (6) Systems-based Practice & Population Health.

Curricular Highlights

Community Service Requirement: Optional.
Research/Thesis Requirement: Optional.

The Tucson and Phoenix educational tracks utilize a similar core structure, while each track contains distinct elements. The first two years of each curriculum are structured in integrated blocks that focus on organs systems or disease states. The second two years consist of required clinical clerkships in key disciplines and significant time for elective work. Basic and clinical science are interwoven with threads, such as behavioral science and humanism, health and society, and interprofessional education. Both curricula emphasize active learning, guided independent learning, working in teams, and early clinical experience. Nearly all students take part in our robust co-curricular activities, including med-

ical student research, rural health and service learning programs.

USMLE

Step 1: Required. Students must record a passing score for graduation, but not promotion.
Step 2: Clinical Skills (CS): Required. Students must only record a score.
Step 2: Clinical Knowledge (CK): Required. Students must record a passing total score to graduate.

Selection Factors

The University of Arizona College of Medicine gives strong preference to residents of Arizona and WICHE applicants from Montana and Wyoming, and Native Americans who reside on reservations contiguous with the State of Arizona. Effective fall 2009, highly qualified nonresident applicants will be considered for up to 25% of the student body. The Admissions Committee considers many factors in evaluating applicants, including the entire academic record, performance on the MCAT, the applicant's personal statement, interviews, and letters of recommendation. Applicants are chosen on the basis of their career goals, motivation, academic ability, integrity, maturity, altruism, communication skills, and leadership abilities. Clinical, research, and community service experiences are viewed favorably. The Admissions Committee strives to accept a student body with diverse backgrounds in order to best meet the medical needs of the people of Arizona. No preference is given to any particular type of undergraduate major. Since many of the patients who receive care at the Arizona Health Sciences Center and its affiliated clinics and hospitals speak Spanish as their primary language, it would be useful for UACOM students to be conversant in Spanish.

Financial Aid

Federal and local scholarships and loans are available to students with financial need. All determinations of need are made after an applicant is accepted for enrollment.

Information about Diversity Programs

We believe in the educational benefits of diversity and actively recruit and admit students with diverse backgrounds and experiences.

Our educational programs include activities where the diversity of the student body contributes to the educational experience. We foster a supportive environment for students of all backgrounds.

Campus Information

Setting

The Tucson campus is adjacent to the campus of The University of Arizona, with all the facilities and services expected of a major university. The College of Medicine is contiguous with University Medical Center and faculty clinics. It is adjacent to the Colleges of Nursing, Pharmacy, and Public Health and to the interdisciplinary Bio5 Research Institute. The University of Arizona College of Medicine-Phoenix in partnership with Arizona State University is located on the Phoenix Biomedical Campus in downtown Phoenix and shares campus with ASU's Department of Biomedical Informatics and the Translational Genomics Research Institute. Within walking distance is ASU's Downtown Campus. Phoenix students train at multiple clinical affiliates throughout the Phoenix metropolitan area. The UACOM has numerous affiliated hospitals and clinical sites and many research affiliations throughout Arizona.

Enrollment

For 2008, total enrollment was: 542

Satellite Campuses/Facilities

The College of Medicine-Phoenix joined in partnership with Arizona State University to expand their two-year clinical experience to a full, four-year curriculum in 2006. In collaboration with Arizona State University, Northern Arizona University and the Translational Genomics Research Institute the educational, research and clinical facilities on the Phoenix Biomedical Campus will be expanded to accommodate a matriculating class of 150 medical students.

Application Process and Requirements 2010–2011

Primary Application Service: AMCAS
Earliest filing date: June 1, 2009
Latest filing date: November 1, 2009

Secondary Application Required?: Yes
Sent to: Selected Applicants
URL: n/a
Fee: Yes, $75
Fee waiver available: Yes
Earliest filing date: July 1, 2009
Latest filing date: January 15, 2010

MCAT® required?: Yes
Latest MCAT® considered: September 2009
Oldest MCAT® considered: 2006

Early Decision Program: School does not have EDP
Applicants notified: n/a
EDP available for: n/a

Regular Acceptance Notice
Earliest date: December 2009
Latest date: Until class is full
Applicant's Response to Acceptance Offer – Maximum Time: Two weeks

Requests for Deferred Entrance Considered: Yes

Deposit to Hold Place in Class: No
Deposit (Resident): n/a
Deposit (Non-resident): n/a
Deposit due: n/a
Applied to tuition: n/a
Deposit refundable: n/a
Refundable by: n/a

Estimated number of new entrants: 158

EDP: n/a, special program: n/a

Start Month/Year: July 2010

Interview Format: Two 30 to 50-minute interviews. Regional interviews are not available.

Other Programs

PREPARATORY PROGRAMS
Postbaccalaureate Program: No
Summer Program: No

COMBINED DEGREE PROGRAMS
Baccalaureate/M.D.: No
M.D./M.P.H.: Yes, Lane Johnson, M.D. , M.P.H., (520) 626-6029, lpj@u.arizona.edu
M.D./M.B.A.: Yes, Tanisha N. Price-Johnson, (520) 626-6214, tanishap@email.arizona.edu
M.D./J.D.: No
M.D./Ph.D.: Yes, Maureen Driscoll, (520) 626-1389, maureend@email.arizona.edu

Premedical Coursework

Course	Req.	Rec.	Lab.	Sems.
Inorganic Chemistry	•			2
Behavioral Sciences				
Biochemistry				
Biology				
Biology/Zoology	•			2
Calculus				
College English	•			2
College Mathematics				

Course	Req.	Rec.	Lab.	Sems.
Computer Science				
Genetics				
Humanities				
Organic Chemistry	•			2
Physics	•			2
Psychology				
Social Sciences				
Other				

Selection Factors: 2008 Accepted Applicants

Proportion of Accepted Applicants with Relevant Experience (Data Self-Reported to AMCAS®)		
Community Service/Volunteer		69%
Medically-Related Work		90%
Research		81%

Shaded bar represents school's accepted scores ranging from the 10th percentile to the 90th percentile. School Median ● National Median ●

Overall GPA 2.0 2.1 2.2 2.3 2.4 2.5 2.6 2.7 2.8 2.9 3.0 3.1 3.2 3.3 3.4 3.5 3.6 (3.7) 3.8 3.9 4.0
Science GPA 2.0 2.1 2.2 2.3 2.4 2.5 2.6 2.7 2.8 2.9 3.0 3.1 3.2 3.3 3.4 3.5 3.6 (3.7) 3.8 3.9 4.0

MCAT® Total Numeric Score 9 10 11 12 13 14 15 16 17 18 19 20 21 22 23 24 25 26 27 28 29 (30) 31 (32) 33 34 35 36 37 38 39 40 41 42 43

Writing Sample		J	K	L	M	N	O	P	(Q)	R	S	T
Verbal Reasoning	3	4	5	6	7	8	9	(10)	11	12	13	14	15
Biological Sciences	3	4	5	6	7	8	9	(10)	(11)	12	13	14	15
Physical Sciences	3	4	5	6	7	8	9	(10)	(11)	12	13	14	15

Acceptance & Matriculation Data for 2008–2009 First Year Class

	Resident	Non-resident	International	Total
Applications	641	206	8	855
Interviewed	553	26	1	579
Deferred	4	0	0	4
Matriculants				
Early Assurance Program	n/a	n/a	n/a	n/a
Early Decision Program	0	0	0	0
Baccalaureate/M.D.	n/a	n/a	n/a	n/a
M.D./Ph.D.	1	0	0	1
Matriculated	156	1	1	**158**

Applications accepted from International Applicants: No

Specialty Choice

2004, 2005, 2006 Graduates, Specialty Choice (As reported by program directors to GME Track™)

Anesthesiology	6%
Emergency Medicine	9%
Family Practice	13%
Internal Medicine	13%
Obstetrics/Gynecology	4%
Orthopaedic Surgery	2%
Pediatrics	18%
Psychiatry	3%
Radiology	5%
Surgery	7%

Matriculant Demographics: 2008–2009 First Year Class

Men: 66   **Women:** 92

Matriculants' Self-Reported Race/Ethnicity

Mexican American	10	Korean	4
Cuban	0	Vietnamese	3
Puerto Rican	2	Other Asian	5
Other Hispanic	5	Total Asian	36
Total Hispanic	16	Native American	1
Chinese	9	Black	4
Asian Indian	14	Native Hawaiian	1
Pakistani	1	White	112
Filipino	1	Unduplicated Number	
Japanese	0	of Matriculants	158

Science and Math Majors: 68%
Matriculants with:
     Baccalaureate degree: 99%
     Graduate degree(s): 15%

Financial Information

Source: 2007–2008 LCME I-B survey and 2008–2009 AAMC TSF questionnaire

	Residents	Non-residents*
Total Cost of Attendance	$40,833	$40,833
Tuition and Fees	$18,776	$18,776
Other (includes living expenses)	$20,513	$20,153
Health Insurance (not applicable)	$1,544	$1,544

*Non-resident tuition rates TBD. See School's Web site.

Average 2008 Graduate Indebtedness: $111,894
% of Enrolled Students Receiving Aid: 91%

Criminal Background Check

This medical school does not require a criminal background check prior to matriculation.

University of Arkansas College of Medicine

Little Rock, Arkansas

Office of the Dean, University of Arkansas for
Medical Sciences College of Medicine
4301 West Markham Street, Slot 551
Little Rock, Arkansas 72205-7199
T 501 686 5354   **F** 501 686 5873

Admissions www.uams.edu/com/applicants/
Main www.uams.edu/com/
Financial www.uams.edu/com/fin-aid/default.asp
E-mail southtomg@uams.edu

Public Institution

Dr. Debra Fiser, Vice Chancellor and Dean

*Dr. Richard P. Wheeler, Executive Associate
Dean, Academic Affairs*

*Tom G. South, Assistant Dean, Admissions
and Financial Aid*

*Dr. Billy R. Thomas, Associate Dean,
Office of Diversity*

Gina Daulton, Director, Student Financial Aid

*Linda DuPuy, Director of Admissions
and Recruitment*

General Information

In 1879, eight visionary physicians had the
foresight to each invest $625 to secure a charter
from the Arkansas Industrial University. On
October 7, 1879, the medical school opened its
doors to 22 eager students. From these humble
beginnings grew the excellence and prestige
now embodied in the College of Medicine.
Today, the College of Medicine has over 1000
full-time and part-time faculty, over 600 residents, and almost 600 medical students. UAMS
is Arkansas' only institution of professional and
graduate education devoted solely to the health
and biological sciences. In fulfilling its educational mission, the College of Medicine, in
conjunction with the UAMS Medical Center,
provides the environment and opportunities
for students and practitioners alike to learn and
maintain the knowledge and skills required in
the 21st century. Comprehensive services are
delivered in an interdisciplinary environment to
all Arkansans, regardless of their ability to pay.
The school is in the planning phase for a major
expansion initiative: a replacement hospital, new
student housing, new psychiatry center, an
addition to both the Jones Eye Institute and the
Outpatient Center, and a new affiliated state
psychiatric hospital. The university's commitment
is to facilitate discovery through applied research
and to teach the best science and compassionate care to tomorrow's caregivers. As much as
the school is proud of its past achievements, it
believes that its best still lies ahead.

Mission Statement

"In relentless pursuit of excellence, every day"
summarizes the essence of the school's fourfold
mission to teach, to heal, to search, and to serve.

Curricular Highlights

Community Service Requirement: Optional.
Research/Thesis Requirement: Optional.

Along with the standard courses in anatomy,
biochemistry, and physiology, the first year
includes a program to introduce the student to
clinical contacts and concepts. This is accomplished with formal lectures in medico-socioe-
conomic topics, small-group discussions, facul-
ty-supervised interviews with patients, and the
extensive use of standardized patients. The
third year is a full 48 weeks with rotation
through the major clinical services. This
expanded clinical year provides substantial
preparation for the predominantly elective
fourth year, which consists of a minimum of
36 weeks to a maximum of 48 weeks of courses
selected with the assistance of a faculty advisor.
On- and off-campus electives are available to
round out preparation for each student's career
goals. Opportunities are provided for students
to engage in research activities and to pursue
graduate courses leading to the M.D./Ph.D.
and M.D./M.P.H. degrees. The number of
M.D./Ph.D. scholarships has increased significantly in recent years. Students are also provided with expanded opportunities through the
M.D./M.B.A. and M.D./J.D. degree programs.

USMLE

Step 1: Required. Students must record a passing
score for promotion.
Step 2: Clinical Skills (CS): Required. Students
must record a passing total score to graduate.
Step 2: Clinical Knowledge (CK): Required.
Students must record a passing total score to
graduate.

Selection Factors

Selection is based on scholastic attainment,
performance on the MCAT, personal interviews
with members of the faculty, and recommendations, particularly evaluations by college preprofessional advisory committees. Applicants

should also demonstrate time and effort devoted to volunteerism and community service.
Selection is made without regard to race, sex,
creed, national origin, age, or handicap.
Unsuccessful applicants may reapply without
prejudice. Non-Arkansas residents who have
strong ties to Arkansas are encouraged to apply.

Financial Aid

An applicant's financial status is not a factor in
selection for admission. The Rural Practice
Programs allow students who commit to practice
primary care medicine in rural communities in
Arkansas to receive loans during medical
school. The student is obligated to return to a
rural community following residency training
and to practice full time for the same number
of years the student was assisted during medical school. For each year of service, one year
of loans is forgiven until the debt is retired. A
unique feature of the Rural Practice Programs
allows Arkansas residents on the Alternate List,
who are willing to practice full-time in a rural
community in Arkansas, to interview with the
Arkansas Rural Medical Practice Student Loan
and Scholarship Board. If the Board approves
the alternate's Rural Practice Program application, the applicant is advanced to the top of
the alternate list. For additional details, contact
the Financial Aid Office.

Information about Diversity Programs

Students from groups underrepresented in
medicine are encouraged to apply. The Office
of Diversity has developed an active recruitment and retention program. The five-week
Summer Science Program offers an introduction to the medical school curriculum, along
with reading and study skill enrichment sessions designed to strengthen students' mastery
of these areas. A pre-matriculation program is
available to all students accepted for admission.

Campus Information

Enrollment

For 2008, total enrollment was: 603

Application Process and Requirements 2010–2011

Primary Application Service: AMCAS
Earliest filing date: July 1, 2009
Latest filing date: November 1, 2009

Secondary Application Required?: Yes
Sent to: All applicants
URL: www.uams.edu
Contact: Tom South, (501) 686-5354
SouthTomG@uams.edu
Fee: Yes, $100
Fee waiver available: Yes
Earliest filing date: July 1, 2009
Latest filing date: November 1, 2009

MCAT® required?: Yes
Latest MCAT® considered: September 2009
Oldest MCAT® considered: April 2007

Early Decision Program: School does not have EDP
Applicants notified: n/a
EDP available for: n/a

Regular Acceptance Notice
Earliest date: December 15, 2009
Latest date: Until class is full
Applicant's Response to Acceptance Offer – Maximum Time: Two weeks

Requests for Deferred Entrance Considered: Yes

Deposit to Hold Place in Class: No
Deposit (Resident): n/a
Deposit (Non-resident): n/a
Deposit due: n/a
Applied to tuition: n/a
Deposit refundable: n/a
Refundable by: n/a

Estimated number of new entrants: 160
EDP: 160, special program: n/a

Start Month/Year: August 2010

Interview Format: Team interviews on scheduled interview dates. All interviews are conducted on campus.

Other Programs

PREPARATORY PROGRAMS
Postbaccalaureate Program: No
Summer Program: Yes, www.uams.edu/physiology/eduadv/main.htm
Dr. James Pasley, (501) 686-5128

COMBINED DEGREE PROGRAMS
Baccalaureate/M.D.: No
M.D./M.P.H.: Yes, www.uams.edu
M.D./M.B.A.: Yes, www.uams.edu
M.D./J.D.: Yes, www.uams.edu
M.D./Ph.D.: Yes, www.uams.edu
William D. Wessinger, PhD

Premedical Coursework

Course	Req.	Rec.	Lab.	Sems.
Inorganic Chemistry	•			2
Behavioral Sciences		•		
Biochemistry		•		
Biology	•			2
Biology/Zoology		•		
Calculus				
College English	•			2
College Mathematics	•			2

Course	Req.	Rec.	Lab.	Sems.
Computer Science		•		
Genetics		•		
Humanities		•		
Organic Chemistry	•			2
Physics	•			2
Psychology		•		
Social Sciences		•		
Spanish & Speech Comm.		•		

Selection Factors: 2008 Accepted Applicants

Proportion of Accepted Applicants with Relevant Experience (Data Self-Reported to AMCAS®)		
Community Service/Volunteer		75%
Medically-Related Work		79%
Research		69%

Shaded bar represents school's accepted scores ranging from the 10th percentile to the 90th percentile.   School Median ●   National Median ●

Overall GPA	2.0	2.1	2.2	2.3	2.4	2.5	2.6	2.7	2.8	2.9	3.0	3.1	3.2	3.3	3.4	3.5	(3.6)	3.7	3.8	3.9	4.0
Science GPA	2.0	2.1	2.2	2.3	2.4	2.5	2.6	2.7	2.8	2.9	3.0	3.1	3.2	3.3	3.4	3.5	(3.6)	3.7	3.8	3.9	4.0

MCAT® Total Numeric Score 9 10 11 12 13 14 15 16 17 18 19 20 21 22 23 24 25 26 27 28 (29) 30 31 (32) 33 34 35 36 37 38 39 40 41 42 43

Writing Sample				J	K	L	M	N	(O)	P	(Q)	R	S	T
Verbal Reasoning	3	4	5	6	7	8	9	(10)	11	12	13	14	15
Biological Sciences	3	4	5	6	7	8	9	(10)	(11)	12	13	14	15
Physical Sciences	3	4	5	6	7	8	(9)	10	(11)	12	13	14	15

Acceptance & Matriculation Data for 2008–2009 First Year Class

	Resident	Non-resident	International	Total
Applications	277	1229	16	1522
Interviewed	260	106	0	366
Deferred	13	5	0	18
Matriculants				
Early Assurance Program	0	0	0	0
Early Decision Program	0	0	0	0
Baccalaureate/M.D.	n/a	n/a	n/a	n/a
M.D./Ph.D.	1	2	0	3
Matriculated	130	24	0	**154**

Applications accepted from International Applicants: No

Matriculant Demographics: 2008–2009 First Year Class

Men: 94   **Women:** 60

Matriculants' Self-Reported Race/Ethnicity

Mexican American	2	**Korean**	0
Cuban	0	**Vietnamese**	2
Puerto Rican	1	**Other Asian**	1
Other Hispanic	2	**Total Asian**	13
Total Hispanic	5	**Native American**	0
Chinese	1	**Black**	14
Asian Indian	6	**Native Hawaiian**	1
Pakistani	2	**White**	124
Filipino	1	**Unduplicated Number**	
Japanese	0	**of Matriculants**	154

Science and Math Majors: 77%
Matriculants with:
Baccalaureate degree: 99%
Graduate degree(s): 18%

Specialty Choice

2004, 2005, 2006 Graduates, Specialty Choice (As reported by program directors to GME Track™)	
Anesthesiology	7%
Emergency Medicine	4%
Family Practice	18%
Internal Medicine	12%
Obstetrics/Gynecology	7%
Orthopaedic Surgery	5%
Pediatrics	7%
Psychiatry	8%
Radiology	5%
Surgery	3%

Financial Information

Source: 2007–2008 LCME I-B survey and 2008–2009 AAMC TSF questionnaire

	Residents	Non-residents
Total Cost of Attendance	$35,072	$51,536
Tuition and Fees	$17,362	$33,826
Other (includes living expenses)	$15,850	$15,850
Health Insurance (can be waived)	$1,860	$1,860

Average 2008 Graduate Indebtedness: $124,841
% of Enrolled Students Receiving Aid: 92%

Criminal Background Check

This medical school requires a criminal background check prior to matriculation.

Keck School of Medicine of the University of Southern California
Los Angeles, California

University of Southern California
Keck School of Medicine, Office of Admissions
1975 Zonal Avenue, KAM 100-C
Los Angeles, California 90089-9021
T 323 442 2552   **F** 323 442 2433

Admissions www.usc.edu/schools/medicine/
education/admissions
Main www.usc.edu/schools/medicine
Financial www.usc.edu/schools/medicine/
education/financial_aid
E-mail medadmit@usc.edu

Private Institution

Dr. Carmen A. Puliafito, Dean

Dr. Erin A. Quinn, Associate Dean for Admissions

Althea Alexander, Assistant Dean for Minority Student Affairs

Gina Camello, Director of Admissions

Alicia M. Rugley, Scholarships and Grants Coordinator

General Information

The Keck School of Medicine of the University of Southern California was established in 1885 as the region's first medical school. All Keck students train at the Los Angeles County+USC Medical Center, one of the largest medical teaching centers in the United States. Through affiliations with over a dozen other private and public hospitals, Keck students have a highly diverse clinical training experience.

Mission Statement

The mission of the Keck School of Medicine is to improve the quality of life for individuals and society by promoting health, preventing and curing disease, advancing biomedical research, and educating tomorrow's physicians and scientists.

Curricular Highlights

Community Service Requirement: Optional.
Research/Thesis Requirement: Optional.

Students are progressively involved with regular patient contact beginning the first week of medical school. An important feature in the curriculum is the Introduction to Clinical Medicine course. The doctor-patient relationship and interviewing are presented during the first year, and physical diagnosis and history-taking are taught in the second. Groups of six to seven students are led by a faculty member who serves as a clinical tutor for their first two years. The curriculum is designed to enhance students' understanding of the basic sciences and their relevance to clinical medicine. Curricular themes are guided by select Pathways and delivered in a case-centered format with the integration of small-group learning

sessions, directed-independent study, and innovative instructional technologies. The first year of the Year I-II continuum begins with 18 weeks of Core Principles of Health and Disease, followed by 49 weeks of organ system review, ending with a 10-week Integrated Case Study section. Each week of the academic year is composed of approximately 20 hours of lecture and small-group sessions, with an additional 20 hours of directed-independent study or Introduction to Clinical Medicine. Examinations in all systems throughout the first two years are graded pass/fail. Dean's Recognition is awarded on the basis of year-end comprehensive examinations and special projects. The final two years are designed as a continuum of two academic calendar years. Each student's program is individually designed to include 50 weeks of required clerkships, 16 weeks of selective clerkships, 16 weeks of elective clerkships, and required senior seminars. Grading for the final two years is on an honors, high pass, pass, and fail basis.

USMLE

Step 1: Required. Students must record a passing score for promotion.
Step 2: Clinical Skills (CS): Required. Students must only record a score.
Step 2: Clinical Knowledge (CK): Required. Students must only record a score.

Selection Factors

The Admissions Committee seriously considers candidates whose academic achievement and MCAT performance indicate the ability to satisfactorily complete the rigorous demands of the medical school curriculum. Also, the committee evaluates various non-academic factors, including personal motivations, evidence of qualities deemed desirable for the study and practice of medicine, significant achievements in extracurricular pursuits, and demonstrated commitment to service and community.

Financial Aid

A variety of university scholarships and loans are available to supplement federal and state programs. Awards are based on need as demonstrated through a financial statement. Merit based awards are also available.

Information about Diversity Programs

The Office of Diversity at the Keck School of Medicine strives to recruit, enroll, and retain students of all socioeconomic, cultural, and ethnic backgrounds. For additional information and opportunities, please visit *www.usc.edu/schools/medicine/school/offices/diversity.html*.

Campus Information

Setting
Located on USC's Health Sciences Campus, the 31-acre medical campus is part of an ethnically diverse community in northeast Los Angeles. The campus is a short drive away from many of the recreational, cultural, and entertainment activities that Los Angeles has to offer.

Enrollment
For 2008, total enrollment was: 679

Special Features
The Keck School of Medicine ranks in the top 25 U.S. medical schools in terms of federal research support. Its affiliations with Los Angeles County Hospital, one of the nation's largest teaching hospitals, and a number of state-of-the-art private hospitals and centers, provide students with an unparalleled hands-on clinical education in a broad range of diseases and settings.

Housing
On-campus housing is available at Seaver Residence Hall. A majority of students live off-campus in nearby communities, many of which are within five miles of campus. During the summer months, the Student Services Office compiles and posts listings of available housing and roommate announcements to assist students in finding housing.

Satellite Campuses/Facilities
Supervised by Keck School faculty, medical students play a key role in patient care in more than a dozen affiliated hospitals, including the adjacent LAC+USC Medical Center.

Application Process and Requirements 2010–2011

Primary Application Service: AMCAS
Earliest filing date: July 1, 2009
Latest filing date: November 1, 2009

Secondary Application Required?: Yes
Sent to: All AMCAS-certified applicants
URL: www.usc.edu/schools/medicine/ksomnfl.html
Fee: Yes, $90
Fee waiver available: Yes
Earliest filing date: July 1, 2009
Latest filing date: December 1, 2009

MCAT® required?: Yes
Latest MCAT® considered: September 2009
Oldest MCAT® considered: 2006

Early Decision Program: School does have EDP
Applicants notified: September 15, 2009
EDP available for: Both Residents
and Non-residents

Regular Acceptance Notice
Earliest date: November 1, 2009
Latest date: Until class is full
Applicant's Response to Acceptance
Offer – Maximum Time: Ten Days

Requests for Deferred
Entrance Considered: Yes

Deposit to Hold Place in Class: Yes
Deposit (Resident): $100
Deposit (Non-resident): $100
Deposit due: Within ten days after
notification of acceptance
Applied to tuition: Yes
Deposit refundable: No
Refundable by: n/a

Estimated number of new entrants: 168
EDP: 10, special program: n/a

Start Month/Year: August 2010

Interview Format: On-campus
interviews only, closed-file.
Regional interviews are not available.

Other Programs

PREPARATORY PROGRAMS
Postbaccalaureate Program: Yes,
http://chem.usc.edu/undergraduate/premed.html
Summer Program: No

COMBINED DEGREE PROGRAMS
Baccalaureate/M.D.: Yes, www.usc.edu/schools/
medicine/ksomnfl.html
M.D./M.P.H.: Yes, www.usc.edu/schools/medicine/
ksomnfl.html
M.D./M.B.A.: Yes, www.usc.edu/schools/
medicine/ksomnfl.html
M.D./J.D.: No
M.D./Ph.D.: Yes, www.usc.edu/schools/medicine/
ksomnfl.html
Master of Science in Clinical & Biomedical
Investigations: Yes, www.usc.edu/schools/
medicine/ksomnfl.html

Premedical Coursework

Course	Req.	Rec.	Lab.	Sems.
Inorganic Chemistry	•		•	2
Behavioral Sciences				
Biochemistry	•			1
Biology	•		•	2
Biology/Zoology				
Calculus		•		
College English	•			
College Mathematics		•		

Course	Req.	Rec.	Lab.	Sems.
Computer Science		•		
Genetics				
Humanities	•			
Organic Chemistry	•		•	1
Physics	•		•	2
Psychology				
Social Sciences	•			
Molecular Biology	•			1

Selection Factors: 2008 Accepted Applicants

Proportion of Accepted Applicants with Relevant Experience (Data Self-Reported to AMCAS®)		
Community Service/Volunteer		71%
Medically-Related Work		89%
Research		88%

Shaded bar represents school's accepted scores ranging from the 10th percentile to the 90th percentile. **School Median** ○ **National Median** ○

Overall GPA	2.0	2.1	2.2	2.3	2.4	2.5	2.6	2.7	2.8	2.9	3.0	3.1	3.2	3.3	3.4	3.5	3.6	(3.7)	3.8	3.9	4.0
Science GPA	2.0	2.1	2.2	2.3	2.4	2.5	2.6	2.7	2.8	2.9	3.0	3.1	3.2	3.3	3.4	3.5	3.6	(3.7)	3.8	3.9	4.0

MCAT® Total Numeric Score 9 10 11 12 13 14 15 16 17 18 19 20 21 22 23 24 25 26 27 28 29 30 31 (32) 33 (34) 35 36 37 38 39 40 41 42 43

	J	K	L	M	N	O	P	Q	R	S	T
Writing Sample					N	O	P	(Q)	R	S	T

Verbal Reasoning	3	4	5	6	7	8	9	(10)	(11)	12	13	14	15
Biological Sciences	3	4	5	6	7	8	9	10	(11)	(12)	13	14	15
Physical Sciences	3	4	5	6	7	8	9	10	(11)	12	13	14	15

Acceptance & Matriculation Data for 2008–2009 First Year Class

	Resident	Non-resident	International	Total
Applications	3539	2773	306	6618
Interviewed	488	214	14	716
Deferred	5	3	1	9
Matriculants				
Early Assurance Program	n/a	n/a	n/a	n/a
Early Decision Program	1	0	0	1
Baccalaureate/M.D.	11	2	0	13
M.D./Ph.D.	2	1	0	3
Matriculated	121	32	6	**159**

Applications accepted from International Applicants: Yes

Matriculant Demographics: 2008–2009 First Year Class

Men: 86   **Women:** 73

Matriculants' Self-Reported Race/Ethnicity

Mexican American	20	**Korean**	3
Cuban	1	**Vietnamese**	4
Puerto Rican	1	**Other Asian**	3
Other Hispanic	6	**Total Asian**	48
Total Hispanic	26	**Native American**	4
Chinese	24	**Black**	9
Asian Indian	10	**Native Hawaiian**	1
Pakistani	1	**White**	88
Filipino	0	**Unduplicated Number**	
Japanese	8	**of Matriculants**	159

Science and Math Majors: 60%
Matriculants with:
Baccalaureate degree: 100%
Graduate degree(s): 12%

Specialty Choice

2004, 2005, 2006 Graduates, Specialty Choice (As reported by program directors to GME Track™)

Anesthesiology	4%
Emergency Medicine	6%
Family Practice	7%
Internal Medicine	16%
Obstetrics/Gynecology	6%
Orthopaedic Surgery	4%
Pediatrics	8%
Psychiatry	7%
Radiology Diagnostic	5%
Surgery General	7%

Financial Information

Source: 2007–2008 LCME I-B survey
and 2008–2009 AAMC TSF questionnaire

	Residents	Non-residents
Total Cost of Attendance	$71,034	$71,034
Tuition and Fees	$44,188	$44,188
Other (includes living expenses)	$22,920	$22,920
Health Insurance (can be waived)	$926	$926

Average 2008 Graduate Indebtedness: $158,872
% of Enrolled Students Receiving Aid: 93%

Criminal Background Check

This medical school does not require a criminal
background check prior to matriculation.

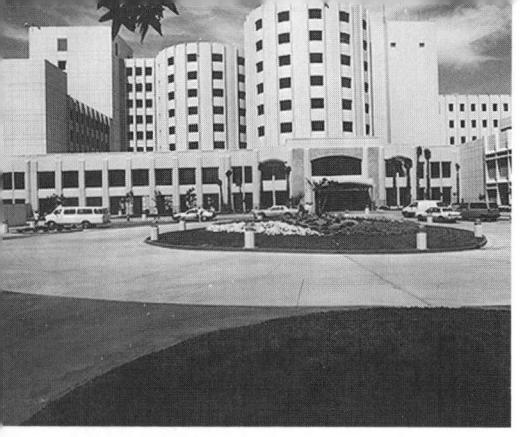

Loma Linda University School of Medicine

Loma Linda, California

Associate Dean for Admissions
Loma Linda University
School of Medicine
Loma Linda, California 92350
T 909 558 4467   **F** 909 558 0359

Admissions www.llu.edu/llu/medicine/
admissions.html
Main www.llu.edu/llu/medicine
Financial www.llu.edu/ssweb/finaid
E-mail admissions.sm@llu.edu

Private Institution

Dr. H. Roger Hadley, Dean

*Dr. Stephen A. Nyirady,
Associate Dean for Admissions*

*Dr. Daisy Deleon, Assistant
to the Dean for Diversity*

Verdell Schaefer, MBA, Financial Aid Director

Lenoa Edwards, Assistant Dean for Admissions

General Information

The School of Medicine was established in 1909. It consists of basic science facilities and the Loma Linda University Medical Center. Also used for clinical instruction are local, regional, county, community, and Veterans Affairs hospitals. The School of Medicine's objectives include providing the student with a solid foundation of medical knowledge, assisting the student to attain professional skills, motivating investigative curiosity, and instilling a desire to participate in the advancement of knowledge. The school reinforces interest in the practical application of Christian principles through service to humanity.

Mission Statement

The school's overriding purpose is the formation of Christian physicians, educated to serve as generalists or specialists and providing whole-person care to individuals, families, and communities.

Curricular Highlights

Community Service Requirement: Optional.
Research/Thesis Requirement: Optional.
Numerous opportunities available

The School of Medicine seeks to prepare students who will be well grounded in the science and art of medicine. The first two years involve an organ systems-based approach to the study of the biomedical sciences, including their application to clinical medicine. The last two years provide clinical rotations in the major areas of medical practice: surgery, internal medicine, pediatrics, obstetrics-gynecology, family medicine, emergency medicine, ambulatory care, psychiatry, and preventive medicine. Elective time is available for additional experience in clinical or research areas. Qualified stu-

dents interested in a career in academic medicine may earn an M.S. or Ph.D. degree along with the M.D. degree in a total of six to eight years. Student performance is evaluated by standard or scaled scores. The grading system is on a pass/fail basis.

USMLE

Step 1: Required. Students must record a passing score for promotion.
Step 2: Clinical Skills (CS): Required. Students must record a passing total score to graduate.
Step 2: Clinical Knowledge (CK): Required. Students must record a passing total score to graduate.

Selection Factors

The MCAT and a minimum of three years (90 semester hours or 135 quarter hours) of collegiate preparation in an accredited college or university in the U.S. or Canada are required. Preference is given to applicants who will have completed the baccalaureate degree prior to matriculation. No specific major is preferred. Demonstrated ability in the sciences is important. CLEP and pass/fail credits are not acceptable for required courses. Applicants are urged to take the MCAT by the spring of the application year. The Admissions Committee seeks candidates who have demonstrated the greatest potential for becoming capable physicians. A strong academic background is needed in preparation for medical studies. While special attention is given to performance in science courses, candidates should also have a solid foundation in the humanities, social sciences, and human behavior. The Admissions Committee seeks applicants who demonstrate problem-solving skills, critical judgment, and the ability to pursue independent study and thinking. For nonacademic qualifications, the committee looks for a commitment to medicine, sound judgment, a positive attitude, the ability to make decisions, participation in meaningful extracurricular activities, emotional stability, and integrity. The School of Medicine is owned and operated by the Seventh-day Adventist Church. While, therefore, preference for admission is given to members of this church, it is a firm policy of the Admissions Committee to admit a number of applicants from other faith traditions who have demonstrated a strong

commitment to Christian principles. No candidate is accepted on the basis of religious affiliation alone. The school does not discriminate on the basis of race, sex, age, or handicap. After receipt of the AMCAS application, each applicant is requested to submit a supplementary form and supply preprofessional faculty evaluations and/or personal letters of recommendation. Invitations for an interview are extended to selected applicants. Applicants with an outstanding academic record and with a particular interest in Loma Linda University School of Medicine are encouraged to apply through the Early Decision Program (EDP). Final selections are made by the Admissions Committee on the basis of overall scholastic record, personal qualities, promise of success as a physician, and commitment to the school's mission.

Financial Aid

The School of Medicine has loan funds available through the Student Finance Office. All aid is awarded on the basis of a uniform needs analysis. Financial aid information is provided to all accepted students. In view of the costs of a medical education, students are urged to plan their financial programs carefully.

Information about Diversity Programs

The School of Medicine encourages applications from persons from groups underrepresented in medicine. The Assistant to the Dean for Diversity works closely with the Office of Admissions to facilitate the admissions process for these applicants.

Campus Information

Enrollment

For 2008, total enrollment was: 718

Application Process and Requirements 2010–2011

Primary Application Service: AMCAS
Earliest filing date: June 1, 2009
Latest filing date: November 1, 2009

Secondary Application Required?: Yes
Sent to: All applicants
URL: Made available upon receipt of verified AMCAS application
Contact: Office of Admissions, (909) 558-4467, admissions.sm@llu.edu
Fee: Yes, $75
Fee waiver available: Yes
Earliest filing date: July 1, 2009
Latest filing date: November 15, 2009

MCAT® required?: Yes
Latest MCAT® considered: September 2009
Oldest MCAT® considered: 2007

Early Decision Program: School does have EDP
Applicants notified: October 1, 2009
EDP available for: Both Residents and Non-residents

Regular Acceptance Notice
Earliest date: December 15, 2009
Latest date: Until class is full
Applicant's Response to Acceptance Offer – Maximum Time: 30 days

Requests for Deferred Entrance Considered: Yes

Deposit to Hold Place in Class: Yes
Deposit (Resident): $100
Deposit (Non-resident): $100
Deposit due: With acceptance offer
Applied to tuition: Yes
Deposit refundable: Yes
Refundable by: May 15, 2010

Estimated number of new entrants: 165
EDP: 10, special program: n/a

Start Month/Year: August 2010

Interview Format: Regional interviews are not available.

Other Programs

PREPARATORY PROGRAMS
Postbaccalaureate Program: No
Summer Program: No

Combined Degree Programs
Baccalaureate/M.D.: No
M.D./M.P.H.: No
M.D./M.B.A.: No
M.D./J.D.: No
M.D./Ph.D.: Yes, www.llu.edu/llu/medicine/basicsciences/msp.html
Lawrence Sowers, PhD, (909) 558-4480, lsowers@llu.edu

Premedical Coursework

Course	Req.	Rec.	Lab.	Hrs.
Inorganic Chemistry	•		•	8
Behavioral Sciences				
Biochemistry		•		
Biology				
Biology/Zoology	•		•	8
Calculus				
College English	•			
College Mathematics				

Course	Req.	Rec.	Lab.	Hrs.
Computer Science		•		
Genetics				
Humanities				
Organic Chemistry	•		•	8
Physics	•		•	8
Psychology				
Social Sciences				
Intro to Basic Statistics		•		

Selection Factors: 2008 Accepted Applicants

Proportion of Accepted Applicants with Relevant Experience (Data Self-Reported to AMCAS)	
Community Service/Volunteer	70%
Medically-Related Work	69%
Research	62%

Shaded bar represents school's accepted scores ranging from the 10th percentile to the 90th percentile. School Median ● National Median ◐

Overall GPA 2.0 2.1 2.2 2.3 2.4 2.5 2.6 2.7 2.8 2.9 3.0 3.1 3.2 3.3 3.4 *3.5 3.6 3.7* (3.8) 3.9 4.0
Science GPA 2.0 2.1 2.2 2.3 2.4 2.5 2.6 2.7 2.8 2.9 3.0 3.1 3.2 3.3 *3.4 3.5 3.6 3.7* (3.8) 3.9 4.0

MCAT® Total Numeric Score 9 10 11 12 13 14 15 16 17 18 19 20 21 22 23 24 *25 26 27 28 29* (30) 31 (32) 33 34 35 36 37 38 39 40 41 42 43

			J	K	L	M	N	O	P	Q	R	S	T
Writing Sample			J	K	L	M	N	O	(P)	(Q)	R	S	T
Verbal Reasoning	3	4	5	6	7	8	9	(10)	11	12	13	14	15
Biological Sciences	3	4	5	6	7	8	9	(10)	(11)	12	13	14	15
Physical Sciences	3	4	5	6	7	8	9	(10)	(11)	12	13	14	15

Acceptance & Matriculation Data for 2008–2009 First Year Class

	Resident	Non-resident	International	Total
Applications	2026	2183	264	4473
Interviewed	193	188	17	398
Deferred	5	12	1	18
Matriculants				
Early Assurance Program	0	0	0	0
Early Decision Program	3	7	0	10
Baccalaureate/M.D.	n/a	n/a	n/a	n/a
M.D./Ph.D.	1	2	3	6
Matriculated	80	76	9	**165**

Applications accepted from International Applicants: Yes

Specialty Choice

2004, 2005, 2006 Graduates, Specialty Choice (As reported by program directors to GME Track™)

Anesthesiology	9%
Emergency Medicine	7%
Family Practice	15%
Internal Medicine	15%
Obstetrics/Gynecology	3%
Orthopaedic Surgery	2%
Pediatrics	5%
Psychiatry	6%
Radiology	2%
Surgery	7%

Matriculant Demographics: 2008–2009 First Year Class

Men: 110 **Women:** 55

Matriculants' Self-Reported Race/Ethnicity

Mexican American	2	Korean	13
Cuban	1	Vietnamese	4
Puerto Rican	2	Other Asian	2
Other Hispanic	13	Total Asian	45
Total Hispanic	17	Native American	3
Chinese	16	Black	10
Asian Indian	6	Native Hawaiian	1
Pakistani	1	White	100
Filipino	7	Unduplicated Number	
Japanese	1	of Matriculants	165

Science and Math Majors: 70%
Matriculants with:
   Baccalaureate degree: 99%
   Graduate degree(s): 4%

Financial Information
Source: 2007–2008 LCME I-B survey and 2008–2009 AAMC TSF questionnaire

	Residents	Non-residents
Total Cost of Attendance	$61,591	$61,591
Tuition and Fees	$37,610	$37,610
Other (includes living expenses)	$22,469	$22,469
Health Insurance (can be waived)	$1,512	$1,512

Average 2008 Graduate Indebtedness: $157,640
% of Enrolled Students Receiving Aid: 92%

Criminal Background Check

This medical school requires a criminal background check prior to matriculation.

Stanford University School of Medicine

Stanford, California

Office of M.D. Admissions
Stanford University School of Medicine
251 Campus Drive, MSOB X301
Stanford, California 94305-5404
T 650 723 6861   F 650 725 7855

Admissions http://med.stanford.edu/md/admissions
Main http://med.stanford.edu
Financial http://med.stanford.edu/md/financial_aid
E-mail mdadmissions@stanford.edu

Private Institution

Dr. Philip A. Pizzo, Dean

Dr. Gabriel Garcia, Associate Dean of Medical School Admissions

Dr. Ronald D. Garcia, Assistant Dean of Minority Affairs

Charlene Hamada, Assistant Dean of Student Affairs

Jonathan Perez, Assistant Director of Medical School Admissions

General Information

The School of Medicine is an integral part of Stanford University. The history of Stanford Medical School begins in 1858 with the founding in San Francisco by Dr. Elias Samuel Cooper of the first medical school on the Pacific Coast. Stanford's School of Medicine is the lineal descendent of this pioneer medical school. In 1908, Stanford University adopted the Cooper Medical College in San Francisco as its medical school and moved it to the university campus in 1959. The Stanford School of Medicine is consistently ranked in the top ten of all research university medical centers in the country.

Mission Statement

Stanford is committed to being a premier research-intensive medical school that improves health through leadership, collaborative discoveries, and innovation in patient care, education, and research. In particular, Stanford seeks individuals whose leadership will result in significant advances in the ability to care for patients. We strive to admit a diverse body of students who are interested in the intellectual substance of medicine and are committed to advancing the field of medicine, broadly defined (i.e. clinical medicine, biomedical sciences, health policy, medical education, and community health).

Curricular Highlights

Community Service Requirement: Optional. Opportunities available and encouraged.
Research/Thesis Requirement: Optional. Opportunities available and encouraged.

Stanford is committed to ensuring that each graduate has fully explored his/her potential as a student and as a scholar. Key goals of the curriculum are the melding of 21st century laboratory and medical sciences, and helping each student build in-depth expertise in an area of personal interest through our Scholarly Concentrations program. While traditional courses and clerkships are required for graduation, the duration of study leading to the M.D. degree may vary from four to six years. All M.D. candidates must satisfactorily complete at least 13 quarters of academic work. Fees for additional quarters are nominal. Courses are graded pass/fail.

USMLE

Step 1: Required. Students must record a passing score for promotion.
Step 2: Clinical Skills (CS): Required. Students must record a passing total score to graduate.
Step 2: Clinical Knowledge (CK): Required. Students must record a passing total score to graduate.

Selection Factors

Stanford does not discriminate on the basis of race, religion, national origin, sex, marital status, age, or disability. The applicant's state of residence is not relevant in the selection process. Applicants whose MCAT scores are below the national mean are highly unlikely to be admitted to the medical school. Transfer Students: For information on the transfer policy, see the Stanford Web site.

Financial Aid

Available grant and loan funds are awarded to students on the basis of demonstrated need. Our generous financial aid program allows our students to graduate with one of the lowest educational debts for any medical school, private or public. For federal aid, students are considered to be independent. For university-based aid, students are considered to be dependent up until the age of 30, and the school will consider the student's parents' ability to contribute to the cost of financing the student's education in determining eligibility for institutional loans and grants. Foreign students must complete a certification of finances reflecting an account of funds to cover the cost of education for the M.D. degree.

Information about Diversity Programs

Stanford takes pride in its highly diverse and exceptionally qualified student body and is committed to increasing the representation of members of groups underrepresented in medicine. A year long program in Leadership in Health Disparities provides all Stanford medical students with the skills, attitudes and knowledge to address the social determinants of health and understand the urgency to provide access to high quality care to all communities.

Campus Information

Setting

The school is located on the 8,800 acre campus of Stanford University (second largest university complex in the world) and is situated in Northern California, approximately 35 miles south of San Francisco and 25 miles north of San Jose.

Enrollment

For 2008, total enrollment was: 465

Special Features

The combination of scientists who pursue basic science research questions and clinicians closely involved in patient care leads to innovative, fruitful collaboration. An example is Bio-X, a unique program designed to promote interdepartmental bioscience research. The program fosters the convergence of leading-edge research in basic, applied and clinical sciences across the spectrum from molecules to organisms. The program involves the schools of Humanities and Sciences, Engineering, and Medicine and is housed in the James H. Clark Center for Biomedical and Engineering Sciences.

Housing

On-campus housing is guaranteed for the first year.

Satellite Campuses/Facilities

Student rotations take place in the major clinical teaching facilities: Stanford Hospital (663 beds), Lucile Packard Children's Hospital (152 beds), Santa Clara County Valley Medical Center (791 beds), the Palo Alto Veterans Affairs Hospital (1,000 beds), and Kaiser Santa Clara Medical Center (327 beds).

Application Process and Requirements 2010–2011

Primary Application Service: AMCAS
Earliest filing date: June 1, 2009
Latest filing date: October 15, 2009

Secondary Application Required?: Yes
Sent to: All applicants
URL: https://med.stanford.edu/aes/
Fee: Yes, $80
Fee waiver available: Yes
Earliest filing date: July 1, 2009
Latest filing date: November 15, 2009

MCAT® required?: Yes
Latest MCAT® considered: September 2009
Oldest MCAT® considered: August 2006

Early Decision Program: School does have EDP
Applicants notified: October 1, 2009
EDP available for: Both Residents and Non-residents

**Regular Acceptance Notice
Earliest date:** December 2009
Latest date: Until class is full
Applicant's Response to Acceptance Offer – Maximum Time: Two weeks

Requests for Deferred Entrance Considered: Yes

Deposit to Hold Place in Class: Yes
Deposit (Resident): $100
Deposit (Non-resident): $100
Deposit due: May 15, 2010
Applied to tuition: Yes
Deposit refundable: Yes
Refundable by: May 15, 2010

Estimated number of new entrants: 86
EDP: 1, special program: n/a

Start Month/Year: August 2010

Interview Format: One faculty and one student interview. Regional interviews are not available.

Other Programs

PREPARATORY PROGRAMS
Postbaccalaureate Program: No
Summer Program: Yes, http://coe.stanford.edu/

COMBINED DEGREE PROGRAMS
Baccalaureate/M.D.: No
M.D./M.P.H.: Yes, http://med.stanford.edu/md-mph/
M.D./M.B.A.: No
M.D./J.D.: No
M.D./Ph.D.: Yes, http://mstp.stanford.edu

Premedical Coursework

Course	Req.	Rec.	Lab.	Sems.
Inorganic Chemistry	•		•	2
Behavioral Sciences		•		
Biochemistry		•		
Biology	•		•	2
Biology/Zoology				
Calculus		•		
College English		•		
College Mathematics				

Course	Req.	Rec.	Lab.	Sems.
Computer Science				
Genetics		•		
Humanities		•		
Organic Chemistry	•		•	2
Physics	•		•	2
Psychology				
Social Sciences		•		
Other 1 & 2		•		

Selection Factors: 2008 Accepted Applicants

Proportion of Accepted Applicants with Relevant Experience (Data Self-Reported to AMCAS®)		
Community Service/Volunteer	67%
Medically-Related Work	88%
Research	98%

Shaded bar represents school's accepted scores ranging from the 10th percentile to the 90th percentile   School Median ●   National Median ●

Overall GPA	2.0	2.1	2.2	2.3	2.4	2.5	2.6	2.7	2.8	2.9	3.0	3.1	3.2	3.3	3.4	3.5	3.6	3.7	(3.8)	3.9	4.0
Science GPA	2.0	2.1	2.2	2.3	2.4	2.5	2.6	2.7	2.8	2.9	3.0	3.1	3.2	3.3	3.4	3.5	3.6	3.7	(3.8)	3.9	4.0

MCAT® Total Numeric Score 9 10 11 12 13 14 15 16 17 18 19 20 21 22 23 24 25 26 27 28 29 30 31 (32) 33 34 (35) 36 37 38 39 40 41 42 43

Writing Sample			J	K	L	M	N	O	P	(Q)	(R)	S	T
Verbal Reasoning	3	4	5	6	7	8	9	(10)	(11)	12	13	14	15
Biological Sciences	3	4	5	6	7	8	9	10	(11)	(12)	13	14	15
Physical Sciences	3	4	5	6	7	8	9	10	(11)	(12)	13	14	15

Acceptance & Matriculation Data for 2008–2009 First Year Class

	Resident	Non-resident	International	Total
Applications	2504	3716	347	6567
Interviewed	178	268	17	463
Deferred	3	3	2	8
Matriculants				
Early Assurance Program	n/a	n/a	n/a	n/a
Early Decision Program	0	0	0	0
Baccalaureate/M.D.	n/a	n/a	n/a	n/a
M.D./Ph.D.	2	8	0	10
Matriculated	33	50	3	**86**

Applications accepted from International Applicants: Yes

Matriculant Demographics: 2008–2009 First Year Class

Men: 40   **Women:** 46

Matriculants' Self-Reported Race/Ethnicity

Mexican American	6	Korean	3
Cuban	3	Vietnamese	2
Puerto Rican	1	Other Asian	6
Other Hispanic	4	Total Asian	30
Total Hispanic	13	Native American	3
Chinese	8	Black	2
Asian Indian	8	Native Hawaiian	0
Pakistani	1	White	46
Filipino	0	Unduplicated Number	
Japanese	2	of Matriculants	86

Science and Math Majors: 71%
Matriculants with:
    Baccalaureate degree: 100%
    Graduate degree(s): 19%

Specialty Choice

2004, 2005, 2006 Graduates, Specialty Choice (As reported by program directors to GME Track™)	
Anesthesiology	6%
Emergency Medicine	6%
Family Practice	7%
Internal Medicine	13%
Obstetrics/Gynecology	3%
Orthopaedic Surgery	5%
Pediatrics	8%
Psychiatry	7%
Radiology	6%
Surgery	6%

Financial Information

Source: 2007–2008 LCME I-B survey and 2008–2009 AAMC TSF questionnaire

	Residents	Non-residents
Total Cost of Attendance	$70,988	$70,988
Tuition and Fees	$43,620	$43,620
Other (includes living expenses)	$25,100	$25,100
Health Insurance (can be waived)	$2,268	$2,268

Average 2008 Graduate Indebtedness: $86,137
% of Enrolled Students Receiving Aid: 79%

Criminal Background Check

This medical school does not require a criminal background check prior to matriculation.

University of California, Davis, School of Medicine
Sacramento, California

Office of Admissions
UC Davis School of Medicine
4610 X Street, Suite 1202
Sacramento California 95817
T 916 734 4800

Admissions www.ucdmc.ucdavis.edu/ome/admissions/
Main www.ucdmc.ucdavis.edu/medschool
Financial www.ucdmc.ucdavis.edu/ome/finaid/
E-mail medadmsinfo@ucdavis.edu

Public Institution

Dr. Claire Pomeroy, Dean

Edward D. Dagang, Director of Admissions

Dr. Mark Henderson, Associate Dean, Admissions

Lauren Snow, Financial Aid Director

Dr. Darin Latimore, Director, Medical Student Diversity

General Information
With a new, state-of-the-art home on the Sacramento campus, the UC Davis School of medicine prides itself in offering a rich and diverse academic environment. The school grooms students for leadership roles in medicine, research, health policy, medical education and management/administration. Distinctions include: ranking in the top 50 schools for research and primary care, strong, dual-degree programs (M.P.H., M.B.A., Ph.D.), and a new five-year program for students interested in telecommunications-enhanced rural medicine. The school admitted its first class in 1968.

Mission Statement
With a mantra of, "Learn. Discover. Share.", the school's educational mission is to create a supportive and collaborative environment which empowers students to develop skills, knowledge and attitudes to become tomorrow's leaders in patient care, public service, research and education. The mission of the larger UC Davis Health System is "discovering and sharing knowledge to advance health."

Curricular Highlights
Community Service Requirement: Optional.
Research/Thesis Requirement: Optional.

UC Davis believes that acquiring and perfecting the skills needed to become a compassionate, culturally-competent and knowledgeable physician requires a combination of hands-on experiences, didactic instruction and problem-based challenges. With an emphasis on self-directed and small group learning, our curriculum is designed to encourage students to evaluate, think and formulate decisions to provide the highest level of patient care. Basic and clinical science courses are designed to illuminate situ-

ations that arise in the clinical setting as well as to spark interest in biomedical research, public health and other areas. A cutting-edge Clinical Skills Center in our new medical education building maximizes technology's role in learning from standardized patients. Finally, our students gain valuable experience through their leadership roles in the community, including our seven student-run free health clinics which benefit various underserved populations in the diverse Sacramento area.

USMLE
Step 1: Required. Students must record a passing score for promotion.
Step 2: Clinical Skills (CS): Required. Students must record a passing total score to graduate.
Step 2: Clinical Knowledge (CK): Required. Students must record a passing total score to graduate.

Selection Factors
Academic strengths in both physical/biological sciences and humanities are valued, as are experiences in both research and clinical care. We look for a broad array of life experiences which align with our institutional values of diversity, equality, community engagement and accessible healthcare.

Financial Aid
Most financial aid is based on demonstrated need, and a wide range of scholarships, fellowships, grants and loans are available. All students are considered for university-awarded, merit and need-based scholarships.

Information about Diversity Programs
Our curriculum's emphasis on cultural competency aligns well with our diverse medical student body, which reflects the diversity of California. The health system often hosts and/or sponsors local, state and regional meetings of medical student organizations including the Latino Medical Student Association and the Student National Medical Association. The UC Davis Health System's Office of Diversity is committed to fostering a supportive environment that maximizes the learning and working experiences for all medical students, residents, faculty and staff.

Campus Information

Setting
The new Medical Education building is located on UC Davis' growing Sacramento campus. The 140-acre campus is adjacent to downtown Sacramento and is home to our level-one trauma teaching hospital (UC Davis Medical Center), our Children's Hospital, our NCI-designate Cancer Center, a leading national autism facility called the MIND Institute, our outpatient clinics, and a variety of research labs. The Sacramento campus will also soon be home to the UC Davis Institute for Regenerative Cures, the UC Davis Betty Irene Moore School of Nursing and the California Telemedicine Resource Center.

Enrollment
For 2008, total enrollment was: 402

Special Features
The school continues to rise quickly in NIH rankings and was awarded one of the first twelve prestigious NIH Clinical and Translational Science Awards in 2006. In 2005, the school won the AAMC's Outstanding Community Service Award.

Housing
Most students reside in communities surrounding the Sacramento campus, including the thriving urban Midtown area. Sacramento residents benefit from a variety of recreational, cultural, political and nightlife activities while living in one of California's more manageable and navigable cities.

Satellite Campuses/Facilities
Most clinical rotations take place at the UC Davis Medical Center in Sacramento and other facilities in the UC Davis Health System. Others take place at Sacramento's Kaiser, Sutter and Methodist hospitals as well as David Grant Medical Center at Travis Air Force Base and San Joaquin General Hospital in Stockton. Students enrolled in our new Rural-PRIME program have opportunities to rotate through our rural hospital network sites and some students gain credit at hospitals and clinics abroad.

Application Process and Requirements 2010–2011

Primary Application Service: AMCAS
Earliest filing date: June 1, 2009
Latest filing date: October 1, 2009

Secondary Application Required?: Yes
Sent to: Screened applicants
Contact: Terri Hall
(916)734-4800, terri.hall@ucdmc.ucdavis.edu
Fee: Yes, $60
Fee waiver available: Yes
Earliest filing date: July 1, 2009
Latest filing date: February 1, 2010

MCAT® required?: Yes
Latest MCAT® considered: September 2009
Oldest MCAT® considered: August 2006

Early Decision Program: School does not have EDP
Applicants notified: n/a
EDP available for: n/a

Regular Acceptance Notice
Earliest date: October 15, 2009
Latest date: Until class is full
Applicant's Response to Acceptance Offer – Maximum Time: Two weeks

Requests for Deferred Entrance Considered: Yes

Deposit to Hold Place in Class: No
Deposit (Resident): n/a
Deposit (Non-resident): n/a
Deposit due: n/a
Applied to tuition: n/a
Deposit refundable: n/a
Refundable by: n/a

Estimated number of new entrants: 105
EDP: n/a, special program: n/a

Start Month/Year: End of July 2010

Interview Format: Open file, two interviews. Regional interviews are not available.

Other Programs

PREPARATORY PROGRAMS
Postbaccalaureate Program: Yes,
www.ucdmc.ucdavis.edu/ome/postbacc/index.html
Summer Program: No

COMBINED DEGREE PROGRAMS
Baccalaureate/M.D.: No
M.D./M.P.H.: Yes, http://mph.ucdavis.edu
Stephen McCurdy, M.D.
(530) 752-8051, samccurdy@ucdavis.edu
M.D./M.B.A.: Yes, www.gsm.ucdavis.edu/students
David L. Woodruff, (530) 752-0515
dlwoodruff@ucdavis.edu
M.D./J.D.: No
M.D./Ph.D.: Yes, http://mdphd.ucdavis.edu
Michael F. Seldin, M.D., Ph.D.
(530) 754-6016, mfseldin@ucdavis.edu

Additional Program: www.ucdmc.ucdavis.edu/
medschool/rural_prime/
Rebecca Miller, (916) 734-4105,
rebecca.miller@ucdmc.ucdavis.edu

Premedical Coursework

Course	Req.	Rec.	Lab.	Qtrs.
Inorganic Chemistry	•		•	3
Behavioral Sciences		•		
Biochemistry		•		1
Biology	•		•	3
Biology/Zoology				
Calculus		•		2
College English	•			3
College Mathematics	•			3
Computer Science				

Course	Req.	Rec.	Lab.	Qtrs.
Genetics		•		1
Humanities		•		
Organic Chemistry	•		•	3
Physics	•		•	3
Psychology				
Social Sciences		•		
College Statistics	•			1
Advanced Biology	•			2
Other				

Selection Factors: 2008 Accepted Applicants

Proportion of Accepted Applicants with Relevant Experience (Data Self-Reported to AMCAS®)		
Community Service/Volunteer	71%
Medically-Related Work	92%
Research	91%

Shaded bar represents school's accepted scores ranging from the 10th percentile to the 90th percentile ▒   **School Median** ●   **National Median** ●

Overall GPA	2.0	2.1	2.2	2.3	2.4	2.5	2.6	2.7	2.8	2.9	3.0	3.1	3.2	3.3	3.4	3.5	3.6	(3.7)	3.8	3.9	4.0
Science GPA	2.0	2.1	2.2	2.3	2.4	2.5	2.6	2.7	2.8	2.9	3.0	3.1	3.2	3.3	3.4	3.5	3.6	(3.7)	3.8	3.9	4.0

MCAT® Total Numeric Score 9 10 11 12 13 14 15 16 17 18 19 20 21 22 23 24 25 26 27 28 29 30 31 (32) 33 (34) 35 36 37 38 39 40 41 42 43

Writing Sample			J	K	L	M	N	O	P	(Q)	R	S	T
Verbal Reasoning	3	4	5	6	7	8	9	(10)	11	12	13	14	15
Biological Sciences	3	4	5	6	7	8	9	10	(11)	12	13	14	15
Physical Sciences	3	4	5	6	7	8	9	10	(11)	12	13	14	15

Acceptance & Matriculation Data for 2008–2009 First Year Class

	Resident	Non-resident	International	Total
Applications	3855	1114	144	5113
Interviewed	517	46	0	563
Deferred	1	0	0	1
Matriculants				
Early Assurance Program	n/a	n/a	n/a	n/a
Early Decision Program	0	0	0	0
Baccalaureate/M.D.	n/a	n/a	n/a	n/a
M.D./Ph.D.	4	0	0	4
Matriculated	94	9	0	**103**

Applications accepted from International Applicants: Yes

Specialty Choice

2004, 2005, 2006 Graduates, Specialty Choice (As reported by program directors to GME Track™)	
Anesthesiology	5%
Emergency Medicine	11%
Family Practice	10%
Internal Medicine	15%
Obstetrics/Gynecology	3%
Orthopaedic Surgery	4%
Pediatrics	14%
Psychiatry	10%
Radiology	6%
Surgery	6%

Matriculant Demographics: 2008–2009 First Year Class

Men: 44   **Women:** 59

Matriculants' Self-Reported Race/Ethnicity

Mexican American	8	**Korean**	3
Cuban	0	**Vietnamese**	7
Puerto Rican	1	**Other Asian**	5
Other Hispanic	1	**Total Asian**	40
Total Hispanic	10	**Native American**	2
Chinese	14	**Black**	5
Asian Indian	8	**Native Hawaiian**	1
Pakistani	3	**White**	57
Filipino	2	**Unduplicated Number**	
Japanese	1	**of Matriculants**	103

Science and Math Majors: 55%
Matriculants with:
Baccalaureate degree: 98%
Graduate degree(s): 13%

Financial Information

Source: 2007–2008 LCME I-B survey
and 2008–2009 AAMC TSF questionnaire

	Residents	Non-residents
Total Cost of Attendance	$45,688	$57,933
Tuition and Fees	$25,908	$38,153
Other (includes living expenses)	$18,274	$18,274
Health Insurance (can be waived)	$1,506	$1,506

Average 2008 Graduate Indebtedness: $118,826
% of Enrolled Students Receiving Aid: 92%

Criminal Background Check

This medical school does not require a criminal background check prior to matriculation.

University of California, Irvine, School of Medicine

Irvine, California

University of California Irvine School of Medicine
Office of Admissions and Outreach
Berk Hall, Room 100
Irvine, California 92697-4089
T 800 824 5388   **F** 949 824 2485

Admissions www.ucihs.uci.edu/admissions
Main www.healthaffairs.uci.edu/som/
Financial www.ofas.uci.edu/content/Medical
Entering.aspx
E-mail medadmit@uci.edu

Public Institution

Dr. David N. Bailey, Vice Chancellor for Health Affairs and Dean

Dr. Ellena M. Peterson, Associate Dean for Admissions and Outreach

Luis Medina, Director of Financial Aid

Gayle Pierce, Director of Admissions and Outreach

General Information

The UC Irvine School of Medicine is located in Orange County between Los Angeles and San Diego. Approximately 425 medical students are enrolled; the faculty includes 650 full-time and 1,500 voluntary members in 25 academic departments. Areas of research emphasis include: neurosciences, oncology, cardiovascular and pulmonary diseases, infectious diseases and molecular biology. Educational facilities are located on the main UC Irvine campus and approximately 10 miles north on the Orange campus is the state of the art UC Irvine University Hospital. Teaching clinical facilities also include off-site outpatient facilities and numerous affiliated hospitals and clinics. Special programs within the medical school include M.D./M.B.A. and M.D./Ph.D. (MSTP) programs and the Program in Medical Education for the Latino Community (PRIME-LC) that incorporates a M.D. and Master's degree emphasizing Latino health care issues.

Mission Statement

The UC Irvine School of Medicine is dedicated to advancing the knowledge and practice of medicine for the benefit of society. This mission will be achieved through programs of excellence in education, research, clinical care, and service to the public.

Curricular Highlights

Community Service Requirement: Optional.
Research/Thesis Requirement: Optional.

The curriculum has been designed not only to provide training in the technical skills necessary to be a competent physician but also to foster the humanistic qualities essential to be a well-rounded, caring and compassionate individual. In addition to the basic sciences in the first two years, substantial clinical material has been integrated into the curriculum through the development of the Clinical Foundations/Introduction to Medicine course. In the first year, students work with standardized patients to develop interview and physical examination skills. These clinical skills are further strengthened in the second year by working in the community with patients. In addition, clinically oriented courses are designed to complement the material covered in basic science courses. During the clinical years, students rotate through the core clinical services of internal medicine, family medicine, surgery, obstetrics and gynecology, psychiatry, pediatrics, emergency medicine, radiology, and neurology. Clinical advisors guide students in the selection of 20 weeks of electives tailored to the students' career goals and educational needs.

USMLE

Step 1: Required. Students must record a passing score for promotion.
Step 2: Clinical Skills (CS): Required. Students must record a passing total score to graduate.
Step 2: Clinical Knowledge (CK): Required. Students must record a passing total score to graduate.

Selection Factors

The Admissions Committee screens for applicants whose academic records indicate that they will be able to handle the medical school curriculum. In addition to scholastic achievement, attributes deemed desirable in prospective students include leadership and participation in extracurricular activities, including exposure to clinical medicine, research, and community service. Consideration is given to applicants from disadvantaged backgrounds. Preference is given to California residents and applicants who are either U.S. citizens or Permanent Residents. The School of Medicine does not accept transfer students.

Financial Aid

The Financial Aid Office coordinates financial aid application materials; reviews and evaluates information provided by applicants; secures, manages, and provides funds in the form of scholarships, grants, and loans to assist in meeting students' educational expenses; and provides debt management counseling.

Information about Diversity Programs

UC Irvine is a multicultural community, composed of individuals from diverse backgrounds. Activities, programs, classes, workshops, lectures, and everyday interactions are enriched by acceptance of one another. The university community strives to create an atmosphere of positive engagement and mutual respect.

Campus Information

Enrollment

For 2008, total enrollment was: 444

Special Features

The new UC Irvine University Hospital opened in 2009 and offers comprehensive acute and general medical care. Also located in the University Hospital complex are a Neuropsychiatric Center, the Chao Family Comprehensive Cancer Center, and a Clinical Research Facility. As part of its focus on family and preventive health, UC Irvine has five neighborhood health centers located throughout Orange County. A new Medical Education Building is scheduled to open on the main UC Irvine campus by Winter 2010. Included in this facility will be a simulation and clinical skills suite, lecture halls and small group teaching rooms, all with telemedicine and video conferencing capability.

Housing

On-campus apartment communities are available to single students as well as married students and their families. Services are also available to assist students looking for off-campus housing.

Application Process and Requirements 2010–2011

Primary Application Service: AMCAS
Earliest filing date: June 1, 2009
Latest filing date: November 1, 2009

Secondary Application Required?: Yes
Sent to: Screened applicants
URL: n/a
Fee: Yes, $60
Fee waiver available: Yes
Earliest filing date: July 15, 2009
Latest filing date: January 15, 2010

MCAT® required?: Yes
Latest MCAT® considered: September 2009
Oldest MCAT® considered: September 2007

Early Decision Program: School does not have EDP
Applicants notified: n/a
EDP available for: n/a

Regular Acceptance Notice
Earliest date: November 15, 2009
Latest date: Until class is full
Applicant's Response to Acceptance Offer – Maximum Time: Two weeks

Requests for Deferred Entrance Considered: Yes

Deposit to Hold Place in Class: No
Deposit (Resident): n/a
Deposit (Non-resident): n/a
Deposit due: n/a
Applied to tuition: n/a
Deposit refundable: n/a
Refundable by: n/a

Estimated number of new entrants: 104
EDP: n/a, special program: n/a

Start Month/Year: August 2010

Interview Format: Selected applicants are interviewed by both a faculty member and a student. Regional interviews are not available.

Other Programs

PREPARATORY PROGRAMS
Postbaccalaureate Program: Yes, outreach@uci.edu, www.som.uci.edu/admissions
Summer Program: No

COMBINED DEGREE PROGRAMS
Baccalaureate/M.D.: No
M.D./M.P.H.: No
M.D./M.B.A.: Yes, mchandle@uci.edu, www.healthaffairs.uci.edu/som/meded/Students/MD_MBA/index.html
M.D./J.D.: No
M.D./Ph.D.: Yes, varrone@uci.edu, http://mstp.uci.edu
Additional Program: Yes, primelc@uci.edu, www.healthaffairs.uci.edu/som/meded/PrimeLC/index.html

Premedical Coursework

Course	Req.	Rec.	Lab.	Sems.
Inorganic Chemistry	•		•	2
Behavioral Sciences		•		
Biochemistry	•			1
Biology	•		•	2
Biology/Zoology				
Calculus	•			1
College English	•			1
College Mathematics				

Course	Req.	Rec.	Lab.	Sems.
Genetics		•		
Humanities		•		
Organic Chemistry	•		•	2
Physics	•			2
Psychology		•		
Social Sciences		•		
Upper Division Biology	•			1
Statistics	•			1

Selection Factors: 2008 Accepted Applicants

Proportion of Accepted Applicants with Relevant Experience (Data Self-Reported to AMCAS®)		
Community Service/Volunteer		67%
Medically-Related Work		93%
Research		93%

Shaded bar represents school's accepted scores ranging from the 10th percentile to the 90th percentile. School Median ● National Median ●

Overall GPA 2.0 2.1 2.2 2.3 2.4 2.5 2.6 2.7 2.8 2.9 3.0 3.1 3.2 3.3 3.4 3.5 3.6 3.7 (3.8) 3.9 4.0
Science GPA 2.0 2.1 2.2 2.3 2.4 2.5 2.6 2.7 2.8 2.9 3.0 3.1 3.2 3.3 3.4 3.5 3.6 (3.7) 3.8 3.9 4.0

MCAT® Total Numeric Score 9 10 11 12 13 14 15 16 17 18 19 20 21 22 23 24 25 26 27 28 29 30 31 (32)(33)34 35 36 37 38 39 40 41 42 43

Writing Sample			J	K	L	M	N	O	P	(Q)	R	S	T
Verbal Reasoning	3	4	5	6	7	8	9	(10)	11	12	13	14	15
Biological Sciences	3	4	5	6	7	8	9	10	(11)	12	13	14	15
Physical Sciences	3	4	5	6	7	8	9	10	(11)	12	13	14	15

Acceptance & Matriculation Data for 2008–2009 First Year Class

	Resident	Non-resident	International	Total
Applications	3824	813	58	4695
Interviewed	486	13	0	499
Deferred	1	0	0	1
Matriculants				
Early Assurance Program	0	0	0	0
Early Decision Program	0	0	0	0
Baccalaureate/M.D.	n/a	n/a	n/a	n/a
M.D./Ph.D.	3	3	0	6
Matriculated	100	4	0	**104**

Applications accepted from International Applicants: No

Matriculant Demographics: 2008–2009 First Year Class

Men: 60   **Women:** 44

Matriculants' Self-Reported Race/Ethnicity

Mexican American	6	Korean	5
Cuban	0	Vietnamese	5
Puerto Rican	1	Other Asian	3
Other Hispanic	6	Total Asian	38
Total Hispanic	13	Native American	0
Chinese	14	Black	4
Asian Indian	9	Native Hawaiian	2
Pakistani	0	White	58
Filipino	1	Unduplicated Number	
Japanese	1	of Matriculants	104

Science and Math Majors: 72%
Matriculants with:
Baccalaureate degree: 100%
Graduate degree(s): 12%

Specialty Choice

2004, 2005, 2006 Graduates, Specialty Choice (As reported by program directors to GME Track™)	
Anesthesiology	6%
Emergency Medicine	9%
Family Practice	9%
Internal Medicine	15%
Obstetrics/Gynecology	8%
Orthopaedic Surgery	3%
Pediatrics	11%
Psychiatry	12%
Radiology	3%
Surgery	7%

Financial Information

Source: 2007-2008 LCME I-B survey and 2008-2009 AAMC TSF questionnaire

	Residents	Non-residents
Total Cost of Attendance	$48,107	$60,352
Tuition and Fees	$23,289	$35,534
Other (includes living expenses)	$22,312	$22,312
Health Insurance (can be waived)	$2,506	$2,506

Average 2008 Graduate Indebtedness: $112,793
% of Enrolled Students Receiving Aid: 92%

Criminal Background Check

This medical school requires a criminal background check prior to matriculation.

University of California, Los Angeles
David Geffen School of Medicine at UCLA

Los Angeles, California

David Geffen School of Medicine at UCLA
Office of Admissions
10833 Le Conte Avenue
Los Angeles, California 90095-7035
T 310 825 6081

Admissions www.medstudent.ucla.edu/ prospective/
Main http://dgsom.healthsciences.ucla.edu/ms-resources
Financial www.medstudent.ucla.edu/current/fao/ ?pgID=210
E-mail somadmiss@mednet.ucla.edu

Public Institution

Dr. Gerald Levey, Dean

Lili Fobert, Director of Admissions

Patricia Pratt, Director of Outreach

Gloria Pinedo, Director of Financial Aid

Dr. Neil Parker, Dean for Admissions and Students

General Information

The David Geffen School of Medicine at UCLA is on the UCLA campus. The University Medical Center, Ambulatory Plaza, Mattel Children's and Neuropsychiatric Hospital and Eye Institute are adjacent. These institutions, together with the Schools of Dentistry, Nursing, and Public Health, are integral parts of the environment. Major affiliations include LA County Harbor and Oliveview Medical Centers, Veterans Affairs Medical Centers West LA and Sepulveda, Cedars-Sinai Medical Center and Kaiser Permanente. The decision of which medical school to attend is extremely important. We provide applicants with critical information through our Web sites. Applicants may check their status on the Admission Web site. Students invited for interviews participate in student tours, meet faculty, students, staff, and members of the Admissions Committee.

Mission Statement

The school seeks students who will be future leaders, have distinguished careers in clinical practice, teaching, research, and public service. The school strives to create an environment in which students prepare for a future where scientific knowledge, societal values and human needs are ever-changing.

Curricular Highlights

Community Service Requirement: Optional. Student-run Clinics are numerous; 80% do service.

Research/Thesis Requirement: Optional. Over 75% participate in research.

The first two years present a thorough grounding in the science basic to medicine. An integrated approach to basic & clinical sciences is enhanced through problem-based learning in small groups. Students are introduced to a holistic approach to patient care from the beginning through the nationally recognized Doctoring course. The first two years center on processes of disease, with emphasis on organ system-oriented instruction. The third year core clerkships encompass internal medicine, surgery, obstetrics and gynecology, pediatrics, psychiatry, family practice, radiology, and neurology. The senior year, through a set of Colleges, provide a unique mentoring and educational experience bringing together student and faculty with similar interests. Senior electives are designed to provide students with a foundation to develop and fulfill personal interests, broaden clinical knowledge, and provide an advantage in securing desired residencies. UCLA has a pass/fail grading system, allowing students to actively participate in school and student-organized activities. There are student run clinics at the Salvation Army Homeless Center, Mobile Clinic, Health Fairs, and activities teaching high school students preventive health, and work with the underserved. Student use summers for research, community work, and international work. The MSTP programs leads to M.D.–Ph.D. degrees for those interested in research. This program requires 3–5 additional years to the M.D. study. Stipends are provided for this program. The school also offers joint M.D.–M.B.A. and M.D.–M.P.H. programs chosen in the junior year. The program is designed for students interested in organization leadership roles. Our Drew program is for those interested in the underserved. Our UCR/UCLA Program is a cooperative venture with the University of California, Riverside. Students spend their first two years at UCR with the same curriculum as UCLA, followed by their final two clinical years at the UCLA School of Medicine.

USMLE

Step 1: Required. Students must record a passing score for promotion.

Step 2: Clinical Skills (CS): Required. Students must record a passing total score to graduate.

Step 2: Clinical Knowledge (CK): Required. Students must record a passing total score to graduate.

Selection Factors

Preference is given to those showing evidence of broad training and high achievement in college education and those who possess those traits of personality and character essential to the success in medicine and the provision of quality, professional and humane medical care. We look for through coursework, school activities, community service and research for evidence of maturity, intellect, scholarship, and service to their communities and to those who are underprivileged and disadvantaged, are culturally aware and are able to speak a second language, especially Spanish. Final selections are made on the basis of individual qualifications and not on the basis of race, ethnicity, sex, age, sexual orientation, national origin or disability.

Financial Aid

Scholarships and loan are available to US citizens and are awarded on the basis of financial need and academics. Every effort is made to provide as much aid as needed.

Information about Diversity Programs

We pride ourselves on the diversity of our student body. Multiple programs to celebrate our diversity are part of student life and are integral to the learning environment.

Campus Information

Setting

We are located on the main UCLA campus offering numerous opportunities for theatre, recreation, athletics and cultural events.

Enrollment

For 2008, total enrollment was: 694

Special Features

A new state of the art medical center opened this year.

Housing

Graduate housing in walking distance is available for the first two years.

Application Process and Requirements 2010–2011

Primary Application Service: AMCAS
Earliest filing date: June 1, 2009
Latest filing date: November 1, 2009

Secondary Application Required?: Yes
Sent to: Screened applicants
URL: Supplied after screening
Fee: Yes, $60
Fee waiver available: Yes
Earliest filing date: n/a
Latest filing date: within 45 days of request

MCAT® required?: Yes
Latest MCAT® considered: September 2009
Oldest MCAT® considered: 2007

Early Decision Program: School does not have EDP
Applicants notified: n/a
EDP available for: n/a

Regular Acceptance Notice
Earliest date: December 15, 2009
Latest date: Until class is full
Applicant's Response to Acceptance Offer – Maximum Time: Two weeks

Requests for Deferred Entrance Considered: Yes

Deposit to Hold Place in Class: No
Deposit (Resident): n/a
Deposit (Non-resident): n/a
Deposit due: n/a
Applied to tuition: n/a
Deposit refundable: n/a
Refundable by: n/a

Estimated number of new entrants: 187
EDP: n/a, special program: n/a

Start Month/Year: August 2010

Interview Format: One-on-one with faculty. Regional interviews are not available.

Other Programs

PREPARATORY PROGRAMS
Postbaccalaureate Program: Yes, www.medstudent.ucla.edu/prospective
Summer Program: Yes, Patrica Pratt (310) 825-5375, ppratt@mednet.ucla.edu

Combined Degree Programs
Baccalaureate/M.D.: No
M.D./M.P.H.: Yes, www.medstudent.ucla.edu/prospective
M.D./M.B.A.: Yes, www.medstudent.ucla.edu/prospective
M.D./J.D.: No
M.D./Ph.D.: Yes, www.medstudent.ucla.edu/prospective
Additional Program: Yes, www.medsch.ucla.edu/uclaprime/program.htm

Premedical Coursework

Course	Req.	Rec.	Lab.	Sems.	Course	Req.	Rec.	Lab.	Sems.
Inorganic Chemistry	•		•	2	Computer Science		•		
Behavioral Sciences					Genetics				
Biochemistry					Humanities		•		
Biology	•		•	2	Organic Chemistry	•		•	2
Biology/Zoology					Physics	•		•	2
Calculus	•			1	Psychology				
College English	•			2	Social Sciences				
College Mathematics	•			2	Other 1 & 2		•		

Selection Factors: 2008 Accepted Applicants

Proportion of Accepted Applicants with Relevant Experience (Data Self-Reported to AMCAS®)		
Community Service/Volunteer		67%
Medically-Related Work		95%
Research		92%

Shaded bar represents school's accepted scores ranging from the 10th percentile to the 90th percentile ● School Median ● National Median

Overall GPA	2.0 2.1 2.2 2.3 2.4 2.5 2.6 2.7 2.8 2.9 3.0 3.1 3.2 3.3 3.4 3.5 3.6 3.7 (3.8) 3.9 4.0
Science GPA	2.0 2.1 2.2 2.3 2.4 2.5 2.6 2.7 2.8 2.9 3.0 3.1 3.2 3.3 3.4 3.5 3.6 3.7 (3.8) 3.9 4.0

MCAT® Total Numeric Score 9 10 11 12 13 14 15 16 17 18 19 20 21 22 23 24 25 26 27 28 29 30 31 32 (33) 34 35 36 37 38 39 40 41 42 43

Writing Sample			J	K	L	M	N	O	P	(Q)	R	S	T
Verbal Reasoning	3	4	5	6	7	8	9	(10)	11	12	13	14	15
Biological Sciences	3	4	5	6	7	8	9	10	(11)	(12)	13	14	15
Physical Sciences	3	4	5	6	7	8	9	10	(11)	(12)	13	14	15

Acceptance & Matriculation Data for 2008–2009 First Year Class

	Resident	Non-resident	International	Total
Applications	5976	2869	289	9134
Interviewed	492	198	0	690
Deferred	4	2	0	6
Matriculants				
Early Assurance Program	0	0	0	0
Early Decision Program	0	0	0	0
Baccalaureate/M.D.	n/a	n/a	n/a	n/a
M.D./Ph.D.	8	3	0	11
Matriculated	162	25	0	**187**

Applications accepted from International Applicants: Yes

Matriculant Demographics: 2008–2009 First Year Class

Men: 96   **Women:** 91

Matriculants' Self-Reported Race/Ethnicity

Mexican American	26	Korean	3
Cuban	1	Vietnamese	8
Puerto Rican	1	Other Asian	7
Other Hispanic	8	Total Asian	60
Total Hispanic	33	Native American	2
Chinese	17	Black	19
Asian Indian	14	Native Hawaiian	2
Pakistani	3	White	82
Filipino	5	Unduplicated Number	
Japanese	5	of Matriculants	187

Science and Math Majors: 70%
Matriculants with:
    Baccalaureate degree: 100%
    Graduate degree(s): 6%

Specialty Choice

2004, 2005, 2006 Graduates, Specialty Choice (As reported by program directors to GME Track™)

Anesthesiology	7%
Emergency Medicine	8%
Family Practice	9%
Internal Medicine	12%
Obstetrics/Gynecology	4%
Orthopaedic Surgery	5%
Pediatrics	10%
Psychiatry	4%
Radiology	7%
Surgery	5%

Financial Information

Source: 2007–2008 LCME I-B survey and 2008–2009 AAMC TSF questionnaire

	Residents	Non-residents
Total Cost of Attendance	$50,213	$62,458
Tuition and Fees	$22,835	$35,080
Other (includes living expenses)	$26,040	$26,040
Health Insurance (can be waived)	$1,338	$1,338

Average 2008 Graduate Indebtedness: $98,677
% of Enrolled Students Receiving Aid: 87%

Criminal Background Check

This medical school requires a criminal background check prior to matriculation.

University of California, San Diego, School of Medicine

La Jolla, California

Office of Admissions, 0621, Medical Teaching Facility
UC San Diego School of Medicine
9500 Gilman Drive
La Jolla, California 92093-0621
T 858 534 3880 **F** 858 534 5282

Admissions http://meded.ucsd.edu/admissions
Main http://meded-portal.ucsd.edu
Financial http://meded.ucsd.edu/hsfao
E-mail somadmissions@ucsd.edu

Public Institution

Dr. David A. Brenner, Vice Chancellor and Dean

Dr. Carolyn Kelly, Associate Dean for Admissions and Student Affairs

Dr. Christine Moutier, Interim Assistant Dean for Diversity & Community Partnerships

Carol Hartupee, Director of Financial Aid

Brian Zeglen, Director of Admissions

General Information

Students at the University of California, San Diego (UCSD) benefit from a diverse faculty and access to a wide variety of research and clinical opportunities.

Mission Statement

The overall objective of the medical school curriculum is to instill graduates with the knowledge, skills, and attributes that will lead to their becoming capable and compassionate physicians. Our educational philosophy is to give students an opportunity to go beyond the core curriculum and pursue electives and independent study that take full advantage of the resources available at UCSD and in the surrounding region, helping them to become expert clinicians and scientists who are aware of, and responsive to, community needs.

Curricular Highlights

Community Service Requirement: Optional. Many community service activities are available.
Research/Thesis Requirement: Optional. Independent Study Project is required.

The goal of the medical curriculum and faculty-student interactions is to develop critical, objective, conscientious physicians prepared for changing conditions of medical practice and continuing self-education. The integrated core curriculum of the first two years provides entering students with an essential understanding of the fundamental disciplines underlying modern medicine. The core curriculum of the last two years is composed of the major clinical specialties taught in hospital and out-patient settings, and relevant extended-care facilities. Elective opportunities are pursued during both the pre-clinical and clinical years. Several com-bined M.D.-Master's degree programs are available. A Program in Medical Education in Health Equity (PRIME-HEq) has been recently developed. The Medical Scientist Training Program provides the opportunity to earn both the M.D. and Ph.D. degrees over a seven to eight-year period of study. A Medical Scholars Program at UCSD (B.S.-M.D.) is available for outstanding California high school seniors planning careers in medicine. A second B.S.-M.D. program is available between UCSD School of Medicine and California Institute of Technology.

USMLE

Step 1: Required. Students must record a passing score for promotion.
Step 2: Clinical Skills (CS): Required. Students must record a passing total score to graduate.
Step 2: Clinical Knowledge (CK): Required. Students must record a passing total score to graduate.

Selection Factors

The Admissions Committee selects applicants who have demonstrated intelligence, maturity, integrity, and dedication to the ideal of service to society. The school is seeking a student body with a broad diversity of backgrounds and interests. The Admissions Committee seeks students with broad training and in-depth achievement in a particular area of knowledge, whether in the humanities, social sciences, or natural sciences. Other evaluation factors include evidence of meaningful involvement in extracurricular activities, performance on the MCAT, letters of recommendation, and personal interviews. The Admissions Committee interview evaluates the applicant's abilities and skills necessary to satisfy the non-academic or technical standards established by the faculty and the personal characteristics necessary to become an effective physician. Preference is afforded to California residents, and consideration is given only to applicants who are either U.S. citizens or permanent residents. The UCSD School of Medicine participates in the WICHE Professional Student Exchange Program. The School of Medicine does not accept transfer students.

Financial Aid

Financial aid in the form of scholarships, grants, loans, and work opportunities is offered to help students in need of financial assistance. Medical Scientist Training Program participants may receive full tuition and stipend support during their combined degree training.

Information about Diversity Programs

The UCSD School of Medicine is committed to expanding the educational opportunities for applicants coming from disadvantaged educational or economic backgrounds. This institutional commitment is expressed through a pre-matriculation summer program, a conditional acceptance program, tutorial support programs, and financial aid assistance.

Campus Information

Setting

UCSD School of Medicine is located in La Jolla, California.

Enrollment

For 2008, total enrollment was: 520

Special Features

UCSD is a hub both for outstanding clinical programs and cutting-edge research. Recognized regional clinical programs include a Level 1 trauma center, an innovative Stroke Center, a leading AIDS/HIV treatment program, and a Regional Burn Center. Other specialized resources include the UCSD Cancer Center, the functional MRI facility, the Institute for Molecular Medicine, and the Stein Institute for Research on Aging. Both the prestigious Ludwig Institute for Cancer Research and the Howard Hughes Medical Institute have significant presences on campus.

Housing

Medical students at UCSD live both in on- and off-campus housing.

Satellite Campuses/Facilities

Clinical rotations are conducted at the UCSD Medical Centers, VA San Diego Healthcare System, San Diego Children's Hospital, Scripps-Mercy Hospital, Balboa Naval Medical Center, and a variety of ambulatory care sites throughout San Diego.

Application Process and Requirements 2010–2011

Primary Application Service: AMCAS
Earliest filing date: June 1, 2009
Latest filing date: November 1, 2009

Secondary Application Required?: Yes
Sent to: Screened applicants,
(858) 534-3880, somadmissions@ucsd.edu
Fee: Yes, $60
Fee waiver available: Yes
Earliest filing date: July 1, 2009
Latest filing date: One month after receiving
Secondary Application invitation

MCAT® required?: Yes
Latest MCAT® considered: September 2009
Oldest MCAT® considered: January 2007

Early Decision Program: School does not have EDP
Applicants notified: n/a
EDP available for: n/a

Regular Acceptance Notice
Earliest date: October 15, 2009
Latest date: Until class is full
Applicant's Response to Acceptance Offer – Maximum Time: Two weeks

Requests for Deferred Entrance Considered: Yes

Deposit to Hold Place in Class: No
Deposit (Resident): n/a
Deposit (Non-resident): n/a
Deposit due: n/a
Applied to tuition: n/a
Deposit refundable: n/a
Refundable by: n/a

Estimated number of new entrants: 125
EDP: n/a, special program: 18

Start Month/Year: August 2010

Interview Format: Two one-hour open-file interviews. Regional interviews are not available.

Other Programs

PREPARATORY PROGRAMS
Postbaccalaureate Program: Yes, http://meded.ucsd.edu/postbac, Saundra Kirk, (858) 534-4171, sjkirk@ucsd.edu
Summer Program: Yes, http://meded.ucsd.edu/somi220/, Carrie Owen, (858) 534-1519, cnowen@ucsd.edu

COMBINED DEGREE PROGRAMS
Baccalaureate/M.D.: Yes, http://meded.ucsd.edu/groups/med-scholars/, Yvonne Coleman, (858) 534-3880, somadmissions@ucsd.edu
M.D./M.P.H.: Yes, http://meded.ucsd.edu/ugme/goddp/
M.D./M.B.A.: No
M.D./J.D.: No
M.D./Ph.D.: Yes, http://meded.ucsd.edu/ugme/goddp/
Additional Program: Yes, http://meded.ucsd.edu/ugme/goddp/

Premedical Coursework

Course	Req.	Rec.	Lab.	Hrs.
Inorganic Chemistry	•			8
Behavioral Sciences		•		
Biochemistry				
Biology	•			8
Biology/Zoology		•		
Calculus		•		
College English		•		
College Mathematics	•			8

Course	Req.	Rec.	Lab.	Hrs.
Computer Science		•		
Genetics		•		
Humanities		•		
Organic Chemistry	•			8
Physics	•			8
Psychology		•		
Social Sciences		•		
Other				

Selection Factors: 2008 Accepted Applicants

Proportion of Accepted Applicants with Relevant Experience (Data Self-Reported to AMCAS®)		
Community Service/Volunteer		63%
Medically-Related Work		89%
Research		91%

Shaded bar represents school's accepted scores ranging from the 10th percentile to the 90th percentile   **School Median** ● **National Median** ●

Overall GPA	2.0	2.1	2.2	2.3	2.4	2.5	2.6	2.7	2.8	2.9	3.0	3.1	3.2	3.3	3.4	3.5	3.6	3.7	③.8	3.9	4.0
Science GPA	2.0	2.1	2.2	2.3	2.4	2.5	2.6	2.7	2.8	2.9	3.0	3.1	3.2	3.3	3.4	3.5	3.6	3.7	③.8	3.9	4.0

MCAT® Total Numeric Score 9 10 11 12 13 14 15 16 17 18 19 20 21 22 23 24 25 26 27 28 29 30 31 ㉜ 33 34 ㉟ 36 37 38 39 40 41 42 43

Writing Sample			J	K	L	M	N	O	P	Ⓠ Ⓡ S	T
Verbal Reasoning	3	4	5	6	7	8	9	⑩ ⑪	12	13	14	15
Biological Sciences	3	4	5	6	7	8	9	10	⑪ ⑫	13	14	15
Physical Sciences	3	4	5	6	7	8	9	10	⑪ ⑫	13	14	15

Acceptance & Matriculation Data for 2008–2009 First Year Class

	Resident	Non-resident	International	Total
Applications	3653	1864	49	5566
Interviewed	562	116	0	676
Deferred	1	0	0	1
Matriculants				
Early Assurance Program	0	0	0	0
Early Decision Program	0	0	0	0
Baccalaureate/M.D.	4	0	0	4
M.D./Ph.D.	3	5	0	8
Matriculated	121	13	0	**134**

Applications accepted from International Applicants: No

Specialty Choice

2004, 2005, 2006 Graduates, Specialty Choice (As reported by program directors to GME Track™)	
Anesthesiology	6%
Emergency Medicine	8%
Family Practice	7%
Internal Medicine	20%
Obstetrics/Gynecology	6%
Orthopaedic Surgery	2%
Pediatrics	11%
Psychiatry	7%
Radiology	4%
Surgery	5%

Matriculant Demographics: 2008–2009 First Year Class

Men: 72   **Women:** 62

Matriculants' Self-Reported Race/Ethnicity

Mexican American	9	**Korean**	2
Cuban	1	**Vietnamese**	9
Puerto Rican	2	**Other Asian**	5
Other Hispanic	2	**Total Asian**	55
Total Hispanic	14	**Native American**	2
Chinese	28	**Black**	1
Asian Indian	12	**Native Hawaiian**	0
Pakistani	0	**White**	68
Filipino	1	**Unduplicated Number**	
Japanese	2	**of Matriculants**	134

Science and Math Majors: 70%
Matriculants with:
Baccalaureate degree: 99%
Graduate degree(s): 6%

Financial Information

Source: 2007–2008 LCME I-B survey and 2008–2009 AAMC TSF questionnaire

	Residents	Non-residents
Total Cost of Attendance	$47,130	$59,375
Tuition and Fees	$23,031	$35,276
Other (includes living expenses)	$22,551	$22,551
Health Insurance (can be waived)	$1,548	$1,548

Average 2008 Graduate Indebtedness: $98,773
% of Enrolled Students Receiving Aid: 88%

Criminal Background Check

This medical school requires a criminal background check prior to matriculation.

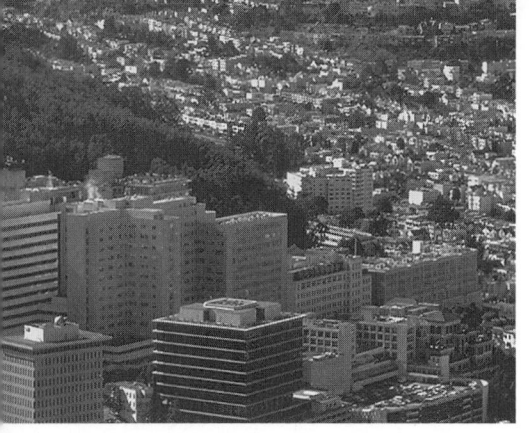

University of California, San Francisco, School of Medicine

San Francisco, California

School of Medicine, Admissions
C-200, Box 0408
University of California, San Francisco
San Francisco, California 94143
T 415 476 4044

Admissions http://medschool.ucsf.edu/admissions
Main http://medschool.ucsf.edu
Financial http://saawww.ucsf.edu/
financial/welcome.htm
E-mail admissions@medsch.ucsf.edu

Public Institution

Dr. Sam Hawgood, Interim Dean

Carrie Steere-Salazar, Director, Student Financial Services

Hallen Chung, Director of Admissions

Dr. David Wofsy, Associate Dean for Admissions

Kathleen Ryan, Admissions Officer

General Information

The UCSF School of Medicine is dedicated to excellence in education, research, and patient care. Woven throughout all of these pursuits is a strong commitment to public service. The UCSF School of Medicine earns its greatest distinction from the quality of its students and its outstanding faculty — including two Nobel laureates, 31 National Academy of Sciences members, 49 American Academy of Arts and Sciences members, 64 Institute of Medicine members, and 17 Howard Hughes Medical Institute investigators.

Mission Statement

The UCSF School of Medicine strives to advance human health through a four-fold mission of education, research, patient care, and public service.

Curricular Highlights

Community Service Requirement: Optional.
Research/Thesis Requirement: Optional.

The first two years consist of integrated core instruction in the basic, behavioral, social, and clinical sciences; clinical experience is introduced within the first week of classes and continues as a longitudinal patient care experience through the Foundations of Patient Care Course. Emphasis is placed on small-group teaching. In the last two years, the various clinical departments provide 54 weeks of Clinical Core, which teach students the basic skills of clinical medicine. The fourth year includes Advanced Studies, which encompass elective rotations, research, and specific fields of inquiry that prepare students for post-graduate training. For more detailed information, visit the School of Medicine Web site at *www.med school.ucsf.edu/curriculum/overview/index.aspx.*

The UCB-UCSF Joint Medical Program is a five-year M.S./M.D. program with the first three years spent at UC Berkeley completing a case-based core medical curriculum, elective coursework and research in support of a health related MS. JMP students then transition to UCSF for their last two years of clinical work. For detailed information, please visit *http://jmp.berkeley.edu.*

USMLE

Step 1: Required. Students must record a passing score for promotion.
Step 2: Clinical Skills (CS): Required. Students must record a passing total score to graduate. *Applies to the graduating class of 2013 and later.
Step 2: Clinical Knowledge (CK): Required. Students must record a passing total score to graduate. *Applies to the graduating class of 2013 and later.

Selection Factors

UCSF students must have demonstrated the ability to perform at a very high level in their prior academic pursuits. Among the many applicants who meet this essential criterion, the school seeks to create a student community that is characterized by diversity in background, extra-curricular talents, academic interests, and career aspirations. There is no single mold that defines a UCSF student. UCSF wants some students who aspire to become terrific doctors, some who will become great scientists, some who will be leaders in health policy, and so on. The goal is to create the most stimulating and enjoyable possible environment in which to live and learn. For further details regarding the admissions process, please visit the School of Medicine's Web site at *www.medschool.ucsf.edu/admissions/apply/index.aspx.*

Financial Aid

Scholarships are awarded to entering students on the basis of scholarship and/or need. General financial support is awarded through the Student Financial Services Office. Aid packages consist of a combination of loans, grants-in-aid, and scholarships. Financial aid is only available to U.S. citizens or permanent residents. For detailed information, please visit *http://saawww.ucsf.edu/financial/welcome.htm.*

Information about Diversity Programs

The School of Medicine welcomes applicants from all ethnic, economic, and cultural backgrounds without discrimination, and has a long-standing commitment to increasing the number of physicians who come from communities that are underserved and/or underrepresented in medicine. As a result, over the last 30 years, UCSF has had one of the highest minority enrollment and graduation rates of any continental U.S. medical school. The curriculum includes both coursework and practical opportunities focused on narrowing health care disparities.

Campus Information

Setting

The main UCSF campus is located in the center of San Francisco, a short walk from Golden Gate Park and no more than 10 minutes from the Pacific Ocean. Downtown San Francisco, easily accessible by car or public transportation, is located approximately two miles from the main campus. Other major UCSF teaching sites include San Francisco General Hospital, the VA Medical Center, the Cancer Center, and the new Mission Bay campus. The surrounding area of northern California provides a natural backdrop and opportunities for recreation that are hard to match.

Enrollment

For 2008, total enrollment was: 594

Special Features

Please visit the UCSF Web site for the latest facts and figures unique to the campus: *www.medschool.ucsf.edu/about/facts.aspx.*

Housing

For detailed information about housing, please visit the UCSF Housing Services Web site at *www.campuslifeservices.ucsf.edu/housing.*

Satellite Campuses/Facilities

Student rotations may be conducted at the UCSF Parnassus Campus, San Francisco General Hospital, UCSF/Mt Zion, SF VA Medical Center, and the UCSF Fresno Medical Education Program, as well as at several other Bay Area affiliated hospitals and clinics.

Application Process and Requirements 2010–2011

Primary Application Service: AMCAS
Earliest filing date: June 1, 2009
Latest filing date: October 15, 2009

Secondary Application Required?: Yes
Sent to: Screened applicants after preliminary review
Contact: UCSF School of Medicine Admissions
(415) 476-4044, admissions@medsch.ucsf.edu
Fee: Yes, $60
Fee waiver available: Yes
Earliest filing date: August 1, 2009
Latest filing date: January 12, 2010

MCAT® required?: Yes
Latest MCAT® considered: September 2009
Oldest MCAT® considered: September 2007

Early Decision Program: School does not have EDP
Applicants notified: n/a
EDP available for: n/a

Regular Acceptance Notice
Earliest date: December 15, 2009
Latest date: Until class is full
Applicant's Response to Acceptance Offer – Maximum Time: Two weeks

Requests for Deferred Entrance Considered: Yes

Deposit to Hold Place in Class: No
Deposit (Resident): n/a
Deposit (Non-resident): n/a
Deposit due: n/a
Applied to tuition: n/a
Deposit refundable: n/a
Refundable by: n/a

Estimated number of new entrants: 168
EDP: n/a, special program: n/a

Start Month/Year: June 2010 (UCB/UCSF Joint Medical Program); September 2010 (UCSF)

Interview Format: Required to interview at UCSF, if invited. Two interviews, 40 minutes to one hour each. Regional interviews are not available.

Other Programs

PREPARATORY PROGRAMS
Postbaccalaureate Program: Yes,
www.medschool.ucsf.edu/outreach
Summer Program: No

COMBINED DEGREE PROGRAMS
Baccalaureate/M.D.: No
M.D./M.P.H.: Yes, www.medschool.ucsf.edu/
admissions/degrees/Curriculum.aspx
M.D./M.B.A.: No
M.D./J.D.: No
M.D./Ph.D.: Yes, http://medschool.ucsf.edu/mstp
Joint Medical Program: Yes,
http://jmp.berkeley.edu/

Premedical Coursework

Course	Req.	Rec.	Lab.	Hrs.	Course	Req.	Rec.	Lab.	Hrs.
Inorganic Chemistry	•		•	12	Computer Science				
Behavioral Sciences					Genetics				
Biochemistry					Humanities				
Biology					Organic Chemistry	•			8
Biology/Zoology	•		•	12	Physics	•		•	12
Calculus					Psychology				
College English					Social Sciences				
College Mathematics					Other				

Selection Factors: 2008 Accepted Applicants

Proportion of Accepted Applicants with Relevant Experience (Data Self-Reported to AMCAS®)		
Community Service/Volunteer		73%
Medically-Related Work		89%
Research		92%

Shaded bar represents school's accepted scores ranging from the 10th percentile to the 90th percentile • School Median ○ National Median ●

Overall GPA 2.0 2.1 2.2 2.3 2.4 2.5 2.6 2.7 2.8 2.9 3.0 3.1 3.2 3.3 3.4 3.5 3.6 3.7 (3.8) 3.9 4.0

Science GPA 2.0 2.1 2.2 2.3 2.4 2.5 2.6 2.7 2.8 2.9 3.0 3.1 3.2 3.3 3.4 3.5 3.6 3.7 (3.8) 3.9 4.0

MCAT® Total Numeric Score 9 10 11 12 13 14 15 16 17 18 19 20 21 22 23 24 25 26 27 28 29 30 31 (32) 33 34 (35) 36 37 38 39 40 41 42 43

Writing Sample			J	K	L	M	N	O	P	(Q)	(R)	S		T
Verbal Reasoning	3	4	5	6	7	8	9	(10)	(11)	12	13	14		15
Biological Sciences	3	4	5	6	7	8	9	10	(11)	(12)	13	14		15
Physical Sciences	3	4	5	6	7	8	9	10	(11)	(12)	13	14		15

Acceptance & Matriculation Data for 2008–2009 First Year Class

	Resident	Non-resident	International	Total
Applications	3179	2746	167	6092
Interviewed	330	173	0	503
Deferred	5	2	0	7
Matriculants				
Early Assurance Program	n/a	n/a	n/a	n/a
Early Decision Program	0	0	0	0
Baccalaureate/M.D.	n/a	n/a	n/a	n/a
M.D./Ph.D.	5	7	0	12
Matriculated	132	35	0	**167**

Applications accepted from International Applicants: Yes

Specialty Choice

2004, 2005, 2006 Graduates, Specialty Choice (As reported by program directors to GME Track™)	
Anesthesiology	8%
Emergency Medicine	10%
Family Practice	4%
Internal Medicine	15%
Obstetrics/Gynecology	6%
Orthopaedic Surgery	2%
Pediatrics	11%
Psychiatry	7%
Radiology	4%
Surgery	6%

Matriculant Demographics: 2008–2009 First Year Class

Men: 71   **Women**: 96

Matriculants' Self-Reported Race/Ethnicity

Mexican American	18	**Korean**	6
Cuban	0	**Vietnamese**	5
Puerto Rican	0	**Other Asian**	6
Other Hispanic	11	**Total Asian**	54
Total Hispanic	29	**Native American**	4
Chinese	25	**Black**	15
Asian Indian	6	**Native Hawaiian**	2
Pakistani	1	**White**	91
Filipino	6	**Unduplicated Number**	
Japanese	3	**of Matriculants**	167

Science and Math Majors: 63%
Matriculants with:
        Baccalaureate degree: 100%
        Graduate degree(s): 11%

Financial Information

Source: 2007–2008 LCME I-B survey and 2008–2009 AAMC TSF questionnaire

	Residents	Non-residents
Total Cost of Attendance	$46,217	$58,462
Tuition and Fees	$22,684	$34,929
Other (includes living expenses)	$21,015	$21,015
Health Insurance (cannot be waived)	$2,518	$2,518

Average 2008 Graduate Indebtedness: $98,398
% of Enrolled Students Receiving Aid: 88%

Criminal Background Check

This medical school does not require a criminal background check prior to matriculation.

University Colorado Denver School of Medicine
Denver, Colorado

Medical School Admissions
University of Colorado Denver School of Medicine
Anschutz Medical Campus, Mail Stop 297
P.O. Box 6508
Aurora, Colorado 80045
T 303 724 8025   **F** 303 724 8028

Admissions www.uchsc.edu/som/admissions/
Main www.uchsc.edu/som
Financial www.uchsc.edu/finaid/
E-mail SOMadmin@uchsc.edu

Public Institution

Dr. Richard D. Krugman, Dean

Dr. Norma Wagoner, Associate Dean for Admissions

Dominic Martinez, Coordinator of Student Outreach and Support

Dr. Robert Winn, Assistant Dean for Admissions

General Information

The University of Colorado Denver School of Medicine (UCDSOM) is a part of the University of Colorado Denver located in Denver and Aurora, Colorado. The Anshutz Medical Campus in Aurora includes the schools of dentistry, nursing, and pharmacy and the graduate school as well as the SOM. Clinical opportunities for medical students are located throughout the Denver metropolitan area and Colorado. The UCDSOM is home to 1,927 full-time and 2,956 volunteer faculty. In addition to educating students and participating in research, the faculty assumes considerable responsibility for patient care. Student research opportunities and a variety of extracurricular activities are available. The UCDSOM moved to the new 217-acre Anschutz Medical Campus in Aurora in January 2008.

Mission Statement

The mission of the University of Colorado School of Medicine is to provide Colorado, the nation, and the world with programs of excellence in: Education – through the provision of educational programs to medical students, allied health students, graduate students and house staff, practicing health professionals, and the public at large; Research – through the development of new knowledge in the basic and clinical sciences, as well as in health policy and health care education; Clinical Care – through state-of-the-art clinical programs, which reflect the unique educational environment of the university, as well as the needs of the patients it serves; and Community Service – through sharing the School's expertise and knowledge to enhance the broader community, including our affiliated institutions, other health care professionals, alumni and other colleagues, and citizens of the state.

Curricular Highlights

Community Service Requirement: Optional. Many community service electives are available.
Research/Thesis Requirement: Required. A scholarly project is required for graduation.

The curriculum is designed to provide the scientific and clinical background to prepare graduates for the practice of medicine. A systems-based curriculum was introduced in 2005. The Essentials block runs for 18 months. The core clinical year runs through April of year 3. The elective year allows students time to do sub-internships, critical care rotations and other courses essential to their career choices. A capstone science course occurs in the spring of year 4. The Foundations of Doctoring curriculum begins in the first block of first year and continues through year 3. Standardized patients are widely used in Foundations.

USMLE

Step 1: Required. Students must record a passing score for promotion.
Step 2: Clinical Skills (CS): Required. Students must record a passing total score to graduate.
Step 2: Clinical Knowledge (CK): Required. Students must record a passing total score to graduate.

Selection Factors

Places are offered to the applicants who are most highly qualified in terms of intelligence, achievement, character, motivation, and maturity. Grades, MCAT scores, recommendations, and personal interviews are assessed. Humanistic qualities, indications of peer collaboration, and professionalism are characteristics of our students. Approximately 75 percent of the class is comprised of Colorado residents. Applicants from rural areas and from groups underrepresented in medicine are encouraged to apply. Wyoming and Montana (WICHE) applicants are treated as in-state. All undergraduate majors are considered acceptable. Excellent performance in the required science courses is essential. The medical school has an active M.D./Ph.D. program for those who wish to combine medical school with intensive laboratory research. The UCDSOM does not discriminate on the basis of race, sex,

creed, national origin, age, or disability. Financial status is not a factor in the selection of applicants.

Financial Aid

The UCSOM participates in federal aid programs and has a number of scholarships which are merit-based. Colorado student grant funds are available for Colorado residents. Financial aid questions should be directed to (303) 556-2886.

Information about Diversity Programs

The UCSOM encourages applications from qualified students from groups underrepresented in American medicine. Detailed information may be obtained from the Office of Diversity at (303) 724-8005.

Campus Information

Setting
The UCDSOM is an urban campus in Aurora, Colorado. In addition to the schools on the campus, the University of Colorado Hospital, The Children's Hospital, the Barbara Davis Center for Childhood Diabetes, and the Ben Nighthorse Campbell Center for Native American Studies are on the Anschutz Medical Campus.

Enrollment
For 2008, total enrollment was: 612

Special Features
In 2007, the total research budget of UCSOM was $406,984,867.

Housing
Rental property and roommate information are available in the Student Assistance Office. Call (303) 724-7684 or visit *www.uchsc.edu/studentassistance.*

Satellite Campuses/Facilities
Besides the hospitals on the Anschutz campus, students rotate through Denver Health Medical Center, National Jewish Hospital, and multiple hospitals throughout Denver and Colorado.

Application Process and Requirements 2010–2011

Primary Application Service: AMCAS
Earliest filing date: June 7, 2009
Latest filing date: November 1, 2009

Secondary Application Required?: Yes
Sent to: All applicants
Willa Buswell, (303) 724-8025,
willa.buswell@ucdenver.edu
URL: n/a
Fee: Yes, $100
Fee waiver available: Yes
Earliest filing date: August 1, 2009
Latest filing date: December 31, 2009

MCAT® required?: Yes
Latest MCAT® considered: September 2009
Oldest MCAT® considered: 2007

Early Decision Program: School does not have EDP
Applicants notified: n/a
EDP available for: n/a

Regular Acceptance Notice
Earliest date: October 16, 2009
Latest date: Until class is full
Applicant's Response to Acceptance Offer – Maximum Time: Two weeks

Requests for Deferred Entrance Considered: Yes

Deposit to Hold Place in Class: Yes
Deposit (Resident): $200
Deposit (Non-resident): $200
Deposit due: Upon acceptance
Applied to tuition: Yes
Deposit refundable: Yes
Refundable by: July 1, 2010

Estimated number of new entrants: 156
EDP: n/a, special program: n/a

Start Month/Year: August 2010

Interview Format: Two one-on-one academically blind interviews. Regional interviews are not available.

Other Programs

PREPARATORY PROGRAMS
Postbaccalaureate Program: Yes, By invitation only
Summer Program: No

COMBINED DEGREE PROGRAMS
Baccalaureate/M.D.: No
M.D./M.P.H.: No
M.D./M.B.A.: No, www.uchsc.edu/sm/sm/mdmbadegree.htm
M.D./J.D.: No
M.D./Ph.D.: Yes, www.uchsc.edu/sm/mstp/

Premedical Coursework

Course	Req.	Rec.	Lab.	Hrs.
Inorganic Chemistry	•		•	8
Behavioral Sciences				
Biochemistry		•		
Biology	•		•	8
Biology/Zoology				
Calculus				
College English	•			9
College Mathematics	•			6

Course	Req.	Rec.	Lab.	Hrs.
Computer Science		•		
Genetics		•		
Humanities		•		
Organic Chemistry	•		•	8
Physics	•		•	8
Psychology				
Social Sciences		•		
Other		•		

Selection Factors: 2008 Accepted Applicants

Proportion of Accepted Applicants with Relevant Experience (Data Self-Reported to AMCAS®)		
Community Service/Volunteer	70%
Medically-Related Work	85%
Research	78%

Shaded bar represents school's accepted scores ranging from the 10th percentile to the 90th percentile. School Median ● National Median ◐

Overall GPA	2.0	2.1	2.2	2.3	2.4	2.5	2.6	2.7	2.8	2.9	3.0	3.1	3.2	3.3	3.4	3.5	3.6	3.7	(3.8)	3.9	4.0
Science GPA	2.0	2.1	2.2	2.3	2.4	2.5	2.6	2.7	2.8	2.9	3.0	3.1	3.2	3.3	3.4	3.5	3.6	3.7	(3.8)	3.9	4.0

MCAT® Total Numeric Score 9 10 11 12 13 14 15 16 17 18 19 20 21 22 23 24 25 26 27 28 29 30 31 (32) 33 (34) 35 36 37 38 39 40 41 42 43

Writing Sample			J	K	L	M	N	O	P	(Q)	R	S	T
Verbal Reasoning	3	4	5	6	7	8	9	(10)	(11)	12	13	14	15
Biological Sciences	3	4	5	6	7	8	9	10	(11)	(12)	13	14	15
Physical Sciences	3	4	5	6	7	8	9	10	(11)	12	13	14	15

Acceptance & Matriculation Data for 2008–2009 First Year Class

	Resident	Non-resident	International	Total
Applications	595	2859	64	3518
Interviewed	308	314	0	622
Deferred	6	3	0	9
Matriculants				
Early Assurance Program	0	0	0	0
Early Decision Program	0	0	0	0
Baccalaureate/M.D.	n/a	n/a	n/a	n/a
M.D./Ph.D.	2	5	0	7
Matriculated	117	38	1	**156**

Applications accepted from International Applicants: Yes

Specialty Choice

2004, 2005, 2006 Graduates, Specialty Choice (As reported by program directors to GME Track™)	
Anesthesiology	8%
Emergency Medicine	7%
Family Practice	14%
Internal Medicine	20%
Obstetrics/Gynecology	4%
Orthopaedic Surgery	4%
Pediatrics	11%
Psychiatry	4%
Radiology	3%
Surgery	5%

Matriculant Demographics: 2008–2009 First Year Class

Men: 79 **Women:** 77

Matriculants' Self-Reported Race/Ethnicity

Mexican American	5	Korean	6
Cuban	2	Vietnamese	5
Puerto Rican	0	Other Asian	2
Other Hispanic	3	Total Asian	17
Total Hispanic	9	Native American	4
Chinese	0	Black	5
Asian Indian	2	Native Hawaiian	0
Pakistani	0	White	126
Filipino	0	Unduplicated Number	
Japanese	2	of Matriculants	156

Science and Math Majors: 67%
Matriculants with:
Baccalaureate degree: 98%
Graduate degree(s): 12%

Financial Information

Source: 2007–2008 LCME I-B survey and 2008–2009 AAMC TSF questionnaire

	Residents	Non-residents
Total Cost of Attendance	$48,130	$72,956
Tuition and Fees	$26,589	$51,415
Other (includes living expenses)	$19,070	$19,070
Health Insurance (can be waived)	$2,471	$2,471

Average 2008 Graduate Indebtedness: $138,352
% of Enrolled Students Receiving Aid: 95%

Criminal Background Check

This medical school requires a criminal background check prior to matriculation.

University of Connecticut School of Medicine
Farmington, Connecticut

Medical Student Affairs
University of Connecticut
School of Medicine
263 Farmington Avenue, Rm. AG-062
Farmington, Connecticut 06030-1906
T 860 679 4306   F 860 679 1282

Admissions http://medicine.uchc.edu/prospective/admissions/
Main http://medicine.uchc.edu
Financial http://medicine.uchc.edu/prospective/financialaid/
E-mail fox@nso1.uchc.edu, sanford@nso1.uchc.edu

Public Institution

Dr. Cato Laurencin, Dean

Dr. Keat Sanford, Assistant Dean for Admissions and Medical Student Affairs

Dr. Marja Hurley, Associate Dean of Minority Affairs

Andrea Devereux, Director of Financial Assistance

Lynda Fox, Administrative Coordinator

Tracy Dieli, Administrative Coordinator

General Information

The School of Medicine occupies the University of Connecticut Health Center complex in Farmington. The Health Center also includes the School of Dental Medicine, graduate programs in Biomedical Sciences and Public Health, the University Hospital and Ambulatory Unit, Research buildings, and Stowe Library. Students receive clinical training in Hartford area-affiliated hospitals.

Mission Statement

The School of Medicine's curriculum is designed to prepare professional men and women to practice medicine in a health care system that is evolving at an accelerated rate. The curriculum will equip students to formulate creative and courageous solutions to health care problems and issues. The primary goal is to develop in all students a fund of knowledge, skills, and attitudes that will enable them to pursue the postgraduate training necessary for their chosen career.

Curricular Highlights

Community Service Requirement: Required. Numerous opportunities available.
Research/Thesis Requirement: Optional. Numerous opportunities available.

The curriculum is based on a multi-departmental, organ-system approach. Normal structure/ function is presented first, followed by pathophysiology and therapeutic approaches. Students learn medical history-taking, physical diagnosis, and other aspects of the physician-patient relationship. They participate in longi-tudinal ambulatory clinical experience all four years. Students rotate through major clinical disciplines in the third year. Students complete a sub-internship, courses in emergent and urgent care, a selective experience, and five elective months in the fourth year. The grading system is pass/fail; grading in year three is hon-ors and pass/fail; no class rank or class stand-ing scales are used.

USMLE

Step 1: Required. Students must record a passing score to for graduation, but not promotion.
Step 2: Clinical Skills (CS): Required. Students must record a passing total score to graduate.
Step 2: Clinical Knowledge (CK): Required. Students must record a passing total score to graduate.

Selection Factors

The University of Connecticut accepts highly qualified Connecticut residents, with special effort to include those who are disadvantaged. Highly qualified out-of-state residents are considered to achieve a diverse class. The Admissions Committee considers the applicant's interests, achievements, abilities, motivation, and character. GPA and MCAT scores are considered, along with academic program difficulty, academic achievement beyond regular course-work, intellectual growth and development, nonacademic activities, and recommendations. UCSOM policy prohibits discrimination in education, in employment, and in the provision of services on account of race, religion, sex, age, marital status, national origin, ancestry, sexual orientation, disabled veteran status, physical or mental disability, mental retardation, other specifically covered mental disabilities, and criminal records that are not job-related, in accordance with provisions of the Civil Rights Act of 1964, Title IX Education Amendments of 1972, the Rehabilitation Act of 1973, the Americans with Disabilities Act, and other existing federal and state laws and executive orders pertaining to equal rights.

Financial Aid

Educational costs are modest and the financial assistance program is strong. Financial need is not considered relevant to the admissions process. Every effort is made to meet each student's financial requirements through scholarships and loans. Entrance, exit, and debt counseling are provided.

Information about Diversity Programs

The UCSOM recruits disadvantaged applicants and applicants from groups underrepresented in medicine through the Admissions Office and the Department of Health Careers Opportunity Programs (HCOP). The Admissions Committee reviews applications from these candidates in the same manner as those of all other candidates. Candidates receive a full and sensitive review and are selected on a competitive basis. Candidates invited for an interview meet with HCOP staff. Summer enrichment programs are available for high school and college students from groups traditionally underrepresented in American medicine. The HCOP Department's telephone number is (860) 679-3483.

Campus Information

Setting

The 162 acre Health Science Complex is seven miles west of Hartford, with panoramic views of rural hills and the Hartford skyline. The John Dempsey University Hospital is onsite. A major research university, extensive research facilities are an integral part of the Health Center's lifeblood.

Enrollment

For 2008, total enrollment was: 325

Special Features

Signature programs include The Pat and Jim Calhoun Cardiology Center, The Carole and Ray Neag Comprehensive Cancer Center, and The Musculoskeletal Institute. Research centers include: International Community Health Studies, Microbial Pathogenesis, Molecular Medicine, Immunotherapy of Cancer and Infectious Diseases, and Women's Health Research.

Housing

The School of Medicine helps students identify housing in the local community.

Satellite Campuses/Facilities

Students rotate through clinical sites to insure a mix of inpatient and ambulatory experiences. Students complete a Continuity Practice experience with a physician in the community.

Application Process and Requirements 2010–2011

Primary Application Service: AMCAS
Earliest filing date: June 1, 2009
Latest filing date: December 15, 2009

Secondary Application Required?: Yes
Sent to: All applicants
Contact: Lynda Fox, (860) 679-4306,
fox@nso1.uchc.edu
Fee: Yes, $85
Fee waiver available: Yes
Earliest filing date: June 1, 2009
Latest filing date: January 30, 2010

MCAT® required?: Yes
Latest MCAT® considered: September 2009
Oldest MCAT® considered: 2006

Early Decision Program: School does have EDP
Applicants notified: October 1, 2009
EDP available for: Both Residents and Non-residents

Regular Acceptance Notice
Earliest date: October 15, 2009
Latest date: Until class is full
Applicant's Response to Acceptance Offer – Maximum Time: Two weeks

Requests for Deferred Entrance Considered: Yes

Deposit to Hold Place in Class: Yes
Deposit (Resident): $100
Deposit (Non-resident): $100
Deposit due: with response to acceptance offer
Applied to tuition: Yes
Deposit refundable: Yes
Refundable by: May 15, 2010

Estimated number of new entrants: 85
EDP: 8, special program: n/a

Start Month/Year: August 2010

Interview Format: One-on-one and group interview session. Some regional interviews are done.

Other Programs

PREPARATORY PROGRAMS

Postbaccalaureate Program: Yes,
http://medicine.uchc.edu/prospective/postbac
Keat Sanford, (860)679-3874, sanford@nso1.uchc.edu
Summer Research Fellowships Program: Yes,
Keat Sanford, (860)679-3874, sanford@nso1.uchc.edu
Medical/Dental Preparatory Program: Yes,
http://medicine.uchc.edu/prospective/
enrichment/collegefellow

COMBINED DEGREE PROGRAMS

Baccalaureate/M.D.: Yes, http://medicine.uchc.
edu/prospective/admissions/babs_md/index.html
Keat Sanford, (860)679-3874, sanford@nso1.uchc.edu
M.D./M.P.H.: Yes, http://publichealth.uconn.edu/
acprgms_mph_combined.php
Keat Sanford, (860)679-3874, sanford@nso1.uchc.edu
M.D./M.B.A.: Yes, http://medicine.uchc.edu/prospective
/admissions/mba_md/index.html
Keat Sanford, (860)679-3874, sanford@nso1.uchc.edu
M.D./J.D.: No
M.D./Ph.D.: Yes, http://medicine.uchc.edu/
prospective/admissions/md_phd/index.html,
Dr. Barbara Kream, (860) 679-3849,
kream@nso1.uchc.edu

Premedical Coursework

Course	Req.	Rec.	Lab.	Hrs.	Course	Req.	Rec.	Lab.	Hrs.
Inorganic Chemistry	•		•	8	Computer Science				
Behavioral Sciences					Genetics		•		
Biochemistry		•			Humanities				
Biology		•			Organic Chemistry	•		•	8
Biology/Zoology	•		•	8	Physics	•		•	8
Calculus		•			Psychology		•		
College English		•			Social Sciences		•		
College Mathematics		•			Physiology		•		

Selection Factors: 2008 Accepted Applicants

Proportion of Accepted Applicants with Relevant Experience (Data Self-Reported to AMCAS®)		
Community Service/Volunteer		70%
Medically-Related Work		84%
Research		87%

Shaded bar represents school's accepted scores ranging from the 10th percentile to the 90th percentile. School Median ● National Median ●

Overall GPA 2.0 2.1 2.2 2.3 2.4 2.5 2.6 2.7 2.8 2.9 3.0 3.1 3.2 3.3 3.4 3.5 3.6 3.7 (3.8) 3.9 4.0

Science GPA 2.0 2.1 2.2 2.3 2.4 2.5 2.6 2.7 2.8 2.9 3.0 3.1 3.2 3.3 3.4 3.5 3.6 (3.7) 3.8 3.9 4.0

MCAT® Total Numeric Score 9 10 11 12 13 14 15 16 17 18 19 20 21 22 23 24 25 26 27 28 29 30 31 (32) 33 34 35 36 37 38 39 40 41 42 43

Writing Sample			J	K	L	M	N	O	P	(Q) R S T
Verbal Reasoning	3	4	5	6	7	8	9	(10)	11	12 13 14 15
Biological Sciences	3	4	5	6	7	8	9	10	(11)	12 13 14 15
Physical Sciences	3	4	5	6	7	8	9	10	(11)	12 13 14 15

Acceptance & Matriculation Data for 2008–2009 First Year Class

	Resident	Non-resident	International	Total
Applications	411	2195	253	2859
Interviewed	249	133	11	393
Deferred	3	2	1	6
Matriculants				
Early Assurance Program	5	0	0	5
Early Decision Program	0	0	0	0
Baccalaureate/M.D.	6	0	0	6
M.D./Ph.D.	0	6	0	6
Matriculated	64	19	2	**85**
Applications accepted from International Applicants: Yes				

Specialty Choice

2004, 2005, 2006 Graduates, Specialty Choice (As reported by program directors to GME Track™)	
Anesthesiology	6%
Emergency Medicine	7%
Family Practice	4%
Internal Medicine	24%
Obstetrics/Gynecology	5%
Orthopaedic Surgery	3%
Pediatrics	15%
Psychiatry	5%
Radiology	5%
Surgery	8%

Matriculant Demographics: 2008–2009 First Year Class

Men: 40   **Women:** 45

Matriculants' Self-Reported Race/Ethnicity

Mexican American	0	Korean	1
Cuban	0	Vietnamese	0
Puerto Rican	1	Other Asian	1
Other Hispanic	2	**Total Asian**	11
Total Hispanic	3	Native American	0
Chinese	2	**Black**	7
Asian Indian	6	Native Hawaiian	0
Pakistani	0	**White**	61
Filipino	0	**Unduplicated Number**	
Japanese	1	**of Matriculants**	85

Science and Math Majors: 69%
Matriculants with:
　　Baccalaureate degree: 100%
　　Graduate degree(s): 11%

Financial Information

Source: 2007-2008 LCME I-B survey and 2008-2009 AAMC TSF questionnaire

	Residents	Non-residents
Total Cost of Attendance	$52,443	$75,090
Tuition and Fees	$25,548	$48,198
Other (includes living expenses)	$24,275	$24,275
Health Insurance (can not be waived)	$2,620	$2,620

Average 2008 Graduate Indebtedness: $116,908
% of Enrolled Students Receiving Aid: 83%

Criminal Background Check

This medical school does not require a criminal background check prior to matriculation.

Yale University School of Medicine
New Haven, Connecticut

Richard A. Silverman, Director of Admissions
Yale University School of Medicine
Edward S. Harkness Hall, 367 Cedar Street
New Haven, Connecticut 06510
T 203 785 2696 **F** 203 785 3234

Admissions http://info.med.yale.edu/education/
admissions/
Main http://info.med.yale.edu/ysm/
Financial www.med.yale.edu/education/
finaid/index.html
E-mail medical.admissions@yale.edu

Private Institution

Dr. Robert J. Alpern, Dean

*Dr. Laura R. Ment, Associate Dean
for Admissions*

*Dr. Forrester A. Lee, Assistant Dean for
Multicultural Affairs*

*Dr. Richard Belitsky, Deputy Dean
for Education*

*Dr. Nancy R. Angoff, Associate Dean
for Student Affairs*

General Information
The Yale University School of Medicine was established in 1810 as the Medical Institution of Yale College. The present-day Yale-New Haven Medical Center includes the School of Medicine, the School of Nursing, and Yale-New Haven Hospital.

Mission Statement
The mission of the Yale University School of Medicine is to educate and inspire scholars and future leaders who will advance the practice of medicine and the biomedical sciences.

Curricular Highlights
Community Service Requirement: Optional. Extensive community service opportunities.
Research/Thesis Requirement: Required. Original thesis required since 1839.

The Yale System of Medical Education is founded on a belief in the maturity and responsibility of students. Highlights of the program are anonymous examinations, the absence of competitive grades, and a required thesis. The ideal Yale physician is schooled in the current state of knowledge of both medical biology and patient care, with a lifelong commitment to learning. The first two years of the curriculum focus on the basic and clinical sciences. The first year emphasizes normal biological form and function, the second year the study of disease. Throughout both years, a pre-clinical clerkship course provides instruction in history, physical examination, and the art of communicating with patients. The third year is largely devoted to clinical clerkships. In the fourth year, students take electives and a primary care clerkship, and complete their thesis.

Required since 1839, the thesis is designed to develop critical thinking, habits of self-education, and application of the scientific method to medicine. Thesis work also gives students an opportunity to work closely with Yale faculty members.

USMLE
Step 1: Required. Students must record a passing score for graduation, but not promotion.
Step 2: Clinical Skills (CS): Required. Students must record a passing total score to graduate.
Step 2: Clinical Knowledge (CK): Required. Students must record a passing total score to graduate.

Selection Factors
The Admissions Committee seeks exceptional students who best suit the educational philosophy of the school. Because of the importance of diversity, applications are encouraged from women and persons from groups underrepresented in medicine. The committee considers each applicant's academic record, MCAT scores, premedical committee evaluations, letters of recommendation, extracurricular and community activities, and personal qualities. In general, the school strives to admit students with the ability to make significant contributions in medicine and a demonstrated capacity for leadership. Interviews are arranged only by invitation of the Admissions Committee. The class of 100 students that enrolled in 2008 includes graduates of 55 undergraduate colleges. The diversity of the student body is also reflected in a wide variety of academic, professional, and personal interests. The Yale School of Medicine does not discriminate on the basis of sex, race, color, religion, age, disability, national or ethnic origin, sexual orientation, or gender identity or expression.

Financial Aid
Financial aid is based primarily on need and is intended to enable any accepted student to attend without unreasonable hardship. All financial aid applicants must submit the FAFSA and the Yale financial aid application, which will be available (online only) on January 1. In addition, those applying for Yale scholarship funds must submit a supplemental needs analysis, which requires student, spouse, and family financial statements.

Information about Diversity Programs
Diversity is important in Yale's collaborative learning environment, and applications are encouraged from individuals from groups underrepresented in medicine. Several student organizations sponsor a range of activities throughout the year, all supported by the Office of Multicultural Affairs.

Campus Information
Setting
In completing their studies near the heart of the Yale University campus, medical students benefit from academic and extracurricular opportunities provided by other Yale schools and by the city of New Haven, a culturally diverse city located 75 miles east of New York.

Enrollment
For 2008, total enrollment was: 394

Special Features
The Anlyan Center is an immense structure for disease-based research, with state-of-the-art teaching space for anatomy and histology. Construction of an enlarged Yale Cancer Center and incorporation of a new "West Campus" are major developments currently underway. Yale was recently honored with a Clinical and Translational Science Award from NIH, reflecting the School's commitment to clinical research. A Master of Health Science degree is now available as a joint degree option for M.D. students who choose to take a tuition-free fifth year. These and other new facilities and programs are part of an unprecedented period of growth at Yale.

Housing
On-campus housing is available for single and married students, and the Yale Housing Office provides access to off-campus apartments in the area.

Satellite Campuses/Facilities
Clinical training occurs at Yale-New Haven Hospital and other nearby hospitals and clinics. In addition, training sites have been established elsewhere in the United States and abroad. International research and community service opportunities are also available.

Application Process and Requirements 2010–2011

Primary Application Service: AMCAS
Earliest filing date: June 1, 2009
Latest filing date: October 15, 2009

Secondary Application Required?: Yes
Sent to: All applicants
URL: http://info.med.yale.edu/education/admissions/
Fee: Yes, $85
Fee waiver available: Yes
Earliest filing date: June 1, 2009
Latest filing date: November 15, 2009

MCAT® required?: Yes
Latest MCAT® considered: September 2009
Oldest MCAT® considered: April 2006

Early Decision Program: School does have EDP
Applicants notified: October 1, 2009
EDP available for: Both Residents and Non-residents

Regular Acceptance Notice
Earliest date: March 15, 2010
Latest date: Until class is full
Applicant's Response to Acceptance
Offer – Maximum Time: Three weeks

Requests for Deferred
Entrance Considered: Yes

Deposit to Hold Place in Class: Yes
Deposit (Resident): $100
Deposit (Non-resident): $100
Deposit due: With response to acceptance offer
Applied to tuition: Yes
Deposit refundable: Yes
Refundable by: May 15, 2010

Estimated number of new entrants: 100
EDP: 2, special program: n/a

Start Month/Year: August 2010

Interview Format: One-on-one, open-file interviews. Regional interviews only available if applicant is unable to come to campus.

Other Programs

PREPARATORY PROGRAMS
Postbaccalaureate Program: No
Summer Program: Yes, http://info.med.yale.edu/omca/programs/mmep.htm
Yale Summer Medical and Dental Education Program: http://info.med.yale.edu/omca/programs/mmep.htm
Biomedical Science Training & Enrichment Program: http://info.med.yale.edu/omca/programs/biostep.htm

COMBINED DEGREE PROGRAMS
Baccalaureate/M.D.: No
M.D./M.P.H.: Yes, http://info.med.yale.edu/ysm/admissions/index.html
M.D./M.B.A.: Yes, http://mba.yale.edu/mba/curriculum/md_mba/index.shtml
M.D./J.D.: Yes, www.law.yale.edu/academics/jointdegrees.asp
M.D./Ph.D.: Yes, http://info.med.yale.edu/mdphd/
Additional Program: Yes, http://info.med.yale.edu/ysm/admissions/index.html

Premedical Coursework

Course	Req.	Rec.	Lab.	Hrs.
Inorganic Chemistry	•		•	6-8
Behavioral Sciences				
Biochemistry				
Biology				
Biology/Zoology	•		•	6-8
Calculus				
College English				
College Mathematics				

Course	Req.	Rec.	Lab.	Hrs.
Computer Science				
Genetics				
Humanities				
Organic Chemistry	•		•	6-8
Physics	•		•	6-8
Psychology				
Social Sciences				
Other				

Selection Factors: 2008 Accepted Applicants

Proportion of Accepted Applicants with Relevant Experience (Data Self-Reported to AMCAS®)	
Community Service/Volunteer	72%
Medically-Related Work	89%
Research	96%

Shaded bar represents school's accepted scores ranging from the 10th percentile to the 90th percentile. **School Median** ● **National Median** ●

Overall GPA	2.0	2.1	2.2	2.3	2.4	2.5	2.6	2.7	2.8	2.9	3.0	3.1	3.2	3.3	3.4	3.5	3.6	3.7	3.8	(3.9)	4.0
Science GPA	2.0	2.1	2.2	2.3	2.4	2.5	2.6	2.7	2.8	2.9	3.0	3.1	3.2	3.3	3.4	3.5	3.6	3.7	3.8	(3.9)	4.0

MCAT® Total Numeric Score 9 10 11 12 13 14 15 16 17 18 19 20 21 22 23 24 25 26 27 28 29 30 31 (32) 33 34 35 (36) 37 38 39 40 41 42 43

Writing Sample			J	K	L	M	N	O	P	(Q)	(R)	S	T
Verbal Reasoning	3	4	5	6	7	8	9	(10)	(11)	12	(13)	14	15
Biological Sciences	3	4	5	6	7	8	9	10	(11)	12	(13)	14	15
Physical Sciences	3	4	5	6	7	8	9	10	(11)	12	(13)	14	15

Acceptance & Matriculation Data for 2008–2009 First Year Class

	Resident	Non-resident	International	Total
Applications	197	4543	432	5172
Interviewed	50	718	58	826
Deferred	1	3	0	4
Matriculants				
Early Assurance Program	n/a	n/a	n/a	n/a
Early Decision Program	0	0	0	0
Baccalaureate/M.D.	n/a	n/a	n/a	n/a
M.D./Ph.D.	3	10	0	13
Matriculated	8	84	8	**100**

Applications accepted from International Applicants: Yes

Matriculant Demographics: 2008–2009 First Year Class

Men: 49   **Women:** 51

Matriculants' Self-Reported Race/Ethnicity

Mexican American	4	Korean	3
Cuban	0	Vietnamese	1
Puerto Rican	0	Other Asian	3
Other Hispanic	5	Total Asian	29
Total Hispanic	8	Native American	1
Chinese	13	Black	10
Asian Indian	9	Native Hawaiian	0
Pakistani	0	White	53
Filipino	1	Unduplicated Number	
Japanese	0	of Matriculants	100

Science and Math Majors: 73%
Matriculants with:
   Baccalaureate degree: 100%
   Graduate degree(s): 8%

Specialty Choice

2004, 2005, 2006 Graduates, Specialty Choice (As reported by program directors to GME Track™)	
Anesthesiology	3%
Emergency Medicine	4%
Family Practice	2%
Internal Medicine	23%
Obstetrics/Gynecology	4%
Orthopaedic Surgery	4%
Pediatrics	7%
Psychiatry	4%
Radiology	6%
Surgery	7%

Financial Information

Source: 2007-2008 LCME I-B survey and 2008-2009 AAMC TSF questionnaire

	Residents	Non-residents
Total Cost of Attendance	$62,210	$62,510
Tuition and Fees	$42,750	$42,750
Other (includes living expenses)	$17,470	$17,770
Health Insurance (can be waived)	$1,990	$1,990

Average 2008 Graduate Indebtedness: $124,135
% of Enrolled Students Receiving Aid: 90%

Criminal Background Check

This medical school does not require a criminal background check prior to matriculation.

The George Washington University School of Medicine and Health Sciences
Washington, District of Columbia

The George Washington University
School of Medicine and Health Sciences
Office of M.D. Admissions
2300 I Street, N.W., Ross Hall 716
Washington, District of Columbia 20037
T 202 994 3506   **F** 202 994 1753

Admissions www.gwumc.edu/edu/admis
Main www.gwumc.edu/smhs
Financial www.gwumc.edu/smhs/Fin-Aid
E-mail medadmit@gwu.edu

Private Institution

Dr. John F. Williams, Provost and Vice President for Health Affairs

Dr. James L. Scott, Dean, School of Medicine and Health Sciences

Diane P. McQuail, Assistant Dean of Admissions

Charles W. Carpenter, Director of Financial Aid

General Information

Founded in 1825, the School of Medicine and Health Sciences is the 11th oldest medical school in the country. The school is housed in Ross Hall, a research, educational and administrative facility located in the nation's capital. Located adjacent to Ross Hall, the new, state-of-the-art GW Hospital opened in August 2002. The facility boasts an Educational Center consisting of a clinical simulation facility, a standardized patient examination facility, a computer resource center, and lounge/conference areas.

Mission Statement

With a vision to be a pre-eminent health institution in the Washington area, GW is committed to providing the highest quality of care and health services to the public; excellence and innovation in education; and research that expands the frontiers of science and knowledge.

Curricular Highlights

Community Service Requirement: Required.
Research/Thesis Requirement: Optional.

The curriculum contains a course entitled "The Practice of Medicine" (POM). This course spans all four years, allowing students to immediately begin clinical training during the first two years while studying the basic sciences. Each first-year student has a physician mentor. Clinical clerkships begin in the third year, and opportunities for international clinical experiences are available during the fourth year. An Honors/Pass/Conditional/Fail system is used for grading. Early Selection Programs are available to sophomores in the spring semester at GW, the University of Maryland-College Park, St. Bonaventure, and George Mason Universities, and Franklin & Marshall, Claremont McKenna, Scripps, Rowan, Knox, Colgate, Lyon, Rhodes, and Hampden-Sydney Colleges. In addition, linkage agree-

ments exist with postbaccalaureate programs at Goucher College, the University of Pennsylvania, Brandeis University, New York University, Scripps College, Johns Hopkins University, and Bryn Mawr College. Transfer information for the second- and third-year classes is available at *www.gwumc.edu/edu/admis/html/admissions/transfer.html*.

USMLE

Step 1: Required. Students must record a passing score for promotion.
Step 2: Clinical Skills (CS): Required. Students must record a passing total score to graduate.
Step 2: Clinical Knowledge (CK): Required. Students must record a passing total score to graduate.

Selection Factors

The initial evaluation is based on data in the AMCAS and GW applications. This evaluation reviews academic performance; MCAT scores; extracurricular, health-related, research, and work experiences; and evidence of non-scholastic accomplishments. The next phase of the selection procedure is based on examination of personal comments and letters of recommendation. The most promising applicants are invited for interview. The last phase includes the review by the Committee on Admissions of the entire dossier. This phase selects academically prepared students with motivational and personal characteristics the Committee considers important in future physicians.

Financial Aid

Information is available at *www.gwumc.edu/mhs/Fin-Aid/*. Merit-based admissions scholarships are available.

Information about Diversity Programs

The School of Medicine is committed to providing an education to students from groups underrepresented in medicine. Applicants are encouraged to meet with students and faculty from groups underrepresented in medicine. There are focused student organizations such as NBLHO and SNMA.

Campus Information

Setting

The Medical Center is on the Foggy Bottom campus of The George Washington University in

Washington, DC. A subway stop sits immediately outside the medical school. The campus is within walking distance of the White House and the National Mall.

Enrollment

For 2008, total enrollment was: 689

Special Features

Students study histology and pathology in a state-of-the-art laboratory, reviewing digital slides on computer monitors. The newly created Office of Student Opportunities serves as a clearinghouse for various research, scholarships, awards, conferences, and study abroad opportunities. The Track Program offers students an opportunity to choose a program of study outside the standard curriculum, *www.gwumc.edu/smhs/students/opportunities*. Electives in first and second years include humanities and ethics. GW operates a Mobile Mammography Program (GW Mammovan), which provides screening mammograms to women in the DC area. The Interdisciplinary Student Community-Oriented Prevention Enhancement Service (ISCOPES) is an interdisciplinary team service-learning experience providing a wide range of health-related services. The student-run Healing Clinic also provides health care to DC's underserved.

Housing

Some graduate student housing is available. The Washington, DC area has abundant off-campus housing options. For information, visit *www.gwumc.edu/edu/admis/html/student/housing.html*.

Satellite Campuses/Facilities

In addition to the GW Hospital, the teaching services of the Children's National Medical Center, Inova Fairfax Hospital, Holy Cross Hospital, National Naval Medical Center, St. Elizabeth's Hospital, Veterans Administration Hospital, and Washington Hospital Center are also available to students. A variety of ambulatory sites in the DC area are also utilized, including neighborhood clinics that serve indigent patients.

Application Process and Requirements 2010–2011

Primary Application Service: AMCAS
Earliest filing date: June 1, 2009
Latest filing date: December 1, 2009

Secondary Application Required?: Yes
Sent to: All applicants
URL: n/a
Fee: Yes, $125
Fee waiver available: Yes
Earliest filing date: June 1, 2009
Latest filing date: January 1, 2010

MCAT® required?: Yes
Latest MCAT® considered: September 2009
Oldest MCAT® considered: April 2007

Early Decision Program: School does have EDP
Applicants notified: October 1, 2009
EDP available for: Both Residents and Non-residents

Regular Acceptance Notice
Earliest date: October 15, 2009
Latest date: Until class is full
Applicant's Response to Acceptance
Offer – Maximum Time: Three weeks

Requests for Deferred
Entrance Considered: Yes

Deposit to Hold Place in Class: Yes
Deposit (Resident): $100
Deposit (Non-resident): $100
Deposit due: May 15, 2010
Applied to tuition: Yes
Deposit refundable: Yes
Refundable by: May 15, 2010

Estimated number of new entrants: 177
EDP: 5, special program: 63

Start Month/Year: August 2010

Interview Format: Two blind interviews with a faculty member and a student. All interviews take place at GW.

Other Programs

PREPARATORY PROGRAMS
Postbaccalaureate Program: No
Summer Program: No

COMBINED DEGREE PROGRAMS
Baccalaureate/M.D.: Yes, 7 year program with George Washington University, http://gwired.gwu.edu/adm/apply/special_prog.html, 8 year program with St. Bonaventure University, www.sbu.edu and www.gwumc.edu
M.D./M.P.H.: Yes, www.gwumc.edu/edu/admis/html/academics/specialprog.html
M.D./M.B.A.: No
M.D./J.D.: No
M.D./Ph.D.: Yes, www.gwumc.edu/edu/admis/html/academics/specialprog.html

Premedical Coursework

Course	Req.	Rec.	Lab.	Hrs.
Inorganic Chemistry	•		•	8
Behavioral Sciences				
Biochemistry				
Biology				
Biology/Zoology	•		•	8
Calculus				
College English	•			6
College Mathematics				

Course	Req.	Rec.	Lab.	Hrs.
Computer Science				
Genetics				
Humanities				
Organic Chemistry	•		•	8
Physics	•		•	8
Psychology				
Social Sciences				
Other				

Selection Factors: 2008 Accepted Applicants

Proportion of Accepted Applicants with Relevant Experience (Data Self-Reported to AMCAS®)	
Community Service/Volunteer	71%
Medically-Related Work	86%
Research	79%

Shaded bar represents school's accepted scores ranging from the 10th percentile to the 90th percentile. School Median ● National Median ●

Overall GPA 2.0 2.1 2.2 2.3 2.4 2.5 2.6 2.7 2.8 2.9 3.0 3.1 3.2 3.3 **3.4 3.5 3.6 (3.7)** 3.8 3.9 4.0
Science GPA 2.0 2.1 2.2 2.3 2.4 2.5 2.6 2.7 2.8 2.9 3.0 3.1 **3.2 3.3 3.4 3.5 (3.6)** 3.7 3.8 3.9 4.0

MCAT® Total Numeric Score 9 10 11 12 13 14 15 16 17 18 19 20 21 22 23 24 25 **26 27 28 29 (30) 31 (32) 33** 34 35 36 37 38 39 40 41 42 43

Writing Sample			J	K	L	**M N O P (Q) R S**	T
Verbal Reasoning	3	4	5	6	7	**8 9 (10) 11** 12	13	14	15
Biological Sciences	3	4	5	6	7	**8 9 (10) (11)** 12	13	14	15
Physical Sciences	3	4	5	6	7	**8 9 (10) (11)** 12	13	14	15

Acceptance & Matriculation Data for 2008–2009 First Year Class

	Resident	Non-resident	International	Total
Applications	44	12738	512	13294
Interviewed	19	1012	7	1038
Deferred	0	4	0	4
Matriculants				
Early Assurance Program	0	31	0	31
Early Decision Program	0	4	1	5
Baccalaureate/M.D.	1	16	0	17
M.D./Ph.D.	0	0	0	0
Matriculated	3	166	8	**177**

Applications accepted from International Applicants: Yes

Specialty Choice

2004, 2005, 2006 Graduates, Specialty Choice (As reported by program directors to GME Track™)	
Anesthesiology	8%
Emergency Medicine	5%
Family Practice	5%
Internal Medicine	22%
Obstetrics/Gynecology	4%
Orthopaedic Surgery	3%
Pediatrics	12%
Psychiatry	7%
Radiology	5%
Surgery	8%

Matriculant Demographics: 2008–2009 First Year Class

Men: 67 **Women:** 110

Matriculants' Self-Reported Race/Ethnicity

Mexican American	0	Korean	3
Cuban	1	Vietnamese	2
Puerto Rican	0	Other Asian	3
Other Hispanic	4	Total Asian	50
Total Hispanic	4	Native American	1
Chinese	5	Black	26
Asian Indian	34	Native Hawaiian	0
Pakistani	1	White	88
Filipino	3	Unduplicated Number	
Japanese	1	of Matriculants	177

Science and Math Majors: 53%
Matriculants with:
Baccalaureate degree: 99%
Graduate degree(s): 15%

Financial Information

Source: 2007–2008 LCME I-B survey and 2008–2009 AAMC TSF questionnaire

	Residents	Non-residents
Total Cost of Attendance	$68,310	$68,310
Tuition and Fees	$46,267	$46,267
Other (includes living expenses)	$22,043	$22,043
Health Insurance (can be waived)	$0	$0

Average 2008 Graduate Indebtedness: $188,205
% of Enrolled Students Receiving Aid: 86%

Criminal Background Check

This medical school currently requires a criminal background check prior to matriculation.

Georgetown University School of Medicine
Washington, District of Columbia

Office of Admissions
Georgetown University School of Medicine
Box 571421
Washington, District of Columbia 20057-1421
T 202 687 1154   **F** 202 687 3079

Admissions http://som.georgetown.edu/prospectivestudents
Main http://som.georgetown.edu
Financial http://som.georgetown.edu/studentservices/financialaid/home/
E-mail medicaladmissions@georgetown.edu

Private Institution

Dr. S. Ray Mitchell, Dean for Medical Education

Brandon C. Schneider, Assistant Dean for Admissions

Joy P. Williams, Associate Dean for Students and Special Programs

David J. Pollock, Assistant Dean for Student Financial Planning

Dr. Russell T. Wall III, Associate Dean for Admissions and Student Services

General Information

The School of Medicine works in association with the 535-bed Georgetown University Hospital, part of the MedStar not-for-profit health care system. The school has affiliations with eight federal and community hospitals in the Washington, DC area. The campus contains a health science library and an integrated learning center with 10 clinical examination rooms. Adjacent to the hospital is the Lombardi Cancer Research Center, which provides both research and clinical care. The school is near the NIH and other internationally prominent health care and research facilities. The Yates Field House offers swimming, jogging tracks, and other athletic programs. The Leavey Center hosts dining establishments and guest quarters.

Mission Statement

Guided by the University's Jesuit tradition of 'cura personalis,' caring for the whole person, Georgetown University School of Medicine will educate, in an integrated way, knowledgeable, skillful, ethical, and compassionate physicians and biomedical scientists, dedicated to the care of others and the health needs of our society. Our educational approach involves the integration of the basic sciences, clinical experiences, and the humanistic disciplines in each systems-based module, reinforcing the learning experience with clinical care skills and patient panels. Students also serve on educational and student affairs committees.

Curricular Highlights

Community Service Requirement: Required.
Research/Thesis Requirement: Research project required.

Georgetown's curriculum in the first two years emphasizes the body's normal and altered structure and functions reinforced with clinically oriented educational experiences, early introduction to patients, the art of advocacy, and the ethical/cultural dimensions of medicine. Small-group teaching in labs, seminars, and at the bedside begins early in the first year. The third year provides comprehensive clinical training to care of patients through clerkships in the major medical specialties. The fourth year gives each student substantial responsibility for the management of patient care through acting internships, elective study, and research. The grading system consists of Honors, High Pass, Pass, and Fail.

USMLE

Step 1: Required. Students must record a passing score for promotion.
Step 2: Clinical Skills (CS): Required. Students must record a passing total score to graduate.
Step 2: Clinical Knowledge (CK): Required. Students must record a passing total score to graduate.

Selection Factors

The Committee on Admissions selects students on the basis of academic achievement, character, maturity, and motivation. The committee evaluates the applicant's entire academic record, performance on the MCAT, college premedical committee evaluations or letters of recommendation, personal essays, and personal interviews. Personal interviews are required and conducted on the medical center campus. Applicants may be invited to interview once all credentials have been reviewed by the Committee. A secondary application and essay are required for all applicants. Applicants are urged to submit their applications and supporting credentials early. The School of Medicine does not discriminate on the basis of race, sex, creed, age, disability, sexual orientation, or national or ethnic origin. The School of Medicine has an Early Assurance Program with its undergraduate institution. Applicants for transfer are only considered from LCME-accredited medical schools.

Financial Aid

The school participates in federal financial aid programs and awards school-administered scholarships and low-interest loans to students on the basis of financial need. Parents' financial information is required for students seeking school-administered aid. Loan indebtedness counseling is an important function of the Office of Student Financial Planning, as a majority of students incur substantial educational debt. Candidates for admission are strongly encouraged to contact the office with questions.

Information about Diversity Programs

The School of Medicine has a diverse student body, with students from groups underrepresented in medicine. Questions about programs may be addressed to the director, Office of Programs for Minority Student Development. The Georgetown Experimental Medical Studies (GEMS) Program is a one-year postbaccalaureate program for qualified disadvantaged students and those from groups underrepresented in medicine. Priority consideration is given to residents of the District of Columbia. For more information, please telephone the GEMS program coordinator at (202) 687-1406.

Campus Information
Setting
On the university campus, in an urban setting.

Enrollment
For 2008, total enrollment was: 779

Special Features
Special features include Georgetown's state-of-the-art Clinical Skills Center, the Lombardi Cancer Center, opportunities for international clerkships following the first year and in the fourth year, and several community outreach programs.

Housing
No on-campus housing is available. The Office of Admissions attempts to assist students in finding housing.

Satellite Campuses/Facilities
Rotations are divided among the university hospital and other hospitals in the metro area. Ambulatory care experiences are within the area.

Application Process and Requirements 2010–2011

Primary Application Service: AMCAS
Earliest filing date: June 1, 2009
Latest filing date: October 31, 2009

Secondary Application Required?: Yes
Sent To: All applicants
URL: http://som.georgetown.edu/prospectivestudents
Fee: $130
Fee Waiver Available: Yes
Earliest filing date: June 15, 2009
Latest filing date: January 5, 2010

MCAT® required?: Yes
Latest MCAT® considered: September 2009
Oldest MCAT® considered: January 2007

Early Decision Program: School does not have EDP
Applicants notified: n/a
EDP available for: n/a

Regular Acceptance Notice
Earliest date: October 15, 2009
Latest date: Until class is full
Applicant's Response to Acceptance
Offer – Maximum Time: Three weeks

Requests for Deferred
Entrance Considered: Yes

Deposit to Hold Place in Class: Yes
Deposit (Resident): $100
Deposit (Non-resident): $100
Deposit due: March 16, 2009. Partial tuition pre-payment due June 1, 2009
Applied to tuition: Yes
Deposit refundable: Yes
Refundable by: May 15, 2010

Estimated number of new entrants: 198
EDP: n/a, special program: n/a

Start Month/Year: August 2010

Interview Format: Interviews are one-on-one. Regional interviews are not available.

Other Programs

PREPARATORY PROGRAMS
Postbaccalaureate Program: Yes, http://gems.georgetown.edu
Summer Program: Yes, http://gsmi.georgetown.edu

COMBINED DEGREE PROGRAMS
Baccalaureate/M.D.: No
M.D./M.P.H.: No

M.D./M.B.A.: Yes, http://msb.georgetown.edu/prospective/graduate/mba/curriculum/enrichment/joint_degree/
M.D./J.D.: No
M.D./Ph.D.: Yes, http://biomedgrad.georgetown.edu/MDPhD/index.html

Premedical Coursework

Course	Req.	Rec.	Lab.	Sems.
Inorganic Chemistry	•		•	2
Behavioral Sciences				
Biochemistry		•		
Biology	•		•	2
Biology/Zoology				
Calculus				
College English	•			2
College Mathematics	•			1

Course	Req.	Rec.	Lab.	Sems.
Computer Science		•		
Genetics		•		
Humanities		•		
Organic Chemistry	•		•	2
Physics	•		•	2
Psychology				
Social Sciences				
Other				

Selection Factors: 2008 Accepted Applicants

Proportion of Accepted Applicants with Relevant Experience (Data Self-Reported to AMCAS®)		
Community Service/Volunteer		73%
Medically-Related Work		89%
Research		86%

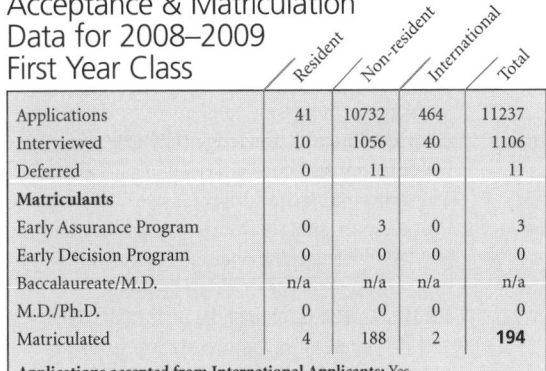

Shaded bar represents school's accepted scores ranging from the 10th percentile to the 90th percentile. School Median ● National Median ●

Overall GPA 2.0 2.1 2.2 2.3 2.4 2.5 2.6 2.7 2.8 2.9 3.0 3.1 3.2 3.3 3.4 3.5 3.6 (3.7) 3.8 3.9 4.0

Science GPA 2.0 2.1 2.2 2.3 2.4 2.5 2.6 2.7 2.8 2.9 3.0 3.1 3.2 3.3 3.4 3.5 3.6 (3.7) 3.8 3.9 4.0

MCAT® Total Numeric Score 9 10 11 12 13 14 15 16 17 18 19 20 21 22 23 24 25 26 27 28 29 30 31 (32) 33 34 35 36 37 38 39 40 41 42 43

	J	K	L	M	N	O	P	Q	R	S	T
Writing Sample	J	K	L	M	N	O	P	(Q)	R	S	T

Verbal Reasoning	3	4	5	6	7	8	9	(10)	11	12	13	14	15
Biological Sciences	3	4	5	6	7	8	9	10	(11)	12	13	14	15
Physical Sciences	3	4	5	6	7	8	9	10	(11)	12	13	14	15

Acceptance & Matriculation Data for 2008–2009 First Year Class

	Resident	Non-resident	International	Total
Applications	41	10732	464	11237
Interviewed	10	1056	40	1106
Deferred	0	11	0	11
Matriculants				
Early Assurance Program	0	3	0	3
Early Decision Program	0	0	0	0
Baccalaureate/M.D.	n/a	n/a	n/a	n/a
M.D./Ph.D.	0	0	0	0
Matriculated	4	188	2	**194**

Applications accepted from International Applicants: Yes

Specialty Choice

2004, 2005, 2006 Graduates, Specialty Choice (As reported by program directors to GME Track™)	
Anesthesiology	8%
Emergency Medicine	7%
Family Practice	6%
Internal Medicine	20%
Obstetrics/Gynecology	4%
Orthopaedic Surgery	8%
Pediatrics	8%
Psychiatry	3%
Radiology	5%
Surgery	8%

Matriculant Demographics: 2008–2009 First Year Class

Men: 101   **Women:** 93

Matriculants' Self-Reported Race/Ethnicity

Mexican American	2	Korean	5
Cuban	2	Vietnamese	5
Puerto Rican	2	Other Asian	4
Other Hispanic	5	Total Asian	49
Total Hispanic	11	Native American	0
Chinese	15	Black	13
Asian Indian	15	Native Hawaiian	1
Pakistani	3	White	125
Filipino	2	Unduplicated Number	
Japanese	1	of Matriculants	194

Science and Math Majors: 65%
Matriculants with:
   Baccalaureate degree: 99%
   Graduate degree(s): 23%

Financial Information

Source: 2007–2008 LCME I-B survey and 2008–2009 AAMC TSF questionnaire

	Residents	Non-residents
Total Cost of Attendance	$67,453	$67,453
Tuition and Fees	$44,444	$44,444
Other (includes living expenses)	$21,299	$21,299
Health Insurance (can be waived)	$1,710	$1,710

Average 2008 Graduate Indebtedness: $163,240
% of Enrolled Students Receiving Aid: 86%

Criminal Background Check

This medical school requires a criminal background check prior to matriculation.

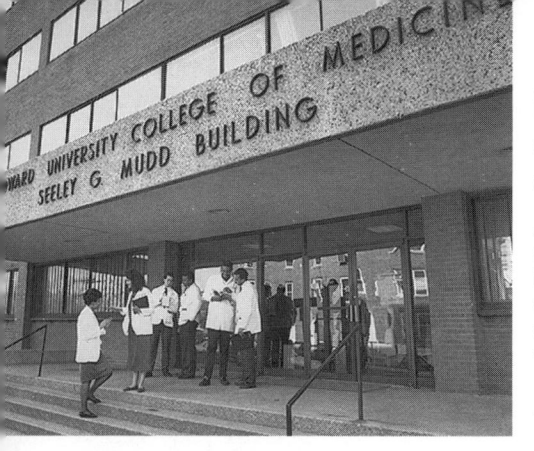

Howard University College of Medicine
Washington, District of Columbia

Office of Admissions, Office of the Dean
Howard University College of Medicine,
520 W Street, N.W., Room 2310
Washington, District of Columbia 20059
T 202 806 6270   **F** 202 265 0048

Admissions http://medicine.howard.edu/students/
prospective/admissions
Main www.medicine.howard.edu
Financial http://medicine.howard.edu/finance/
overview.htm
E-mail hucmadmissions@howard.edu

Private Institution

Dr. Robert E. Taylor, Dean

Judith M. Walk, Director of Admissions

Dr. Dawn L. Cannon, Associate Dean for Student Affairs and Admissions

Ann Finney, Admissions Officer

General Information
The Howard University College of Medicine is the oldest and largest historically black medical school in the United States and the 36th oldest of all 130 medical schools in this country. The medical department's primary goal at inception remains the college's goal today: to train students to become competent, compassionate physicians who will provide care in medically underserved communities. The college has more than 4,000 living alumni, including approximately 25 percent of all black practicing physicians in this country. The 321-bed Howard University Hospital is the college's primary teaching hospital for medical students and is used for postgraduate training in the various specialties of medicine. Medical students also serve clerkships at the Children's National Medical Center, INOVA Fairfax Hospital, St. Elizabeth's Hospital, the Washington Veterans Affairs Medical Center, Providence Hospital, the Washington Hospital Center, and Prince George's Hospital Center.

Mission Statement
Howard University College of Medicine provides students of high academic potential with a medical education of exceptional quality and prepares physicians and other health care professionals to serve the underserved. Particular focus is on the education of disadvantaged students for careers in medicine.

Curricular Highlights
Community Service Requirement: Optional.
Research/Thesis Requirement: Optional.

An integrated curriculum was implemented in August 2001. Students in the first year complete curriculum blocks in Molecules and Cells, Structure and Function, and Medicine and Society. In year two, pathophysiology, pathology and pharmacology are integrated according to organ systems. The Medicine and Society block continues throughout the second year, and blocks in Physical Diagnosis and Introduction to Clinical Medicine are also included in year two. The third and fourth years consist of blocks of instruction in a continuum of clerkships and examinations in core clinical disciplines. During the fourth year, opportunity is available for additional clinical or research experience through 24 or 28 weeks of required electives. Grades in the College of Medicine are reported as H (honors), S (satisfactory), or U (unsatisfactory).

USMLE
Step 1: Required. Students must record a passing score for promotion.
Step 2: Clinical Skills (CS): Required. Students must record a passing total score to graduate.
Step 2: Clinical Knowledge (CK): Required. Students must record a passing total score to graduate.

Selection Factors
There are four major criteria used in the selection of applicants for admission to the College of Medicine: (1) character and discernible motivation for a career in medicine, (2) scholastic record, (3) results of the MCAT, and (4) letters of recommendation from pre-professional advisors and faculty. Candidates for admission and alternates are selected from among those applicants who satisfy the criteria and who are most likely to serve in communities needing physician services. An invitation for an interview may be extended to an applicant after the Committee on Admissions has made a preliminary examination of the applicant's credentials and has decided that an interview is desirable. Although the total student is evaluated, the Committee on Admissions gives strongest consideration to those who have GPAs of 3.0 and above. There are no residence restrictions. All applicants will be evaluated regardless of the applicants sex, race, religion, national or ethnic origin, age, marital status, or disability. A $100 (refundable) deposit and a $300 (non-refundable) enrollment fee (due with response to acceptance) is required of accepted applicants who have never previously enrolled at Howard University.

Financial Aid
Nearly all of the students enrolled in the College of Medicine receive some sort of financial assistance. Financial aid applicants must submit the FAFSA. Students with demonstrated need may receive school-based scholarships and loans, and those who qualify are recommended for federally guaranteed and private educational loans. Some merit awards are offered to outstanding entering first-year students and for exceptional academic performance in the medical curriculum. Some students receive scholarships funded by the National Health Service Corps or by the military.

Campus Information

Setting
The location of the campus in Washington, D.C., provides a cosmopolitan setting with a diversity of population and activities. The campus is Metrorail and Metrobus-accessible, and within walking distance of the hospital.

Enrollment
For 2008, total enrollment was: 464

Housing
Limited on-campus housing is available for graduate and professional students. Most medical students live off-campus within a short commute to the university.

Satellite Campuses/Facilities
Student rotations are divided between Howard University Hospital and several hospitals, ambulatory centers, and private physicians' offices in the metropolitan area.

Application Process and Requirements 2010–2011

Primary Application Service: AMCAS
Earliest filing date: June 1, 2009
Latest filing date: December 15, 2009

Secondary Application Required?: Yes, http://medicine.howard.edu/students/prospective/admissions/process.htm
Sent to: All applicants
Contact: Ms. Judith Walk
(202) 806-6279, jwalk@howard.edu
Fee: Yes, $75
Fee waiver available: No
Earliest filing date: August 15, 2009
Latest filing date: January 30, 2010 or thirty days after receipt of secondary e-mail

MCAT® required?: Yes
Latest MCAT® considered: September 2009
Oldest MCAT® considered: August 2007

Early Decision Program: School does not have EDP
Applicants notified: n/a
EDP available for: n/a

Regular Acceptance Notice
Earliest date: October 15, 2009
Latest date: Until class is full
Applicant's Response to Acceptance
Offer – Maximum Time: 30 days, until April 15, 2010

Requests for Deferred
Entrance Considered: Yes

Deposit to Hold Place in Class: Yes
Deposit (Resident): $100
Deposit (Non-resident): $100
Deposit due: With acceptance offer, accompanied by non-refundable enrollment fee
Applied to tuition: Yes
Deposit refundable: Yes
Refundable by: April 15, 2010

Estimated number of new entrants: 115
EDP: n/a, special program: n/a

Start Month/Year: July 2010

Interview Format: One-on-one interview with admissions committee member. Regional interviews are not available.

Other Programs

PREPARATORY PROGRAMS
Postbaccalaureate Program: No
Summer Program: Yes, www.founders.howard.edu/preprof/enrichmentprog.htm
Summer Medical and Dental Education Program (SMDEP): www.med.howard.edu/lloyd/HUCM_Information_06-07.pdf

COMBINED DEGREE PROGRAMS
Baccalaureate/M.D.: Yes, www.founders.howard.edu/preprof/BSMD-Brochure.pdf
M.D./M.P.H.: No
M.D./M.B.A.: Yes, Dr. Sheik N. Hassan, (202) 806-9494, shassan@howard.edu
M.D./J.D.: No
M.D./Ph.D.: Yes, Dr. Verle Headings, (202) 806-6100, vheadings@howard.edu

Premedical Coursework

Course	Req.	Rec.	Lab.	Hrs.
Inorganic Chemistry	•		•	8
Behavioral Sciences				
Biochemistry		•		4
Biology	•		•	8
Biology/Zoology				
Calculus				
College English	•			6
College Mathematics	•			6

Course	Req.	Rec.	Lab.	Hrs.
Computer Science				
Genetics		•		4
Humanities	•			6
Organic Chemistry	•		•	8
Physics	•		•	8
Psychology				
Social Sciences				
Other				

Selection Factors: 2008 Accepted Applicants

Proportion of Accepted Applicants with Relevant Experience (Data Self-Reported to AMCAS®)		
Community Service/Volunteer	71%
Medically-Related Work	74%
Research	72%

Shaded bar represents school's accepted scores ranging from the 10th percentile to the 90th percentile. **School Median** ● **National Median** ●

Overall GPA 2.0 2.1 2.2 2.3 2.4 2.5 2.6 2.7 2.8 2.9 3.0 **3.1 3.2 3.3 3.4 (3.5) 3.6 3.7 3.8 3.9** 4.0
Science GPA 2.0 2.1 2.2 2.3 2.4 2.5 2.6 2.7 **2.8 2.9 3.0 3.1 3.2 3.3 (3.4)** 3.5 3.6 3.7 3.8 3.9 4.0

MCAT® Total Numeric Score 9 10 11 12 13 14 15 16 17 18 19 20 21 **22 23 24 (25) 26 27 28 29 30 31 (32)** 33 34 35 36 37 38 39 40 41 42 43

Writing Sample			J	K	L	**M**	**N**	**(O)**	**P**	**(Q)**	**R**	S	T
Verbal Reasoning	3	4	5	**6**	**7**	**(8)**	**9**	**(10)**	**11**	12	13	14	15
Biological Sciences	3	4	5	6	**7**	**8**	**(9)**	**10**	**(11)**	12	13	14	15
Physical Sciences	3	4	5	6	**7**	**(8)**	**9**	**10**	**(11)**	12	13	14	15

Acceptance & Matriculation Data for 2008–2009 First Year Class

	Resident	Non-resident	International	Total
Applications	19	5093	523	5635
Interviewed	5	323	16	344
Deferred	0	2	0	2
Matriculants				
Early Assurance Program	0	0	0	0
Early Decision Program	0	0	0	0
Baccalaureate/M.D.	0	0	0	0
M.D./Ph.D.	0	0	0	0
Matriculated	2	102	10	**114**

Applications accepted from International Applicants: Yes

Matriculant Demographics: 2008–2009 First Year Class

Men: 49   **Women:** 65

Matriculants' Self-Reported Race/Ethnicity

Mexican American	3	Korean	1
Cuban	1	Vietnamese	2
Puerto Rican	3	Other Asian	1
Other Hispanic	4	Total Asian	19
Total Hispanic	11	Native American	2
Chinese	1	Black	80
Asian Indian	12	Native Hawaiian	0
Pakistani	1	White	8
Filipino	1	Unduplicated Number	
Japanese	0	of Matriculants	114

Science and Math Majors: 72%
Matriculants with:
  Baccalaureate degree: 89%
  Graduate degree(s): 15%

Specialty Choice

2004, 2005, 2006 Graduates, Specialty Choice (As reported by program directors to GME Track™)

Anesthesiology	4%
Emergency Medicine	4%
Family Practice	9%
Internal Medicine	20%
Obstetrics/Gynecology	10%
Orthopaedic Surgery	3%
Pediatrics	9%
Psychiatry	5%
Radiology	3%
Surgery	10%

Financial Information

Source: 2007-2008 LCME I-B survey and 2008-2009 AAMC TSF questionnaire

	Residents	Non-residents
Total Cost of Attendance	$54,364	$54,364
Tuition and Fees	$34,081	$34,0816
Other (includes living expenses)	$20,283	$20,283
Health Insurance	$0	$0

Average 2008 Graduate Indebtedness: $149,862
% of Enrolled Students Receiving Aid: 96%

Criminal Background Check

This medical school requires a criminal background check prior to matriculation.

Florida International University College of Medicine

Miami, Florida

Office of Admissions
Florida International University
College of Medicine
11200 S.W 8th Street – HLSII 660 W2
Miami, Florida 33199
T 305 348 0644   **F** 305 348 0650

Admissions http://medicine.fiu.edu/admissions.php
Main http://medicine.fiu.edu
Financial: http://medicine.fiu.edu/admissions.php?ss=finaid-intro
E-mail med.admissions@fiu.edu

Public Institution

Dr. John Rock, Founding Dean and Senior VP for Medical Affairs

Dr. Sanford Markham, Executive Associate Dean for Student Affairs

Dr. Robert Dollinger, Assistant Dean, Student Affairs, Counseling and Communities

Dr. Barbra Roller, Assistant Dean, Student Affairs, Admissions and Records

Betty L. Monfort, MPH, Director, Admissions and Records

Charlotte Rhine, MEd, Associate Director, Admissions and Records

Pemra Cetin, MBA, Director, Financial Aid

General Information

In August 2009, the College of Medicine welcomes the inaugural class. The four year program, leading to the M.D. degree, involves in-depth exposure and training in all areas of medical education with specific focus on family and community medicine. Unique to the College is the hands-on experience each student receives in observing and caring for families who have little or no access to medical care. Key in the medical training is the focus on the importance of the doctor-patient relationship in diverse patient populations.

Mission Statement

The Mission of the College of Medicine at Florida International University is to serve as a model for the next generation of medical education and to elevate the level of care available to the Florida community. Our goals are to: (1) Educate culturally competent physicians to serve diverse populations; (2) Provide South Florida students greater access to medical education, admitting a student body that reflects the rich diversity of the region; (3) Develop a curriculum focused on community medicine, elevating the quality of medical care; and (4) Develop basic, translational and clinical research programs that will ensure state of the art care and will substantially expand the economic growth potential of the region.

General Information

Curricular Highlights

Community Service Requirement: Required. Community Service is an integral part of our mission and innovative curriculum.
Research/Thesis Requirement: Optional.

The emphasis is community-based, patient-centered learning with the development of an understanding of personal, cultural, and social factors affecting health care. Students will develop competencies in a full range of medical specialties. The College has created a new curriculum that is community based and emphasizes patient-centered learning with a focus on developing an understanding of personal, cultural and social factors in healthcare. Organized as a four year integration of studies, the curriculum has five strands: Clinical Medicine, Disease, Illness and Injury (pathological approaches), Human Biology (basic medical sciences), Medicine and Society, and Professional Development (statistical and evidence based medicine). Curricular innovations include the Medicine and Society strand, the goal of which is to enable students to gain an understanding of factors that affect personal and community health care. As part of our signature program, Neighborhood HELP, students work with individuals, families and communities in interdisciplinary student teams from Public Health, Nursing and Social Work. This strand integrates ethics, public health, cultural competency and sustained community experiences. Cases will be used throughout the curriculum as a context for learning. Small class sizes will provide individualized attention. Small group learning and independent study are emphasized; research is encouraged as an option. The founding faculty have been selected for their excellence in teaching; the learning format is focused on individual student achievement.

USMLE

Step 1: Required. Students must record a passing score for promotion.
Step 2: Clinical Skills (CS): Required. Students must only record a score.
Step 2: Clinical Knowledge (CK): Required. Students must only record a score.

Selection Factors

The Admissions Committee uses AMCAS, a secondary application, letters of recommendation and interview feedback to select applicants who have demonstrated a well-rounded, rigorous academic preparation, character and maturity and who best suit our mission. Applicants must show a strong interest in medicine, a record of personal experiences suggesting medical care exposure, research, altruism, integrity, community service, and leadership with the ability and desire to pursue lifelong learning and the personal attributes necessary to be a competent, compassionate physician. See *http://medicine.fiu.edu*

Financial Aid

Financial Aid is awarded on the basis of demonstrated financial need. Scholarships, institutional grants, federal and private student loans are available for eligible students.

Information about Diversity Programs

FIU takes pride in its commitment to diversity as exemplified among our students, faculty and staff.

Campus Information

Setting

Located in Miami, a major international and cultural center, FIU is an urban research university serving South Florida, the state, the nation and the international community. The 344-acre University Park campus, where the College of Medicine is housed, offers a wealth of services and access to many living and learning communities and is only minutes from Miami International Airport, the Port of Miami, cultural centers, outdoor recreation, sporting events, schools, shopping and beautiful beaches.

Enrollment

For 2008, total enrollment was n/a.

Housing

Apartment-style on-campus housing is available, complimented by a supportive Residential Life program. A list of affordable off-campus housing near the FIU campus is also available.

Satellite Campuses/Facilities

Clinical training will be integrated throughout the South Florida medical community. Students will rotate through a vast array of excellent hospitals and clinics including Jackson North, Mt. Sinai, Mercy and Miami Children's Hospital.

Application Process and Requirements 2010–2011

Primary Application Service: AMCAS
Earliest filing date: June 1, 2009
Latest filing date: December 1, 2009

Secondary Application Required?: Yes
URL: n/a
Name: Betty L. Monfort, (305) 348-0644
med.admissions@fiu.edu
Sent to: Applicants with minimum required scores
Fee: Yes, $30.00
Fee Waiver Available: Yes, (if waived by AMCAS)
Earliest filing date: June 2009
Latest filing date: December 15, 2009

MCAT® required?: Yes
Latest MCAT® considered: September 2009
Oldest MCAT® considered: 2007

Early Decision Program: School does have EDP
Applicants notified: October 1, 2009
EDP available for: All qualified applicants

Regular Acceptance Notice
Earliest date: October 15, 2009
Latest date: Varies
Applicant's Response to Acceptance
Offer – Maximum Time: 4 weeks from date of offer

Requests for deferred entrance considered: No

Deposit to Hold Place in Class: Yes
Deposit (Resident): $200
Deposit (Non-resident): $200
Deposit due: with offer acceptance
Applied to tuition: Yes
Deposit refundable: No
Refundable by: n/a

Estimated number of new entrants: 40
EDP: n/a, **special program:** n/a

Start month/year: August 2010

Interview format: Two committee members will interview invited applicants. Regional interviews are not available.

Other Programs

PREPARATORY PROGRAMS
Postbaccalaureate Program: No
Summer Program: No

COMBINED DEGREE PROGRAMS
Baccalaureate/M.D.: No
M.D./M.P.H.: No
M.D./M.B.A.: No
M.D./J.D.: No
M.D./Ph.D.: No

Premedical Coursework

Course	Req.	Rec.	Lab.	Sems.
Inorganic Chemistry	•		•	2
Behavioral Sciences		•		
Biochemistry		•		
Biology	•		•	2
Biology/Zoology				
Calculus	•			2
College English	•			2
College Mathematics		•		

Course	Req.	Rec.	Lab.	Sems.
Computer Science		•		
Genetics		•		
Humanities		•		
Organic Chemistry	•		•	2
Physics	•		•	2
Psychology				
Social Sciences		•		
Cell Biology		•		

Selection Factors: 2008 Accepted Applicants

Proportion of Accepted Applicants with Relevant Experience (Data Self-Reported to AMCAS®)	Community Service/Volunteer Medically-Related Work Research	DATA NOT AVAILABLE

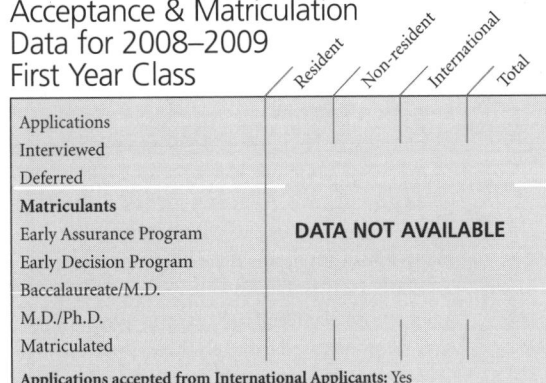

Shaded bar represents school's accepted scores ranging from the 10th percentile to the 90th percentile. School Median ● National Median ●

Overall GPA 2.0 2.1 2.2 2.3 2.4 2.5 2.6 2.7 2.8 2.9 3.0 3.1 3.2 3.3 3.4 3.5 3.6 (3.7) 3.8 3.9 4.0
Science GPA 2.0 2.1 2.2 2.3 2.4 2.5 2.6 2.7 2.8 2.9 3.0 3.1 3.2 3.3 3.4 3.5 (3.6) 3.7 3.8 3.9 4.0

MCAT® Total Numeric Score 9 10 11 12 13 14 15 16 17 18 19 20 21 22 23 24 25 26 27 28 29 30 3(32)33 34 35 36 37 38 39 40 41 42 43

Writing Sample J K L M N O P (Q) R S T
Verbal Reasoning 3 4 5 6 7 8 9 (10) 11 12 13 14 15
Biological Sciences 3 4 5 6 7 8 9 10 (11) 12 13 14 15
Physical Sciences 3 4 5 6 7 8 9 10 (11) 12 13 14 15

Acceptance & Matriculation Data for 2008–2009 First Year Class

	Resident	Non-resident	International	Total
Applications				
Interviewed				
Deferred				
Matriculants				
Early Assurance Program		DATA NOT AVAILABLE		
Early Decision Program				
Baccalaureate/M.D.				
M.D./Ph.D.				
Matriculated				

Applications accepted from International Applicants: Yes

Matriculant Demographics: 2008–2009 First Year Class

Men: n/a   **Women:** n/a

Matriculants' Self-Reported Race/Ethnicity

Mexican American   Korean
Cuban   Vietnamese
Puerto Rican   Other Asian
Oth...   ...
Tot...
Chi...   DATA NOT AVAILABLE
Asi...
Pak...
Fili...   ...ber
Japanese   of Matriculants

Science and Math Majors: 57%
Matriculants with:
   Baccalaureate degree: 99%
   Graduate degree(s): 4%

Specialty Choice

2004, 2005, 2006 Graduates, Specialty Choice
(As reported by program directors to GME Track™)

Anesthesiology
Emergency Medicine
Family Practice
Internal Medicine
Obstetrics/Gynecology   DATA NOT
Orthopaedic Surgery   AVAILABLE
Pediatrics
Psychiatry
Radiology
Surgery

Financial Information

Source: 2007-2008 LCME I-B survey and 2008-2009 AAMC TSF questionnaire

	Residents	Non-residents
Total Cost of Attendance	$49,607	$81,117
Tuition and Fees	$21,000	$51,000
Other (includes living expenses)	$26,807	$28,317
Health Insurance (can be waived)	$1,800	$1,800

Average 2008 Graduate Indebtedness: n/a
% of Enrolled Students Receiving Aid: n/a

Criminal Background Check

This medical school requires a criminal background check prior to matriculation.

Florida State University College of Medicine

Tallahassee, Florida

Office of Student Affairs and Admissions
Florida State University College of Medicine
Administration Building, Room 1110-F
Tallahassee, Florida 32306-4300
T 850 644 7904 **F** 850 645 2846

Admissions www.med.fsu.edu/admission/md
Main www.med.fsu.edu
Financial www.med.fsu.edu/StudentAffairs/finaid
E-mail medadmissions@med.fsu.edu

Public Institution

Dr. John P. Fogarty, Dean

Dr. Graham A. Patrick, Assistant Dean for Admissions

Dr. Eugene Trowers, Assistant Dean for Diversity and Outreach

Billy Auguste. Student Financial Specialist

Dana Urrutia, Admissions Coordinator

Melinda McDaniel, Enrollment Services Coordinator

General Information

The Florida State University College of Medicine was created in July 2000 by a legislative act to train physicians with a focus on serving medically underserved populations in rural and inner-city areas and the growing geriatric population in the state. The FSU College of Medicine is located in Tallahassee, with regional medical campuses, where students complete third and fourth-year clerkships, in Pensacola, Orlando, Sarasota, Tallahassee, Daytona Beach, and Fort Pierce.

Mission Statement

The mission of the FSU College of Medicine is to educate and develop exemplary physicians who practice patient-centered health care, discover and advance knowledge, and respond to community needs, especially through service to elder, rural, and other medically underserved populations.

Curricular Highlights

Community Service Requirement: Optional.
Research/Thesis Requirement: Optional.

The academic program includes instruction in the biopsychosocial sciences and community-based health care. The first and second-year integrated curriculum uses a combination of lecture and case-based and problem-based learning in small-group discussions and simulated standardized-patient interviews. A three-year doctoring course, composed of lecture, small-group discussion, patient encounters, clinical skills instruction, and preceptorships, provides application models to complement

years 1, 2, and 3. The third year and part of the fourth year consist of required rotations in internal medicine, surgery, pediatrics, obstetrics-gynecology, family medicine/rural medicine, geriatrics, emergency medicine, advanced medicine (critical care unit), advanced family practice, and psychiatry. Students may spend up to 24 weeks in electives designed to provide a foundation on which to develop and fulfill personal interests, broaden clinical knowledge, and prepare for postgraduate medical training.

USMLE

Step 1: Required. Students must record a passing score for promotion.
Step 2: Clinical Skills (CS): Required. Students must record a passing total score to graduate.
Step 2: Clinical Knowledge (CK): Required. Students must record a passing total score to graduate.

Selection Factors

Although scholastic aptitude is necessary to complete studies in medical school, neither high GPAs nor high MCAT scores alone or in combination are adequate to obtain admission. International applicants must have a permanent resident visa. Applicants who have grades and test scores predictive of success in medical school, have demonstrated through their experiences a high degree of motivation for medicine and a strong commitment to the service of others, and have a likelihood of practicing medicine with medically underserved populations will be invited to interview. The committee evaluates all aspects of the applicant's academic record, including trends in scholastic performance.

Financial Aid

Scholarships and loan funds from private, state, and federal sources are available to qualified students and are awarded on the basis of need and/or scholarship.

Information about Diversity Programs

Because of the mission of the College of Medicine and the educational value of admitting a diverse class, Florida State University College of Medicine developed a Postbaccalaureate Bridge Program to provide opportunities for applicants from groups underrepresented in medicine. Applicants from

these groups who embody the characteristics valued by the college are selected for the Bridge year, which is used to develop and enhance study, time management, and test-taking skills; psychosocial and basic science backgrounds; and clinical experiences. If these students meet all requirements established for the year, they are admitted to the next year's medical school class. Students may contact Eugene Trowers, MD, at (850) 644-4607 for more information.

Campus Information

Setting

The main medical school campus is located on the Florida State University campus in a newly constructed $65 million dollar medical school complex. Each regional campus is located near affiliated hospitals in its respective community and includes study and resource areas. Applicants are invited to take a virtual tour of the campus at *www.med.fsu.edu*.

Enrollment

For 2008, total enrollment was: 416

Special Features

The FSU College of Medicine utilizes a state of the art Clinical Learning Center on the main campus and community resources to ensure that students receive a significant amount of one-on-one training with physician preceptors. The College of Medicine has affiliation agreements with over 20 hospitals across the state of Florida, as well as affiliations with nearby rural community hospitals. A wide range of elective opportunities is available in the fourth year at each of the regional sites, as well as at other accredited institutions both nationally and internationally.

Housing

On-campus housing is available. A list of affordable housing within Tallahassee and at each of the regional campuses is maintained.

Satellite Campuses/Facilities

Student rotations in the third year occur at one of the regional campuses. Rural learning opportunities are also available within driving distance of each site.

Application Process and Requirements 2010–2011

Primary Application Service: AMCAS
Earliest filing date: June 1, 2009
Latest filing date: December 14, 2009

Secondary Application Required?: Yes
Sent to: Screened applicants
Contact: Dana Urrutia, (850) 644-1857, dana.urrutia@med.fsu.edu
Fee: No
Fee waiver available: No
Earliest filing date: June 1, 2009
Latest filing date: December 31, 2009

MCAT® required?: Yes
Latest MCAT® considered: September 2009
Oldest MCAT® considered: 2007

Early Decision Program: School does have EDP
Applicants notified: October 1, 2009
EDP available for: Both Residents and Non-residents

**Regular Acceptance Notice
Earliest date:** October 15, 2009
Latest date: Until Class is Full
**Applicant's Response to Acceptance
Offer – Maximum Time:** Two weeks

**Requests for Deferred
Entrance Considered:** Yes

Deposit to Hold Place in Class: Yes
Deposit (Resident): $30
Deposit (Non-resident): $30
Deposit due: Within two weeks of receipt of letter of acceptance
Applied to tuition: No
Deposit refundable: No
Refundable by: n/a

Estimated number of new entrants: 120
EDP: 15, special program: 10

Start Month/Year: May 2010

Interview Format: Two committee members interview invited applicants. Regional interviews are not available.

Other Programs

PREPARATORY PROGRAMS
Postbaccalaureate Program: Yes, www.med.fsu.edu/StudentAffairs/outreach/bridge.asp

COMBINED DEGREE PROGRAMS
Baccalaureate/M.D.: No
M.D./M.P.H.: No
M.D./M.B.A.: No
M.D./J.D.: No
M.D./Ph.D.: No

Additional Program: Yes, http://med.fsu.edu/admission/MedicalScholars.pdf

Premedical Coursework

Course	Req.	Rec.	Lab.	Hrs.
Inorganic Chemistry	•		•	8
Behavioral Sciences		•		
Biochemistry	•			3
Biology	•		•	8
Biology/Zoology				
Calculus				
College English	•			6
College Mathematics	•			6

Course	Req.	Rec.	Lab.	Hrs.
Computer Science				
Genetics		•		3
Humanities				
Organic Chemistry	•		•	8
Physics	•		•	8
Psychology		•		3
Social Sciences				
Spanish		•		6

Selection Factors: 2008 Accepted Applicants

Proportion of Accepted Applicants with Relevant Experience (Data Self-Reported to AMCAS)	
Community Service/Volunteer	70%
Medically-Related Work	93%
Research	71%

Shaded bar represents school's accepted scores ranging from the 10th percentile to the 90th percentile. School Median ● National Median ●

Overall GPA	2.0	2.1	2.2	2.3	2.4	2.5	2.6	2.7	2.8	2.9	3.0	3.1	3.2	3.3	3.4	3.5	3.6	(3.7)	3.8	3.9	4.0
Science GPA	2.0	2.1	2.2	2.3	2.4	2.5	2.6	2.7	2.8	2.9	3.0	3.1	3.2	3.3	3.4	3.5	3.6	(3.7)	3.8	3.9	4.0

MCAT® Total Numeric Score 9 10 11 12 13 14 15 16 17 18 19 20 21 22 23 24 25 26 27 28 (29) 30 31 (32) 33 34 35 36 37 38 39 40 41 42 43

Writing Sample			J	K	L	M	N	(O)	P	(Q)	R	S	T
Verbal Reasoning	3	4	5	6	7	8	(9)	(10)	11	12	13	14	15
Biological Sciences	3	4	5	6	7	8	9	(10)	(11)	12	13	14	15
Physical Sciences	3	4	5	6	7	8	(9)	10	(11)	12	13	14	15

Acceptance & Matriculation Data for 2008–2009 First Year Class

	Resident	Non-resident	International	Total
Applications	1588	758	23	2369
Interviewed	368	4	0	372
Deferred	1	0	0	1
Matriculants				
Early Assurance Program	0	0	0	0
Early Decision Program	14	0	0	14
Baccalaureate/M.D.	n/a	n/a	n/a	0
M.D./Ph.D.	n/a	n/a	n/a	0
Matriculated	116	2	0	**118**

Applications accepted from International Applicants: No

Specialty Choice

2004, 2005, 2006 Graduates, Specialty Choice (As reported by program directors to GME Track™)	
Anesthesiology	1%
Emergency Medicine	10%
Family Practice	13%
Internal Medicine	6%
Obstetrics/Gynecology	7%
Orthopaedic Surgery	4%
Pediatrics	4%
Psychiatry	1%
Radiology	2%
Surgery	8%

Matriculant Demographics: 2008–2009 First Year Class

Men: 57   **Women:** 61

Matriculants' Self-Reported Race/Ethnicity

Mexican American	1	Korean	1
Cuban	10	Vietnamese	3
Puerto Rican	1	Other Asian	1
Other Hispanic	9	Total Asian	24
Total Hispanic	19	Native American	0
Chinese	0	Black	9
Asian Indian	15	Native Hawaiian	0
Pakistani	1	White	81
Filipino	3	Unduplicated Number	
Japanese	1	of Matriculants	118

Science and Math Majors: 57%
Matriculants with:
　　Baccalaureate degree: 99%
　　Graduate degree(s): 4%

Financial Information

Source: 2007–2008 LCME I-B survey and 2008–2009 AAMC TSF questionnaire

	Residents	Non-residents
Total Cost of Attendance	$48,026	$83,185
Tuition and Fees	$18,610	$53,769
Other (includes living expenses)	$29,416	$29,416
Health Insurance (cannot be waived)	$0	$0

Average 2008 Graduate Indebtedness: $147,597
% of Enrolled Students Receiving Aid: 88%

Criminal Background Check

This medical school requires a criminal background check prior to matriculation.

University of Central Florida College of Medicine

Orlando, Florida

12201 Research Parkway, 3rd Floor
PO Box 160116
Orlando, FL, 32816-0116
T 407 823 4244 **F** 407 823 4048

Admissions www.med.ucf.edu/admissions
Main www.med.ucf.edu
Financial www.med.ucf.edu/academics/financial_aid/index.asp
E-mail mdadmissions@mail.ucf.edu

Public Institution

Dr. Deborah C. German, Dean

REL Larkin, Director of Admissions

Ruthanne Madsen, Director of Student Financial Services

Teresa Lyons-Oten, Registrar

Dr. Randy Manning, Associate Dean for Student Affairs

General Information

UCF COM will be the premier medical school born in the 21st century. Enrolling our charter class in August 2009, UCF COM will be fully integrated into the Central Florida community's healthcare and medical research infrastructure. By partnering with Orlando Health and Florida Hospital systems, the new Orlando VA Medical Center and Nemours Children's Clinic Orlando, students will have the opportunity for clinical training in all specialties of medicine at 17 major facilities. The Central Florida community has embraced UCF COM's future physicians with their financial contributions; local doctors comprise over 700 volunteer clinical faculty. We will capitalize on UCF's existing strengths in biomedical sciences, modeling and simulation, and optics and photonics. The UCF Burnett School of Biomedical Sciences, conducts research in cancer, cardiovascular diseases, neurological diseases and infectious diseases and is an important part of the COM.

Mission Statement

The University of Central Florida College of Medicine educates and inspires individuals to be exemplary physicians and scientists, leaders in medicine, scholars in discovery, and adopters of innovative technology to improve the health and well-being of all. Our patient-centered mission is achieved by outstanding medical care and services, groundbreaking research, and leading edge medical and biotechnical education.

Curricular Highlights

Community Service Requirement: Required.
Research/Thesis Requirement: Required.

The curriculum is a unique and exciting blend of state-of-the-art technology, virtual patients, clinical and laboratory experiences, research, directed small group sessions, and interactive didactic lectures. The first two years of the curriculum are structured into instructional modules. The first year focuses on how basic science relates to the human body and disease; the second year is an organ system-based approach, applying first-year knowledge to the study of clinical disease, pathological processes, diagnosis, and treatment. Numerous clinical experiences occur throughout the first two years that also include a Focused Individualized Study and Research module. Third and fourth year curriculum is devoted to clinical experience through core clerkships and electives in our affiliated hospital facilities. Avatar patient technology will be used extensively throughout all four years to support learning objectives.

USMLE

Step 1: Required. Students must record a passing score for graduation, but not promotion.
Step 2: Clinical Skills (CS): Required. Students must only record a score.
Step 2: Clinical Knowledge (CK): Required. Students must only record a score.

Selection Factors

Supplemental applications are available to all qualified U.S. citizens, permanent residents, and those granted asylum upon verification of their AMCAS application providing that the applicant meets the minimum GPA/MCAT requirements. Applicants chosen for an interview will be highly motivated, capable, passionate, academically proven, and have diverse skills, talents, and life experiences that will benefit the program, community, and fellow classmates.

Financial Aid

The financial status of the applicant is not considered in the admissions process. Student Financial Services staff assist M.D. students in obtaining funding resources and also provide counseling for many financial and debt management topics.

Information about Diversity Programs

Increasing diversity and inclusiveness is one of the central goals of UCF. Minorities account for nearly 20 percent of UCF faculty, and an aggressive minority recruitment plan continues to be a priority for the university.

Campus Information

Setting

The College of Medicine will spend its entire first year adjacent to the UCF main campus in Orlando, only a short ride from the Space Coast and Daytona Beach. The COM will move to a new building in the UCF Health Sciences Campus at Lake Nona in the spring of 2010. This new medical campus will initially include the College of Medicine Medical Education and Burnett Biomedical Sciences buildings, with additional buildings in the health sciences planned in the future. Adjacent to the campus will be a new Veterans Affairs Hospital, Burnham Institute for Medical Research, Nemours Children's Hospital, and many additional clinical and research facilities in our new medical city at Lake Nona. The rapidly growing complex also includes single and multi-family housing, retail areas, schools, and spacious parks.

Enrollment

For 2008, total enrollment was: n/a

Special Features

All facilities from the classrooms to the numerous study areas are equipped with the latest communication and teaching technologies. Students will enjoy the latest developments in medical simulation and clinical cases. Clinical experiences will be fully integrated into all four years of the program and into the community allowing participation in rural or urban medicine at multiple hospitals and clinics in the Central Florida area.

Housing

On-campus housing is not available. A list of affordable housing near the UCF campus in Orlando as well as the Lake Nona area is available.

Application Process and Requirements 2010–2011

Primary Application Service: AMCAS
Earliest filing date: June 1, 2009
Latest filing date: December 1, 2009

Secondary Application required?
URL: Provided to qualified applicants via e-mail
Sent to: Screened Applicants
Fee: Yes, $30
Fee Waiver Available: Yes
Earliest filing date: July 1, 2009
Latest filing date: January 15, 2010

MCAT® required?: Yes
Latest MCAT® considered: September 2009
Oldest MCAT® considered: 2007

Early Decision Program: School does have EDP
Applicants notified: October 1, 2009
EDP available for: Both Residents and Non-residents

Regular Acceptance Notice
Earliest date: October 15, 2009
Latest date: Until Class is Full
Applicant's Response to Acceptance Offer – Maximum Time: 2 weeks

Requests for deferred entrance considered: Yes

Deposit to Hold Place in Class: None
Deposit (Resident): n/a
Deposit (Non-resident): n/a
Deposit due: n/a
Applied to tuition: n/a
Deposit refundable: n/a
Refundable by: n/a

Estimated number of new entrants: 60
EDP: 4, special program: n/a

Start month/year: August 2010

Interview format: Two partially closed interviews by COM faculty. Regional interviews are not available.

Other Programs

PREPARATORY PROGRAMS
Postbaccalaureate Program: No
Summer Program: No

COMBINED DEGREE PROGRAMS
Baccalaureate/M.D.: No
M.D./M.P.H.: No
M.D./M.B.A.: No
M.D./J.D.: No
M.D./Ph.D.: No

Premedical Coursework

Course	Req.	Rec.	Lab.	Hrs.
Inorganic Chemistry	•		•	8
Behavioral Sciences				
Biochemistry		•		
Biology	•		•	8
Biology/Zoology				
Calculus/Statistics		•		
College English	•			6
College Mathematics	•			6
Computer Science				

Course	Req.	Rec.	Lab.	Hrs.
Genetics		•		
Humanities		•		
Organic Chemistry	•		•	8
Physics	•		•	8
Psychology				
Social Sciences				
Molecular Biology		•		
Statistics		•		
Cell Biology		•		

Selection Factors: 2008 Accepted Applicants

Proportion of Accepted Applicants with Relevant Experience (Data Self-Reported to AMCAS®)	DATA NOT AVAILABLE

Shaded bar represents school's accepted scores ranging from the 10th percentile to the 90th percentile ▪   School Median ● National Median ●

Overall GPA	DATA NOT AVAILABLE
Science GPA	

MCAT® Total Numeric Score 9 10 11 12 13 14 15 16 17 18 19 20 21 22 23 24 25 26 27 28 29 30 31 32 33 34 35 36 37 38 39 40 41 42 43

Writing Sample	
Verbal Reasoning	DATA NOT AVAILABLE
Biological Sciences	
Physical Sciences	

Acceptance & Matriculation Data for 2008–2009 First Year Class

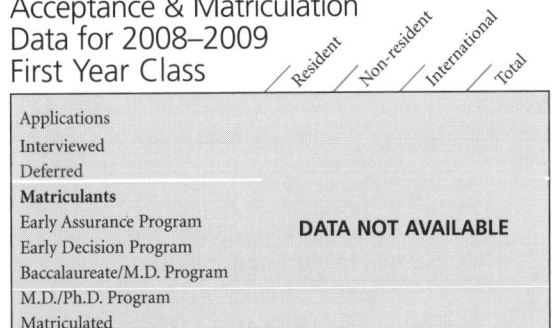

	Resident	Non-resident	International	Total
Applications				
Interviewed				
Deferred				
Matriculants		DATA NOT AVAILABLE		
Early Assurance Program				
Early Decision Program				
Baccalaureate/M.D. Program				
M.D./Ph.D. Program				
Matriculated				

Applications accepted from International Applicants:

Specialty Choice

2004, 2005, 2006 Graduates, Specialty Choice (As reported by program directors to GME Track™)
Anesthesiology
Emergency Medicine
Family Practice
Internal
Obstetrics
Orthopedics DATA NOT AVAILABLE
Pediatrics
Psychiatry
Radiology
Surgery

Matriculant Demographics: 2008–2009 First Year Class

Men: n/a   **Women:** n/a

Matriculants' Self-Reported Race/Ethnicity

Mexican American   Korean
Cuban   Vietnamese
Puerto Rican   Other Asian
Othe
Total
Chine   **DATA NOT AVAILABLE**
Asiar
Pakis
Filipino   **Unduplicated Number**
Japanese   **of Matriculants**

Science Majors: n/a
Matriculants with:
Baccalaureate Degree: n/a
Graduate Degree(s): n/a

Financial Information (Estimated)

Source: 2007–2008 LCME I-B survey and 2008–2009 AAMC TSF questionnaire

	Residents	Non-residents
Total Cost of Attendance	$48,425	$75,625
Tuition and Fees	$23,800	$51,000
Other (includes living expenses)	$22,825	$23,125
Health Insurance (can be waived)	$1,800	$2,000

Average 2008 Graduate Indebtedness: n/a
% of Enrolled Students Receiving Aid: n/a

Criminal Background Check

This medical school requires a criminal background check prior to matriculation.

University of Florida College of Medicine
Gainesville, Florida

Director, Office of Admissions
PO Box 100216, UF Health Sciences Center
Univ. of Florida College of Medicine
Gainesville, Florida 32610-0216
T 352 273 7990   **F** 352 392 1307

Admissions www.med.ufl.edu/oea/admiss
Main www.med.ufl.edu
Financial www.med.ufl.edu/oea/finaid
E-mail med-admissions@ufl.edu

Public Institution

Dr. Michael L. Good, Dean

Denise Chichester, Director of Admissions

*Dr. Donna M. Parker, Assistant Dean
for Minority Affairs*

Eileen M. Parris, Coordinator of Financial Aid

*Dr. Ira H. Gessner, Chair, Medical Selection
Committee*

General Information

The College of Medicine of the University of
Florida (UF) Health Science Center admitted
its first class in September 1956. Located on the
2,000-acre campus of UF, the College of Medicine
enjoys strong ties with other university programs
and other Health Science Center colleges. The
HSC complex also includes the Chandler A.
Stetson Medical Science Building, Communicore
Building, Academic Research Building, Nursing
and Health Professions Building, Cancer and
Genetics Research Building, Shands at UF
Hospital, Brain Institute, and Veterans
Administration Medical Center. The Cancer
Hospital opens in November 2009. The UF
Health Science Center Jacksonville is our urban
campus and includes one of the few Proton
Beam facilities in the world. Formal educational
affiliations have also been established in Ft.
Lauderdale, Miami, Orlando, and Pensacola.

Mission Statement

To educate medical students in humanistic, scientific and practical principles of medicine to
become, and remain, exemplary practitioners,
academicians and leaders. To educate scientists
for research, teaching or industry careers. To
provide compassionate, skilled and innovative
healthcare. To foster discovery, promote health,
prevent disease, and so educate the public. To
promote the professional and personal growth
of faculty and staff.

Curricular Highlights

Community Service Requirement: Required.
Consistent health care experience preferred.
Research/Thesis Requirement: Optional.

The four years are divided into three blocks of
time – Preclinical Coursework (2 years), Clinical

Clerkships (1 year), and Post-clerkship Electives
and Required Courses (1 year). Preclinical
coursework provides students with essential basic
science and general clinical information necessary
for clinical training. The third year is devoted to
clinical clerkships. Required clerkships include
family medicine, medicine, neurology, pediatrics,
psychiatry, obstetrics/gynecology, and surgery.
Students spend 10-12 weeks participating in
clerkships at UF Health Science Center
Jacksonville. During clerkships, students become
integral members of the medical team and have
direct responsibility for assigned patients. The
fourth year includes seven elective periods and
three required courses: anesthesiology, emergency
medicine, and either senior medicine, community
medicine, or pediatrics. An eleventh period is
available for accomplishing residency interviews.
For students who have already chosen a specialty,
fourth-year programs may be designed to provide
career choice-related experiences.

USMLE

Step 1: Required. Students must record a passing
score for promotion.
Step 2: Clinical Skills (CS): Required. Students
must only record a score.
Step 2: Clinical Knowledge (CK): Required.
Students must only record a score.

Selection Factors

We appraise applicants on personal attributes,
academic record, activities, MCAT, and recommendations. A personal interview is required
and is granted at the discretion of the Medical
Selection Committee. The school does not discriminate on the basis of race, sex, age, disability,
creed, or national origin. Florida residents are
given preference and exceptionally well qualified
non-residents are considered each year. The COM
welcomes applicants from members of groups
underrepresented in medicine and from persons
who demonstrate a clear commitment to
underserved populations.

Financial Aid

Financial assistance is available to all enrolled
students who show need. The college has
scholarships and low interest loans available.
Applications are mailed to all accepted applicants.
Summer and school-year research fellowships
are also available.

Information about Diversity Programs

There are summer research programs offered
by the Office of Minority Affairs.

Campus Information

Setting

The Gainesville campus lies midway between
the Atlantic Ocean and the Gulf of Mexico in
the lush beauty of north central Florida. The
surrounding area includes fresh water springs,
wild prairies, and many parks exhibiting a
great diversity of wildlife. Arts and culture
abound in Gainesville. The Phillips Center for
the Performing Arts features world-class enter-
tainers from all genres. The Harn Art Museum
houses some of the finest art in the world. The
Florida Natural History Museum now includes
the McGuire Butterfly Center. Gainesville hosts
many professional Arts groups including the
Hippodrome Theatre, Dance Alive (Ballet) and
the Gainesville Chamber Orchestra each performing regularly throughout the year.

Enrollment

For 2008, total enrollment was: 467

Special Features

Several new facilities under construction
include the Nanotechnology Center and the
Emerging Pathogens Center.

Housing

On-campus housing is not available.

Satellite Campuses/Facilities

UF Health Sciences Center, Jacksonville includ-
ing the Proton Beam Facility; Lake City VA
Hospital; Sacred Heart Hospital in Pensacola,
Shands at Alachua General Hospital in
Gainesville, Malcolm Randall VA Hospital,
McKnight Brain Institute, Cancer & Genetics
Institute and Shands Cancer Hospital all in
proximity to The Shands Hospital at the
University of Florida, our primary hospital
facility in Gainesville. Several out-patient facil-
ities exist in Gainesville.

Application Process and Requirements 2010–2011

Primary Application Service: AMCAS
Earliest filing date: June 1, 2009
Latest filing date: December 1, 2009

Secondary Application Required?: Yes
Sent to: Applicants of interest
URL: n/a
Contact: Denise Chichester, (352) 273-7990, med-admission@ufl.edu
Fee: No
Fee waiver available: n/a
Earliest filing date: July 15, 2009
Latest filing date: January 15, 2010

MCAT® required?: Yes
Latest MCAT® considered: September 2009
Oldest MCAT® considered: August 2007

Early Decision Program: School does not have EDP
Applicants notified: n/a
EDP available for: n/a

Regular Acceptance Notice
Earliest date: October 16, 2009
Latest date: Until class is full
Applicant's Response to Acceptance
Offer – Maximum Time: Two weeks

Requests for Deferred
Entrance Considered: Yes

Deposit to Hold Place in Class: Yes
Deposit (Resident): $200
Deposit (Non-resident): $200
Deposit due: Two weeks after notice of acceptance
Applied to tuition: Yes
Deposit refundable: Yes
Refundable by: May 15, 2010

Estimated number of new entrants: 135
EDP: n/a, special program: 12

Start Month/Year: August 2010

Interview Format: Two open-file interviews at COM. Regional interviews are not available.

Other Programs

PREPARATORY PROGRAMS
Postbaccalaureate Program: No
Summer Program: Yes,
www.med.ufl.edu/oma/srp.shtml
Office of Minority Affairs, (352) 273-6656

COMBINED DEGREE PROGRAMS
Baccalaureate/M.D.: Yes,
http://medinfo.ufl.edu/students/jhmp
M.D./M.P.H.: Yes, www.mph.ufl.edu/programs/collaborative/md.htm
M.D./M.B.A.: Yes, www.med.ufl.edu/oea/osa/cat-research_option.shtml
M.D./J.D.: Yes, www.med.ufl.edu/oea/osa/cat-research_option.shtml
M.D./Ph.D.: Yes, www.med.ufl.edu/md-phd
Additional Program: Yes, www.msrp.med.ufl.edu

Premedical Coursework

Course	Req.	Rec.	Lab.	Hrs.
Inorganic Chemistry	•		•	8
Behavioral Sciences				
Biochemistry	•		•	4
Biology				
Biology/Zoology	•		•	8
Calculus				
College English				
College Mathematics				

Course	Req.	Rec.	Lab.	Hrs.
Computer Science				
Genetics				
Humanities				
Organic Chemistry	•		•	4
Physics	•		•	8
Psychology				
Social Sciences				
Other				

Selection Factors: 2008 Accepted Applicants

Proportion of Accepted Applicants with Relevant Experience (Data Self-Reported to AMCAS)		Community Service/Volunteer	60%
		Medically-Related Work	84%
		Research	85%

Shaded bar represents school's accepted scores ranging from the 10th percentile to the 90th percentile   School Median ●   National Median ●

Overall GPA	2.0	2.1	2.2	2.3	2.4	2.5	2.6	2.7	2.8	2.9	3.0	3.1	3.2	3.3	3.4	3.5	3.6	3.7	(3.8)	3.9	4.0
Science GPA	2.0	2.1	2.2	2.3	2.4	2.5	2.6	2.7	2.8	2.9	3.0	3.1	3.2	3.3	3.4	3.5	3.6	3.7	(3.8)	3.9	4.0

MCAT® Total Numeric Score 9 10 11 12 13 14 15 16 17 18 19 20 21 22 23 24 25 26 27 28 29 30 31 (32) 33 34 35 36 37 38 39 40 41 42 43

			J	K	L	M	N	O	P	(Q)	R	S	T
Writing Sample			J	K	L	M	N	O	P	(Q)	R	S	T
Verbal Reasoning	3	4	5	6	7	8	9	(10)	11	12	13	14	15
Biological Sciences	3	4	5	6	7	8	9	10	(11)	12	13	14	15
Physical Sciences	3	4	5	6	7	8	9	10	(11)	12	13	14	15

Acceptance & Matriculation Data for 2008–2009 First Year Class

	Resident	Non-resident	International	Total
Applications	1489	1251	44	2784
Interviewed	334	38	0	372
Deferred	4	0	0	4
Matriculants				
Early Assurance Program	n/a	n/a	n/a	n/a
Early Decision Program	0	0	0	0
Baccalaureate/M.D.	12	0	0	12
M.D./Ph.D.	0	0	0	0
Matriculated	128	8	0	**132**

Applications accepted from International Applicants: No

Specialty Choice

2004, 2005, 2006 Graduates, Specialty Choice (As reported by program directors to GME Track™)	
Anesthesiology	7%
Emergency Medicine	6%
Family Practice	5%
Internal Medicine	16%
Obstetrics/Gynecology	6%
Orthopaedic Surgery	3%
Pediatrics	12%
Psychiatry	8%
Radiology	7%
Surgery	6%

Matriculant Demographics: 2008–2009 First Year Class

Men: 68   **Women:** 64

Matriculants' Self-Reported Race/Ethnicity

Mexican American	0	Korean	1
Cuban	7	Vietnamese	1
Puerto Rican	0	Other Asian	3
Other Hispanic	8	Total Asian	22
Total Hispanic	14	Native American	0
Chinese	5	Black	8
Asian Indian	10	Native Hawaiian	0
Pakistani	1	White	103
Filipino	3	Unduplicated Number	
Japanese	0	of Matriculants	132

Science and Math Majors: 69%
Matriculants with:
   Baccalaureate degree: 99%
   Graduate degree(s): 6%

Financial Information

Source: 2007-2008 LCME I-B survey and 2008-2009 AAMC TSF questionnaire

	Residents	Non-residents
Total Cost of Attendance	$44,443	$73,683
Tuition and Fees	$26,514	$55,754
Other (includes living expenses)	$16,526	$16,526
Health Insurance (can be waived)	$1,403	$1,403

Average 2008 Graduate Indebtedness: $107,589
% of Enrolled Students Receiving Aid: 87%

Criminal Background Check

This medical school does not require a criminal background check prior to matriculation.

University of Miami
Miller School of Medicine
Miami, Florida

Office of Admissions
University of Miami Miller School of Medicine
P.O. Box 016159
Miami, Florida 33101
T 305 243 3234   F 305 243 6548

Admissions www.miami.edu/medical-admissions
Main www.med.miami.edu
Financial www.mededu.miami.edu/OSFA
E-mail med.admissions@miami.edu

Private Institution
Dr. Pascal Goldschmidt, Dean

Dr. Richard S. Weisman, Associate Dean for Admissions

Dr. Astrid Mack, Associate Dean for Minority Affairs

Laura L. Kasperski, Assistant Dean for Student Financial Assistance

General Information
The University of Miami Miller School of Medicine is the largest and oldest medical school in the state of Florida. Six hospitals containing nearly 3,000 beds are located on the medical campus and provide a complete spectrum of clinical experiences. Specialty centers at the Miller School of Medicine include The Bascom Palmer Eye Institute and Anne Bates Leach Eye Hospital, the Ambulatory Care Center, the Diabetes Research Institute, the Lois Pope Life Center (which houses The Miami Project to Cure Spinal Cord Paralysis), the Bachelor Children's Research Institute, the Ryder Trauma Center, and the Sylvester Comprehensive Cancer Center.

Mission Statement
The Miller School of Medicine has four interrelated missions: patient care, teaching, research, and community service.

Curricular Highlights
Community Service Requirement: Optional.
Research/Thesis Requirement: Optional.

The curriculum is an integrated program that requires students to be active and responsible learners. It emphasizes faculty and student-led small-group experiences wherein basic science concepts are introduced and assimilated in light of common disease states and clinical relevance. It also includes material not traditionally emphasized: professionalism, humanism and ethics, population medicine, prevention and screening, quality and outcome assessment, medical informatics, geriatrics, alternative medicine, nutrition, medical economics, and end-of-life care. An over-arching theme throughout all four years is the continuous acquisition and refinement of clinical skills

through expert teaching and patient encounters, starting in the first weeks of the first year of the curriculum.

USMLE
Step 1: Required. Students must record a passing score for promotion.
Step 2: Clinical Skills (CS): Required. Students must only record a score.
Step 2: Clinical Knowledge (CK): Required. Students must only record a score.

Selection Factors
Secondary applications are sent to all U.S. citizens and permanent residents who submit a verified AMCAS application. In deciding whether to return secondary materials, applicants are reminded that the last entering class had an average undergraduate cumulative GPA of 3.7 and an average composite MCAT score of 32. Factors assessed by the committee to rate all completed applications include: preparedness to study medicine, diversity of life experiences, meaningfulness of direct patient contact experiences, and quality of letters of recommendation. Applicants with the highest ratings are invited for an interview. Applicants' files are reviewed without regard to race, creed, sex, national origin, age, or handicap.

Financial Aid
In 2008-2009, the amount of financial aid awarded totaled about $22 million. The school participates in all major federal and state programs. A number of scholarships are awarded each year for merit and for life diversity and financial need. Information concerning financial assistance and student budgets may be obtained on the Office of Financial Assistance web site at *www.mededu.miami.edu/OSFA* or by calling 305-243-6211.

Information about Diversity Programs
The school sponsors a special seven-week summer program that provides pre-medical undergraduates with opportunities to gain first-hand knowledge of the requirements of a medical education. Applications and information may be obtained by calling 305-243-5998.

Campus Information
Setting
The School of Medicine is at the heart of the Miami Health District, located in the Civic Center area of Miami, about midway between Miami International Airport and downtown Miami. The regional medical campus is located in Boca Raton, Florida, on the campus of Florida Atlantic University, about 50 miles north of the parent campus.

Enrollment
For 2008, total enrollment was: 728

Special Features
The entire medical campus is completely "wireless," and lectures are now podcasted, both in audio and in video formats. Numerous opportunities exist for students to participate in community medicine, outreach programs, and international medicine to study the root causes of medical inequalities at multiple sites in the Caribbean, Russia, Central America, and Africa.

Housing
Many medical students live in two apartment buildings adjacent to campus. The Medical Campus is served by Metro Rail, an elevated light railway, which has made large areas of Miami accessible to medical students.

Satellite Campuses/Facilities
The School of Medicine has a regional medical campus in Boca Raton on the campus of Florida Atlantic University. Up to 64 students each year will start and complete their medical educations at the regional campus. While the Medical Campus and regional campus curricula are identical in their missions, they have different emphases. Students at the regional campus gain their clinical training at John F. Kennedy (JFK) Community Hospital and other local hospitals and clinics in a patient-centered environment.

Application Process and Requirements 2010–2011

Primary Application Service: AMCAS
Earliest filing date: June 1, 2009
Latest filing date: December 1, 2009

Secondary Application Required?: Yes
Sent to: All U.S. citizens and permanent residents
Contact: Richard S. Weisman, (305) 243-3234, med.admissions@miami.edu
Fee: Yes, $75
Fee waiver available: Yes
Earliest filing date: June 15, 2009
Latest filing date: January 31, 2010

MCAT® required?: Yes
Latest MCAT® considered: September 2009
Oldest MCAT® considered: 2007

Early Decision Program: School does not have EDP
Applicants notified: n/a
EDP available for: n/a

Regular Acceptance Notice
Earliest date: October 15, 2009
Latest date: Until class is full
Applicant's Response to Acceptance
Offer – Maximum Time: Two weeks

Requests for Deferred
Entrance Considered: Yes

Deposit to Hold Place in Class: Yes
Deposit (Resident): $100
Deposit (Non-resident): $100
Deposit due: response to acceptance letter
Applied to tuition: Yes
Deposit refundable: No
Refundable by: May 15, 2010

Estimated number of new entrants: 206
EDP: 0, special program: 25

Start Month/Year: August 2010

Interview Format: Open file, structured, one hour interviews. Regional interviews are not available.

Other Programs

PREPARATORY PROGRAMS
Postbaccalaureate Program: Yes
www.miami.edu, Eva Alonso, (305) 284-5176
Summer Program: Yes, www.miami.edu/medical-admissions
Astrid Mack, Ph.D. , (305) 284-5998

COMBINED DEGREE PROGRAMS
Baccalaureate/M.D.: Yes
www.miami.edu/medical-admissions
M.D./M.P.H.: Yes, http://spider.med.miami.edu/grad/phd.html
Dr. Jay Wilkinson, (305) 243-2209
M.D./M.B.A.: Yes
M.D./J.D.: No
M.D./Ph.D.: Yes, http://chroma.med.miami.edu/mdphd. Dr. Sandra Lemmon, (305) 243-1094

Premedical Coursework

Course	Req.	Rec.	Lab.	Hrs.
Inorganic Chemistry	•		•	8
Behavioral Sciences				
Biochemistry		•		
Biology				
Biology/Zoology	•		•	6
Calculus				
College English	•			6
College Mathematics				

Course	Req.	Rec.	Lab.	Hrs.
Computer Science				
Genetics		•		
Humanities				
Organic Chemistry	•		•	8
Physics	•		•	8
Psychology				
Social Sciences				
Additional Sciences		•		6

Selection Factors: 2008 Accepted Applicants

Proportion of Accepted Applicants with Relevant Experience (Data Self-Reported to AMCAS)	
Community Service/Volunteer	71%
Medically-Related Work	88%
Research	83%

Shaded bar represents school's accepted scores ranging from the 10th percentile to the 90th percentile   School Median ○   National Median ●

Overall GPA	2.0	2.1	2.2	2.3	2.4	2.5	2.6	2.7	2.8	2.9	3.0	3.1	3.2	3.3	3.4	3.5	3.6	3.7	(3.8)	3.9	4.0
Science GPA	2.0	2.1	2.2	2.3	2.4	2.5	2.6	2.7	2.8	2.9	3.0	3.1	3.2	3.3	3.4	3.5	3.6	3.7	(3.8)	3.9	4.0

MCAT® Total Numeric Score 9 10 11 12 13 14 15 16 17 18 19 20 21 22 23 24 25 26 27 28 29 30 31 (32) 33 34 35 36 37 38 39 40 41 42 43

Writing Sample				J	K	L	M	N	O	P	(Q)	R	S	T
Verbal Reasoning	3	4	5	6	7	8	9	(10)	11	12	13	14	15
Biological Sciences	3	4	5	6	7	8	9	10	(11)	12	13	14	15
Physical Sciences	3	4	5	6	7	8	9	10	(11)	12	13	14	15

Acceptance & Matriculation Data for 2008–2009 First Year Class

	Resident	Non-resident	International	Total
Applications	1508	3087	43	4638
Interviewed	312	171	0	483
Deferred	2	2	0	4
Matriculants				
Early Assurance Program	0	0	0	0
Early Decision Program	0	0	0	0
Baccalaureate/M.D.	12	8	0	20
M.D./Ph.D.	4	3	0	7
Matriculated	137	57	0	**194**

Applications accepted from International Applicants: No

Matriculant Demographics: 2008–2009 First Year Class

Men: 103   **Women:** 91

Matriculants' Self-Reported Race/Ethnicity

Mexican American	0	Korean	4
Cuban	24	Vietnamese	1
Puerto Rican	1	Other Asian	5
Other Hispanic	5	Total Asian	34
Total Hispanic	28	Native American	0
Chinese	6	Black	14
Asian Indian	12	Native Hawaiian	1
Pakistani	3	White	143
Filipino	5	Unduplicated Number	
Japanese	0	of Matriculants	194

Science and Math Majors: 65%
Matriculants with:
    Baccalaureate degree: 99%
    Graduate degree(s): 12%

Specialty Choice

2004, 2005, 2006 Graduates, Specialty Choice (As reported by program directors to GME Track™)	
Anesthesiology	10%
Emergency Medicine	4%
Family Practice	4%
Internal Medicine	21%
Obstetrics/Gynecology	6%
Orthopaedic Surgery	2%
Pediatrics	7%
Psychiatry	4%
Radiology	7%
Surgery	5%

Financial Information
Source: 2007–2008 LCME I-B survey and 2008–2009 AAMC TSF questionnaire

	Residents	Non-residents
Total Cost of Attendance	$53,955	$63,661
Tuition and Fees	$30,048	$39,254
Other (includes living expenses)	$21,910	$22,410
Health Insurance (can be waived)	$1,997	$1,997

Average 2008 Graduate Indebtedness: $155,328
% of Enrolled Students Receiving Aid: 87%

Criminal Background Check

This medical school does not require a criminal background check prior to matriculation.

University of South Florida College of Medicine

Tampa, Florida

Office of Admissions/MDC-3
University of South Florida College of Medicine
12901 Bruce B. Downs Boulevard
Tampa, Florida 33612-4799
T 813 974 2229   **F** 813 974 4990

Admissions www.hsc.usf.edu/nocms/medicine/
mdadmissions
Main http://health.usf.edu/medicine/home.html
Financial http://hsc.usf.edu/medicine/studentaffairs/
financial_aid/index.htm
E-mail md-admissions@health.usf.edu

Public Institution

Dr. Stephen K. Klasko, Dean College of Medicine and VP for USF Health

Dr. Alicia Monroe, Vice Dean for Educational Affairs

Suzanne Jackson, Director of Student Diversity and Enrichment

Michelle Williamson, Director of Financial Aid

General Information

The College of Medicine, along with the Colleges of Public Health and Nursing and the School of Physical Therapy compose USF Health and offers students unique opportunities for inter-professional relationships and experiences. The College of Medicine admitted the first class of medical students in 1971. The M.D. curriculum carefully integrates basic science learning with early clinical training. Located in Tampa, the College offers medical students a rich and diverse set of patients in nationally-ranked clinical sites.

Mission Statement

The mission of the College of Medicine is to provide for the education of students and professionals of the health and biomedical sciences through the creation of a scholarly environment that fosters excellence in the lifelong goals of education, research, and compassionate care.

Curricular Highlights

Community Service Requirement: Required.
Research/Thesis Requirement: Optional.

The faculty at the COM strive to create a four-year curriculum that is dynamic and forward-looking, reflecting a health care system that is ever-changing and increasingly global in its scope. It is designed to permit the student to learn the fundamental principles of medicine, to acquire skills of critical judgment based on evidence and experience, and to develop an ability to use principles and skills wisely in solving problems of health and disease. Areas of study include the sciences basic to medicine, the major clinical disciplines, and other significant elements such as behavioral science, medical ethics, and human values. The preclinical

curriculum (years 1 and 2) utilizes an integrated, systems-based approach with an emphasis on early clinical experiences. In the major clinical years (years 3 and 4), students participate in direct patient care using both ambulatory and hospital settings across a number of excellent clinical facilities, gaining exposure to a vast array of patient populations. Required clerkships emphasize a patient-centered, interdisciplinary approach to care. Students are given increasing responsibility for patient care in preparation for graduate medical education residencies.

USMLE

Step 1: Required. Students must record a passing score for promotion.
Step 2: Clinical Skills (CS): Required. Students must record a passing total score to graduate.
Step 2: Clinical Knowledge (CK): Required. Students must record a passing total score to graduate.

Selection Factors

Applicants are selected for interviews based on academic achievement, demonstrated motivation to practice medicine and humanism, and leadership. The Admissions Committee reviews all materials including evaluation of the interviews and letters of recommendations, course load and types of courses taken. The majority of the matriculating class are Florida residents, but highly qualified non-Florida residents are also considered. Applicants are encouraged to apply early and complete their applications as soon as possible.

Financial Aid

The financial status of applicants does not affect their acceptance. Limited funds are available for loans and scholarships. First-year students are not permitted to engage in outside employment. There are employment opportunities in Tampa and the surrounding area for spouses. Contact our Office of Financial Aid at (813) 974-2068.

Information about Diversity Programs

The Office of Student Diversity and Enrichment (OSDE) works closely with the Office of M.D. Admissions and the rest of USF Health to recruit and support a diverse student body. Events, activities, programs, and facilities of the University

of South Florida are available to all. For specific information about specific programs and services offered call (813) 974-4707 or visit *http://health.usf.edu/medicine/osde/index.htm.*

Campus Information

Setting

The USF M.D. Program is located in the nation's fifth most diverse large city area and is partners with an array of medical training hospitals in the Tampa Bay and central Florida area. The diversity of the patient population and medical training facilities contribute to an extraordinary clinical training program.

Enrollment

For 2008, total enrollment was: 480

Special Features

The College of Medicine's community training partners include the nation's 12th busiest transplant hospital and Level 1 Trauma/Burn Centers at Tampa General Hospital, All Children's Hospital (ranked among the top 10 children's hospitals), the Moffitt Cancer Center (3rd busiest outpatient cancer hospital in the nation and Florida's only NCI-accredited comprehensive cancer hospital and research center), two very large Veterans Affairs hospitals (the J.A. Haley VA is the busiest outpatient VA facility in the nation), and Florida's only Shriner's Hospital, as well as many other large local hospitals and rural clinics.

Housing

While on-campus student housing is limited, there are many student-centered complexes within close proximity. In addition, the M.D. Student Peer Advisory Council provides an unofficial housing directory to new students in the spring of their matriculation year.

Satellite Campuses/Facilities

Since clinical training at USF is integrated into the entire Tampa Bay medical community, students may rotate through a vast array of excellent hospitals and clinics in both city and rural environments.

Application Process and Requirements 2010–2011

Primary Application Service: AMCAS
Earliest filing date: June 1, 2009
Latest filing date: December 1, 2009

Secondary Application Required?: Yes
Sent to: Screened applicants
URL: www.hsc.usf.edu/nocms/medicine/mdadmissions/
Contact: Admissions office, (813) 974-2229, md-admissions@health.usf.edu
Fee: Yes, $30
Fee waiver available: Yes
Earliest filing date: June 1, 2009
Latest filing date: January 15, 2010

MCAT® required?: Yes
Latest MCAT® considered: October 2009
Oldest MCAT® considered: 2007

Early Decision Program: School does have EDP
Applicants notified: October 1, 2009
EDP available for: Both Residents and Non-residents

Regular Acceptance Notice
Earliest date: October 15, 2009
Latest date: Until class is full
Applicant's Response to Acceptance Offer – Maximum Time: Two weeks

Requests for Deferred Entrance Considered: Yes

Deposit to Hold Place in Class: Yes
Deposit (Resident): $100
Deposit (Non-resident): $100
Deposit due: Within two weeks of acceptance.
Applied to tuition: Yes
Deposit refundable: Yes
Refundable by: May 15, 2010

Estimated number of new entrants: 120
EDP: 15, special program: 15

Start Month/Year: August 2010

Interview Format: Partial open file. Regional interviews are not available.

Other Programs

PREPARATORY PROGRAMS
Postbaccalaureate Program: No
Summer Program: Yes, http://health.usf.edu/medicine/osde/programs.htm
Pre-Matriculation Program: Yes, http://health.usf.edu/medicine/osde/programs.htm

COMBINED DEGREE PROGRAMS
Baccalaureate/M.D.: Yes, www.hsc.usf.edu/medicine/mdadmissions/special_programs.htm
M.D./M.P.H.: Yes, www.hsc.usf.edu/medicine/mdadmissions/special_programs.htm
M.D./M.B.A.: Yes, www.hsc.usf.edu/medicine/mdadmissions/special_programs.htm
M.D./J.D.: Yes, www.hsc.usf.edu/medicine/mdadmissions/special_programs.htm
M.D./Ph.D.: Yes, www.hsc.usf.edu/medicine/mdadmissions/special_programs.htm

Premedical Coursework

Course	Req.	Rec.	Lab.	Sems.
Inorganic Chemistry	•		•	2
Behavioral Sciences				
Biochemistry		•		2
Biology	•		•	2
Biology/Zoology				
Calculus				
College English	•			2
College Mathematics	•			2

Course	Req.	Rec.	Lab.	Sems.
Computer Science				
Genetics				
Humanities		•		
Organic Chemistry	•		•	2
Physics	•		•	2
Psychology				
Social Sciences		•		
Other				

Selection Factors: 2008 Accepted Applicants

Proportion of Accepted Applicants with Relevant Experience (Data Self-Reported to AMCAS®)		
Community Service/Volunteer		71%
Medically-Related Work		91%
Research		82%

Shaded bar represents school's accepted scores ranging from the 10th percentile to the 90th percentile   School Median ●   National Median ●

Overall GPA	2.0	2.1	2.2	2.3	2.4	2.5	2.6	2.7	2.8	2.9	3.0	3.1	3.2	3.3	3.4	3.5	3.6	3.7	(3.8)	3.9	4.0
Science GPA	2.0	2.1	2.2	2.3	2.4	2.5	2.6	2.7	2.8	2.9	3.0	3.1	3.2	3.3	3.4	3.5	3.6	3.7	(3.8)	3.9	4.0

MCAT® Total Numeric Score 9 10 11 12 13 14 15 16 17 18 19 20 21 22 23 24 25 26 27 28 29 30 (31) 32 33 34 35 36 37 38 39 40 41 42 43

Writing Sample				J	K	L	M	N	O	(P)	(Q)	R	S	T
Verbal Reasoning	3	4	5	6	7	8	9	(10)	11	12	13	14	15
Biological Sciences	3	4	5	6	7	8	9	10	(11)	12	13	14	15
Physical Sciences	3	4	5	6	7	8	9	10	(11)	12	13	14	15

Acceptance & Matriculation Data for 2008–2009 First Year Class

	Resident	Non-resident	International	Total
Applications	1677	1170	33	2880
Interviewed	401	59	0	460
Deferred	3	0	0	3
Matriculants				
Early Assurance Program	n/a	n/a	n/a	n/a
Early Decision Program	5	0	0	5
Baccalaureate/M.D.	15	0	0	15
M.D./Ph.D.	0	0	0	0
Matriculated	109	11	0	**120**
Applications accepted from International Applicants: No				

Matriculant Demographics: 2008–2009 First Year Class

Men: 57   **Women:** 63

Matriculants' Self-Reported Race/Ethnicity

Mexican American	1	**Korean**	1
Cuban	2	**Vietnamese**	1
Puerto Rican	4	**Other Asian**	1
Other Hispanic	1	**Total Asian**	25
Total Hispanic	7	**Native American**	2
Chinese	3	**Black**	10
Asian Indian	15	**Native Hawaiian**	1
Pakistani	3	**White**	84
Filipino	0	**Unduplicated Number**	
Japanese	2	**of Matriculants**	120

Science and Math Majors: 65%
Matriculants with:
> **Baccalaureate degree:** 98%
> **Graduate degree(s):** 19%

Specialty Choice

2004, 2005, 2006 Graduates, Specialty Choice (As reported by program directors to GME Track™)	
Anesthesiology	6%
Emergency Medicine	8%
Family Practice	11%
Internal Medicine	19%
Obstetrics/Gynecology	4%
Orthopaedic Surgery	2%
Pediatrics	11%
Psychiatry	7%
Radiology	7%
Surgery	6%

Financial Information

Source: 2007–2008 LCME I-B survey and 2008–2009 AAMC TSF questionnaire

	Residents	Non-residents
Total Cost of Attendance	$44,390	$75,067
Tuition and Fees	$22,456	$53,133
Other (includes living expenses)	$21,934	$21,934
Health Insurance (can be waived)	$0	$0

Average 2008 Graduate Indebtedness: $119,021
% of Enrolled Students Receiving Aid: 87%

Criminal Background Check

This medical school requires a criminal background check prior to matriculation.

Emory University School of Medicine

Atlanta, Georgia

Emory University School of Medicine
Office of Admissions
1648 Pierce Drive NE, Suite 231
Atlanta, Georgia 30322-4510
T 404 727 5660   **F** 404 727 5456

Admissions www.med.emory.edu
Main www.med.emory.edu
Financial www.emory.edu/FINANCIAL_AID
E-mail medadmiss@emory.edu

Private Institution

Dr. Thomas J. Lawley, Dean

Dr. Ira K. Schwartz, Associate Dean for Medical Education/Student Affairs, Director of Admissions

Dr. Robert Lee, Associate Dean and Director, Office of Multicultural Affairs

Michael Behler, Associate Director of Financial Aid

Dr. J. William Eley, Executive Associate Dean for Medical Education/Student Affairs

General Information

Located six miles east of Atlanta, the Emory University School of Medicine was founded in 1915, resulting from several reorganizations dating from 1854 when the Atlanta Medical College was founded. Student clinical experiences are in numerous teaching hospitals, which provide more than 3,000 beds and large outpatient clinics. The university has close ties with Grady Memorial Hospital, the Centers for Disease Control and Prevention, the Carter Center of Emory University, and other affiliated institutions.

Mission Statement

Emory University School of Medicine is committed to providing leadership in medicine and science through the development of recognized programs of excellence and innovation in medical education, biomedical research, and patient care.

Curricular Highlights

Community Service Requirement: Optional. Encouraged.
Research/Thesis Requirement: Optional.

In 2007, EUSM implemented a progressive new curriculum which coincided with the opening of our new state-of-the-art medical education building. The new curriculum features a hybrid of lectures, small groups, and enhanced clinical exposure throughout the first 18 months of training. Students begin 12 months of clinical rotations midway through the second year, followed by a 5 month Discovery Phase which allows time for clinical

or bench research, international experience, or other academic inquiry. The curriculum offers flexibility to allow students to take advantage of all of Emory's diverse opportunities. The fourth year is highlighted by a capstone experience which helps further prepare students for entering residency.

USMLE

Step 1: Required. Students must record a passing score for promotion.
Step 2: Clinical Skills (CS): Required. Students must only record a score.
Step 2: Clinical Knowledge (CK): Required. Students must record a passing total score to graduate.

Selection Factors

Students are selected on the basis of scholastic achievement and personal qualifications, without regard to race, sex, sexual orientation, age, disability, creed, veteran status, or national origin. In addition to the AMCAS application, all applicants must (a) present a very high level of scholarship; (b) take the MCAT within four years of the matriculating year; (c) complete the Emory supplemental application form and fee (available on-line upon Emory's receipt of the AMCAS application); (d) have the required evaluation(s) submitted; and (e) appear for a personal interview, if invited. Students from foreign schools must have completed at least one year of academic work in an accredited U.S. or Canadian institution. Anyone enrolled in a graduate degree program should complete all required work for the degree by the date of matriculation. Only students enrolled in U.S. LCME-accredited medical schools with a similar curriculum are eligible to apply for transfer. Advanced standing is not given for work completed in other professional or graduate schools.

Financial Aid

Those who show documented need are eligible to receive funding in the form of scholarships and loans. Parental financial information is necessary to determine need-based funding. Each year, Emory awards 5 entering students merit-based Woodruff Fellowships, which provide full tuition and stipend for all four years.

Information about Diversity Programs

EUSM is strongly committed to increasing diversity in medicine. The Office of Multicultural Affairs works in conjunction with the Admission Committee and the Office of Student Affairs in the recruitment, selection, and retention of qualified students from groups underrepresented in medicine.

Campus Information

Setting

EUSM is located on the main university campus, situated on 631 acres of land in the historic neighborhood of Druid Hills. Emory is positioned along the Clifton Corridor, which also includes the U.S. Centers for Disease Control and Prevention.

Enrollment

For 2008, total enrollment was: 498

Special Features

Emory's clinical facilities provide for an extraordinary variety of training opportunities with diverse patient populations. Students are trained at the Emory University Hospital, Emory Crawford Long Hospital, Wesley Woods Geriatric Center, Children's Healthcare of Atlanta at Egleston and at Hughes Spalding, The Emory Clinic, Winship Cancer Center, Atlanta VA Medical Center, Grady Memorial Hospital, and numerous out-patient clinical sites. Grady Memorial Hospital is one of the largest hospitals in the U.S. Students have opportunities to volunteer in clinics, conduct research, and spend elective time abroad.

Housing

Off-campus apartments and houses are plentiful and affordable. New graduate housing will open in August 2009, offering all the modern amenities of luxury apartment complexes.

Application Process and Requirements 2010–2011

Primary Application Service: AMCAS
Earliest filing date: June 1, 2009
Latest filing date: October 15, 2009

Secondary Application Required?: Yes
Sent to: All applicants
Contact: Medical School Admissions,
(404) 727-5660, medadmiss@emory.edu
Fee: Yes, $100
Fee waiver available: Yes
Earliest filing date: August 1, 2009
Latest filing date: December 1, 2009

MCAT® required?: Yes
Latest MCAT® considered: September 2009
Oldest MCAT® considered: 2006

Early Decision Program: School does not have EDP
Applicants notified: n/a
EDP available for: n/a

Regular Acceptance Notice
Earliest date: October 29, 2009
Latest date: Until class is full
Applicant's Response to Acceptance Offer – Maximum Time: Two weeks

Requests for Deferred Entrance Considered: Yes

Deposit to Hold Place in Class: No
Deposit (Resident): n/a
Deposit (Non-resident): n/a
Deposit due: n/a
Applied to tuition: n/a
Deposit refundable: n/a
Refundable by: n/a

Estimated number of new entrants: 132
EDP: n/a, special program: n/a

Start Month/Year: August 2010

Interview Format: Group interview and individual interview. Regional interviews are not available.

Other Programs

PREPARATORY PROGRAMS
Postbaccalaureate Program: No
Summer Program: No

COMBINED DEGREE PROGRAMS
Baccalaureate/M.D.: No
M.D./M.P.H.: Yes, www.med.emory.edu
John E. McGowan, Jr., M.D.
jmcgowa@sph.emory.edu
M.D./M.B.A.: No
M.D./J.D.: No
M.D./Ph.D.: Yes, www.med.emory.edu
Mary Horton, MPH, MA
(404) 727-6977, mdphd@emory.edu
Additional Program: Yes, www.med.emory.edu, Cheryl Sroka, MD/MSCR Program, csroka@emory.edu

Premedical Coursework

Course	Req.	Rec.	Lab.	Qtrs.
Inorganic Chemistry	•		•	8
Behavioral Sciences	•			
Biochemistry		•		
Biology	•		•	8
Biology/Zoology				
Calculus				
College English	•			6
College Mathematics				

Course	Req.	Rec.	Lab.	Qtrs.
Computer Science				
Genetics				
Humanities	•			18
Organic Chemistry	•		•	8
Physics	•		•	8
Psychology				
Social Sciences	•			
Other				

Selection Factors: 2008 Accepted Applicants

Proportion of Accepted Applicants with Relevant Experience (Data Self-Reported to AMCAS®)		Community Service/Volunteer	76%
		Medically-Related Work	81%
		Research	87%

Shaded bar represents school's accepted scores ranging from the 10th percentile to the 90th percentile ▓   School Median ● National Median ●

Overall GPA	2.0	2.1	2.2	2.3	2.4	2.5	2.6	2.7	2.8	2.9	3.0	3.1	3.2	3.3	3.4	3.5	3.6	3.7	(3.8)	3.9	4.0
Science GPA	2.0	2.1	2.2	2.3	2.4	2.5	2.6	2.7	2.8	2.9	3.0	3.1	3.2	3.3	3.4	3.5	3.6	3.7	(3.8)	3.9	4.0

MCAT® Total Numeric Score 9 10 11 12 13 14 15 16 17 18 19 20 21 22 23 24 25 26 27 28 29 30 31 (32) 33 34 (35) 36 37 38 39 40 41 42 43

Writing Sample			J	K	L	M	N	O	P	(Q)	R	S	T
Verbal Reasoning	3	4	5	6	7	8	9	(10)	(11)	12	13	14	15
Biological Sciences	3	4	5	6	7	8	9	10	(11)	(12)	13	14	15
Physical Sciences	3	4	5	6	7	8	9	10	(11)	(12)	13	14	15

Acceptance & Matriculation Data for 2008–2009 First Year Class

	Resident	Non-resident	International	Total
Applications	635	5102	318	6055
Interviewed	151	499	28	678
Deferred	3	4	0	7
Matriculants				
Early Assurance Program	n/a	n/a	n/a	n/a
Early Decision Program	0	0	0	0
Baccalaureate/M.D.	n/a	n/a	n/a	n/a
M.D./Ph.D.	3	8	1	12
Matriculated	45	78	5	**128**

Applications accepted from International Applicants: Yes

Matriculant Demographics: 2008–2009 First Year Class

Men: 62   **Women:** 66

Matriculants' Self-Reported Race/Ethnicity

Mexican American	1	**Korean**	5
Cuban	0	**Vietnamese**	0
Puerto Rican	0	**Other Asian**	4
Other Hispanic	1	**Total Asian**	17
Total Hispanic	2	**Native American**	0
Chinese	3	**Black**	13
Asian Indian	6	**Native Hawaiian**	0
Pakistani	1	**White**	90
Filipino	0	**Unduplicated Number**	
Japanese	0	**of Matriculants**	128

Science and Math Majors: 62%
Matriculants with:
Baccalaureate degree: 100%
Graduate degree(s): 6%

Specialty Choice

2004, 2005, 2006 Graduates, Specialty Choice (As reported by program directors to GME Track™)	
Anesthesiology	5%
Emergency Medicine	7%
Family Practice	4%
Internal Medicine	21%
Obstetrics/Gynecology	3%
Orthopaedic Surgery	3%
Pediatrics	8%
Psychiatry	4%
Radiology	6%
Surgery	8%

Financial Information

Source: 2007–2008 LCME I-B survey and 2008–2009 AAMC TSF questionnaire

	Residents	Non-residents
Total Cost of Attendance	$70,466	$70,466
Tuition and Fees	$41,476	$41,476
Other (includes living expenses)	$26,992	$26,992
Health Insurance (can be waived)	$1,998	$1,998

Average 2008 Graduate Indebtedness: $146,824
% of Enrolled Students Receiving Aid: 84%

Criminal Background Check

This medical school does not require a criminal background check prior to matriculation.

Medical College of Georgia
School of Medicine

Augusta, Georgia

Dr. Geoffrey H. Young
Associate Dean for Admissions
Medical College of Georgia
School of Medicine
Augusta, Georgia 30912-4760
T 706 721 3186   F 706 721 0959

Admissions www.mcg.edu/careers/medicine.htm
Main www.mcg.edu
Financial www.mcg.edu/students/finaid
E-mail stdadmin@mail.mcg.edu

Public Institution

Dr. D. Douglas Miller, Dean

Dr. Geoffrey H. Young, Associate Dean for Admissions

Wilma A. Sykes-Brown, M.A., Assistant Dean for Educational Outreach and Partnerships

Dr. Beverly Ann Boggs, Director of Student Financial Aid

Linda R. DeVaughn, Director of Admissions

General Information

The School of Medicine of the Medical College of Georgia was founded in 1828 and is the nation's 13th oldest medical school. The institution is a separate university under the University System of Georgia. It consists of five schools: medicine, allied health, dentistry, graduate studies, and nursing.

Mission Statement

The Medical College of Georgia is committed to a supportive campus climate, necessary services, and leadership and development opportunities, all to educate the whole person and meet the needs of students, faculty, and staff; cultural, ethnic, racial, and gender diversity supported by practices that embody the ideals of an open democratic and global society; technology to advance education; collaborative relationships with other System institutions, state agencies, local schools and technical institutes, and industry, sharing physical, human, and information resources to enhance services available to the citizens of Georgia.

Curricular Highlights

Community Service Requirement: Optional.
Research/Thesis Requirement: Optional.

During the pre-clinical years, students acquire the building blocks that underlie medical practice. The modular content of the curriculum is taught in lectures and labs with integrated clinical conferences and small-group activities. In the first semester, the Cellular and Systems Structures module introduces Gross Anatomy, Histology, and Development. In the second semester, Biochemistry, Genetics, and Physiology are taught, while the Brain and Behavior mod-

ule covers Psychiatry and Neuroscience. The Essentials of Clinical Medicine (ECM) is a two-year sequence emphasizing patient care skills. In year two, the year-long Cellular and Systems Disease States module exposes students to Microbiology, Pathology, and Pharmacology in the context of clinical medicine. Clinical Training: Patient contact begins in year one in the ECM course that extends through year two. Year three consists of required clerkships in Family Medicine, Internal Medicine, Neurology, OB/Gyn, Pediatrics, Psychiatry, and Surgery. During year four, students complete rotations in Emergency Medicine, Critical Care, Ambulatory Medicine, and an acting internship, with the remainder of the year for electives that can include research.

USMLE

Step 1: Required. Students must record a passing score for promotion.
Step 2: Clinical Skills (CS): Required. Students must record a passing total score to graduate.
Step 2: Clinical Knowledge (CK): Required. Students must record a passing total score to graduate.

Selection Factors

Applicants for admission are evaluated on a competitive basis. Information used includes, but is not limited to, the applicant's responsibilities prior to application; activities; shadowing physicians; ethnic, socioeconomic, and cultural background; region of residence with respect to its health professional needs; commitment to practice in an underserved area; references; motivation and potential for serving as a physician; interviews; MCAT performance; and grades. In addition, students must meet specified technical standards to participate effectively in the medical education program and in the practice of medicine. Preference is given to Georgia residents. See *www.mcg.edu/SOM/admit/* for more information.

Financial Aid

The Office of Financial Aid coordinates programs of assistance available to students. Information may be obtained at *www.mcg.edu/students/finaid.*

Information about Diversity Programs

The Medical College of Georgia seeks to encourage applications from qualified students from groups underrepresented in medicine. A summer program is designed for disadvantaged college students who show academic promise and who desire to practice medicine. Students may apply by writing to: Wilma A. Sykes-Brown, M.A., Assistant Dean for Educational Outreach and Partnerships, CB-1801, Medical College of Georgia, Augusta, GA 30912-1900.

Campus Information

Setting

The medical school is located in Augusta, GA, the second-largest city in Georgia, which is located on the south bank of the Savannah River, midway between the Great Smokey Mountains and the Atlantic Ocean. Augusta is a thriving city and a leading health care center, with nine area hospitals.

Enrollment

For 2008, total enrollment was: 750

Special Features

MCG Children's Medical Center is dedicated to serving the health care needs of children, from newborns to teenagers. The 149-bed modern center recognizes the importance of family involvement in a child's healing process and embraces the philosophy of family-centered care. A new $54 million Cancer Research Center opened in 2006. The campus has a new student Wellness Center.

Housing

A variety of on-campus living environments are available.

Satellite Campuses/Facilities

Core clerkships take place at the MCG Hospitals and Clinics, the Children's Medical Center, and affiliated hospitals and community-based teaching sites throughout Georgia. The Medical College of Georgia in partnership with the University of Georgia is seeking accreditation to matriculate students to the Medical College of Georgia/ University of Georgia Medical Partnership Campus in Athens in 2010. The medical partnership campus would be a four year curriculum campus.

Application Process and Requirements 2010–2011

Primary Application Service: AMCAS
Earliest filing date: June 1, 2009
Latest filing date: November 1, 2009

Secondary Application Required?: Yes
Sent to: All Georgia residents; others are screened
URL: Provided by school
Contact: (706) 721-3186
Fee: No
Fee waiver available: n/a
Earliest filing date: June 1, 2009
Latest filing date: Two weeks after receipt and must be in the student file by December 1, 2009

MCAT® required?: Yes
Latest MCAT® considered: September 2009
Oldest MCAT® considered: 2007

Early Decision Program: School does have EDP
Applicants notified: October 1, 2009
EDP available for: Residents only

Regular Acceptance Notice
Earliest date: October 2009
Latest date: Until class is full
Applicant's Response to Acceptance Offer – Maximum Time: Two weeks

Requests for Deferred Entrance Considered: Yes

Deposit to Hold Place in Class: Yes
Deposit (Resident): $100
Deposit (Non-resident): $100
Deposit due: With response to acceptance offer
Applied to tuition: Yes
Deposit refundable: Yes
Refundable by: May 15, 2010

Estimated number of new entrants: 230
EDP: 60, special program: 6

Start Month/Year: August 2010

Interview Format: One individual interview with committee member. Regional interviews are not available.

Other Programs

PREPARATORY PROGRAMS
Postbaccalaureate Program: No
Summer Program: Yes, mcg.edu/careers/specop/
Wilma A. Sykes-Brown, MA, 706-721-2522, wsykes@mail.mcg.edu
Summer Student Training and Research (STAR) Program: www.mcg.edu/star

COMBINED DEGREE PROGRAMS
Baccalaureate/M.D.: No
M.D./M.P.H.: No
M.D./M.B.A.: No
M.D./J.D.: No
M.D./Ph.D.: Yes, www.mcg.edu/som/mdphd/geninfo.htm, Edward Inscho, PhD, 706-721-5615, einscho@mcg.edu

Premedical Coursework

Course	Req.	Rec.	Lab.	Sems.
Inorganic Chemistry	•		•	2
Behavioral Sciences				
Biochemistry		•		
Biology				
Biology/Zoology	•		•	2
Calculus				
College English	•			2
College Mathematics				
Computer Science				

Course	Req.	Rec.	Lab.	Sems.
Genetics				
Humanities				
Organic Chemistry	•		•	1
Physics	•		•	2
Psychology				
Social Sciences				
Advanced Chemistry	•			1
Cellular Biology		•		
Statistics		•		

Selection Factors: 2008 Accepted Applicants

Proportion of Accepted Applicants with Relevant Experience (Data Self-Reported to AMCAS)		
Community Service/Volunteer		71%
Medically-Related Work		81%
Research		75%

Shaded bar represents school's accepted scores ranging from the 10th percentile to the 90th percentile   School Median ●   National Median ●

Overall GPA	2.0	2.1	2.2	2.3	2.4	2.5	2.6	2.7	2.8	2.9	3.0	3.1	3.2	3.3	3.4	3.5	3.6	3.7	(3.8)	3.9	4.0
Science GPA	2.0	2.1	2.2	2.3	2.4	2.5	2.6	2.7	2.8	2.9	3.0	3.1	3.2	3.3	3.4	3.5	3.6	(3.7)	3.8	3.9	4.0

MCAT® Total Numeric Score 9 10 11 12 13 14 15 16 17 18 19 20 21 22 23 24 25 26 27 28 29 30 (31) 32 33 34 35 36 37 38 39 40 41 42 43

Writing Sample		J	K	L	M	N	O	(P)	(Q)	R	S	T
Verbal Reasoning	3	4	5	6	7	8	9	(10)	11	12	13	14	15
Biological Sciences	3	4	5	6	7	8	9	10	(11)	12	13	14	15
Physical Sciences	3	4	5	6	7	8	9	(10)	(11)	12	13	14	15

Acceptance & Matriculation Data for 2008–2009 First Year Class

	Resident	Non-resident	International	Total
Applications	1054	984	64	2102
Interviewed	553	16	0	569
Deferred	3	0	0	3
Matriculants				
Early Assurance Program	0	0	0	0
Early Decision Program	77	0	0	77
Baccalaureate/M.D.	n/a	n/a	n/a	n/a
M.D./Ph.D.	3	0	0	3
Matriculated	188	2	0	**190**

Applications accepted from International Applicants: Only Canadian

Matriculant Demographics: 2008–2009 First Year Class

Men: 107   **Women:** 83

Matriculants' Self-Reported Race/Ethnicity

Mexican American	1	**Korean**	6
Cuban	2	**Vietnamese**	1
Puerto Rican	0	**Other Asian**	4
Other Hispanic	1	**Total Asian**	45
Total Hispanic	4	**Native American**	1
Chinese	7	**Black**	15
Asian Indian	25	**Native Hawaiian**	0
Pakistani	1	**White**	128
Filipino	0	**Unduplicated Number**	
Japanese	1	**of Matriculants**	190

Science and Math Majors: 74%
Matriculants with:
    Baccalaureate degree: 100%
    Graduate degree(s): 8%

Specialty Choice

2004, 2005, 2006 Graduates, Specialty Choice (As reported by program directors to GME Track™)	
Anesthesiology	9%
Emergency Medicine	6%
Family Practice	8%
Internal Medicine	18%
Obstetrics/Gynecology	6%
Orthopaedic Surgery	5%
Pediatrics	17%
Psychiatry	1%
Radiology	4%
Surgery	6%

Financial Information

Source: 2007–2008 LCME I-B survey and 2008–2009 AAMC TSF questionnaire

	Residents	Non-residents
Total Cost of Attendance	$39,295	$55,379
Tuition and Fees	$15,604	$31,688
Other (includes living expenses)	$22,492	$22,492
Health Insurance (can be waived)	$1,199	$1,199

Average 2008 Graduate Indebtedness: $107,017
% of Enrolled Students Receiving Aid: 80%

Criminal Background Check

This medical school does not require a criminal background check prior to matriculation.

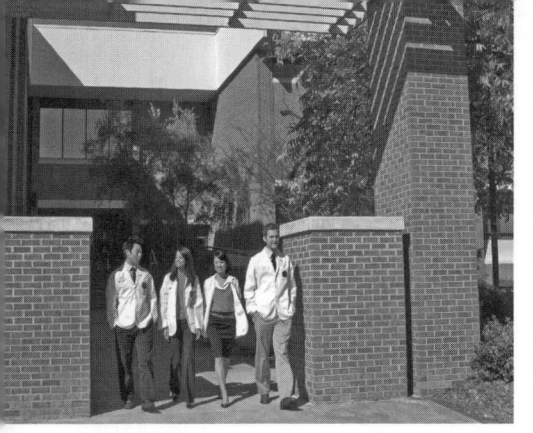

Mercer University School of Medicine

Macon, Georgia

Office of Admissions and Student Affairs
Mercer University School of Medicine
1550 College Street
Macon, Georgia 31207
T 478 301 2542   **F** 478 301 2547

Admissions http://medicine.mercer.edu/admissions
Main http://medicine.mercer.edu
Financial http://medicine.mercer.edu/Admissions/admissions_financial
E-mail admissions@med.mercer.edu

Private Institution

Dr. William F. Bina, Interim Dean

Dr. Maurice S. Clifton, Associate Dean for Admissions and Student Affairs

Youvette D. Hudson, Registrar/Director for Financial Aid Planning

Mary G. Scott, Associate Director of Financial Planning

Mary C. Putnam, Assistant Director of Admissions and Student Affairs

General Information

Mercer University School of Medicine was founded in 1982 to improve health care access to the residents of Georgia. A private institution with strong state support, MUSM has been a leader in educating physicians who practice in the state after their training. MUSM also offers multiple graduate degrees including a Masters in Public Health.

Mission Statement

The mission of Mercer University School of Medicine (MUSM) is to educate physicians and health professionals to meet the primary care and health care needs of rural and medically underserved areas of Georgia.

Curricular Highlights

Community Service Requirement: Required. Numerous volunteer opportunities are available
Research/Thesis Requirement: Optional.

One of the first schools to adopt an all Problem-Based-Learning curriculum, there are no lectures and students take responsibility for their own learning. This open-ended nature requires and generates maturity and confidence not seen in traditional curricula. Learning must go well beyond the basic facts in that students are called upon to integrate and demonstrate verbally their basic science knowledge base to explain clinical findings. In addition, students are evaluated in areas related to group and interpersonal, problem-solving, information-gathering and evaluation skills. Students interview and examine actual and standardized patients early in the first year. The Community Medicine program provides a continuity experience in the clinical aspects of a community-oriented primary care medical practice during the first, second and fourth years. The third year consists of required clinical rotations in internal medicine, surgery, pediatrics, obstetrics-gynecology, family medicine, and psychiatry. The fourth year includes required clerkships in acute and critical care and community medicine.

USMLE

Step 1: Required. Students must record a passing score for promotion.
Step 2: Clinical Skills (CS): Required. Students must only record a score.
Step 2: Clinical Knowledge (CK): Required. Students must record a passing total score to graduate.

Selection Factors

The Admissions Committee only accepts applicants who are legal residents of Georgia. Each applicant must show promise of learning effectively in Mercer's curriculum and strong potential for practice in a medical specialty commensurate with the health care needs of rural and other underserved areas of Georgia. Most counties in Georgia have underserved status by the federal government, and the specialties that are needed include the primary care specialties of Internal Medicine, Pediatrics and Family Medicine, but also Surgery, and Obstetrics and Gynecology. Interviews are by invitation only and are held at both the Macon and Savannah campuses. In making the final decisions for acceptance or rejection, the Admissions Committee considers all criteria, but emphasizes strongly an applicant's demonstrated desire to fulfill the mission of the institution. The committee does not discriminate on the basis of race, sex, creed, national origin, age, or handicap.

Financial Aid

Financial aid in the form of loans and scholarships is available to incoming accepted students. Financial need is determined by a federally approved need analysis and awards are made on the basis of need and merit. Most scholarships are based on need and mission compliance. The Office of Student Financial Planning provides easy access to information about all financial aid programs available and financial planning and debt management thru financial management conferences and workshops.

Information about Diversity Programs

MUSM embraces the position that promoting and supporting diversity among the student body is central to the mission of the school. A diverse student body enriches professional education by providing a multiplicity of views and prospective that enhances learning within this highly interactive, student centered curriculum. For additional information and opportunities, please contact diversity@med.mercer.edu.

Special Features

The assessment system includes oral exams which foster integration of basic science knowledge base to explain clinical findings. Our students participate in a wide variety of leadership and community service programs, and many in international outreach programs in Africa, Central and South America.

Campus Information

Setting

There are two branch campuses, the Macon campus at Mercer University and at the Medical Center of Central Georgia, and the Savannah campus at the Memorial Health University Medical Center. Clinical teaching is also provided at several rural hospitals and clinics throughout Georgia.

Enrollment

For 2008, total enrollment was: 279

Housing

The Office of Student Affairs maintains a housing list of available apartments/houses and a list of those students who wish to secure roommates.

Satellite Campuses/Facilities

Students may study all four years on either the Macon or Savannah campus with a limited number of spaces for students to complete the first two years in Macon, and the clinical years in Savannah. There are many sites available for the Community Medicine program, and most students are able to return to a location near their home.

Application Process and Requirements 2010–2011

Primary Application Service: AMCAS
Earliest filing date: June 1, 2009
Latest filing date: November 1, 2009

Secondary Application Required?: Yes
Sent to: Screened applicants
Contact: Gail Coleman, (478) 301-2524, admissions@mercer.edu
Fee: Yes, $50
Fee waiver available: Yes
Earliest filing date: June 2009
Latest filing date: January 15, 2010

MCAT® required?: Yes
Latest MCAT® considered: September 2009
Oldest MCAT® considered: 2007

Early Decision Program: School does have EDP
Applicants notified: October 1, 2009
EDP available for: Residents only

Regular Acceptance Notice
Earliest date: November 2009
Latest date: Until class is full
Applicant's Response to Acceptance Offer – Maximum Time: Two weeks

Requests for Deferred Entrance Considered: Yes

Deposit to Hold Place in Class: Yes
Deposit (Resident): $100
Deposit (Non-resident): n/a
Deposit due: With response to acceptance offer
Applied to tuition: Yes
Deposit refundable: Yes
Refundable by: May 15, 2010

Estimated number of new entrants: 90
EDP: 40, special program: n/a

Start Month/Year: August 2010

Interview Format: Two, one-hour interviews.

Other Programs

PREPARATORY PROGRAMS
Postbaccalaureate Program: No
Summer Program: Yes, Admissions@med.mercer.edu

COMBINED DEGREE PROGRAMS
Baccalaureate/M.D.: No
M.D./M.P.H.: No
M.D./M.B.A.: No
M.D./J.D.: No
M.D./Ph.D.: No

Premedical Coursework

Course	Req.	Rec.	Lab.	Sems.
Inorganic Chemistry	•		•	2
Behavioral Sciences				
Biochemistry		•		
Biology	•		•	2
Biology/Zoology				
Calculus				
College English				
College Mathematics				

Course	Req.	Rec.	Lab.	Sems.
Computer Science				
Genetics				
Humanities				
Organic Chemistry	•		•	2
Physics	•		•	2
Psychology				
Social Sciences				
Other				

Selection Factors: 2008 Accepted Applicants

Proportion of Accepted Applicants with Relevant Experience (Data Self-Reported to AMCAS®)	
Community Service/Volunteer	72%
Medically-Related Work	75%
Research	65%

Shaded bar represents school's accepted scores ranging from the 10th percentile to the 90th percentile. School Median ● National Median ●

Overall GPA 2.0 2.1 2.2 2.3 2.4 2.5 2.6 2.7 2.8 2.9 3.0 3.1 3.2 3.3 3.4 3.5 (3.6) 3.7 3.8 3.9 4.0
Science GPA 2.0 2.1 2.2 2.3 2.4 2.5 2.6 2.7 2.8 2.9 3.0 3.1 3.2 3.3 3.4 (3.5) 3.6 3.7 3.8 3.9 4.0

MCAT® Total Numeric Score 9 10 11 12 13 14 15 16 17 18 19 20 21 22 23 24 25 26 (27) 28 29 30 31 (32) 33 34 35 36 37 38 39 40 41 42 43

Writing Sample		J	K	L	M	N	(O)	P	(Q) R S T
Verbal Reasoning	3	4	5	6	7	8	(9)	(10) 11	12 13 14 15
Biological Sciences	3	4	5	6	7	8	9	(10) (11)	12 13 14 15
Physical Sciences	3	4	5	6	7	8	(9)	10 (11)	12 13 14 15

Acceptance & Matriculation Data for 2008–2009 First Year Class

	Resident	Non-resident	International	Total
Applications	770	1	2	773
Interviewed	295	0	0	295
Deferred	4	0	0	4
Matriculants				
Early Assurance Program	n/a	n/a	n/a	n/a
Early Decision Program	27	0	0	27
Baccalaureate/M.D.	n/a	n/a	n/a	n/a
M.D./Ph.D.	n/a	n/a	n/a	n/a
Matriculated	90	0	0	**90**

Applications accepted from International Applicants: No

Matriculant Demographics: 2008–2009 First Year Class

Men: 46   **Women:** 44

Matriculants' Self-Reported Race/Ethnicity

Mexican American	0	**Korean**	2
Cuban	0	**Vietnamese**	1
Puerto Rican	0	**Other Asian**	3
Other Hispanic	1	**Total Asian**	10
Total Hispanic	1	**Native American**	0
Chinese	2	**Black**	1
Asian Indian	2	**Native Hawaiian**	0
Pakistani	0	**White**	79
Filipino	1	**Unduplicated Number**	
Japanese	1	**of Matriculants**	90

Science and Math Majors: 70%
Matriculants with:
Baccalaureate degree: 100%
Graduate degree(s): 7%

Specialty Choice

2004, 2005, 2006 Graduates, Specialty Choice (As reported by program directors to GME Track™)	
Anesthesiology	3%
Emergency Medicine	4%
Family Practice	8%
Internal Medicine	22%
Obstetrics/Gynecology	7%
Orthopaedic Surgery	3%
Pediatrics	18%
Psychiatry	1%
Radiology	8%
Surgery	15%

Financial Information

Source: 2007–2008 LCME I-B survey and 2008–2009 AAMC TSF questionnaire

	Residents	Non-residents
Total Cost of Attendance	$60,900	n/a
Tuition and Fees	$37,230	n/a
Other (includes living expenses)	$22,924	n/a
Health Insurance (can be waived)	$746	n/a

Average 2008 Graduate Indebtedness: $152,591
% of Enrolled Students Receiving Aid: 94%

Criminal Background Check

This medical school requires a criminal background check prior to matriculation.

Morehouse School of Medicine
Atlanta, Georgia

Admissions and Student Affairs
Morehouse School of Medicine
720 Westview Drive, S.W.
Atlanta, Georgia 30310-1495
T 404 752 1650 **F** 404 752 1512

Admissions www.msm.edu/educational/
mdprogram.htm
Main www.msm.edu/
Financial www.msm.edu/admissions/fa/financial_aid.htm
E-mail mdadmissions@msm.edu

Private Institution

Dr. Eve J. Higginbotham, Dean and Senior Vice President for Academic Affairs

Dr. Ngozi Anachebe, Assistant Dean for Student Affairs

Dr. Cynthia Handy, Director of Student Fiscal Affairs

Dr. Sterling Roaf, Director of Admissions

General Information

Established in 1975 as the School of Medicine at Morehouse College, Morehouse School of Medicine became independent from its founding institution in 1981. MSM is a member of the Atlanta University Center Consortium Inc.- a consortium of five Historically Black Colleges and Universities. Through our affiliations with Atlanta-based Grady Health System, Children's Healthcare of Atlanta at Hughes Spalding, South Fulton Medical Center and the Atlanta Medical Center, our students and residents are able to experience a broad patient population and engage in the opportunity for the best training experience possible.

Mission Statement

Morehouse School of Medicine is dedicated to improving the health and well-being of individuals and communities; increasing the diversity of the health professional and scientific workforce; and addressing primary health-care needs through programs in education, research, and service, with emphasis on people of color and the underserved urban and rural populations in Georgia and the nation.

Curricular Highlights

Community Service Requirement: Optional.
Research/Thesis Requirement: Optional.

The first two years of the curriculum emphasize an understanding of the principles, concepts, and major factual background of the basic medical sciences. Exposure to clinical medicine begins in the first year through assignment to a preceptor and increases in the second year with introduction to clinical medicine. Clinical education is continued through core clerkships during the third and fourth years, with 20 weeks of electives in the senior year. Student performance is evaluated primarily by letter grades. Learning resources and other support services are available to all students throughout their four years.

USMLE

Step 1: Required. Students must record a passing score for promotion.
Step 2: Clinical Skills (CS): Required. Students must record a passing total score to graduate.
Step 2: Clinical Knowledge (CK): Required. Students must record a passing total score to graduate.

Selection Factors

Selection of students for admission is made after careful consideration of many factors. These include MCAT scores, the academic record, the extent of academic improvement, balance and depth of academic program, difficulty of courses taken, and other indicators of maturation of learning ability. Additional factors considered are extracurricular activities, hobbies, the need to work, research projects and experiences, evidence of activities that indicate concurrence with the school's mission, and evidence of pursuing interests and talents in depth. Finally, the committee looks for evidence of those traits of personality and character essential to succeed in medicine: compassion, integrity, motivation, and perseverance. All information available about each applicant is considered without assigning priority to any single factor. Students are admitted on the basis of individual qualifications regardless of sex, age, race, creed, national origin, or handicap. Preferential consideration is given to qualified applicants who are residents of the state of Georgia. Foreign applicants must have a permanent resident visa. Technical standards have been established as a prerequisite for admission and graduation from the MSM. A candidate for the M.D. degree must have aptitude, abilities, and skills in five areas: observation, communication, motor, conceptual integrative and quantitative, and behavioral and social. Applicants are not considered for admission who have been dismissed from another medical school for academic or disciplinary reasons. Transfer applications are considered only from students in good standing at an LCME-accredited U.S. or Canadian medical school; transfers from foreign medical schools or osteopathic, veterinary, or dental schools are not accepted. Transfers are accepted into the second year only on a space-available basis. The transfer application deadline is May 1.

Financial Aid

In addition to federal loan programs, a number of scholarships and grants are available.

Campus Information

Setting

Morehouse School of Medicine is situated five minutes from downtown Atlanta within the Atlanta University Center (AUC) in the historic West End. Atlanta is also home to the Centers for Disease Control and Prevention (CDC), over 20 major medical centers, the Carter Presidential Library, the Martin Luther King Center for Nonviolent Social Change, and a plethora of educational, entertainment, and cultural opportunities. Atlanta's sports teams consist of the Atlanta Braves, Atlanta Falcons, and the Atlanta Hawks. Home to one of the busiest airports in the world, Hartsfield-Jackson Atlanta International Airport, the city is a major international transportation hub. A premier city for the 21st century, Atlanta is a bustling, progressive metropolis with an energy all its own.

Enrollment

For 2008, total enrollment was: 216

Housing

On-campus housing is not available. Students seeking assistance in their relocation can access the school's very useful Web site at *http://web. msm.edu/relocation_guide/housing.htm.*

Application Process and Requirements 2010–2011

Primary Application Service: AMCAS
Earliest filing date: June 1, 2009
Latest filing date: December 1, 2009

Secondary Application Required?: Yes
Sent to: All eligible applicants after preliminary screening
URL: URL given to invited applicants only
Fee: Yes, $50
Fee waiver available: Yes
Earliest filing date: July 15, 2009
Latest filing date: January 8, 2010

MCAT® required?: Yes
Latest MCAT® considered: December 2009
Oldest MCAT® considered: 2007

Early Decision Program: School does have EDP
Applicants notified: October 1, 2009
EDP available for: Residents only

Regular Acceptance Notice
Earliest date: November 2009
Latest date: Until class is full
Applicant's Response to Acceptance Offer – Maximum Time: 14 days

Requests for Deferred Entrance Considered: Yes

Deposit to Hold Place in Class: Yes
Deposit (Resident): $100
Deposit (Non-resident): $100
Deposit due: 14 days from acceptance offer
Applied to tuition: Yes
Deposit refundable: Yes
Refundable by: May 15, 2010

Estimated number of new entrants: 56
EDP: 2, special program: n/a

Start Month/Year: July 2010

Interview Format: Two one-on-one interviews. Regional interviews are not available.

Other Programs

PREPARATORY PROGRAMS
Postbaccalaureate Program: No
Summer Program: Yes
www.applyweb.com/apply/mhsum/index.html

COMBINED DEGREE PROGRAMS
Baccalaureate/M.D.: No
M.D./M.P.H.: Yes, Sterling Roaf, M.D.
(404) 752-1650, sroaf@msm.edu
M.D./M.B.A.: No
M.D./J.D.: No
M.D./Ph.D.: Yes

Premedical Coursework

Course	Req.	Rec.	Lab.	Sems.
Inorganic Chemistry	•		•	2
Behavioral Sciences		•		1
Biochemistry		•	•	1
Biology	•		•	2
Biology/Zoology				
Calculus				
College English	•			2
College Mathematics	•			2

Course	Req.	Rec.	Lab.	Sems.
Computer Science				
Genetics		•	•	1
Humanities				
Organic Chemistry	•		•	2
Physics	•		•	2
Psychology				
Social Sciences				
Other				

Selection Factors: 2008 Accepted Applicants

Proportion of Accepted Applicants with Relevant Experience (Data Self-Reported to AMCAS®)		
Community Service/Volunteer	76%
Medically-Related Work	71%
Research	76%

Shaded bar represents school's accepted scores ranging from the 10th percentile to the 90th percentile. School Median ○ National Median ●

Overall GPA 2.0 2.1 2.2 2.3 2.4 2.5 2.6 2.7 2.8 2.9 **3.0 3.1 3.2 3.3 3.4 (3.5) 3.6 3.7 3.8 3.9** 4.0
Science GPA 2.0 2.1 2.2 2.3 2.4 2.5 2.6 **2.7 2.8 2.9 3.0 3.1 3.2 (3.3) 3.4 3.5 3.6 3.7 3.8 3.9** 4.0

MCAT® Total Numeric Score 9 10 11 12 13 14 15 16 17 18 19 20 21 22 23 **24 25 26 (27) 28 29 30 31 (32)** 33 34 35 36 37 38 39 40 41 42 43

Writing Sample			J	K	L	**M N (O) P (Q) R**	S	T
Verbal Reasoning	3	4	5	6	**7 8 (9) (10) 11**	12	13	14	15
Biological Sciences	3	4	5	6	7	**8 9 (10) (11)**	12	13	14	15
Physical Sciences	3	4	5	6	**7 8 (9) 10 (11)**	12	13	14	15

Acceptance & Matriculation Data for 2008–2009 First Year Class

	Resident	Non-resident	International	Total
Applications	438	3213	102	3753
Interviewed	113	135	0	248
Deferred	1	2	0	3
Matriculants				
Early Assurance Program	0	0	0	0
Early Decision Program	0	0	0	0
Baccalaureate/M.D.	n/a	n/a	n/a	n/a
M.D./Ph.D.	n/a	n/a	n/a	n/a
Matriculated	34	22	0	**56**

Applications accepted from International Applicants: No

Specialty Choice

2004, 2005, 2006 Graduates, Specialty Choice (As reported by program directors to GME Track™)	
Anesthesiology	3%
Emergency Medicine	7%
Family Practice	13%
Internal Medicine	14%
Obstetrics/Gynecology	8%
Orthopaedic Surgery	1%
Pediatrics	19%
Psychiatry	7%
Radiology	2%
Surgery	5%

Matriculant Demographics: 2008–2009 First Year Class

Men: 22 **Women:** 34

Matriculants' Self-Reported Race/Ethnicity

Mexican American	0	Korean	3
Cuban	0	Vietnamese	0
Puerto Rican	0	Other Asian	2
Other Hispanic	0	Total Asian	11
Total Hispanic	0	Native American	0
Chinese	1	Black	42
Asian Indian	3	Native Hawaiian	0
Pakistani	2	White	3
Filipino	0	Unduplicated Number	
Japanese	0	of Matriculants	56

Science and Math Majors: 73%
Matriculants with:
    Baccalaureate degree: 100%
    Graduate degree(s): 18%

Financial Information

Source: 2007–2008 LCME I-B survey and 2008–2009 AAMC TSF questionnaire

	Residents	Non-residents
Total Cost of Attendance	$60,611	$60,611
Tuition and Fees	$30,328	$30,328
Other (includes living expenses)	$20,135	$20,135
Health Insurance (can be waived)	$2,148	$2,148

Average 2008 Graduate Indebtedness: $167,388
% of Enrolled Students Receiving Aid: 95%

Criminal Background Check

This medical school requires a criminal background check prior to matriculation.

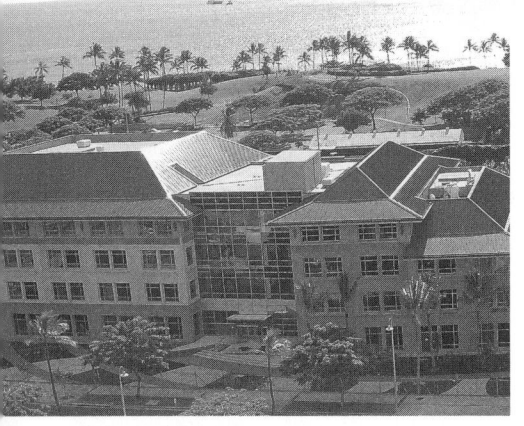

University of Hawai'i
John A. Burns School of Medicine
Honolulu, Hawaii

Office of Student Affairs - Admissions
Medical Education Building
University of Hawai'i, John A. Burns
School of Medicine
651 Ilalo Street
Honolulu, Hawai'i 96813-5534
T 808 692 1000 **F** 808 692 1251

Admissions http://jabsom.hawaii.edu/
Main http://jabsom.hawaii.edu
Financial http://jabsom.hawaii.edu/
E-mail mnishiki@hawaii.edu

Public Institution

Dr. Jerris R. Hedges, Dean

Dr. Satoru Izutsu, Senior Associate Dean

Gail C. Koki, Student Liaison, Financial Aid and Scholarships

Marilyn M. Nishiki, Admissions Officer & Registrar

General Information

The University of Hawai'i at Manoa John A. Burns School of Medicine is in the College of Health Sciences and Social Welfare. The School of Medicine is located in Kaka'ako.
It also has teaching facilities in affiliated community hospitals and primary care clinics throughout the state.

Mission Statement

To educate outstanding physicians, scientists, biomedical students, and allied health professionals for Hawai'i and the Pacific, and to conduct both clinical and basic research, education, and community service of specific interest to our region and community. Its student body mirrors the rich diversity of the state's population.

Curricular Highlights
Community Service Requirement: Optional.
Research/Thesis Requirement: Optional.

The school utilizes a problem-based learning curriculum (PBL), in which basic sciences are learned in the context of the study of health care problems and supplemented by selected lecture and laboratory sessions. Clinical skills and community health activities are prominent, and begin in the first year of the curriculum. Special features include an emphasis on PBL as the primary instructional method in the pre-clinical years; early introduction of clinical training, community service, and research experiences; rural health training opportunities; a longitudinal, interdisciplinary clerkship opportunity in the third-year; and opportunities for training experiences in various communities throughout Hawai'i, the Pacific, and Asia.

USMLE

Step 1: Required. Students must record a passing score for promotion.
Step 2: Clinical Skills (CS): Required. Students must record a passing total score to graduate.
Step 2: Clinical Knowledge (CK): Required. Students must record a passing total score to graduate.

Selection Factors

Applicants are considered without discrimination as to age, sex, race, creed, national origin, religion, or handicap. The school admits 62 students to its first-year class. A priority is to admit applicants with strong ties to the State of Hawai'i. Applications go through a screening process. The first screen determines an applicant's ties to the State of Hawai'i: legal residence, birthplace, high school graduated, college attended, parent's legal residence, and legacy. Three of the six categories are required to be a resident for application purposes. Applicants who pass the second academic screen will be invited for interviews and asked to submit letters of recommendation. Applicants are responsible for scheduling three one-on-one interviews to be conducted in Hawai'i. Acceptance, alternate, and rejection letters are emailed in early April.

Financial Aid

Financial status is not a factor in considering applicants for acceptance. Efforts are made to assist medical students in obtaining loans and scholarships, wherever possible. Loan funds from federal sources are available only to U.S. citizens and permanent residents. In general, students are discouraged from engaging in outside employment. Applicants are referred to the Student Liaison-Financial Aid and Scholarships, Office of Student Affairs at the John A. Burns School of Medicine or to the University of Hawai'i at Manoa Financial Aid Services Office.

Information about Diversity Programs

The student body and faculty are culturally diverse. The school is actively involved in the recruitment, admission, and retention of students from disadvantaged backgrounds who have potential and are interested in pursuing an M.D. degree. Dr. Mary Ann Antonelli

(mantonel@hawaii.edu, or 808- 692-1000), Director of Student Affairs, is the Diversity contact person at the John A. Burns School of Medicine. The Imi Ho'ola Post-Baccalaureate Program is for students from socially, educationally, or economically disadvantaged backgrounds who have demonstrated a strong commitment to serve areas of need in Hawai'i and the U.S.-Affiliated Pacific Islands. For more information, contact Dr. Nanette L.K. Judd, Imi Ho'ola Post-Baccalaureate Program Director (judd@hawaii.edu or 808-692-1030).

Campus Information
Setting
The School of Medicine is located at a 10.5-acre state-owned parcel in Kaka'ako, on the water's edge, between Waikiki and downtown Honolulu. It is an environment conducive to the school's goal of becoming a top-ranked research-intensive medical school with the opportunity to attract world-class research scientists to join the school's faculty.

Enrollment
For 2008, total enrollment was: 253

Special Features
The school's problem-based learning curriculum has been in place since 1989. For the past several years, emphasis has been placed on promoting biomedical research. Recruitment of world-class scientists has resulted in an increase of research funding. It is envisioned that these research areas will be further developed at the new quarters in Kaka'ako.

Housing
Medical students and candidates for graduate degrees in the medical school are expected to make their own living arrangements. The University of Hawai'i at Manoa campus provides limited dormitory and apartment facilities.

Satellite Campuses/Facilities
Clinical activities of the school's curriculum are conducted in affiliated community hospitals and clinics. There is no university hospital connected to the school of medicine.

Application Process and Requirements 2010–2011

Primary Application Service: AMCAS
Earliest filing date: June 1, 2009
Latest filing date: November 1, 2009

Secondary Application Required?: Yes
Sent to: Screened applicants who minimally achieve the required cut-off scores.
Contact: Marilyn Nishiki, (808) 692-1000, mnishiki@hawaii.edu
Fee: Yes, $50
Fee waiver available: No
Earliest filing date: School-specific deadlines
Latest filing date: School-specific deadlines

MCAT® required?: Yes
Latest MCAT® considered: September 2009
Oldest MCAT® considered: 2007

Early Decision Program: School does have EDP
Applicants notified: October 1, 2009
EDP available for: Residents only

Regular Acceptance Notice
Earliest date: October 15, 2009
Latest date: Until class is full
Applicant's Response to Acceptance Offer – Maximum Time: Two weeks

Requests for Deferred Entrance Considered: Yes

Deposit to Hold Place in Class: No
Deposit (Resident): n/a
Deposit (Non-resident): n/a
Deposit due: n/a
Applied to tuition: n/a
Deposit refundable: n/a
Refundable by: n/a

Estimated number of new entrants: 62
EDP: 1, special program: 10

Start Month/Year: July 2010

Interview Format: One-on-one interviews. Regional interviews are not available.

Other Programs

PREPARATORY PROGRAMS
Postbaccalaureate Program: Yes, http://jabsom.hawaii.edu
Nanette K. Judd, PhD, MPH, RN
(808) 692-1030, judd@hawaii.edu
Summer Program: No

COMBINED DEGREE PROGRAMS
Baccalaureate/M.D.: No
M.D./M.P.H.: No
M.D./M.B.A.: No
M.D./J.D.: No
M.D./Ph.D.: No

Premedical Coursework

Course	Req.	Rec.	Lab.	Hrs.
Inorganic Chemistry	•		•	8
Behavioral Sciences				
Biochemistry	•			3
Biology	•		•	8
Biology/Zoology		•		
Calculus				
College English				
College Mathematics		•		

Course	Req.	Rec.	Lab.	Hrs.
Computer Science				
Genetics		•		
Humanities		•		
Organic Chemistry	•		•	8
Physics	•		•	8
Psychology		•		
Social Sciences				
Cell and Molecular Bio				3

Selection Factors: 2008 Accepted Applicants

Proportion of Accepted Applicants with Relevant Experience (Data Self-Reported to AMCAS®)		
Community Service/Volunteer		67%
Medically-Related Work		89%
Research		83%

Shaded bar represents school's accepted scores ranging from the 10th percentile to the 90th percentile.
School Median ● National Median ●

Overall GPA	2.0	2.1	2.2	2.3	2.4	2.5	2.6	2.7	2.8	2.9	3.0	3.1	3.2	3.3	3.4	3.5	3.6	(3.7)	3.8	3.9	4.0
Science GPA	2.0	2.1	2.2	2.3	2.4	2.5	2.6	2.7	2.8	2.9	3.0	3.1	3.2	3.3	3.4	3.5	3.6	(3.7)	3.8	3.9	4.0

MCAT® Total Numeric Score 9 10 11 12 13 14 15 16 17 18 19 20 21 22 23 24 25 26 27 28 29 30 (31) 32 33 34 35 36 37 38 39 40 41 42 43

Writing Sample			J	K	L	M	N	O	P	(Q)	R	S	T
Verbal Reasoning	3	4	5	6	7	8	9	(10)	11	12	13	14	15
Biological Sciences	3	4	5	6	7	8	9	10	(11)	12	13	14	15
Physical Sciences	3	4	5	6	7	8	9	10	(11)	12	13	14	15

Acceptance & Matriculation Data for 2008–2009 First Year Class

	Resident	Non-resident	International	Total
Applications	177	1606	112	1895
Interviewed	146	72	13	231
Deferred	0	0	0	0
Matriculants				
Early Assurance Program	0	0	0	0
Early Decision Program	0	0	0	0
Baccalaureate/M.D.	n/a	n/a	n/a	n/a
M.D./Ph.D.	n/a	n/a	n/a	n/a
Matriculated	51	9	2	**62**

Applications accepted from International Applicants: Yes

Specialty Choice

2004, 2005, 2006 Graduates, Specialty Choice (As reported by program directors to GME Track™)	
Anesthesiology	6%
Emergency Medicine	6%
Family Practice	7%
Internal Medicine	23%
Obstetrics/Gynecology	7%
Orthopaedic Surgery	2%
Pediatrics	8%
Psychiatry	5%
Radiology	3%
Surgery	5%

Matriculant Demographics: 2008–2009 First Year Class

Men: 28   **Women:** 34

Matriculants' Self-Reported Race/Ethnicity

Mexican American	0	Korean	4
Cuban	0	Vietnamese	1
Puerto Rican	0	Other Asian	3
Other Hispanic	0	Total Asian	45
Total Hispanic	0	Native American	0
Chinese	18	Black	0
Asian Indian	0	Native Hawaiian	6
Pakistani	0	White	17
Filipino	2	Unduplicated Number	
Japanese	27	of Matriculants	62

Science and Math Majors: 60%
Matriculants with:
Baccalaureate degree: 100%
Graduate degree(s): 16%

Financial Information

Source: 2007–2008 LCME I-B survey and 2008–2009 AAMC TSF questionnaire

	Residents	Non-residents
Total Cost of Attendance	$50,322	$73,314
Tuition and Fees	$22,928	$45,920
Other (includes living expenses)	$25,141	$25,141
Health Insurance (can be waived)	$2,253	$2,253

Average 2008 Graduate Indebtedness: $61,687
% of Enrolled Students Receiving Aid: 79%

Criminal Background Check

This medical school requires a criminal background check prior to matriculation.

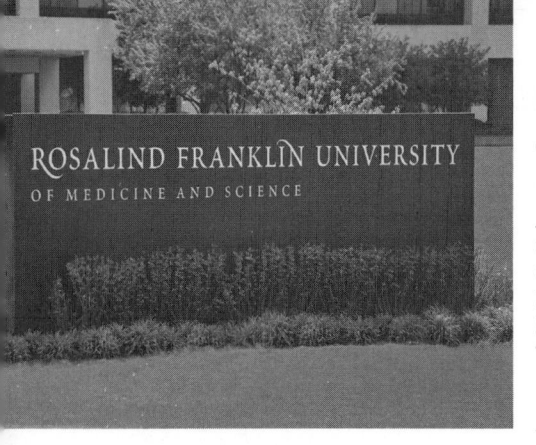

Rosalind Franklin University of Medicine and Science Chicago Medical School

North Chicago, Illinois

Rosalind Franklin University of Medicine and Science
Office of Medical School Admissions
3333 Green Bay Road
North Chicago, Illinois 60064
T 847 578 3204

Admissions www.rosalindfranklin.edu/tabid/1629/default.aspx
Main www.rosalindfranklin.edu/tabid/363/default.aspx
Financial www.rosalindfranklin.edu/tabid/1942/default.aspx
E-mail cms.admissions@rosalindfranklin.edu

Private Institution

Dr. Arthur J. Ross III, M.B.A., Dean

Maryann DeCaire, Associate Vice President of Enrollment Services

Dr. Cathy Lazarus, Senior Associate Dean for Student Affairs and Medical Education

Rebecca Durkin, Associate Vice President, Office of Student Development

General Information

Founded in 1912, The Chicago Medical School has been dedicated to excellence in medical education for nearly a century. The Chicago Medical School has educated thousands of professionals with recognized innovation in health education, excellence in the creation of knowledge and scientific discovery focused on prediction and prevention of disease, outstanding clinical programs, and compassionate community service. Major hospital affiliates include Advocate Christ Medical Center, Advocate Illinois Masonic, Advocate Lutheran General Hospital, John H. Stroger, Jr., Hospital of Cook County, Mount Sinai Hospital and Medical Center, and the North Chicago Veterans Affairs Medical Center (NCVAMC).

Mission Statement

The Chicago Medical School educates physicians and scientists dedicated to providing exemplary, compassionate patient care and excellence in scientific discovery within an inter-professional environment.

Curricular Highlights

Community Service Requirement: Optional.
Research/Thesis Requirement: Optional.

The Chicago Medical School's curriculum offers a strong grounding in the sciences basic to medicine along with assuring competency in skills necessary for the practice of medicine. The CMS curriculum features a unique inter-professional approach, with interaction among a broad range of health professional students and practitioners. The curriculum is a mix of lectures, labs, small-group discussions, team-based learning, and opportunities for peer-to-peer learning. The educational information system, Desire to Learn (D2L), provides 24-hour-a-day access to learning materials. Students have early clinical experiences in the state-of-the-art evaluation and education center, as well as opportunities to connect with physician preceptors. The required junior clinical clerkships include medicine, ambulatory care, surgery, family medicine, obstetrics/gynecology, psychiatry, medCore, pediatrics, neurology, and emergency medicine. The senior requirements include four weeks in a medicine or pediatrics subinternship, plus 32 weeks of approved electives (14 of which must be completed at one of the school's primary affiliated sites). The elective period gives students an opportunity, through both intramural and extramural experiences, to explore and strengthen their personal career interests.

USMLE

Step 1: Required. Students must record a passing score for promotion.
Step 2: Clinical Skills (CS): Required. Students must record a passing total score to graduate.
Step 2: Clinical Knowledge (CK): Required. Students must record a passing total score to graduate.

Selection Factors

Students are selected on the basis of various criteria, including scholarship, character, motivation, and educational background. A student's potential for the study and practice of medicine will be evaluated on the basis of academic achievement, MCAT results, appraisals by a preprofessional advisory committee or individual instructors, and a personal interview, if requested by the Student Admissions Committee. To fulfill the mission of The Chicago Medical School, admissions policies are designed to ensure that the selection process matriculates a class made up of individuals capable of meeting the needs of current and future patients. Applicants will be evaluated not only for educational potential, but with the aim of providing diverse educational experience for other members of the class.

Financial Aid

The Financial Aid Office is committed to helping students secure the funding needed to pursue their educational endeavors. Financial Aid is available in the form of loans, scholarships, and work-study. For more information, contact the Financial Aid Office at (847) 578-3217.

Information about Diversity Programs

The school maintains an extensive recruitment and retention program for students from groups underrepresented in medicine.

Campus Information

Setting

Rosalind Franklin University of Medicine and Science is situated in the northern suburbs of Chicago, with easy access to downtown Chicago and the surrounding areas by car or public transportation. State-of-the-art facilities include a recently completed $10 million research wing expansion; multimedia classrooms and gross anatomy laboratory; and an Education and Evaluation Center for physical examination skills training. Recreational facilities include an exercise room, game room, and the Student Union (home to the University Bookstore, Union Café, and dedicated e-mail stations).

Enrollment

For 2008, total enrollment was: 755

Housing

On-campus housing is available at Rosalind Franklin University. Each of the University's three apartment buildings has five floors and consists of 60 one and two-bedroom apartments. Individual apartments feature a variety of amenities, such as kitchen appliances (range, refrigerator, dishwasher, and microwave), fully networked Internet connectivity, and washer/dryer hookups. Each apartment building also includes study and lounge areas, shared laundry facilities on every floor, and individual storage units. For more information about student housing, contact the Office of Student Housing at (847) 578-8350 or campus.housing@rosalindfranklin.edu.

Application Process and Requirements 2010–2011

Primary Application Service: AMCAS
Earliest filing date: June 1, 2009
Latest filing date: November 1, 2009

Secondary Application Required?: Yes
Sent to: All applicants
URL: n/a
Fee: Yes, $100
Fee waiver available: Yes
Earliest filing date: July 1, 2009
Latest filing date: December 15, 2009

MCAT® required?: Yes
Latest MCAT® considered: September 2009
Oldest MCAT® considered: 2007

Early Decision Program: School does have EDP
Applicants notified: October 1, 2009
EDP available for: Both Residents and Non-residents

Regular Acceptance Notice
Earliest date: October 15, 2009
Latest date: Until class is full
Applicant's Response to Acceptance Offer – Maximum Time: Two weeks

Requests for Deferred Entrance Considered: Yes

Deposit to Hold Place in Class: Yes
Deposit (Resident): $100
Deposit (Non-resident): $100
Deposit due: With acceptance offer
Applied to tuition: Yes
Deposit refundable: Yes
Refundable by: May 15, 2010

Estimated number of new entrants: 185
EDP: 3, special program: n/a

Start Month/Year: August 2010

Interview Format: Two open-file interviews with committee members, faculty, staff, and/or fourth-year students. Regional interviews are not available.

Other Programs

PREPARATORY PROGRAMS
Postbaccalaureate Program: No
Summer Program: No

COMBINED DEGREE PROGRAMS
Baccalaureate/M.D.: No
M.D./M.P.H.: No
M.D./M.B.A.: No
M.D./J.D.: No
M.D./Ph.D.: Yes, www.rosalindfranklin.edu/tabid/710/default.aspx

Premedical Coursework

Course	Req.	Rec.	Lab.	Sems.
Inorganic Chemistry	•	•		2
Behavioral Sciences				
Biochemistry				
Biology				
Biology/Zoology	•	•		2
Calculus				
College English				
College Mathematics				

Course	Req.	Rec.	Lab.	Sems.
Computer Science				
Genetics				
Humanities				
Organic Chemistry	•		•	2
Physics	•		•	2
Psychology				
Social Sciences				
Other				

Selection Factors: 2008 Accepted Applicants

Proportion of Accepted Applicants with Relevant Experience (Data Self-Reported to AMCAS®)		
Community Service/Volunteer		69%
Medically-Related Work		89%
Research		83%

Shaded bar represents school's accepted scores ranging from the 10th percentile to the 90th percentile ▬   School Median ● National Median ●

Overall GPA	2.0	2.1	2.2	2.3	2.4	2.5	2.6	2.7	2.8	2.9	3.0	3.1	3.2	3.3	3.4	3.5	3.6	3.7	(3.8)	3.9	4.0
Science GPA	2.0	2.1	2.2	2.3	2.4	2.5	2.6	2.7	2.8	2.9	3.0	3.1	3.2	3.3	3.4	3.5	3.6	3.7	(3.8)	3.9	4.0

MCAT® Total Numeric Score 9 10 11 12 13 14 15 16 17 18 19 20 21 22 23 24 25 26 27 28 29 30 (31) 32 33 34 35 36 37 38 39 40 41 42 43

Writing Sample			J		K		L	M	N	O	P	(Q)	R	S	T
Verbal Reasoning	3	4	5	6	7	8	9	(10)	11	12	13	14	15
Biological Sciences	3	4	5	6	7	8	9	10	(11)	12	13	14	15
Physical Sciences	3	4	5	6	7	8	9	10	(11)	12	13	14	15

Acceptance & Matriculation Data for 2008–2009 First Year Class

	Resident	Non-resident	International	Total
Applications	1145	8522	721	10388
Interviewed	274	418	40	732
Deferred	2	1	1	4
Matriculants				
Early Assurance Program	0	0	0	0
Early Decision Program	0	1	0	1
Baccalaureate/M.D.	n/a	n/a	n/a	n/a
M.D./Ph.D.	0	0	3	3
Matriculated	81	97	9	**187**

Applications accepted from International Applicants: Yes

Specialty Choice

2004, 2005, 2006 Graduates, Specialty Choice (As reported by program directors to GME Track™)	
Anesthesiology	6%
Emergency Medicine	10%
Family Practice	8%
Internal Medicine	23%
Obstetrics/Gynecology	4%
Orthopaedic Surgery	4%
Pediatrics	11%
Psychiatry	3%
Radiology	4%
Surgery	6%

Matriculant Demographics: 2008–2009 First Year Class

Men: 95   **Women:** 92

Matriculants' Self-Reported Race/Ethnicity

Mexican American	2	Korean	12
Cuban	0	Vietnamese	3
Puerto Rican	0	Other Asian	4
Other Hispanic	2	Total Asian	61
Total Hispanic	3	Native American	0
Chinese	10	Black	13
Asian Indian	26	Native Hawaiian	0
Pakistani	6	White	104
Filipino	2	Unduplicated Number	
Japanese	1	of Matriculants	187

Science and Math Majors: 67%
Matriculants with:
      Baccalaureate degree: 98%
      Graduate degree(s): 24%

Financial Information

Source: 2007–2008 LCME I-B survey and 2008–2009 AAMC TSF questionnaire

	Residents	Non-residents
Total Cost of Attendance	$61,443	$61,443
Tuition and Fees	$41,687	$41,687
Other (includes living expenses)	$17,956	$17,956
Health Insurance (can be waived)	$1,800	$1,800

Average 2008 Graduate Indebtedness: $201,834
% of Enrolled Students Receiving Aid: 85%

Criminal Background Check

This medical school requires a criminal background check prior to matriculation.

Loyola University Chicago Stritch School of Medicine

Maywood, Illinois

Loyola University Chicago Stritch School of Medicine
Office of Admissions
2160 South First Avenue
Maywood, Illinois 60153
T 708 216 3229

Admissions www.meddean.luc.edu/admissions/admissions.htm
Main www.stritch.luc.edu
Financial www.meddean.luc.edu\financialaid
E-mail SSOM-admissions@lumc.edu

Private Institution

Dr. John M. Lee, Dean

Adrian Jones, J.D., Assistant Dean for Admissions & Recruitment

Donna J. Sobie, Director, Financial Aid

General Information

Loyola University Chicago, founded in 1870 by the Jesuits, is one of the largest Catholic universities in the United States. By 1909, the university had organized several small medical colleges into a new medical school and, in 1948, the school was named in honor of Samuel Cardinal Stritch, Archbishop of Chicago. In 1969 the university opened the Loyola University Medical Center, built on land given by the Veterans Administration, in Maywood, a suburban community located 12 miles west of downtown Chicago. The medical center is home to the Stritch School of Medicine, Loyola University Hospital, Cardinal Bernardin Cancer Center, and Loyola Outpatient Center. Students receive their clinical training at the 570-bed Loyola University Hospital, 248-bed Hines Veterans Affairs Hospital, and other affiliated hospitals in the Chicago area.

Curricular Highlights

Community Service Requirement: Optional. Highly desirable.
Research/Thesis Requirement: Optional.

The primary purpose of the Stritch School of Medicine is to train physicians who will care for their patients with skill, respect, and compassion. The personal and intellectual development of each student is promoted through close contact with faculty members and the administration. Students are exposed to the operation of a large academic medical center, as well as to VA and community offices and hospitals, where they learn in an atmosphere of cooperation and mutual assistance. The first year of the curriculum concentrates on the basic principles and processes related to the normal structure, function, and regulation of the human body. In addition, the first year includes instruction in health promotion/disease prevention, health care finance and access, medical ethics and the doctor/patient

relationship. The second year of the curriculum focuses on basic science principles related to the mechanisms of human disease, neuroscience, and the therapeutic approach to disease. Additionally, students have the opportunity to continue to develop their knowledge about human behavioral science, physical examination skills, basic clinical skills, evidence-based clinical decision-making, and medical ethics and humanities. During the first and second year students have early clinical experience through a physician mentor program in ambulatory settings and the peer mentor program which couples first and third year students for clinical learning opportunities. The third and fourth years are organized into clinical clerkships which include up to 34 weeks of elective time during the fourth year. Special curricular features include an emphasis on bioethics and professionalism and intensive training in history-taking, physical examination, and communication skills using the extensive Clinical Skills Center and Human Simulation Center, which combines the latest in educational technology and patient simulation activities. We also offer a three year Honors Program in Bioethics and Professionalism.

USMLE

Step 1: Required. Students must record a passing score for graduation, but not promotion.
Step 2: Clinical Skills (CS): Required. Students must record a passing total score to graduate.
Step 2: Clinical Knowledge (CK): Required. Students must record a passing total score to graduate.

Selection Factors

A bachelor's degree and the MCAT taken no later than September of the year of application, are required. Any undergraduate major is acceptable. Applicants must be U.S. citizens or hold a permanent resident visa. As a rule, applicants are limited to applying no more than twice. Applicants enrolled in advanced degree programs must expect to complete their degrees prior to matriculation. Applicants who present academic credentials that indicate they are capable of succeeding in the rigorous medical education program will be evaluated for evidence of the personal qualifications they

can bring to the medical profession. Essential characteristics include an interest in learning, integrity, compassion, and the ability to assume responsibility. Of particular concern will be an applicant's exploration of the field of medicine and the nature of the motivation to enter this profession. Early submission of the AMCAS application and prompt return of all supporting material will enhance an applicant's chance of being offered a place in the class. Loyola University does not discriminate on the basis of race, religion, national origin, sex, age, or disability.

Financial Aid

Financial aid is primarily in the form of loans, but limited scholarship and grant money is also available. Applicants should receive a preliminary financial aid award prior to May 15.

Information about Diversity Programs

The Summer Enrichment Program (SEP) at Loyola University Chicago Stritch School of Medicine is a six-week experience for pre-medical students. The program's mission is to offer students a variety of educational experiences and service activities to enhance their preparation for a career in medicine. The program targets students who have the potential to enrich the diversity of the medical student community.

Campus Information

Enrollment

For 2008, total enrollment was: 563

Application Process and Requirements 2010–2011

Primary Application Service: AMCAS
Earliest filing date: June 1, 2009
Latest filing date: November 15, 2009

Secondary Application Required?: Yes
Sent to: Screened applicants
URL: n/a
Fee: Yes, $75
Fee waiver available: Yes
Earliest filing date: June 2009
Latest filing date: February 2010

MCAT® required?: Yes
Latest MCAT® considered: September 2009
Oldest MCAT® considered: 2006

Early Decision Program: School does not have EDP
EDP available for: n/a
Applicants notified: n/a

Regular Acceptance Notice
Earliest date: October 16, 2009
Latest date: Until class is full
Applicant's Response to Acceptance Offer – Maximum Time: Two weeks

Requests for Deferred Entrance Considered: Yes

Deposit to Hold Place in Class: No
Deposit (Resident): n/a
Deposit (Non-resident): n/a
Deposit due: n/a
Applied to tuition: n/a
Deposit refundable: n/a
Refundable by: n/a

Estimated number of new entrants: 145
EDP: n/a, special program: n/a

Start Month/Year: July 2010

Interview Format: Semi-open file with admission committee members. Regional interviews are not available.

Other Programs

PREPARATORY PROGRAMS
Postbaccalaureate Program: No
Summer Program: Yes, Office of Student Affairs, (708) 216-3220, kcalhoun@lumc.edu

COMBINED DEGREE PROGRAMS
Baccalaureate/M.D.: No
M.D./M.P.H.: Yes
M.D./M.B.A.: No
M.D./J.D.: No
M.D./Ph.D.: Yes, www.meddean.luc.edu/ prospective/mdphd/index.htm
Additional Program: Yes, http://bioethics. lumc.edu/education/MD_MA_Program.html

Premedical Coursework

Course	Req.	Rec.	Lab.	Sems.	Course	Req.	Rec.	Lab.	Sems.
Inorganic Chemistry	•		•	2	Computer Science				
Behavioral Sciences					Genetics		•		
Biochemistry		•			Humanities		•		
Biology					Organic Chemistry	•		•	2
Biology/Zoology	•		•	2	Physics	•		•	2
Calculus					Psychology				
College English					Social Sciences				
College Mathematics					Molecular Biology		•		

Selection Factors: 2008 Accepted Applicants

Proportion of Accepted Applicants with Relevant Experience (Data Self-Reported to AMCAS®)		
Community Service/Volunteer		76%
Medically-Related Work		89%
Research		87%

Shaded bar represents school's accepted scores ranging from the 10th percentile to the 90th percentile. School Median ● National Median ●

Overall GPA	2.0	2.1	2.2	2.3	2.4	2.5	2.6	2.7	2.8	2.9	3.0	3.1	3.2	3.3	3.4	3.5	3.6	(3.7)	3.8	3.9	4.0
Science GPA	2.0	2.1	2.2	2.3	2.4	2.5	2.6	2.7	2.8	2.9	3.0	3.1	3.2	3.3	3.4	3.5	(3.6)	3.7	3.8	3.9	4.0

MCAT® Total Numeric Score 9 10 11 12 13 14 15 16 17 18 19 20 21 22 23 24 25 26 27 28 29 30 (31) 32 33 34 35 36 37 38 39 40 41 42 43

Writing Sample			J	K	L	M	N	O	P	(Q)	R	S	T
Verbal Reasoning	3	4	5	6	7	8	9	(10)	11	12	13	14	15
Biological Sciences	3	4	5	6	7	8	9	10	(11)	12	13	14	15
Physical Sciences	3	4	5	6	7	8	9	(10)	(11)	12	13	14	15

Acceptance & Matriculation Data for 2008–2009 First Year Class

	Resident	Non-resident	International	Total
Applications	1423	8700	19	10142
Interviewed	168	404	0	572
Deferred	0	2	0	2
Matriculants				
Early Assurance Program	n/a	n/a	n/a	n/a
Early Decision Program	0	0	0	0
Baccalaureate/M.D.	n/a	n/a	n/a	n/a
M.D./Ph.D.	2	1	0	3
Matriculated	65	80	0	**145**

Applications accepted from International Applicants: No

Specialty Choice

2004, 2005, 2006 Graduates, Specialty Choice (As reported by program directors to GME Track™)	
Anesthesiology	5%
Emergency Medicine	9%
Family Practice	10%
Internal Medicine	23%
Obstetrics/Gynecology	4%
Orthopaedic Surgery	5%
Pediatrics	12%
Psychiatry	2%
Radiology	3%
Surgery	6%

Matriculant Demographics: 2008–2009 First Year Class

Men: 73 **Women:** 72

Matriculants' Self-Reported Race/Ethnicity

Mexican American	3	Korean	4
Cuban	1	Vietnamese	0
Puerto Rican	1	Other Asian	2
Other Hispanic	2	Total Asian	19
Total Hispanic	6	Native American	1
Chinese	3	Black	10
Asian Indian	6	Native Hawaiian	2
Pakistani	0	White	111
Filipino	2	Unduplicated Number	
Japanese	2	of Matriculants	145

Science and Math Majors: 52%
Matriculants with:
Baccalaureate degree: 100%
Graduate degree(s): 12%

Financial Information

Source: 2007–2008 LCME I-B survey and 2008–2009 AAMC TSF questionnaire

	Residents	Non-residents
Total Cost of Attendance	$58,756	$59,256
Tuition and Fees	$38,732	$38,732
Other (includes living expenses)	$18,201	$18,701
Health Insurance (can be waived)	$1,823	$1,823

Average 2008 Graduate Indebtedness: $161,976
% of Enrolled Students Receiving Aid: 90%

Criminal Background Check

This medical school requires a criminal background check prior to matriculation.

Northwestern University Feinberg School of Medicine

Chicago, Illinois

Office of Admissions
Northwestern University
Feinberg School of Medicine
303 East Chicago Avenue, Morton I-606
Chicago, Illinois 60611-3008
T 312 503 8206   **F** 312 503 0550

Admissions www.feinberg.northwestern.edu/
admissions/md/index.html
Main www.feinberg.northwestern.edu
Financial http://chicagofinancialaid.
northwestern.edu
E-mail med-admissions@northwestern.edu

Private Institution

Dr. J. Larry Jameson, Dean

*Dr. Warren H. Wallace, Associate Dean
for Admissions*

*Dr. John E. Franklin, Associate Dean for
Minority and Cultural Affairs*

General Information

Northwestern University's Feinberg School of Medicine (FSM), founded in 1859, continues to educate today's students at a premier medical school and in outstanding hospitals: Northwestern Memorial, Children's Memorial, Prentice Women's, the Rehabilitation Institute of Chicago, and the Jesse Brown VA Medical Center. Students have translational and clinical research options as well as the opportunitiy to engage the cultural life of Chicago and work with its diverse population.

Mission Statement

The mission of the Feinberg School of Medicine is to educate physicians and physician-scientists who will excel both scientifically and clinically. We expect our students to take leadership roles in medicine and to serve the people of our increasingly diverse communities.

Curricular Highlights

Community Service Requirement: Optional. Multiple free clinics are available.
Research/Thesis Requirement: Optional. This option includes summer and senior selectives.

We strive to provide a student centered environment where adult learners employ their own questions as the starting point for inquiry. The first two years of the curriculum feature an integrated, organ-system based approach to the essential basic sciences. Small group "Problem Based Learning" sessions augment the concepts developed in lectures and laboratory sessions. The psychosocial foundations of medicine are emphasized in "Patient, Physician and Society (PPS)": students develop clinical skills and study the many ways in which medicine interacts with the larger society. Three short blocks are devoted to medical decision-making where students hone their ability to analyze and to manage the information

required for effective clinical decision-making. During the third year clerkships, students continue the PPS curriculum by returning to the medical school each month for discussion of topics common to all clerkships. A sub-internship, ICU and ER rotations, and several electives round out the curriculum in the fourth year.

USMLE

Step 1: Required. Students must record a passing score for graduation, but not promotion.
Step 2: Clinical Skills (CS): Required. Students must record a passing score in each section to graduate.
Step 2: Clinical Knowledge (CK): Required. Students must record a passing score in each section to graduate.

Selection Factors

The Committee on Admissions looks for evidence of academic excellence, mature motivation for a career in medicine, altruism, and character. A premium is placed on the breadth and depth of academic and life experiences, as well as clinical and research exposure. Applicants should be liberally educated men and women whose studies have gone beyond the conventional premedical courses. We seek a diverse class and do not discriminate on the basis of race, religion, national origin, gender, sexual orientation, age, or disability. The Illinois Medical School Matriculant Criminal History Records Act requires each entering medical student to submit to a criminal history records check prior to matriculation.

Financial Aid

Financial considerations do not influence admissions decisions. Feinberg makes every effort to ensure that accepted students receive a competitive financial aid package, including support through national and university loan programs, scholarships, and grants. Students receive financial management counseling, and we offer a loan program to international students who have a credit-worthy U.S. loan co-signer.

Information about Diversity Programs

FSM strives to admit a student body whose diversity mirrors that of our society. The Office of Minority and Cultural Affairs supports the

broad array of student groups involved in community outreach and offers programming in the formal curriculum, lunchtime speakers, dialogue groups and a film series on health disparities and social justice.

Campus Information

Setting

Located in the Streeterville section of downtown Chicago, the medical school is adjacent to beautiful Lake Michigan and within easy walking distance of apartments, museums, restaurants, athletic facilities, and retailers. Public and university transportation makes Chicago's diverse neighborhoods and cultural opportunities even more readily accessible.

Enrollment

For 2008, total enrollment was: 700

Special Features

The Medical School offers numerous research centers, institutes and programs including Lurie Comprehensive Cancer Center, Feinberg Cardiovascular Research Center, Institute for Genetic Medicine, Northwestern University Clinical and Translationl Sciences Institute, and Institute for Women's Health among many others (please see *www.feinberg.northwestern. edu/directory/centers.html*). New clinical facilities include the recently completed Prentice Women's Hospital. The new Children's Memorial Hospital building is currently under construction on the downtown campus. The Jesse Brown Medical Center has recently completed a new in-patient bed tower.

Housing

Most students live in high-rise apartments near the medical center although excellent public transportation makes commuting from city neighborhoods or Chicago's suburbs feasible.

Satellite Campuses/Facilities

Students do required clinical rotations in Chicago at Northwestern Hospitals and the Jesse Brown VA. Senior away rotations are available at affiliated institutions in Latin America, Africa, Europe, and Asia.

Application Process and Requirements 2010–2011

Primary Application Service: AMCAS
Earliest filing date: June 1, 2009
Latest filing date: November 1, 2009

Secondary Application Required?: Yes
Sent to: AMCAS
URL: https://medicalapp.northwestern.edu
Fee: Yes, $75
Fee waiver available: Yes
Earliest filing date: July 15, 2009
Latest filing date: Varies

MCAT® required?: Yes
Latest MCAT® considered: September 2009
Oldest MCAT® considered: 2007

Early Decision Program: School does have EDP
Applicants notified: Winter 2010
EDP available for: Both residents and non-residents

Regular Acceptance Notice
Earliest date: November 2009
Latest date: Until class is full
Applicant's Response to Acceptance Offer – Maximum Time: Two weeks

Requests for Deferred Entrance Considered: Yes

Deposit to Hold Place in Class: No
Deposit (Resident): n/a
Deposit (Non-resident): n/a
Deposit due: n/a
Applied to tuition: n/a
Deposit refundable: n/a
Refundable by: n/a

Estimated number of new entrants: 170
EDP: n/a, special program: n/a

Start Month/Year: August 2010

Interview Format: Individual and panel interview. Regional interviews are not available.

Other Programs

PREPARATORY PROGRAMS
Postbaccalaureate Program: No
Summer Program: No

COMBINED DEGREE PROGRAMS
Baccalaureate/M.D.: Yes,
www.feinberg.northwestern.edu/hpme/index.html
M.D./M.P.H.: Yes, www.publichealth.
northwestern.edu/admissions_mdmph.htm
M.D./M.B.A.: No
M.D./J.D.: No
M.D./Ph.D.: Yes, www.mstp.northwestern.edu
MD/MA-Medical Humanities & Bioethics: Yes,
www.bioethics.northwestern.edu/masters/
feinbergma.html

Premedical Coursework

Course	Req.	Rec.	Lab.	Sems.
Inorganic Chemistry	•	•		2
Behavioral Sciences				
Biochemistry				
Biology	•		•	2
Biology/Zoology				
Calculus				
College English		•		
College Mathematics				

Course	Req.	Rec.	Lab.	Sems.
Computer Science				
Genetics		•		
Humanities		•		2
Organic Chemistry	•		•	2
Physics	•		•	2
Psychology		•		
Social Sciences				
Statistics				2

Selection Factors: 2008 Accepted Applicants

Proportion of Accepted Applicants with Relevant Experience (Data Self-Reported to AMCAS)		Community Service/Volunteer	68%
		Medically-Related Work	81%
		Research	92%

Shaded bar represents school's accepted scores ranging from the 10th percentile to the 90th percentile   School Median ●   National Median ●

Overall GPA	2.0	2.1	2.2	2.3	2.4	2.5	2.6	2.7	2.8	2.9	3.0	3.1	3.2	3.3	3.4	3.5	3.6	3.7	3.8	(3.9)	4.0
Science GPA	2.0	2.1	2.2	2.3	2.4	2.5	2.6	2.7	2.8	2.9	3.0	3.1	3.2	3.3	3.4	3.5	3.6	3.7	3.8	(3.9)	4.0

MCAT® Total Numeric Score 9 10 11 12 13 14 15 16 17 18 19 20 21 22 23 24 25 26 27 28 29 30 31 (32) 33 34 35 (36) 37 38 39 40 41 42 43

Writing Sample			J	K	L	M	N	O	P	(Q)	R	S	T
Verbal Reasoning	3	4	5	6	7	8	9	(10)	(11)	12	13	14	15
Biological Sciences	3	4	5	6	7	8	9	10	(11)	12	(13)	14	15
Physical Sciences	3	4	5	6	7	8	9	10	(11)	12	(13)	14	15

Acceptance & Matriculation Data for 2008–2009 First Year Class

	Resident	Non-resident	International	Total
Applications	943	6028	441	7412
Interviewed	130	693	40	863
Deferred	2	7	0	9
Matriculants				
Early Assurance Program	4	1	0	5
Early Decision Program	0	0	0	0
Baccalaureate/M.D.	9	35	1	45
M.D./Ph.D.	4	8	2	14
Matriculated	50	112	7	**169**

Applications accepted from International Applicants: Yes

Specialty Choice

2004, 2005, 2006 Graduates, Specialty Choice (As reported by program directors to GME Track™)	
Anesthesiology	4%
Emergency Medicine	8%
Family Practice	2%
Internal Medicine	25%
Obstetrics/Gynecology	5%
Orthopaedic Surgery	5%
Pediatrics	10%
Psychiatry	2%
Radiology	5%
Surgery	7%

Matriculant Demographics: 2008–2009 First Year Class

Men: 95   **Women:** 74

Matriculants' Self-Reported Race/Ethnicity

Mexican American	2	**Korean**	9
Cuban	2	**Vietnamese**	1
Puerto Rican	1	**Other Asian**	3
Other Hispanic	7	**Total Asian**	69
Total Hispanic	10	**Native American**	0
Chinese	25	**Black**	1
Asian Indian	28	**Native Hawaiian**	1
Pakistani	2	**White**	84
Filipino	1	**Unduplicated Number**	
Japanese	1	**of Matriculants**	169

Science and Math Majors: 64%
Matriculants with:
     Baccalaureate degree: 98%
     Graduate degree(s): 7%

Financial Information

Source: 2007–2008 LCME I-B survey and 2008–2009 AAMC TSF questionnaire

	Residents	Non-residents
Total Cost of Attendance	$68,788	$68,788
Tuition and Fees	$41,926	$41,926
Other (includes living expenses)	$24,501	$24,501
Health Insurance (can be waived)	$2,361	$2,361

Average 2008 Graduate Indebtedness: $151,978
% of Enrolled Students Receiving Aid: 75%

Criminal Background Check

This medical school requires a criminal background check prior to matriculation.

Rush Medical College of Rush University

Chicago, Illinois

Rush Medical College of Rush University
Office of Admissions, Suite 524
600 South Paulina Street
Chicago, Illinois 60612
T 312 942 6915 **F** 312 942 2333

Admissions www.rushu.rush.edu/
medcol/admissions.html
Main www.rushu.rush.edu/medcol
Financial www.rushu.rush.edu/finaid
E-mail RMC_Admissions@rush.edu

Private Institution

Dr. Thomas A. Deutsch, Dean

*Dr. Cynthia Boyd, Recruitment
Team Leader*

David Nelson, Director of Student Financial Aid

Dr. Susan K. Jacob, Associate Dean

*Jill M. Volk, Director of Recruitment
and Special Programs*

General Information

Rush Medical College, founded in 1837, is the oldest component of Rush University. Through an academic and health care network of more than a dozen affiliated hospitals and a neighborhood health center, Rush University Medical Center serves 1.5 to 2 million people annually. Thus, students train in urban and suburban areas in a variety of socioeconomic and ethnic settings.

Mission Statement

Rush educates students as practitioners, scientists, and teachers who will become leaders in advancing health care and furthering the advancement of knowledge through research. The university integrates patient care, education, and research through the practitioner-teacher model. Rush encourages the growth of its students by committing itself to the pursuit of excellence, dedication to community service, free inquiry, and the highest intellectual and ethical standards.

Curricular Highlights

Community Service Requirement: Optional.
Research/Thesis Requirement: Optional.

Rush provides a firm background in the science of medicine and a balanced introduction to the practice of clinical medicine in a four-year curriculum designed to provide educational flexibility. The faculty have created an environment that fosters commitments to competent and compassionate patient care and to attitudes of inquiry and life-long learning. Preclinical Curriculum – The primary objective of the first year (M1) is to provide students with exposure to the vocabulary and fundamental concepts upon which clinical

medicine is based. The courses utilize lecture, laboratory, small group and workshop formats. The M2 curriculum centers on the causes and effects of disease and therapeutics. Several courses utilize a case-based approach integrating basic sciences into the context of clinical medicine. The Physicianship Program is an integrated and multi-disciplinary program that spans the M1 and M2 years and is designed to provide students with a foundation of clinical knowledge, skills, attitudes and behaviors so students are prepared for clinical experiences where physician skills are practiced in the context of patient care. Clinical Curriculum – the third and fourth years provide students with training in clinical skills, diagnosis and patient management in a variety of clinical settings. The third year is comprised of required core clerkships, while the fourth year provides students with the opportunity to pursue areas of special interest. Students complete the majority of their required clinical rotations at Rush University Medical Center or the John H. Stroger, Jr. Hospital.

USMLE

Step 1: Required. Students must record a passing score for promotion.
Step 2: Clinical Skills (CS): Required. Students must only record a score.
Step 2: Clinical Knowledge (CK): Required. Students must only record a score.

Selection Factors

The Committee on Admissions considers both the academic and non-academic qualifications of applicants in making its decisions and places strong emphasis on the applicant's humanistic concerns, unique experiences and demonstrated motivation for a career in medicine. All applicants are invited to complete the supplemental application and submit letters of recommendation. The Committee looks for objective evidence that the applicant will be able to handle the academic demands of the curriculum. Health-care-related experiences and social service activities are measures of how an applicant pursues their values, engages in activities that move them outside of their usual boundaries and expands their horizons. Academic achievement, letters of recommendation, MCAT performance, health care experience

and interviews are considered in the final evaluation of all applicants. Only U.S. citizens or permanent residents are considered for admission.

Financial Aid

Financial aid awards are made after acceptance into medical school. Rush University grant eligibility is based on both student and parent resources, regardless of the student's age or status. Students are awarded financial aid packages, grants, scholarships and loans to meet 100 percent of the demonstrated financial need during each year of their medical education.

Information about Diversity Programs

Rush seeks to attract a diverse student body that is more representative of the national population and more informed about multicultural determinants of health and the socioeconomic problems affecting the delivery of care.

Campus Information

Setting

Rush Medical College is located on the near west side of Chicago; the John H. Stroger, Jr. Hospital of Cook County, a major teaching affiliate, is two blocks away. The community is thriving and culturally diverse, with easy access by public transportation.

Enrollment

For 2008, total enrollment was: 533

Special Features

The Rush Community Service Initiatives Program creates a network of community programs that matches students' interest and initiative with the social and healthcare needs of Chicago's underserved population. Students have the opportunity to participate in clinical and non-clinical programs.

Housing

Student housing is available in the Center Court Garden Apartments, located on block from campus.

Application Process and Requirements 2010–2011

Primary Application Service: AMCAS
Earliest filing date: June 1, 2009
Latest filing date: November 1, 2009

Secondary Application Required?: Yes
Sent to: All applicants
URL: www.rushsupp.com
Contact: RMC_Admissions@rush.edu
Fee: Yes, $75
Fee waiver available: Yes
Earliest filing date: July 31, 2009
Latest filing date: December 31, 2009

MCAT® required?: Yes
Latest MCAT® considered: October 2009
Oldest MCAT® considered: January 2008

Early Decision Program: School does not have EDP
Applicants notified: n/a
EDP available for: n/a

Regular Acceptance Notice
Earliest date: November 2009
Latest date: Varies
Applicant's Response to Acceptance Offer – Maximum Time: Six weeks

Requests for Deferred Entrance Considered: Yes

Deposit to Hold Place in Class: Yes
Deposit (Resident): $100
Deposit (Non-resident): $100
Deposit due: With acceptance offer
Applied to tuition: Yes
Deposit refundable: Yes
Refundable by: May 15, 2010

Estimated number of new entrants: 128
EDP: n/a, special program: n/a

Start Month/Year: August/September 2010

Interview Format: Two individual interviews with faculty. Regional interviews are not available.

Other Programs

PREPARATORY PROGRAMS
Postbaccalaureate Program: No
Summer Program: No

COMBINED DEGREE PROGRAMS
Baccalaureate/M.D.: No
M.D./M.P.H.: No
M.D./M.B.A.: No
M.D./J.D.: No
M.D./Ph.D.: Yes, RMC_Admissions@rush.edu

Premedical Coursework

Course	Req.	Rec.	Lab.	Hrs.	Course	Req.	Rec.	Lab.	Hrs.
Inorganic Chemistry	•			8	Computer Science				
Behavioral Sciences					Genetics				
Biochemistry					Humanities				
Biology	•			8	Organic Chemistry	•			8
Biology/Zoology					Physics	•			8
Calculus					Psychology				
College English					Social Sciences				
College Mathematics					Other				

Selection Factors: 2008 Accepted Applicants

Proportion of Accepted Applicants with Relevant Experience (Data Self-Reported to AMCAS)		
Community Service/Volunteer		69%
Medically-Related Work		87%
Research		80%

Shaded bar represents school's accepted scores ranging from the 10th percentile to the 90th percentile. School Median ● National Median ●

Overall GPA 2.0 2.1 2.2 2.3 2.4 2.5 2.6 2.7 2.8 2.9 3.0 3.1 3.2 3.3 **3.4 3.5 (3.6) 3.7 3.8** 3.9 4.0
Science GPA 2.0 2.1 2.2 2.3 2.4 2.5 2.6 2.7 2.8 2.9 3.0 3.1 **3.2 3.3 3.4 3.5 (3.6) 3.7 3.8** 3.9 4.0

MCAT® Total Numeric Score 9 10 11 12 13 14 15 16 17 18 19 20 21 22 23 24 25 26 27 **28 29 30 (31) 32 33 34 35** 36 37 38 39 40 41 42 43

Writing Sample			J	K	L	M	N	O	P	(Q)	R	S	T
Verbal Reasoning	3	4	5	6	7	8	9	(10)	11	12	13	14	15
Biological Sciences	3	4	5	6	7	8	9	(10)	(11)	12	13	14	15
Physical Sciences	3	4	5	6	7	8	9	(10)	(11)	12	13	14	15

Acceptance & Matriculation Data for 2008–2009 First Year Class

	Resident	Non-resident	International	Total
Applications	1422	5009	45	6476
Interviewed	287	112	0	399
Deferred	5	1	0	6
Matriculants				
Early Assurance Program	n/a	n/a	n/a	n/a
Early Decision Program	0	0	0	0
Baccalaureate/M.D.	n/a	n/a	n/a	n/a
M.D./Ph.D.	0	0	0	0
Matriculated	96	34	0	**130**

Applications accepted from International Applicants: No

Specialty Choice

2004, 2005, 2006 Graduates, Specialty Choice (As reported by program directors to GME Track™)	
Anesthesiology	6%
Emergency Medicine	7%
Family Practice	8%
Internal Medicine	22%
Obstetrics/Gynecology	5%
Orthopaedic Surgery	4%
Pediatrics	8%
Psychiatry	2%
Radiology	5%
Surgery	9%

Matriculant Demographics: 2008–2009 First Year Class

Men: 60 **Women:** 70

Matriculants' Self-Reported Race/Ethnicity

Mexican American	3	Korean	3
Cuban	0	Vietnamese	1
Puerto Rican	0	Other Asian	3
Other Hispanic	7	Total Asian	36
Total Hispanic	10	Native American	0
Chinese	8	Black	4
Asian Indian	16	Native Hawaiian	1
Pakistani	3	White	89
Filipino	2	Unduplicated Number	
Japanese	5	of Matriculants	130

Science and Math Majors: 61%
Matriculants with:
Baccalaureate degree: 99%
Graduate degree(s): 8%

Financial Information
Source: 2007–2008 LCME I-B survey and 2008–2009 AAMC TSF questionnaire

	Residents	Non-residents
Total Cost of Attendance	$63,318	$63,318
Tuition and Fees	$44,928	$44,928
Other (includes living expenses)	$18,390	$18,390
Health Insurance (cannot be waived)	$0	$0

Average 2008 Graduate Indebtedness: $172,780
% of Enrolled Students Receiving Aid: 89%

Criminal Background Check

This medical school requires a criminal background check prior to matriculation.

Southern Illinois University School of Medicine

Springfield, Illinois

Office of Admissions
Southern Illinois University
School of Medicine, P.O. Box 19624
Springfield, Illinois 62794-9624
T 217 545 6013   F 217 545 5538

Admissions www.siumed.edu/studentaffairs/
admissions/home.html
Main www.siumed.edu
Financial www.siumed.edu/studentaffairs
E-mail admissions@siumed.edu

Public Institution

Dr. J. Kevin Dorsey, Dean and Provost

*Dr. Erik J. Constance,
Associate Dean for Student Affairs*

*Dr. Wesley Robinson-McNeese, Executive
Assistant to the Dean for Diversity*

Nancy Calvert, Director of Financial Aid

Evan Wilson, Director of Admissions

General Information

Southern Illinois University School of Medicine was established in 1969 and graduated its first class in 1975. Students spend the first 12 months of the program at the medical education facilities on the Carbondale campus and the remaining three years at the Medical Center in Springfield.

Mission Statement

The mission of the SIU School of Medicine is to assist the people of central and southern Illinois in meeting their health care needs through education, patient care, research and service to the community.

Curricular Highlights

Community Service Requirement: Optional. Highly recommended.
Research/Thesis Requirement: Optional.

The overall focus of the first two years of the curriculum is on case-based, student-directed learning in a small-group setting supported by lectures/resource sessions. Close integration of basic science and clinical information takes place throughout the four-year course of study. Clinical training begins in the first year with simulated patients and real patients. An increased emphasis on issues such as community health care and the psychosocial issues of medicine continues SIU School of Medicine's emphasis on caring while curing and treating patients as people rather than medical conditions. The third year consists of a series of multidisciplinary clinical rotations, with emphasis on both hospital-based and ambulatory practice. The fourth year comprises a series of electives designed to help students with final preparations for residency and offers

opportunities for off-campus training. The grading system is honors/pass/fail. The school also offers a six-year M.D.-J.D. program.

USMLE

Step 1: Required. Students must record a passing score for graduation, but not promotion.
Step 2: Clinical Skills (CS): Required. Students must only record a score.
Step 2: Clinical Knowledge (CK): Required. Students must only record a score.

Selection Factors

Applications for the M.D. program are accepted from Illinois residents who are U.S. citizens or possess a permanent resident visa. Completion of a minimum of 90 semester hours of undergraduate work in an accredited degree-granting college or university is required. Foreign students are advised to have completed at least 60 semester hours of coursework in the United States. The M.D.–J.D. program is open to non-Illinois residents. All applicants are expected to have a strong foundation in the natural sciences, social sciences, and humanities; they must demonstrate facility in writing and speaking the English language, as well as achieve competitive MCAT scores. Preference is given to those with sufficient recent academic activity to demonstrate the potential for successful completion of the rigorous educational program and to those who demonstrate the necessary noncognitive characteristics of a successful medical student and physician. Applicants are invited for interviews according to their strengths in academics, extracurricular activities, employment and volunteer experiences, and area of residence, with preference given to central and southern Illinois residents. The School of Medicine does not discriminate on the basis of race, religion, age, sex, handicap, or national or ethnic origin in administration of its education policies, admissions policies, scholarship and loan programs, or other school-administered programs.

Financial Aid

The School participates in all major federal student aid programs. Students receive aid on the basis of need as calculated on the FAFSA. Scholarship and grant aid are generally limited to students who demonstrate exceptional need.

Information about Diversity Programs

An effort is made to recruit qualified applicants from groups that have been underrepresented in the medical profession. The school has several active minority student organizations. For more information, contact the Office of Diversity at 217-545-7334. The School of Medicine also sponsors the Medical/Dental Education Preparatory Program (MEDPREP), a non-degree granting program in Carbondale for disadvantaged undergraduate or postbaccalaureate students, as well as underrepresented, rural, or low-income students (*www.siumed.edu/medprep/*).

Campus Information

Setting

SIU School of Medicine holds the first year of medical school in a small-town, collegiate environment on the main quad at SIU-Carbondale, an institution serving over 20,000 undergraduate, graduate, and professional students. The remaining three years take place at the SIU medical campus in the north central residential/commercial region of Springfield (pop. 115,000), the state capital. The facilities in Springfield are located in one of downstate Illinois' largest and fastest growing medical districts. The main medical instructional buildings are adjacent to Memorial Medical Center. A second affiliated hospital, St. John's, and additional clinics are situated within blocks of the main campus.

Enrollment

For 2008, total enrollment was: 292

Housing

Carbondale and Springfield: off-campus housing. Monthly rates for apartments in both locations: $450 to $600 per month.

Satellite Campuses/Facilities

Students receive training in affiliated clinical locations throughout central and southern Illinois.

Application Process and Requirements 2010–2011

Primary Application Service: AMCAS
Earliest filing date: June 1, 2009
Latest filing date: November 15, 2009

Secondary Application Required?: Yes
Sent to: Selected applicants
Contact: Evan Wilson, (217)-545-6013, admissions@siumed.edu
Fee: Yes, $50
Fee waiver available: Yes
Earliest filing date: July 1, 2009
Latest filing date: February 1, 2010

MCAT® required?: Yes
Latest MCAT® considered: September 2009
Oldest MCAT® considered: January 2007

Early Decision Program: School does not have EDP
Applicants notified: n/a
EDP available for: n/a

Regular Acceptance Notice
Earliest date: October 15, 2009
Latest date: Until class is full
**Applicant's Response to Acceptance
Offer – Maximum Time:** Two weeks

**Requests for Deferred
Entrance Considered:** Yes

Deposit to Hold Place in Class: Yes
Deposit (Resident): $100
Deposit (Non-resident): $100
Deposit due: With receipt of acceptance offer
Applied to tuition: Yes
Deposit refundable: Yes
Refundable by: May 15, 2010

Estimated number of new entrants: 72
EDP: n/a, special program: 2

Start Month/Year: August 2010

Interview Format: M.D. two one-on-one interviews; M.D./J.D. three one-on-one. Regional interviews are not available.

Other Programs

PREPARATORY PROGRAMS
Postbaccalaureate Program: Yes, www.siumed.edu/medprep/
Summer Program: No

COMBINED DEGREE PROGRAMS
Baccalaureate/M.D.: No
M.D./M.P.H.: No
M.D./M.B.A.: No
M.D./J.D.: Yes, www.siumed.edu/medhum/ mdjdprog.htm
M.D./Ph.D.: No

Premedical Coursework

Course	Req.	Rec.	Lab.	Sems.
Inorganic Chemistry		•	•	2
Behavioral Sciences				
Biochemistry		•		1
Biology		•	•	2
Biology/Zoology				
Calculus				
College English		•		2
College Mathematics		•		2
Computer Science				

Course	Req.	Rec.	Lab.	Sems.
Genetics		•		
Humanities		•		
Organic Chemistry		•	•	2
Physics		•	•	2
Psychology		•		
Social Sciences		•		
Advanced Level Biology		•		1
Other2				
Other3				

Selection Factors: 2008 Accepted Applicants

Proportion of Accepted Applicants with Relevant Experience (Data Self-Reported to AMCAS®)		
Community Service/Volunteer		68%
Medically-Related Work		83%
Research		77%

Shaded bar represents school's accepted scores ranging from the 10th percentile to the 90th percentile. School Median ● National Median ●

Overall GPA 2.0 2.1 2.2 2.3 2.4 2.5 2.6 2.7 2.8 2.9 3.0 3.1 3.2 3.3 3.4 3.5 (3.6) 3.7 3.8 3.9 4.0

Science GPA 2.0 2.1 2.2 2.3 2.4 2.5 2.6 2.7 2.8 2.9 3.0 3.1 3.2 3.3 3.4 (3.5) 3.6 3.7 3.8 3.9 4.0

MCAT® Total Numeric Score 9 10 11 12 13 14 15 16 17 18 19 20 21 22 23 24 25 26 27 28 (29) 30 31 (32) 33 34 35 36 37 38 39 40 41 42 43

				J	K	L	M	N	(O)	P	(Q)	R	S	T
Writing Sample				J	K	L	M	N	(O)	P	(Q)	R	S	T
Verbal Reasoning	3	4	5	6	7	8	(9)	(10)	11	12	13	14	15
Biological Sciences	3	4	5	6	7	8	9	(10)	(11)	12	13	14	15
Physical Sciences	3	4	5	6	7	8	9	(10)	(11)	12	13	14	15

Acceptance & Matriculation Data for 2008–2009 First Year Class

	Resident	Non-resident	International	Total
Applications	1052	118	4	1174
Interviewed	273	1	0	274
Deferred	6	0	0	6
Matriculants				
Early Assurance Program	0	0	0	0
Early Decision Program	0	0	0	0
Baccalaureate/M.D.	n/a	n/a	n/a	n/a
M.D./Ph.D.	n/a	n/a	n/a	n/a
Matriculated	72	0	0	**72**

Applications accepted from International Applicants: No

Matriculant Demographics: 2008–2009 First Year Class

Men: 40   **Women:** 32

Matriculants' Self-Reported Race/Ethnicity

Mexican American	0	**Korean**	2
Cuban	1	**Vietnamese**	0
Puerto Rican	0	**Other Asian**	1
Other Hispanic	2	**Total Asian**	8
Total Hispanic	2	**Native American**	1
Chinese	0	**Black**	11
Asian Indian	1	**Native Hawaiian**	0
Pakistani	1	**White**	54
Filipino	3	**Unduplicated Number**	
Japanese	1	**of Matriculants**	72

Science and Math Majors: 74%
Matriculants with:
Baccalaureate degree: 100%
Graduate degree(s): 15%

Specialty Choice

2004, 2005, 2006 Graduates, Specialty Choice (As reported by program directors to GME Track™)	
Anesthesiology	4%
Emergency Medicine	10%
Family Practice	14%
Internal Medicine	15%
Obstetrics/Gynecology	7%
Orthopaedic Surgery	6%
Pediatrics	14%
Psychiatry	1%
Radiology Diagnostic	4%
Surgery General	7%

Financial Information

Source: 2007–2008 LCME I-B survey and 2008–2009 AAMC TSF questionnaire

	Residents	Non-residents
Total Cost of Attendance	$38,616	$83,036
Tuition and Fees	$24,714	$69,134
Other (includes living expenses)	$13,416	$13,416
Health Insurance (can be waived)	$486	$486

Average 2008 Graduate Indebtedness: $127,247
% of Enrolled Students Receiving Aid: 93%

Criminal Background Check

This medical school requires a criminal background check prior to matriculation.

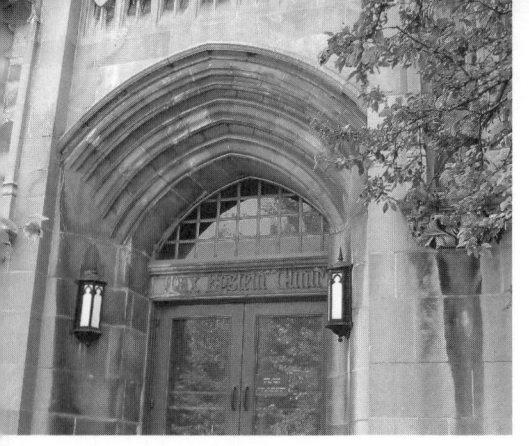

University of Chicago Division of the Biological Sciences, The Pritzker School of Medicine

Chicago, Illinois

Office of Admissions, University of Chicago
Pritzker School of Medicine
924 E. 57th Street, BSLC 104W
Chicago, Illinois 60637-5416
T 773 702 1937 **F** 773 834 5412

Admissions http://pritzker.bsd.uchicago.edu
Main http://pritzker.bsd.uchicago.edu
Financial http://pritzker.bsd.uchicago.edu
E-mail pritzkeradmissions@bsd.uchicago.edu

Private Institution

Dr. Holly J. Humphrey,
Dean for Medical Education

Sylvia Robertson, Assistant Dean
for Admissions and Financial Aid

Dr. William McDade, Associate Dean
for Multicultural Affairs

Dr. Herbert Abelson, Associate Dean
for Admissions

General Information

The Pritzker School of Medicine is unique among medical schools in that it is a part of the academic Division of the Biological Sciences. As an integral part of a world-class university, it offers medical students opportunities for interdisciplinary learning, clinical training, and research in a setting where recognized experts from all disciplines contribute to the development of physicians-in-training.

Mission Statement

At the University of Chicago, in an atmosphere of interdisciplinary scholarship and discovery, the Pritzker School of Medicine is dedicated to inspiring diverse students of exceptional promise to become leaders and innovators in science and medicine for the betterment of humanity.

Curricular Highlights

Community Service Requirement: Optional. Students have an impressive record of service.
Research/Thesis Requirement: Optional. Research is encouraged and supported.

The basic competencies which underlie the curriculum at Pritzker are grouped into four areas: the scientific basis of medicine; the scientific basis of diagnosis, prevention, and treatment of disease; interpersonal communication and teaching; and professional growth and development. Significant programs are devoted to helping students excel in these educational objectives. The library provides a comprehensive set of on-line medical and scientific materials with off-site access by students and faculty. This complements a Web-based curriculum that includes multimedia presentations and searchable text. A Clinical Performance Center uses standardized patients

and videotaped performance to educate students in taking a history, performing a physical examination, and clinical decision-making. The scientific foundation of medicine is achieved through lectures, labs, case-based problem-solving, and computer-based guided self-study and assessment. The clinical biennium consists of eight clinical clerkships and electives taught entirely by full-time clinical faculty and by selected residents who are trained in the humanistic teaching of medical students.

USMLE

Step 1: Required. Students must only record a score.
Step 2: Clinical Skills (CS): Required. Students must only record a score.
Step 2: Clinical Knowledge (CK): Required. Students must only record a score.

Selection Factors

A supplementary application is made available to everyone who submits an AMCAS application to the Pritzker School of Medicine. The Committee on Admissions reviews an application once the supplementary application is returned and the required letters of evaluation are received. About 600 applicants are invited to interview on the university campus from September through February. Offers of admission are extended on a rolling basis from October through April. Offers of admission are made solely on the basis of ability, achievement, motivation, and humanistic qualities. Outstanding personal characteristics and a strong career commitment are as important as excellence in academics.

Financial Aid

Scholarships and low-interest loans are made available to all students who have demonstrated need. There are both federally subsidized loans and low-interest loans from the university. Merit scholarships are available for a limited number of exceptionally well-qualified students. Individual counseling and debt management programs are available to all students. Financial aid packets are mailed to all accepted applicants after January 1. Financial aid resources for international applicants are extremely limited.

Information about Diversity Programs

Pritzker is particularly interested in providing a diverse educational experience for its students. Medical students from groups underrepresented in medicine who have attended Pritzker often assume strong leadership roles, both within their class and at the national level.

Campus Information

Setting

The University of Chicago is located on the south side of Chicago in the ethnically diverse community of Hyde Park, just minutes by train from downtown Chicago. The resources of this world-class city and its extraordinary lake-front are at the campus doorstep. The University of Chicago Medical Center campus, including its 21 buildings with 22 acres of space for research, teaching, and patient care, are within easy walking distance of Pritzker's libraries, classrooms, and labs.

Enrollment

For 2008, total enrollment was: 457

Special Features

The University of Chicago is made up predominantly of graduate and professional students participating in four major academic divisions and six professional schools, all sharing one campus. In this environment, graduates acquire superb skills in medical reasoning, problem-solving, team-building, and life-long learning, which help them assume leadership roles in residency training programs and as faculty in academic medicine. Pritzker students engage in some form of scholarly activity prior to completing their M.D. degree, and approximately 20 percent pursue combined degrees.

Housing

As a part of an extensive orientation program, students are guided in their housing search. Rents average $800/month.

Application Process and Requirements 2010–2011

Primary Application Service: AMCAS
Earliest filing date: June 1, 2009
Latest filing date: October 15, 2009

Secondary Application Required?: Yes
Sent to: All applicants
Contact: Sylvia Robertson, (773) 702-1937, pritzkeradmissions@bsd.uchicago.edu
Fee: Yes, $75
Fee waiver available: Yes
Earliest filing date: July 1, 2009
Latest filing date: December 1, 2009

MCAT® required?: Yes
Latest MCAT® considered: September 2009
Oldest MCAT® considered: 2007

Early Decision Program: School does have EDP
Applicants notified: October 1, 2009
EDP available for: Both Residents and Non-residents

Regular Acceptance Notice
Earliest date: October 15, 2009
Latest date: Until class is full
Applicant's Response to Acceptance
Offer – Maximum Time: On or before May 15, 2010

Requests for Deferred
Entrance Considered: Yes

Deposit to Hold Place in Class: No
Deposit (Resident): n/a
Deposit (Non-resident): n/a
Deposit due: n/a
Applied to tuition: n/a
Deposit refundable: n/a
Refundable by: n/a

Estimated number of new entrants: 88
EDP: 2, special program: n/a

Start Month/Year: August 2010

Interview Format: Three individual interviews. On-campus interviews only.

Other Programs

PREPARATORY PROGRAMS
Postbaccalaureate Program: No
Summer Program: Yes, http://pritzker.bsd.uchicago.edu/about/diversity/pipeline/psomer.shtml

COMBINED DEGREE PROGRAMS
Baccalaureate/M.D.: No
M.D./M.P.H.: No
M.D./M.B.A.: Yes, http://pritzker.bsd.uchicago.edu/jointdegrees/
M.D./J.D.: Yes, http://pritzker.bsd.uchicago.edu/jointdegrees/
M.D./Ph.D.: Yes, http://pritzker.bsd.uchicago.edu/jointdegrees/

Premedical Coursework

Course	Req.	Rec.	Lab.	Sems.	Course	Req.	Rec.	Lab.	Sems.
Inorganic Chemistry	•		•	2	Computer Science				
Behavioral Sciences					Genetics		•		
Biochemistry		•	•		Humanities				
Biology	•		•	2	Organic Chemistry	•		•	2
Biology/Zoology					Physics	•		•	2
Calculus		•			Psychology				
College English		•			Social Sciences		•		
College Mathematics					Other				

Selection Factors: 2008 Accepted Applicants

Proportion of Accepted Applicants with Relevant Experience (Data Self-Reported to AMCAS²)		
Community Service/Volunteer		74%
Medically-Related Work		87%
Research		91%

Shaded bar represents school's accepted scores ranging from the 10th percentile to the 90th percentile   School Median ● National Median ●

Overall GPA	2.0	2.1	2.2	2.3	2.4	2.5	2.6	2.7	2.8	2.9	3.0	3.1	3.2	3.3	3.4	3.5	3.6	3.7	3.8	(3.9)	4.0
Science GPA	2.0	2.1	2.2	2.3	2.4	2.5	2.6	2.7	2.8	2.9	3.0	3.1	3.2	3.3	3.4	3.5	3.6	3.7	3.8	(3.9)	4.0

MCAT® Total Numeric Score 9 10 11 12 13 14 15 16 17 18 19 20 21 22 23 24 25 26 27 28 29 30 31 ③② 33 34 35 ㊱ 37 38 39 40 41 42 43

Writing Sample			J	K	L	M	N	O	P	Ⓠ	R	S	T
Verbal Reasoning	3	4	5	6	7	8	9	⑩	⑪	12	13	14	15
Biological Sciences	3	4	5	6	7	8	9	10	⑪	12	⑬	14	15
Physical Sciences	3	4	5	6	7	8	9	10	⑪	12	⑬	14	15

Acceptance & Matriculation Data for 2008–2009 First Year Class

	Resident	Non-resident	International	Total
Applications	919	5930	465	7314
Interviewed	108	597	30	735
Deferred	0	3	0	3
Matriculants				
Early Assurance Program	n/a	n/a	n/a	n/a
Early Decision Program	0	0	0	0
Baccalaureate/M.D.	n/a	n/a	n/a	n/a
M.D./Ph.D.	1	6	0	7
Matriculated	28	68	4	**100**

Applications accepted from International Applicants: Yes

Matriculant Demographics: 2008–2009 First Year Class

Men: 51   **Women:** 49

Matriculants' Self-Reported Race/Ethnicity

Mexican American	5	Korean	5
Cuban	0	Vietnamese	3
Puerto Rican	0	Other Asian	1
Other Hispanic	0	Total Asian	26
Total Hispanic	5	Native American	1
Chinese	10	Black	11
Asian Indian	7	Native Hawaiian	0
Pakistani	1	White	60
Filipino	0	Unduplicated Number	
Japanese	0	of Matriculants	100

Science and Math Majors: 62%
Matriculants with:
Baccalaureate degree: 99%
Graduate degree(s): 12%

Specialty Choice

2004, 2005, 2006 Graduates, Specialty Choice (As reported by program directors to GME Track™)	
Anesthesiology	5%
Emergency Medicine	6%
Family Practice	3%
Internal Medicine	20%
Obstetrics/Gynecology	3%
Orthopaedic Surgery	5%
Pediatrics	13%
Psychiatry	4%
Radiology	6%
Surgery	9%

Financial Information

Source: 2007–2008 LCME I-B survey and 2008–2009 AAMC TSF questionnaire

	Residents	Non-residents
Total Cost of Attendance	$63,409	$63,409
Tuition and Fees	$38,239	$38,239
Other (includes living expenses)	$22,912	$22,912
Health Insurance (can be waived)	$2,258	$2,258

Average 2008 Graduate Indebtedness: $167,677
% of Enrolled Students Receiving Aid: 89%

Criminal Background Check

This medical school requires a criminal background check prior to matriculation.

University of Illinois at Chicago College of Medicine

Chicago, Peoria, Rockford, and Urbana, Illinois

Medical College Admissions
UIC College of Medicine
808 South Wood St., Room 165 CME M/C 783
Chicago, Illinois 60612-7302
T 312 996 5635   **F** 312 996 6693

Admissions www.medicine.uic.edu/admissions
Main www.medicine.uic.edu
Financial www.uic.edu/depts/mcam/finaid/index.shtml
E-mail medadmit@uic.edu

Public Institution

Dr. Joseph A. Flaherty, Dean

Dr. Jorge A. Girotti, Associate Dean and Director

Dr. Javette Orgain, Assistant Dean Urban Health Program

Tara Haddadin, Assistant Director of Financial Aid

Linda Singleton, Associate Director of Admissions

General Information

The college opened in 1882 as a private institution and joined the University of Illinois in 1913. Since 1982, the programs leading to the M.D. degree are conducted at four geographic sites. The Chicago site is located in the Medical Center of the university. The Urbana-Champaign site offers a four-year curriculum integrated with the programs of a comprehensive campus. The Peoria site includes facilities in each of the hospitals in that community and a modern downtown campus. The Rockford site has a centrally located campus and conducts programs in each of the Rockford hospitals and in several nearby smaller communities.

Mission Statement

The mission of the UIC College of Medicine is to enhance the health of the citizens of Illinois through the education of physicians and biomedical scientists, the advancement of our understanding and knowledge of health and disease, and the provision of health care in a setting of education and research. In pursuit of this mission, the college is committed to the goal of achieving excellence in teaching, research, and service in the science, art, and practice of medicine. This goal is best attained by applying valid educational principles, demonstrating high-quality patient care, and establishing a spirit of inquiry leading to scholarly achievement in basic and clinical research.

Curricular Highlights

Community Service Requirement: Optional.
Research/Thesis Requirement: Optional.

The college offers a generalist curriculum whose goal is to graduate physicians who are well grounded in basic and clinical sciences, oriented and competent as beginning general physicians, capable of entering graduate training in either generalist specialties or subspecialties, and able to function in an ever changing health care environment. We offer several special programs that allow students to combine medicine with doctoral degrees, business and public health, and independent study options to carry out in-depth studies of topics of their choosing.

USMLE

Step 1: Required. Students must record a passing score for promotion.
Step 2: Clinical Skills (CS): Required. Students must only record a score.
Step 2: Clinical Knowledge (CK): Required. Students must record a passing total score to graduate.

Selection Factors

The college selects applicants with the best combination of academic and extracurricular achievement, maturity, integrity, and motivation. Selection of students is based on an individualized evaluation of all available data and a personal interview. We consider the quality of work in all subject areas, breadth of education, and experiences that demonstrate initiative and creativity. The college gives preference to Illinois residents and does not discriminate on the basis of race, creed, sex, religion, national origin, age, disability, or status as a disabled veteran.

Financial Aid

Students are encouraged to apply early for loans and scholarships. Financial aid information is available by calling (312) 413-0127.

Information about Diversity Programs

The College has programs to encourage applicants from medically underserved areas of Illinois, a program for candidates interested in practicing in an urban area, and has staff to provide guidance to students from groups underrepresented in medicine.

Campus Information

Setting

UIC offers high-quality education to medical and graduate students at four sites across Illinois. Chicago is the largest of the college's four programs, and is located in the heart of the Illinois Medical District, about two miles west of downtown Chicago. The Urbana/Champaign campus is a complete four-year program leading to the M.D.. The first-year basic science program at Urbana also serves students who will complete their last three years of medical school at Peoria or Rockford. Peoria has a greater metropolitan population of over 356,000, Peoria offers the best of both urban and country living. Rockford is the third largest city in Illinois, and offers the appeal of a small town with the advantages of a large city.

Enrollment

For 2008, total enrollment was: 1,385

Special Features

UIC offers first-rate research facilities and resources. UIC is one of only 88 institutions of higher education nationally to receive the prestigious Research I designation from the Carnegie Foundation for the Advancement of Teaching. Attracting more than $250 million in research funding each year, the College of Medicine faculty and professional staff provide a wealth of expertise. The Molecular Biology Research Building (MBRB), which opened in 1995, is a 230,000 square feet state-of-the-art research facility. The building houses 56 Principal Investigators and 108 laboratories. Researchers from both basic and clinical science departments conduct individual and collaborative research at the MBRB. The campus houses a 9.4 Tesla magnet, which is the world's strongest magnetic field for human imaging. Finally, a new 300,000 square feet Research Building opened in summer 2005. The building is one of the most modern, architecturally innovative facilities in the country, with laboratory space for over 100 investigators.

Housing

On-campus housing is available at Chicago and Urbana. All campuses have private housing available nearby.

Application Process and Requirements 2010–2011

Primary Application Service: AMCAS
Earliest filing date: June 1, 2009
Latest filing date: November 15, 2009

Secondary Application Required?: Yes
Sent to: UIC College of Medicine – Admissions
Contact: Admissions Office, (312) 996-5635, medadmit@uic.edu
Fee: Yes, $70
Fee waiver available: Yes
Earliest filing date: June 15, 2009
Latest filing date: January 15, 2010

MCAT® required?: Yes
Latest MCAT® considered: September 2009
Oldest MCAT® considered: 2007

Early Decision Program: School does have EDP
Applicants notified: October 1, 2009
EDP available for: Both Residents and Non-resident

Regular Acceptance Notice
Earliest date: October 14, 2009
Latest date: Until class is full
Applicant's Response to Acceptance Offer – Maximum Time: Two weeks

Requests for Deferred Entrance Considered: Yes

Deposit to Hold Place in Class: Yes
Deposit (Resident): $100
Deposit (Non-resident): $100
Deposit due: With response to acceptance offer
Applied to tuition: Yes
Deposit refundable: Yes
Refundable by: May 14, 2010

Estimated number of new entrants: 300
EDP: 5, special program: 25

Start Month/Year: August 2010

Interview Format: Individual or panel. Regional interviews are offered in Rockford, Ill or Peoria, Ill.

Other Programs

PREPARATORY PROGRAMS
Postbaccalaureate Program: www.uic.edu/depts/mcam/uhp/, Dr. Javette Orgain, (312)996-6491, uhpcom@uic.edu
Summer Program: www.uic.edu/depts/mcam/uhp/, Dr. Javette Orgain, (312)996-6491, uhpcom@uic.edu

COMBINED DEGREE PROGRAMS
Baccalaureate/M.D.: www.iuic.edu/depts/oaa/spec_prog/gppa
Josephine Volpe, (312) 355-2477, gppa@uic.edu
M.D./M.P.H.: http://chicago.medicine.uic.edu/departments_programs
Susan S. O'Keefe, (312) 996-6920, sokeefe@uic.edu
M.D./M.B.A.: http://chicago.medicine.uic.edu/departments_programs
Susan S. O'Keefe, (312)996-6920, sokeefe@uic.edu
M.D./J.D.: www.med.uiuc.edu/msp/mdjd.asp
James Hall or Nora Few, (217) 333-8146, mspo@uiuc.edu
M.D./Ph.D.: www.chicago.medicine.uic.edu/mstp
Roberta Bernstein, (312) 996-7473, roberta@uic.edu
Verbal Reasoning Program: www.uic.edu/depts/mcam/uhp/
Dr. Javette Orgain, (312) 996-6491, uhpcom@uic.edu
Additional Program: www.uic.edu/depts/mcam/uhp/
Susan S. O'Keefe, (312) 996-6920, sokeefe@uic.edu

Premedical Coursework

Course	Req.	Rec.	Lab.	Sems.
Inorganic Chemistry	•		•	2
Behavioral Sciences				
Biochemistry				
Biology	•		•	2
Biology/Zoology				
Calculus				
College English				
College Mathematics				

Course	Req.	Rec.	Lab.	Sems.
Computer Science				
Genetics		•		
Humanities				
Organic Chemistry	•		•	2
Physics	•		•	2
Psychology	•			2
Social Sciences				
Anthropology or Sociology	•			1
Advanced Level Biology	•			1

Selection Factors: 2008 Accepted Applicants

Proportion of Accepted Applicants with Relevant Experience (Data Self-Reported to AMCAS®)		
Community Service/Volunteer	68%
Medically-Related Work	86%
Research	81%

Shaded bar represents school's accepted scores ranging from the 10th percentile to the 90th percentile. **School Median** ● **National Median** ●

Overall GPA 2.0 2.1 2.2 2.3 2.4 2.5 2.6 2.7 2.8 2.9 3.0 3.1 3.2 3.3 3.4 3.5 (3.6) 3.7 3.8 3.9 4.0
Science GPA 2.0 2.1 2.2 2.3 2.4 2.5 2.6 2.7 2.8 2.9 3.0 3.1 3.2 3.3 3.4 (3.5) 3.6 3.7 3.8 3.9 4.0

MCAT® Total Numeric Score 9 10 11 12 13 14 15 16 17 18 19 20 21 22 23 24 25 26 27 28 29 30 (31) 32 33 34 35 36 37 38 39 40 41 42 43

Writing Sample			J	K	L	M	N	O	P	(Q) R S T
Verbal Reasoning	3	4	5	6	7	8	9	(10)	11	12 13 14 15
Biological Sciences	3	4	5	6	7	8	9	10	(11)	12 13 14 15
Physical Sciences	3	4	5	6	7	8	9	10	(11)	12 13 14 15

Acceptance & Matriculation Data for 2008–2009 First Year Class

	Resident	Non-resident	International	Total
Applications	1633	5012	65	6710
Interviewed	547	300	0	874
Deferred	11	2	0	13
Matriculants				
Early Assurance Program	0	0	0	0
Early Decision Program	5	0	0	5
Baccalaureate/M.D.	24	0	0	24
M.D./Ph.D.	8	12	0	20
Matriculated	217	91	0	**308**

Applications accepted from International Applicants: No

Matriculant Demographics: 2008–2009 First Year Class

Men: 144 **Women:** 164

Matriculants' Self-Reported Race/Ethnicity

Mexican American	23	**Korean**	15
Cuban	3	**Vietnamese**	2
Puerto Rican	4	**Other Asian**	13
Other Hispanic	23	**Total Asian**	91
Total Hispanic	51	**Native American**	3
Chinese	17	**Black**	28
Asian Indian	34	**Native Hawaiian**	2
Pakistani	5	**White**	162
Filipino	6	**Unduplicated Number**	
Japanese	1	**of Matriculants**	308

Science and Math Majors: 67%
Matriculants with:
Baccalaureate degree: 99%
Graduate degree(s): 19%

Specialty Choice

2004, 2005, 2006 Graduates, Specialty Choice (As reported by program directors to GME Track™)	
Anesthesiology	9%
Emergency Medicine	8%
Family Practice	8%
Internal Medicine	16%
Obstetrics/Gynecology	3%
Orthopaedic Surgery	4%
Pediatrics	10%
Psychiatry	4%
Radiology	6%
Surgery	8%

Financial Information

Source: 2007–2008 LCME I-B survey and 2008–2009 AAMC TSF questionnaire

	Residents	Non-residents
Total Cost of Attendance	$49,265	$79,607
Tuition and Fees	$29,564	$59,906
Other (includes living expenses)	$18,899	$18,899
Health Insurance (can be waived)	$802	$802

Average 2008 Graduate Indebtedness: $149,248
% of Enrolled Students Receiving Aid: 85%

Criminal Background Check

This medical school requires a criminal background check prior to matriculation.

Indiana University School of Medicine
Indianapolis, Indiana

Medical School Admissions Office,
Indiana University School of Medicine
1120 South Drive, Fesler Hall 213
Indianapolis, Indiana 46202-5113
T 317 274 3772

Admissions www.medicine.iu.edu/body.cfm?id=166
Main www.medicine.iu.edu
Financial http://msaa.iusm.iu.edu/FinancialAid/finaidtxt.html
E-mail inmedadm@iupui.edu

Public Institution

Dr. D. Craig Brater, Dean

Robert M. Stump Jr., Director of Admissions

Jose Espada, Director, Student Financial Services

Karen Smartt, Associate Director of Admissions

Dr. Stephen B. Leapman, Executive Associate Dean and Chair, Admissions Committee

General Information
Indiana University School of Medicine, founded in 1903, is the sole institution responsible for providing medical education in the state of Indiana and operates the Indiana Statewide Medical Education System. In addition to its responsibilities in teaching, patient care, and service, Indiana University School of Medicine is a major academic research center. In conducting its medical educational programs, Indiana University School of Medicine utilizes six teaching hospitals on or near the medical center campus, as well as other affiliated hospitals in Indianapolis and throughout the state.

Mission Statement
The goal of the Indiana University School of Medicine is the education of physicians, scientists, and other health professionals in an intellectually rich environment with research as its scientific base. In education, we are committed to imparting a fundamental understanding of both clinical practice and the basic scientific knowledge upon which it rests, to provide a firm foundation for lifelong learning. In research, we are committed to the advancement of knowledge. In patient care, we are committed to the highest standards of medical practice in an atmosphere of respect and empathy for our patients. Education, research, and delivery of health care are inseparable components of our mission. Excellence can only be achieved when all components are of highest quality, well integrated, and mutually supportive.

Curricular Highlights
Community Service Requirement: Optional, but expected.
Research/Thesis Requirement: Optional.

The School of Medicine's faculty have adopted a competency-based curriculum which equips students with excellent clinical skills balanced by the development of interpersonal and professional skills. The basic medical sciences are presented in the first two years. In addition, an intensive multidisciplinary course, Introduction to Clinical Medicine, spans both years. The faculty utilizes small problem-based learning groups throughout the first two years. A 12-month clinical clerkship program at the medical center in Indianapolis occupies the third year. In the fourth year, students complete three clerkships, and select seven one-month electives. Students may arrange elective experiences around the country and abroad. Students pursuing the M.D. degree may simultaneously pursue graduate degrees in a variety of disciplines, or elect to participate in the five-year Physician Scholar Program which incorporates a year of research into the M.D. degree program.

USMLE
Step 1: Required. Students must record a passing score for graduation, but not promotion.
Step 2: Clinical Skills (CS): Required. Students must record a passing total score to graduate.
Step 2: Clinical Knowledge (CK): Required. Students must record a passing total score to graduate.

Selection Factors
Students are offered places in the class on the basis of scholarship, character, personality, references, residence, interview, and performance on the MCAT. In addition, the medical school faculty has specified non-academic criteria (technical standards), which all applicants must meet in order to participate effectively in the medical education program and the practice of medicine. The School of Medicine is state-assisted, and the Admissions Committee shows preference to Indiana residents. Nevertheless, a number of nonresidents are offered acceptances each year (179 for 2008). The applications of nonresidents who have significant ties to the state of Indiana may be given greater consideration. The School of Medicine does not discriminate on the basis of age, color, disability, ethnicity, gender, marital status, national origin, race, religion, sexual orientation, or veteran status.

Financial Aid
Both merit and need-based scholarships are available, as are need-based loans. There are scholarships for Indiana residents who commit to practicing primary care medicine in a medically underserved location in Indiana.

Information about Diversity Programs
Information about diversity programs may be found at *http://faculty.medicine.iu.edu/body.cfm?id=12.*

Campus Information
Setting
The Indiana University Medical Center campus covers some 85 acres within one mile of the center of Indianapolis and is part of the 30,000 student Indiana University-Purdue University at Indianapolis. The medical center is also host to outstanding schools of dentistry and nursing.

Enrollment
For 2008, total enrollment was: 1,205

Special Features
A Physician Scholars Program permits students to take up to a year off to pursue research or other medically-related interests. The Kenya Program allows students to work with IU faculty at Moi University to provide medical care for Kenyans. Similar programs in Latin America are under development.

Housing
On-campus housing is limited, but there is an abundance of available housing within 5-20 minutes of campus.

Satellite Campuses/Facilities
First- and second-year students may be enrolled at host higher education campuses in Bloom-ington, Evansville, Fort Wayne, Gary, Lafayette, Muncie, South Bend, and Terre Haute, in addition to Indianapolis. A new Rural Health Program was implemented at Terre Haute in 2008. The school will expand opportunities for third-year clerkships throughout the state beginning in 2009.

Application Process and Requirements 2010–2011

Primary Application Service: AMCAS
Earliest filing date: June 1, 2009
Latest filing date: December 15, 2009

Secondary Application Required?: No
Contact: Admissions Office, (317) 274-3772, inmedadm@iupui.edu
URL: n/a
Fee: Yes, $60
Fee waiver available: No
Earliest filing date:
Latest filing date:

MCAT® required?: Yes
Latest MCAT® considered: September 2009
Oldest MCAT® considered: August 2006

Early Decision Program: School does have EDP
Applicants notified: October 1, 2009
EDP available for: Both Residents and Non-residents

Regular Acceptance Notice
Earliest date: October 15, 2009
Latest date: Until class is full
Applicant's Response to Acceptance Offer – Maximum Time: Three weeks

Requests for Deferred Entrance Considered: Yes

Deposit to Hold Place in Class: No
Deposit (Resident): n/a
Deposit (Non-resident): n/a
Deposit due: n/a
Applied to tuition: n/a
Deposit refundable: n/a
Refundable by: n/a

Estimated number of new entrants: 336
EDP: 30, special program: n/a

Start Month/Year: August 2010

Interview Format: Individual interviews. Regional interviews are not available.

Other Programs

PREPARATORY PROGRAMS
Postbaccalaureate Program: Yes, www.msms.iu.edu
Summer Program: No
Additional Program: Master of Science in Medical Science, www.msms.iu.edu

COMBINED DEGREE PROGRAMS
Baccalaureate/M.D.: No
M.D./M.P.H.: Yes, http://grad.medicine.iu.edu/body.cfm?id=1853
M.D./M.B.A.: Yes, http://grad.medicine.iu.edu/body.cfm?id=1852
M.D./J.D.: No
M.D./Ph.D.: Yes, http://grad.medicine.iu.edu/body.cfm?id=1851
Additional Program: Yes, http://grad.medicine.iu.edu/body.cfm?id=1854

Premedical Coursework

Course	Req.	Rec.	Lab.	Sems.
Inorganic Chemistry				
Behavioral Sciences				
Biochemistry				
Biology	•		•	2
Biology/Zoology				
Calculus				
College English				
College Mathematics				

Course	Req.	Rec.	Lab.	Sems.
Computer Science				
Genetics				
Humanities				
Organic Chemistry	•		•	2
Physics	•		•	2
Psychology				
Social Sciences				
General Chemistry	•		•	2

Selection Factors: 2008 Accepted Applicants

Proportion of Accepted Applicants with Relevant Experience (Data Self-Reported to AMCAS®)		
Community Service/Volunteer		76%
Medically-Related Work		77%
Research		75%

Shaded bar represents school's accepted scores ranging from the 10th percentile to the 90th percentile ▬   **School Median** ●   **National Median** ●

Overall GPA	2.0	2.1	2.2	2.3	2.4	2.5	2.6	2.7	2.8	2.9	3.0	3.1	3.2	3.3	3.4	3.5	3.6	3.7	(3.8)	3.9	4.0
Science GPA	2.0	2.1	2.2	2.3	2.4	2.5	2.6	2.7	2.8	2.9	3.0	3.1	3.2	3.3	3.4	3.5	3.6	3.7	(3.8)	3.9	4.0

MCAT® Total Numeric Score 9 10 11 12 13 14 15 16 17 18 19 20 21 22 23 24 25 26 27 28 29 30 31 (32) 33 34 35 36 37 38 39 40 41 42 43

Writing Sample			J	K	L	M	N	O	P	(Q)	R	S	T
Verbal Reasoning	3	4	5	6	7	8	9	(10)	11	12	13	14	15
Biological Sciences	3	4	5	6	7	8		10	(11)	12	13	14	15
Physical Sciences	3	4	5	6	7	8	9	10	(11)	12	13	14	15

Acceptance & Matriculation Data for 2008–2009 First Year Class

	Resident	Non-resident	International	Total
Applications	670	2626	273	3569
Interviewed	563	320	29	912
Deferred	3	1	0	4
Matriculants				
Early Assurance Program	0	0	0	0
Early Decision Program	17	0	0	17
Baccalaureate/M.D.	n/a	n/a	n/a	n/a
M.D./Ph.D.	3	3	0	6
Matriculated	259	43	6	**308**

Applications accepted from International Applicants: Yes

Matriculant Demographics: 2008–2009 First Year Class

Men: 173   **Women:** 135

Matriculants' Self-Reported Race/Ethnicity

Mexican American	3	Korean	5
Cuban	0	Vietnamese	1
Puerto Rican	0	Other Asian	4
Other Hispanic	7	Total Asian	44
Total Hispanic	10	Native American	3
Chinese	14	Black	16
Asian Indian	17	Native Hawaiian	0
Pakistani	3	White	237
Filipino	1	Unduplicated Number	
Japanese	0	of Matriculants	308

Science and Math Majors: 71%
Matriculants with:
    Baccalaureate degree: 98%
    Graduate degree(s): 18%

Specialty Choice

2004, 2005, 2006 Graduates, Specialty Choice (As reported by program directors to GME Track™)	
Anesthesiology	10%
Emergency Medicine	7%
Family Practice	11%
Internal Medicine	14%
Obstetrics/Gynecology	4%
Orthopaedic Surgery	5%
Pediatrics	10%
Psychiatry	3%
Radiology	5%
Surgery	6%

Financial Information

Source: 2007–2008 LCME I-B survey and 2008–2009 AAMC TSF questionnaire

	Residents	Non-residents
Total Cost of Attendance	$58,427	$73,406
Tuition and Fees	$27,965	$42,944
Other (includes living expenses)	$27,886	$27,886
Health Insurance (can be waived)	$2,576	$2,576

Average 2008 Graduate Indebtedness: $45,141
% of Enrolled Students Receiving Aid: 80%

Criminal Background Check

This medical school requires a criminal background check prior to matriculation.

University of Iowa Roy J. and Lucille A. Carver College of Medicine

Iowa City, Iowa

Medical Student Admissions, University of Iowa
Roy J. & Lucille A. Carver College of Medicine
1213 Medical Education and Research Facility
Iowa City, Iowa 52242
T 319 335 8052   **F** 319 335 8049

Admissions www.medicine.uiowa.edu/osac/admissions
Main www.medicine.uiowa.edu
Financial www.medicine.uiowa.edu/osac/
financial/index.html
E-mail medical-admissions@uiowa.edu

Public Institution

Dr. Paul Rothman, Dean

Catherine M. Solow,
Assistant Dean of Student Affairs

Barbara E. Barlow, Recruitment Coordinator
and Minority Affairs Coordinator

Linda G. Bissell, Director of Financial Services

Judith D. Lehman,
Admissions Process Coordinator

General Information

The college is part of a major health center serving the state and region. The health sciences campus includes the University of Iowa Hospitals and Clinics; Veterans Affairs Hospital; Hardin Health Sciences Library; and medical college, basic sciences, dental, nursing, and pharmacy buildings. The Medical Education and Research Facility opened in 2001.

Mission Statement

The Carver College of Medicine has three inextricably linked missions: education, research, and service. The college aspires to be responsive to the needs of society, and in particular the citizens of Iowa, through the excellence of its educational programs in the health professions and biomedical sciences, by the outstanding quality of its research, and through the provision of innovative and comprehensive health care and other services.

Curricular Highlights

Community Service Requirement: Optional.
Research/Thesis Requirement: Optional.

Case-based and self-directed learning, clinical correlation, computer-based learning, small-group activities, and vertical integration of material are emphasized in the curriculum. Year 1: investigation of the normal structure and function of the human body. Year 2: investigation of abnormal structure and function. Patient contact, introduction to medical history-taking and physical diagnosis, and coverage of emerging topic areas are presented in Foundations of Clinical Practice, a course that runs the first two years of the curriculum. In the fourth semester, this course provides stu-

dents with a foundation in clinical medicine that will prepare them to perform in the clinical arena. The two clinical years of the curriculum afford a broad base of training to provide the student with the essential skills and knowledge required to enter residency training. A generalist core is a feature of the clinical years. Ample time for electives is provided.

USMLE

Step 1: Required. Students must record a passing score for promotion.
Step 2: Clinical Skills (CS): Required. Students must record a passing score in each section to graduate.
Step 2: Clinical Knowledge (CK): Required. Students must record a passing score in each section to graduate.

Selection Factors

The Admissions Committee selects applicants best qualified for the study and practice of medicine. To be eligible for admission, the applicant must attain at least a 2.5 GPA (based on a 4.0 scale) for all college work undertaken. Factors considered: 1. Overall undergraduate academic record. 2. Science GPA. 3. MCAT Scores. 4. Residence: Preference given to Iowa residents with high scholastic standing. Consideration also given to outstanding non-residents. 5. Personal characteristics: Evaluated through letters of recommendation, information on the AMCAS application, interview and information on the supplemental form. 6. Onsite personal interview. Applications for transfer are not considered.

Financial Aid

Applicants are selected without consideration of their ability to meet the cost of medical school. Students receive financial aid on the basis of need as calculated using the FAFSA. Scholarship and grant assistance are available. Students are responsible for their own financial support, but the college provides information on locating funding sources. Loan and grant funds from private, state, collegiate, and federal sources are available.

Information about Diversity Programs

The college is committed to the recruitment, selection, and retention of a diverse student body. Financial and academic assistance is provided to disadvantaged students and those from groups underrepresented in American medicine. Financial aid packages are designed on the basis of need, and grant and scholarship assistance are available. The application fee and admission deposit may be waived for financially disadvantaged students upon request.

Campus Information

Setting

The college is on the 1,900-acre campus of a major research institution, the University of Iowa, and is located in a community of 60,000. University Hospitals and Clinics, one of the largest university-owned teaching hospitals, is adjacent. Cultural activities, Big 10 sports, shopping and nearby parks provide outlets for recreation and services.

Enrollment

For 2008, total enrollment was: 583

Special Features

The college provides opportunities in international and domestic cross-cultural sites. Courses are offered in global health and U.S. health policy issues. The writing program provides consultation on personal statements, CVs, and creative writing. The program coordinates activities for medical students involving literature, music, and the visual and performing arts.

Housing

On-campus housing is generally not available. The university offers a clearinghouse to help students find housing. Rents range from $350-1,600/month. There are two coed medical fraternities with rents ranging from $295-$475/month.

Satellite Campuses/Facilities

The major satellite campus is the Des Moines Medical Education Consortium, a cooperative venture of several Des Moines hospitals, where some students complete required clerkships. Some ambulatory care clerkships are completed with adjunct faculty across the state.

Application Process and Requirements 2010–2011

Primary Application Service: AMCAS
Earliest filing date: June 1, 2009
Latest filing date: November 1, 2009

Secondary Application Required?: Yes
Sent to: Screened applicants
URL: www.medicine.uiowa.edu/osac/admissions
Fee: Yes, $60
Fee waiver available: Yes
Earliest filing date: July 1, 2009
Latest filing date: December 15, 2009

MCAT® required?: Yes
Latest MCAT® considered: September 2009
Oldest MCAT® considered: April 2004

Early Decision Program: School does have EDP
Applicants notified: October 1, 2009
EDP available for: Both Residents and Non-residents

Regular Acceptance Notice
Earliest date: October 15, 2008
Latest date: Until class is full
Applicant's Response to Acceptance Offer – Maximum Time: Two weeks from date of letter

Requests for Deferred Entrance Considered: Yes

Deposit to Hold Place in Class: Yes
Deposit (Resident): $50
Deposit (Non-resident): $50
Deposit due: March 1, 2010, or within 3 weeks after acceptance offer if after March 1, 2010
Applied to tuition: Yes
Deposit refundable: Yes
Refundable by: June 15, 2010

Estimated number of new entrants: 148
EDP: 5, special program: n/a

Start Month/Year: August 19, 2010
(first day of orientation)

Interview Format: Candidates interviewed by two faculty members in one room. Regional interviews are not available.

Other Programs

PREPARATORY PROGRAMS
Postbaccalaureate Program: No
Summer Program: No
Prematriculation Summer Program (for admitted candidates): Yes, www.medicine.uiowa.edu/osac/medical_education/index.html

COMBINED DEGREE PROGRAMS
Baccalaureate/M.D.: No
M.D./M.P.H.: Yes, www.public-health.uiowa.edu/mph/about/combined_degrees/md_mph.html
M.D./M.B.A.: Yes, www.medicine.uiowa.edu/osac/registrar/combined_degrees.html
M.D./J.D.: Yes, www.medicine.uiowa.edu/osac/programsrecords/CombinedDegrees.htm
M.D./Ph.D.: Yes, www.healthcare.uiowa.edu/mstp/

Premedical Coursework

Course	Req.	Rec.	Lab.	Sems.
Inorganic Chemistry	•		•	2
Behavioral Sciences				
Biochemistry		•		
Biology	•		•	2
Biology/Zoology				
Calculus				
College English	•			2
College Mathematics	•			1
Computer Science				

Course	Req.	Rec.	Lab.	Sems.
Genetics		•		
Humanities				
Organic Chemistry	•		•	2
Physics	•		•	2
Psychology				
Social Sciences				
Advanced Biology				1
Social, Behavioral Sciences/Humanities	•			4

Selection Factors: 2008 Accepted Applicants

Proportion of Accepted Applicants with Relevant Experience (Data Self-Reported to AMCAS)		
Community Service/Volunteer		73%
Medically-Related Work		87%
Research		86%

Shaded bar represents school's accepted scores ranging from the 10th percentile to the 90th percentile. School Median ● National Median ●

Overall GPA	2.0	2.1	2.2	2.3	2.4	2.5	2.6	2.7	2.8	2.9	3.0	3.1	3.2	3.3	3.4	3.5	3.6	3.7	(3.8)	3.9	4.0
Science GPA	2.0	2.1	2.2	2.3	2.4	2.5	2.6	2.7	2.8	2.9	3.0	3.1	3.2	3.3	3.4	3.5	3.6	3.7	(3.8)	3.9	4.0

MCAT® Total Numeric Score 9 10 11 12 13 14 15 16 17 18 19 20 21 22 23 24 25 26 27 28 29 30 31 (32) 33 34 35 36 37 38 39 40 41 42 43

Writing Sample			J	K	L	M	N	O	P	(Q)	R	S	T
Verbal Reasoning	3	4	5	6	7	8	9	(10)	11	12	13	14	15
Biological Sciences	3	4	5	6	7	8	9	10	(11)	12	13	14	15
Physical Sciences	3	4	5	6	7	8	9	10	(11)	12	13	14	15

Acceptance & Matriculation Data for 2008–2009 First Year Class

	Resident	Non-resident	International	Total
Applications	365	2527	2	2894
Interviewed	268	397	0	665
Deferred	5	0	0	5
Matriculants				
Early Assurance Program	0	0	0	0
Early Decision Program	4	0	0	4
Baccalaureate/M.D.	n/a	n/a	n/a	n/a
M.D./Ph.D.	2	8	0	10
Matriculated	98	50	0	**148**

Applications accepted from International Applicants: No

Matriculant Demographics: 2008–2009 First Year Class

Men: 77 **Women:** 71

Matriculants' Self-Reported Race/Ethnicity

Mexican American	9	Korean	3
Cuban	0	Vietnamese	3
Puerto Rican	0	Other Asian	1
Other Hispanic	1	Total Asian	21
Total Hispanic	10	Native American	1
Chinese	4	Black	6
Asian Indian	10	Native Hawaiian	1
Pakistani	0	White	112
Filipino	0	Unduplicated Number	
Japanese	0	of Matriculants	148

Science and Math Majors: 65%
Matriculants with:
  Baccalaureate degree: 99%
  Graduate degree(s): 5%

Specialty Choice

2004, 2005, 2006 Graduates, Specialty Choice (As reported by program directors to GME Track™)	
Anesthesiology	9%
Emergency Medicine	7%
Family Practice	11%
Internal Medicine	14%
Obstetrics/Gynecology	6%
Orthopaedic Surgery	5%
Pediatrics	10%
Psychiatry	2%
Radiology	6%
Surgery	6%

Financial Information

Source: 2007–2008 LCME I-B survey and 2008–2009 AAMC TSF questionnaire

	Residents	Non-residents
Total Cost of Attendance	$43,605	$59,419
Tuition and Fees	$26,712	$42,526
Other (includes living expenses)	$15,876	$15,876
Health Insurance (can be waived)	$1,017	$1,017

Average 2008 Graduate Indebtedness: $124,440
% of Enrolled Students Receiving Aid: 94%

Criminal Background Check

This medical school requires a criminal background check prior to matriculation.

University of Kansas School of Medicine
Kansas City, Kansas

Associate Dean for Admissions
University of Kansas School of Medicine
Mail Stop 1049, 3901 Rainbow Boulevard
Kansas City, Kansas 66160
T 913 588 5245   **F** 913 588 5259

Admissions www.kumc.edu/som/prospective
students.html
Main www.kumc.edu/som/
Financial www.kumc.edu/studentcenter/
financialaid.html
E-mail premedinfo@kumc.edu

Public Institution

*Dr. Barbara F. Atkinson, Executive Vice
Chancellor and Executive Dean*

*Sandra J. McCurdy, Associate Dean
for Admissions*

*Dr. Patricia A. Thomas, Associate Dean for
Cultural Enhancement and Diversity*

Sara Honeck, Director of Student Financial Aid

General Information

Since the establishment of the University of
Kansas School of Medicine in 1905, its students and faculty have built upon a tradition
of excellence. Through exceptional medical
education, patient care, service, and research,
the medical faculty and staff are dedicated to
preparing students for the future of medicine
by providing the innovative education and
training needed to practice in today's ever-
changing health care delivery system.

Mission Statement

The School of Medicine commits to enhance
the quality of life and to serve our community
through the discovery of knowledge, the education of health professionals, and improving
the health of the public.

Curricular Highlights

Community Service Requirement: Optional.
Research/Thesis Requirement: Optional.

The interdisciplinary curriculum promotes
self-directed, active learning to facilitate students' mastery of the knowledge, skills, attitudes, and behaviors required to become highly competent and compassionate healers. In
preparation for lifelong acquisition and synthesis of new discoveries and knowledge, students become critical thinkers who can analyze
difficult problems, formulate effective action
plans, and provide optimal clinical care. Years
one and two consist of 13 sequential modules
organized around central themes or organ systems, with didactic instruction and self-directed learning balanced between lectures and
small-group activities. Each student uses a
tablet computer to access course management,
learning, and research systems. Beginning in
the first semester, each student is paired with a

mentoring physician in a longitudinal ambulatory clinical experience. Several summer programs are offered for clinical credit to students
who have completed their first year. For core
clinical rotations, students rotate through hospitals and community-based clinics located in
Kansas City, Wichita, or select sites throughout
the state. Students may also choose the Rural
Track, a multidisciplinary clinical training program. Clinical electives may be taken locally,
across the country, or at more than 20
approved international locations.

USMLE

Step 1: Required. Students must record a passing
score for promotion.
Step 2: Clinical Skills (CS): Required. Students
must record a passing total score to graduate.
Step 2: Clinical Knowledge (CK): Required.
Students must record a passing total score to
graduate.

Selection Factors

Applicants are encouraged to submit their
AMCAS applications by September 1.
Qualified Kansas residents receive strong first
preference for secondary applications, interviews, and admission; successful nonresident
applicants will have significant Kansas ties
and/or add breadth to the class. Academic performance, MCAT scores, application materials,
letters of recommendation, impressions gained
from interviews, and nonacademic activities
are assessed throughout the admissions
process. Transfer applications are considered
only if a position is available in the third-year
class; Kansas residents with a compelling need
to transfer receive priority.

Financial Aid

Loans and scholarships are available, with the
FAFSA used to determine recipients of need-
based aid. A major source of assistance for
selected students is the Kansas Medical Loan
Program, which provides payment of tuition
and a stipend of up to $2,000 per month.
Recipients receive loan forgiveness by practicing primary care or emergency medicine in an
underserved county in Kansas.

Information about Diversity Programs

The University of Kansas and the School of

Medicine believe the intentional creation of a
diverse learning environment is essential to
achieving their educational missions. Diversity
and quality in medical education and health
care delivery are ensured through programs
that recruit, enroll, and graduate a diverse population of students; train culturally competent
physicians; recruit a diverse faculty; institu-
tionalize measures that develop and retain
minority academic physicians; and expand
research on health care issues affecting disadvantaged and underserved populations.

Campus Information

Setting
The School of Medicine is located at the tip of
the popular 39th Street West district and just
north of historic Westport and the Country
Club Plaza. The metropolitan area is well-
known for its award-winning parks system and
an abundance of venues for athletic events and
the visual and performance arts.

Enrollment
For 2008, total enrollment was: 707

Special Features
Student educational resources include a high-
tech clinical skills teaching laboratory, a computer testing center, and a newly renovated
medical library. A new heart hospital and biomedical research center opened in 2006.
Medical students provide medical care to uninsured patients through student-operated
JayDoc Clinics in Kansas City and Wichita.

Housing
All housing is off-campus, with affordable
housing readily available in the two-county area.

Satellite Campuses/Facilities
Approximately one-third of each class completes clinical training on the KU School of
Medicine-Wichita campus. This premier community-based program of medical education,
patient care, and research is centered upon a
partnership with four hospitals that offer a
total capacity of more than 3,000 licensed beds.

Application Process and Requirements 2010–2011

Primary Application Service: AMCAS
Earliest filing date: June 1, 2009
Latest filing date: October 15, 2009

Secondary Application Required?: Yes
Sent to: All Residents and selected Non-resident applicants
URL: https://www2.kumc.edu/som/meds/login.aspx
Fee: Yes, $50
Fee waiver available: Yes
Earliest filing date: July 1, 2009
Latest filing date: November 15, 2009

MCAT® required?: Yes
Latest MCAT® considered: September 2009
Oldest MCAT® considered: January 2007

Early Decision Program: School does have EDP
Applicants notified: October 1, 2009
EDP available for: Both Residents and Non-residents

Regular Acceptance Notice
Earliest date: November 15, 2009
Latest date: Varies
Applicant's Response to Acceptance Offer – Maximum Time: Two weeks

Requests for Deferred Entrance Considered: Yes

Deposit to Hold Place in Class: Yes
Deposit (Resident): $50
Deposit (Non-resident): $50
Deposit due: With response to acceptance offer
Applied to tuition: Yes
Deposit refundable: Yes
Refundable by: May 15, 2010

Estimated number of new entrants: 175
EDP: 45, special program: 25

Start Month/Year: July 2010

Interview Format: Two individual interviews, one open-file with a committee member. Regional interviews are not available.

Other Programs

PREPARATORY PROGRAMS
Postbaccalaureate Program: Yes, www2.kumc.edu/oced/hcpp.htm
Summer Program: Yes, www2.kumc.edu/oced/hcpp.htm
Primary Care Workshops: www.kumc.edu/som/primarycareworkshop.html
Premedical Student Conference: www.kumc.edu/som/psc.html

COMBINED DEGREE PROGRAMS
Baccalaureate/M.D.: No
M.D./M.P.H.: Yes, http://mph.kumc.edu/
M.D./M.B.A.: No
M.D./J.D.: No
M.D./Ph.D.: Yes, www3.kumc.edu/mdphd/
Additional Program: Yes, www.kumc.edu/hpm

Premedical Coursework

Course	Req.	Rec.	Lab.	Sems.
Inorganic Chemistry	•		•	2
Behavioral Sciences		•		
Biochemistry		•		
Biology	•		•	2
Biology/Zoology				
Calculus				
College English	•			2
College Mathematics	•			1

Course	Req.	Rec.	Lab.	Sems.
Computer Science				
Genetics		•		
Humanities		•		
Organic Chemistry	•		•	2
Physics	•		•	2
Psychology		•		
Social Sciences				
Other				

Selection Factors: 2008 Accepted Applicants

Proportion of Accepted Applicants with Relevant Experience (Data Self-Reported to AMCAS®)		
Community Service/Volunteer		72%
Medically-Related Work		78%
Research		59%

Shaded bar represents school's accepted scores ranging from the 10th percentile to the 90th percentile. School Median ● National Median ●

Overall GPA 2.0 2.1 2.2 2.3 2.4 2.5 2.6 2.7 2.8 2.9 3.0 3.1 3.2 3.3 **3.4 3.5 3.6 3.7** (3.8) 3.9 4.0
Science GPA 2.0 2.1 2.2 2.3 2.4 2.5 2.6 2.7 2.8 2.9 3.0 3.1 **3.2 3.3 3.4 3.5 3.6** (3.7) 3.8 3.9 4.0

MCAT® Total Numeric Score 9 10 11 12 13 14 15 16 17 18 19 20 21 **22 23 24 25 26 27** (28) 29 30 31 (32) 33 34 35 36 37 38 39 40 41 42 43

Writing Sample			J	K	L	M	N	O	P	Q	R	S	T
Verbal Reasoning	3	4	5	6	7	8	9	(10)	11	12	13	14	15
Biological Sciences	3	4	5	6	7	8	9	(10)	(11)	12	13	14	15
Physical Sciences	3	4	5	6	7	8	(9)	10	(11)	12	13	14	15

Acceptance & Matriculation Data for 2008–2009 First Year Class

	Resident	Non-resident	International	Total
Applications	441	1588	18	2047
Interviewed	350	106	0	456
Deferred	6	1	0	7
Matriculants				
Early Assurance Program	6	0	0	6
Early Decision Program	41	1	0	42
Baccalaureate/M.D.	n/a	n/a	n/a	n/a
M.D./Ph.D.	3	2	0	5
Matriculated	154	21	0	**175**

Applications accepted from International Applicants: No

Matriculant Demographics: 2008–2009 First Year Class

Men: 90   **Women:** 85

Matriculants' Self-Reported Race/Ethnicity

Mexican American	7	**Korean**	0
Cuban	0	**Vietnamese**	5
Puerto Rican	0	**Other Asian**	4
Other Hispanic	1	**Total Asian**	21
Total Hispanic	8	**Native American**	4
Chinese	4	**Black**	11
Asian Indian	10	**Native Hawaiian**	0
Pakistani	0	**White**	138
Filipino	1	**Unduplicated Number**	
Japanese	0	**of Matriculants**	175

Science and Math Majors: 75%
Matriculants with:
Baccalaureate degree: 100%
Graduate degree(s): 9%

Specialty Choice

2004, 2005, 2006 Graduates, Specialty Choice (As reported by program directors to GME Track™)	
Anesthesiology	6%
Emergency Medicine	6%
Family Practice	19%
Internal Medicine	14%
Obstetrics/Gynecology	8%
Orthopaedic Surgery	3%
Pediatrics	8%
Psychiatry	2%
Radiology	5%
Surgery	8%

Financial Information

Source: 2007–2008 LCME I-B survey and 2008–2009 AAMC TSF questionnaire

	Residents	Non-residents
Total Cost of Attendance	$47,935	$66,282
Tuition and Fees	$24,199	$42,546
Other (includes living expenses)	$22,738	$22,738
Health Insurance (can be waived)	$998	$998

Average 2008 Graduate Indebtedness: $123,309
% of Enrolled Students Receiving Aid: 92%

Criminal Background Check

This medical school requires a criminal background check prior to matriculation.

University of Kentucky College of Medicine

Lexington, Kentucky

University of Kentucky College of Medicine
Office of Admissions
138 Leader Avenue
Lexington, Kentucky 40506-9983
T 859 323 6161   **F** 859 257 3633

Admissions www.mc.uky.edu/meded/admissions/index.asp
Main www.mc.uky.edu/medicine
Financial www.mc.uky.edu/meded/financialaid/index.asp
E-mail kymedap@uky.edu

Public Institution
Dr. Jay Perman, Dean

Dr. Carol L. Elam,
Assistant Dean for Admissions
and Institutional Advancement

Julie McDaniel, Financial Aid Director

General Information

The University of Kentucky College of Medicine admitted its first class in 1960. The College of Medicine is part of the University of Kentucky Academic Medical Center located on the university campus in Lexington. The medical center comprises six colleges: medicine, nursing, pharmacy, dentistry, health sciences, and public health. The majority of on-site clinical teaching occurs at the University of Kentucky Chandler Hospital, the Veterans Affairs Medical Center, and the Kentucky Clinic. Hospitals in Lexington and across the Commonwealth hold affiliation agreements with the college for clinical teaching and patient service. Basic science teaching areas for lecture, laboratory, and small-group instruction, and the Medical Center Library, are located in the Willard Medical Sciences Building.

Mission Statement

Our mission is to assume a leadership role in addressing the health care needs of the Commonwealth of Kentucky and to be preeminent among medical schools in selected areas of education, research, and service.

Curricular Highlights

Community Service Requirement: Required. Interprofessional & underserved exposure required.
Research/Thesis Requirement: Optional.

In a curriculum that integrates basic and clinical sciences, students are taught fundamental problems of human biology, how to recognize causes of these problems, and how to prevent disease and treat patients. Year 1 of the curriculum focuses on normal function of the human body (human structure, cellular structure and function, neurosciences, and human function). First-year students receive early exposure and experience in patient care through the study of interviewing, history-taking, physical exam skills, and clinical decision-making using both standardized and real patients in a longitudinal care experience. In the first two years, students explore principles of prevention and assess the impact of social, ethical, legal, economic, and psychological factors using case study discussions. Year 2 exposes students to abnormal functions of the human body. Coursework is designed to integrate studies of infectious disease, immunology, pathology, pharmacology, and psychiatry. Computer-based instruction and simulation reinforce basic science studies and provide linkages to clinical applications. Clinical students work with patients in both inpatient and outpatient settings and are required to take medical histories, perform physical exams, and monitor laboratory tests. Year 3 includes integrated internal medicine and emergency care clerkships, along with pediatrics, OB/GYN, neurosciences, family and community medicine, and surgery. Year 4 includes clinical pharmacology, rural medicine experiences, 2 acting internships, and a 4-month elective period. A specialized Rural Track provides clinical education at rural sites.

USMLE

Step 1: Required. Students must record a passing score for promotion.
Step 2: Clinical Skills (CS): Required. Students must record a passing total score to graduate.
Step 2: Clinical Knowledge (CK): Required. Students must record a passing total score to graduate.

Selection Factors

The UKCOM gives preference to qualified applicants who are Kentucky residents. Determination of state residence is made by the registrar's office. Secondary applications are sent to all Kentucky residents and to nonresidents with competitive undergraduate GPAs and MCAT scores. Selected candidates are invited for interviews conducted at the UKCOM. Necessary personal attributes of applicants include time management abilities, interpersonal skills, leadership, and demonstrated service to others. Admission decisions are based upon review of academic and nonacademic factors, including scholastic excellence, MCAT performance, personal attributes, exposure to the profession, premed-ical recommendations, and admission interviews. Transfers from LCME-accredited schools are considered on a space-available basis. The UKCOM does not discriminate on the basis of race, sex, creed, national origin, age, or handicap.

Financial Aid

A limited number of scholarships are awarded to selected students with exceptional achievement. Institutional loan/scholarship assistance is available for eligible resident and nonresident students. The Financial Aid Office provides counseling and assists students in applying for aid. A guaranteed tuition plan locks tuition and fees for each entering class.

Information about Diversity Programs

The UKCOM is committed to the recruitment and retention of disadvantaged students and students from groups underrepresented in medicine. Interested applicants are encouraged to contact the admissions office.

Campus Information

Setting
The UKCOM is located on the University campus in Lexington.

Enrollment
For 2008, total enrollment was: 424

Special Features
Adjacent to UKCOM are Chandler Medical Center, UK Children's Hospital, VA Hospital, Markey Cancer Center, Sanders-Brown Center on Aging, University Health Service, the Gill Heart Institute and biomedical research centers. A new bed tower is under construction.

Housing
Housing is available close to campus. Rents average $600 to $800 per month.

Satellite Campuses/Facilities
Students participate in rural health electives throughout Kentucky through the Area Health Education Centers.

Application Process and Requirements 2010–2011

Primary Application Service: AMCAS
Earliest filing date: June 1, 2009
Latest filing date: November 1, 2009

Secondary Application Required?: Yes
Sent to: Screened applicants
Contact: Kim Scott, (859) 323-6161, kstahlma@email.uky.edu
Fee: Yes, $50
Fee waiver available: Yes
Earliest filing date: July 1, 2009
Latest filing date: January 15, 2010

MCAT® required?: Yes
Latest MCAT® Considered: September 2009
Oldest MCAT® considered: January 2007

Early Decision Program: School does have EDP
Applicants notified: October 1, 2009
EDP available for: Both Residents and Non-residents

Regular Acceptance Notice
Earliest date: October 15, 2009
Latest date: Until class is full
Applicant's Response to Acceptance Offer – Maximum Time: Two weeks

Requests for Deferred Entrance Considered: Yes

Deposit to Hold Place in Class: Yes
Deposit (Resident): $100
Deposit (Non-resident): $100
Deposit due: With response to acceptance offer
Applied to tuition: Yes
Deposit refundable: Yes
Refundable by: May 15, 2010

Estimated number of new entrants: 113
EDP: 20, special program: n/a

Start Month/Year: August 2010

Interview Format: Two individual interviews. Regional interviews are not available.

Other Programs

PREPARATORY PROGRAMS
Postbaccalaureate Program: No
Summer Program: No

COMBINED DEGREE PROGRAMS
Baccalaureate/M.D.: Yes, www.mc.uky.edu/meded/bsmd/index.asp
Marlene Sauer, (859) 323-6437, msauer1@email.uky.edu
M.D./M.P.H.: Yes, Kim Scott,(859) 323-6161, kstahlma@email.uky.edu
M.D./M.B.A.: No
M.D./J.D.: No
M.D./Ph.D.: Yes, www.mc.uky.edu/mdphd/
Marlene Sauer, (859) 323-6437, msauer1@email.uky.edu

Premedical Coursework

Course	Req.	Rec.	Lab.	Sems.	Course	Req.	Rec.	Lab.	Sems.
Inorganic Chemistry	•		•	2	Computer Science				
Behavioral Sciences					Genetics				
Biochemistry		•			Humanities		•		
Biology	•		•	2	Organic Chemistry	•		•	2
Biology/Zoology					Physics	•		•	2
Calculus					Psychology				
College English	•			2	Social Sciences		•		
College Mathematics					Other				

Selection Factors: 2008 Accepted Applicants

Proportion of Accepted Applicants with Relevant Experience (Data Self-Reported to AMCAS)		
Community Service/Volunteer	70%
Medically-Related Work	81%
Research	73%

Acceptance & Matriculation Data for 2008–2009 First Year Class

	Resident	Non-resident	International	Total
Applications	450	1619	150	2219
Interviewed	266	115	16	397
Deferred	2	0	0	2
Matriculants				
Early Assurance Program	n/a	n/a	n/a	n/a
Early Decision Program	21	0	0	21
Baccalaureate/M.D.	4	0	0	4
M.D./Ph.D.	2	0	0	2
Matriculated	89	19	5	**113**

Applications accepted from International Applicants: Yes

Specialty Choice

2004, 2005, 2006 Graduates, Specialty Choice (As reported by program directors to GME Track™)

Anesthesiology	4%
Emergency Medicine	4%
Family Practice	11%
Internal Medicine	18%
Obstetrics/Gynecology	5%
Orthopaedic Surgery	1%
Pediatrics	8%
Psychiatry	5%
Radiology	5%
Surgery	5%

Matriculant Demographics: 2008–2009 First Year Class

Men: 67   **Women:** 46

Matriculants' Self-Reported Race/Ethnicity

Mexican American	0	Korean	2
Cuban	0	Vietnamese	1
Puerto Rican	0	Other Asian	1
Other Hispanic	2	Total Asian	7
Total Hispanic	2	Native American	0
Chinese	2	Black	4
Asian Indian	2	Native Hawaiian	0
Pakistani	0	White	95
Filipino	0	Unduplicated Number	
Japanese	0	of Matriculants	113

Science and Math Majors: 75%
Matriculants with:
 Baccalaureate degree: 99%
 Graduate degree(s): 6%

Financial Information

Source: 2007–2008 LCME I-B survey and 2008–2009 AAMC TSF questionnaire

	Residents	Non-residents
Total Cost of Attendance	$47,131	$69,971
Tuition and Fees	$26,345	$49,220
Other (includes living expenses)	$19,891	$19,856
Health Insurance (can be waived)	$895	$895

Average 2008 Graduate Indebtedness: $135,834
% of Enrolled Students Receiving Aid: 93%

Criminal Background Check

This medical school requires a criminal background check prior to matriculation.

University of Louisville School of Medicine

Louisville, Kentucky

Office of Admissions, School of Medicine
Abell Administration Center
323 East Chestnut, University of Louisville
Louisville, Kentucky 40202-3866
T 502 852 5193 **F** 502 852 0302

Admissions www.louisville.edu/medschool/admissions
Main www.louisville.edu/medschool
Financial www.louisville.edu/medschool/finaid
E-mail medadm@louisville.edu

Public Institution

Dr. Edward C. Halperin, Dean

Pamela D. Osborne, Director, Medical School Admissions

Mary Joshua, Associate Director, Office of Minority and Rural Affairs

Leslie Kaelin, Director, Financial Aid

Dr. Stephen F. Wheeler, Associate Dean, Medical School Admissions

Dr. V. Faye Jones, Associate Dean, Office of Minority and Rural Affairs

General Information

The School of Medicine was established at the Louisville Medical Institute in 1833 and became affiliated with the University of Louisville in 1846. In 1970 the university became a member of the state system of higher education.

Mission Statement

The University of Louisville School of Medicine's mission is to excel in the education of physicians and scientists for careers in teaching, research, patient care and service, to bring our fundamental discoveries to the bedside, and to be a vital component in the University's quest to become a premier, nationally recognized metropolitan research university.

Curricular Highlights

Community Service Requirement: Optional.
Research/Thesis Requirement: Optional.

The University of Louisville School of Medicine is committed to training physicians who are humanistically oriented and patient-centered and who will meet the diverse health care needs of Kentucky's citizens. The curriculum is focused on providing comprehensive exposure to the fundamental aspects of medicine while retaining sufficient flexibility for effective development of an individual student's abilities and interests. It emphasizes a learning environment that enables students to maximize their success and prepares them to achieve their professional goals. Four goals drive the design, development, implementation and evaluation of our curriculum: Integration of basic and clinical sciences, within courses and clinical rotations; Expanded use of non-lecture teaching and learning modalities such as directed self-learning, small-group activities, and case-based learning; Expanded use of technology to support teaching and learning such as course and clerkship Web sites and patient simulations; and Development of course and clerkship learning objectives that support the overall goals and Educational Objectives for the Undergraduate Medical Education Program.

USMLE

Step 1: Required. Students must record a passing score for promotion.
Step 2: Clinical Skills (CS): Required. Students must only record a score.
Step 2: Clinical Knowledge (CK): Required. Students must record a passing total score to graduate.

Selection Factors

The ULSOM is a state institution which gives preference to residents of Kentucky. International applicants are only considered if they have both strong Kentucky ties and a pending permanent residency application. Applicants are selected on the basis of their individual merits without bias concerning sex, race, creed, national origin, age, or handicap. Applicants are chosen on the basis of intellect, integrity, maturity, and interpersonal sensitivity. Consideration is given to the past academic record, college pre-professional committee evaluations/faculty letters of recommendations, extracurricular activities, and personal interviews held at the medical school and the Trover Campus.

Financial Aid

Financial needs of the applicant are not a consideration in the selection process. Scholarships are available on a limited basis and are granted according to demonstrated financial need, and scholastic and professional promise.

Information about Diversity Programs

Applications from disadvantaged individuals and members of groups underrepresented in medicine are encouraged. Applicants are reviewed by the full Admissions Committee, which accepts students on an individual basis. Selected admitted students have the option to participate in a summer pre-matriculation program offered through the Office of Minority & Rural Affairs.

Campus Information

Setting

The ULSOM is located in the heart of downtown Louisville's medical center. The major acute and trauma care clinical teaching activities take place in the 404-bed University Hospital. Within two blocks are three formally affiliated hospitals: Kosair Children's Hospital, the only full-service children's hospital in the state of Kentucky; Jewish Hospital; and Norton Hospital. Other facilities include the world-renowned Kentucky Lions Eye Research Institute; James Graham Brown Cancer Center; the Veterans Affairs Medical Center; the Child Evaluation Center; Frazier Rehab Institute; and the ULSOM Trover Campus, located in Madisonville, Kentucky.

Enrollment

For 2008, total enrollment was: 600

Special Features

The ULSOM patient simulation center provides students hands-on, risk free learning, realistic patient encounters and interactive self-directed learning. All of the educational campus is WI-FI. Additionally, we offer students the opportunity to complete clinical training in a rural setting at the ULSOM Trover Campus in Madisionville, Kentucky.

Housing

The U of L medical-dental dormitory/apartment building is on campus. Non-university housing listings are available from the Office of Faculty and Student Advocacy, (502) 852-6185.

Satellite Campuses/Facilities

Students rotate at five primary hospital sites; four sites are within walking distance of the Health Science Center campus. Interested candidates may apply for dedicated admission to complete clinical training at the ULSOM Trover Campus in Madisonville, Kentucky.

Application Process and Requirements 2010–2011

Primary Application Service: AMCAS
Earliest filing date: June 1, 2009
Latest filing date: October 15, 2009

Secondary Application Required?: Yes
Sent to: Screened applicants
Contact: medadm@louisville.edu
Fee: Yes, $75
Fee waiver available: Yes
Earliest filing date: July 1, 2009
Latest filing date: December 31, 2009

MCAT® required?: Yes
Latest MCAT® considered: September 2009
Oldest MCAT® considered: 2007

Early Decision Program: School does have EDP
Applicants notified: October 1, 2009
EDP available for: Both Residents and Non-residents

Regular Acceptance Notice
Earliest date: October 16, 2009
Latest date: Varies
Applicant's Response to Acceptance Offer – Maximum Time: Two weeks

Requests for Deferred Entrance Considered: Yes

Deposit to Hold Place in Class: Yes
Deposit (Resident): $100
Deposit (Non-resident): $100
Deposit due: With acceptance letter
Applied to tuition: Yes
Deposit refundable: Yes
Refundable by: May 15, 2010

Estimated number of new entrants: 160
EDP: 4, special program: 10

Start Month/Year: August 2010

Interview Format: Academically blind interview with two committee members. Regional interviews are not available.

Other Programs

PREPARATORY PROGRAMS
Postbaccalaureate Program: No
Summer Program: Yes, www.louisville.edu/medschool/ahec/special.programs/ Mary Joshua, (502) 852-7159, specprog@louisville.edu

COMBINED DEGREE PROGRAMS
Baccalaureate/M.D.: No
M.D./M.P.H.: Yes, http://louisville.edu/medschool/dualdegree
M.D./M.B.A.: Yes, http://louisville.edu/medschool/dualdegree, Toni Ganzel, M.D., M.B.A., (502) 852-5192, medstuaf@gwise.louisville.edu
M.D./J.D.: No
M.D./Ph.D.: Yes, http://louisville.edu/medschool/dualdegree
Additional Program: Yes, www.louisville.edu/bioethicsma

Premedical Coursework

Course	Req.	Rec.	Lab.	Sems.
Inorganic Chemistry	•		•	2
Behavioral Sciences				
Biochemistry		•		1
Biology	•		•	2
Biology/Zoology				
Calculus	•			1
College English	•			2
College Mathematics		•		2

Course	Req.	Rec.	Lab.	Sems.
Computer Science				
Genetics		•		1
Humanities				
Organic Chemistry	•		•	2
Physics	•		•	2
Psychology				
Social Sciences				
Physiology		•		1
Statistics		•		1

Selection Factors: 2008 Accepted Applicants

Proportion of Accepted Applicants with Relevant Experience (Data Self-Reported to AMCAS®)		
Community Service/Volunteer		75%
Medically-Related Work		76%
Research		72%

Shaded bar represents school's accepted scores ranging from the 10th percentile to the 90th percentile. **School Median** ● **National Median** ●

Overall GPA	2.0	2.1	2.2	2.3	2.4	2.5	2.6	2.7	2.8	2.9	3.0	3.1	3.2	3.3	3.4	3.5	3.6	(3.7)	3.8	3.9	4.0
Science GPA	2.0	2.1	2.2	2.3	2.4	2.5	2.6	2.7	2.8	2.9	3.0	3.1	3.2	3.3	3.4	3.5	(3.6)	3.7	3.8	3.9	4.0

MCAT® Total Numeric Score 9 10 11 12 13 14 15 16 17 18 19 20 21 22 23 24 25 26 27 28 29 (30) 31 (32) 33 34 35 36 37 38 39 40 41 42 43

Writing Sample			J	K	L	M	N	O	(P)	(Q)	R	S	T
Verbal Reasoning	3	4	5	6	7	8	9	(10)	11	12	13	14	15
Biological Sciences	3	4	5	6	7	8	9	(10)	(11)	12	13	14	15
Physical Sciences	3	4	5	6	7	8	9	(10)	(11)	12	13	14	15

Acceptance & Matriculation Data for 2008–2009 First Year Class

	Resident	Non-resident	International	Total
Applications	423	1902	23	2348
Interviewed	276	107	3	386
Deferred	3	0	0	3
Matriculants				
Early Assurance Program	4	0	0	4
Early Decision Program	0	0	0	0
Baccalaureate/M.D.	n/a	n/a	n/a	n/a
M.D./Ph.D.	2	0	0	2
Matriculated	116	37	2	**155**

Applications accepted from International Applicants: Yes

Specialty Choice

2004, 2005, 2006 Graduates, Specialty Choice (As reported by program directors to GME Track™)	
Anesthesiology	7%
Emergency Medicine	5%
Family Practice	8%
Internal Medicine	19%
Obstetrics/Gynecology	4%
Orthopaedic Surgery	4%
Pediatrics	12%
Psychiatry	5%
Radiology	6%
Surgery	6%

Matriculant Demographics: 2008–2009 First Year Class

Men: 87 **Women:** 68

Matriculants' Self-Reported Race/Ethnicity

Mexican American	2	Korean	0
Cuban	1	Vietnamese	1
Puerto Rican	0	Other Asian	2
Other Hispanic	1	Total Asian	19
Total Hispanic	4	Native American	2
Chinese	4	Black	13
Asian Indian	9	Native Hawaiian	0
Pakistani	0	White	118
Filipino	3	Unduplicated Number	
Japanese	1	of Matriculants	155

Science and Math Majors: 77%
Matriculants with:
Baccalaureate degree: 99%
Graduate degree(s): 8%

Financial Information

Source: 2007–2008 LCME I-B survey and 2008–2009 AAMC TSF questionnaire

	Residents	Non-residents
Total Cost of Attendance	$44,316	$62,638
Tuition and Fees	$25,103	$43,425
Other (includes living expenses)	$17,663	$17,663
Health Insurance (can be waived)	$1,550	$1,550

Average 2008 Graduate Indebtedness: $135,354
% of Enrolled Students Receiving Aid: 94%

Criminal Background Check

This medical school requires a criminal background check prior to matriculation.

Louisiana State University School of Medicine in New Orleans

New Orleans, Louisiana

Admissions Office, Louisiana State University
School of Medicine in New Orleans
1901 Perdido Street, Box P3-4
New Orleans, Louisiana 70112-1393
T 504 568 6262   **F** 504 568 7701

Admissions www.medschool.lsuhsc.edu/admissions
Main www.medschool.lsuhsc.edu
Financial www.lsuhsc.edu/no/students/financialaid/
E-mail ms-admissions@lsuhsc.edu

Public Institution

Dr. Steve Nelson, Dean

Dr. Sam G. McClugage Jr.,
Associate Dean for Admissions

Dr. Edward Helm, Associate Dean, Office of
Community and Minority Health Education

Patrick Gorman, Director of
Student Financial Aid

General Information

LSU School of Medicine in New Orleans was
established in 1931 in downtown New Orleans.
During the past two decades, several new
buildings have been erected, including a state-
of-the-art Student Learning Center which
includes procedural and simulation labs, a
computer lounge, and large and small-group
meeting rooms. A new residence facility,
Stanislaus Hall, containing a comprehensive
fitness center, is among the more recent additions to the campus.

Mission Statement

The LSUSOM is dedicated to providing the
opportunity for an excellent medical education
to all Louisiana applicants who are prepared to
benefit from its curriculum and instruction. To
this end, the Admissions Committee will strive
to recruit and admit residents from Louisiana
from every geographic, economic, social, and
cultural dimension of the state of Louisiana.

Curricular Highlights

Community Service Requirement: Required.
Research/Thesis Requirement: Optional.

The first two years of the medical school curriculum emphasize several basic sciences and
their relevance to clinical medicine. Clinical
experiences begin in the first year in courses
such as Science and Practice of Medicine. The
second year of medical school utilizes an integrated approach to the teaching of basic science and pre-clinical courses within an environment that fosters an early exposure to
patient care. Clerkships begin in the third year
where students rotate through the various clinical disciplines. In the fourth year, students are
given several months for electives in addition
to required rotations in Ambulatory Medicine,

Acting Internships, etc. Some of these rotations
can be completed at the institutions associated
with the LSU School of Medicine throughout
the state or at other approved institutions outside the state or country. Computer-assisted
instruction is an important component of the
curriculum. Entering students are required to
purchase laptop computers.

USMLE

Step 1: Required. Students must record a passing
score for promotion.
Step 2: Clinical Skills (CS): Required. Students
must record a passing total score to graduate.
Step 2: Clinical Knowledge (CK): Required.
Students must record a passing total score to
graduate.

Selection Factors

Candidates are encouraged to contact the
Office of Admissions for a brochure which
summarizes the selection process for LSU
School of Medicine in New Orleans.

Financial Aid

Financial assistance is available for students
through several different methods. There are
direct scholarship programs, scholarships for
disadvantaged students, state and federal loan
programs, work-study programs, and employment opportunities in the New Orleans area for
students in their third and fourth years. Financial
assistance information is available from the
Student Financial Aid Office at (504) 568-4820.

Information about Diversity Programs

Members of groups underrepresented in medicine are encouraged to apply. The School of
Medicine's Office of Community and Minority
Health Education actively recruits students
from groups underrepresented in medicine
and provides counseling for high school and
college students. Further information may be
obtained by contacting Dr. Edward Helm,
Associate Dean for Community and Minority
Health Education, at (504) 568-8501.

Campus Information

Setting

LSU School of Medicine is located in downtown New Orleans in a medical corridor which
is within walking distance of the historic

French Quarter, museums, shopping districts,
and two sports arenas for professional football
and basketball teams.

Enrollment

For 2008, total enrollment was: 691

Special Features

The interdisciplinary Science and Practice of
Medicine course and the Isidore Cohn Learning
Center were both created to provide a more
innovative way for the clinical teaching of students beginning in the first year. The Learning
Center includes over 14,000 square feet of
space, small-group teaching rooms, simulation
laboratories, a computer center, and meeting
rooms. More information is available at
www.medschool.lsuhsc.edu/learning_center/.

Housing

Two recently renovated student housing facilities
are available. Furnished and unfurnished apartments are available for married (with or without
children) and single students. Many students
choose to rent apartments in New Orleans or
the surrounding metropolitan area. Lists of
available apartments are supplied upon request.

Satellite Campuses/Facilities

LSU School of Medicine rotates its students
among one of several public hospitals, mainly in
New Orleans, Baton Rouge, or Lafayette, LA, as
well as several private hospitals such as Children's
Hospital in the city of New Orleans. The LSU
Health Care Services Division has oversight for
eight public teaching hospitals in the State of
Louisiana in which many LSUSOM medical
students, residents and fellows receive training.
Several clinics in the metropolitan area and
around the state are also similarly used for the
training of health care professionals.

Application Process and Requirements 2010–2011

Primary Application Service: AMCAS
Earliest filing date: June 1, 2009
Latest filing date: November 30, 2009

Secondary Application Required?: Yes
Sent to: All applicants
URL: www.medschool.lsuhsc.edu/admissions/secondary_application
Fee: Yes, $50
Fee waiver available: Yes
Earliest filing date: June 15, 2009
Latest filing date: January 15, 2010

MCAT® required?: Yes
Latest MCAT® considered: September 2009
Oldest MCAT® considered: 2006

Early Decision Program: School does have EDP
Applicants notified: October 1, 2009
EDP available for: Both Residents and Non-residents

Regular Acceptance Notice
Earliest date: October 15, 2009
Latest date: Varies
Applicant's Response to Acceptance Offer – Maximum Time: Two weeks

Requests for Deferred Entrance Considered: Yes

Deposit to Hold Place in Class: Yes
Deposit (Resident): $100
Deposit (Non-resident): $100
Deposit due: Due with acceptance offer
Applied to tuition: Yes
Deposit refundable: Yes
Refundable by: May 15, 2010

Estimated number of new entrants: 180
EDP: 15, special program: 8

Start Month/Year: August 2010

Interview Format: Three one-on-one interviews. Regional interviews are not available.

Other Programs

PREPARATORY PROGRAMS
Postbaccalaureate Program: No
Summer Program: Yes, Dr. Edward Helm, (504) 568-8501

COMBINED DEGREE PROGRAMS
Baccalaureate/M.D.: No
M.D./M.P.H.: Yes, http://publichealth.lsuhsc.edu/
M.D./M.B.A.: No
M.D./J.D.: No
M.D./Ph.D.: Yes, http://graduatestudies.lsuhsc.edu/
Additional Program: Yes, Rural Scholars' Track
Cathie Stuckey, (504) 568-6262, ms-admissions@lsuhsc.edu

Premedical Coursework

Course	Req.	Rec.	Lab.	Hrs.
Inorganic Chemistry	•		•	8
Behavioral Sciences		•		
Biochemistry		•		
Biology		•		
Biology/Zoology	•		•	8
Calculus		•		
College English	•			6
College Mathematics				

Course	Req.	Rec.	Lab.	Hrs.
Computer Science		•		
Genetics		•		
Humanities		•		
Organic Chemistry	•		•	8
Physics	•		•	8
Psychology		•		
Social Sciences		•		
Other				

Selection Factors: 2008 Accepted Applicants

Proportion of Accepted Applicants with Relevant Experience (Data Self-Reported to AMCAS®)		
Community Service/Volunteer	71%
Medically-Related Work	81%
Research	64%

Shaded bar represents school's accepted scores ranging from the 10th percentile to the 90th percentile. School Median ● National Median ●

Overall GPA 2.0 2.1 2.2 2.3 2.4 2.5 2.6 2.7 2.8 2.9 3.0 3.1 3.2 3.3 3.4 3.5 3.6 (3.7) 3.8 3.9 4.0

Science GPA 2.0 2.1 2.2 2.3 2.4 2.5 2.6 2.7 2.8 2.9 3.0 3.1 3.2 3.3 3.4 3.5 3.6 (3.7) 3.8 3.9 4.0

MCAT® Total Numeric Score 9 10 11 12 13 14 15 16 17 18 19 20 21 22 23 24 25 26 27 28 (29) 30 31 (32) 33 34 35 36 37 38 39 40 41 42 43

Writing Sample			J	K	L	M	N	(O)	P	(Q)	R	S	T
Verbal Reasoning	3	4	5	6	7	8	9	(10)	11	12	13	14	15
Biological Sciences	3	4	5	6	7	8	9	(10)	(11)	12	13	14	15
Physical Sciences	3	4	5	6	7	8	9	(10)	(11)	12	13	14	15

Acceptance & Matriculation Data for 2008–2009 First Year Class

	Resident	Non-resident	International	Total
Applications	631	335	24	990
Interviewed	387	16	0	403
Deferred	3	1	0	4
Matriculants				
Early Assurance Program	0	0	0	0
Early Decision Program	11	0	0	11
Baccalaureate/M.D.	n/a	n/a	n/a	n/a
M.D./Ph.D.	1	4	0	5
Matriculated	168	11	0	**179**

Applications accepted from International Applicants: No

Matriculant Demographics: 2008–2009 First Year Class

Men: 100   **Women:** 79

Matriculants' Self-Reported Race/Ethnicity

Mexican American	2	Korean	0
Cuban	1	Vietnamese	4
Puerto Rican	0	Other Asian	2
Other Hispanic	8	Total Asian	17
Total Hispanic	10	Native American	1
Chinese	5	Black	10
Asian Indian	6	Native Hawaiian	1
Pakistani	0	White	146
Filipino	1	Unduplicated Number	
Japanese	0	of Matriculants	179

Science and Math Majors: 83%
Matriculants with:
    Baccalaureate degree: 98%
    Graduate degree(s): 15%

Specialty Choice

2004, 2005, 2006 Graduates, Specialty Choice (As reported by program directors to GME Track™)	
Anesthesiology	6%
Emergency Medicine	7%
Family Practice	8%
Internal Medicine	15%
Obstetrics/Gynecology	7%
Orthopaedic Surgery	4%
Pediatrics	8%
Psychiatry	3%
Radiology	6%
Surgery	7%

Financial Information

Source: 2007–2008 LCME I-B survey and 2008–2009 AAMC TSF questionnaire

	Residents	Non-residents
Total Cost of Attendance	$35,340	$49.488
Tuition and Fees	$12,866	$27,014
Other (includes living expenses)	$20,722	$20,722
Health Insurance (can be waived)	$1,752	$1,752

Average 2008 Graduate Indebtedness: $127,113
% of Enrolled Students Receiving Aid: 88%

Criminal Background Check

This medical school requires a criminal background check prior to matriculation.

Louisiana State University Health Sciences Center School of Medicine in Shreveport

Shreveport, Louisiana

Office of Student Admissions
Louisiana State University Health Sciences Center
School of Medicine in Shreveport,
P.O. Box 33932, Shreveport, Louisiana 71130-3932
T 318 675 5190   **F** 318 675 8690

Admissions www.admissions.lsuhsc.edu
Main www.sh.lsuhsc.edu/index.html
Financial http://sh-aux.lsuhsc.edu/financialaid/
E-mail shvadm@lsuhsc.edu

Public Institution

Dr. Andrew Chesson,
Acting Chancellor and Dean

Dr. F. Scott Kennedy, Assistant Dean
for Student Admissions

Shirley Roberson, Director for
Multicultural Affairs

Sherry Gladney, Director of
Student Financial Aid

Warren E. Cockerham, Registrar

Jacquline Hatcher, Coordinator of
Student Admissions

General Information

The LSU Health Sciences Center in Shreveport (LSUHSC-S) provides education, research, patient care services, and community outreach. Educating health professionals and scientists at all levels, its major responsibility includes the advancement and dissemination of knowledge in medicine and the basic sciences. It also provides vital public service through its hospital and clinics.

Mission Statement

LSUHSC-S has a dual mission: to assure the availability of acute and primary health care services to the uninsured, to the underinsured, and to others with problems of access to medical care, and to serve as the principal site for the clinical education of future doctors and other health care professionals.

Curricular Highlights

Community Service Requirement: Optional. Community service is highly desirable.
Research/Thesis Requirement: Optional. Desirable, but not required.

The modern curriculum thoroughly integrates medical issues and applications in the first two years, during which the basic sciences are emphasized. Recently, didactic lecture hours were cut dramatically, and small-group, active-learning experiences were dramatically increased. The overall effect was decreased contact hours and increased self-directed learning. All essential basic-science concepts

traditionally taught in the first two years are now integrated with clinical examples, clinical cases and standardized patient experiences. The required clerkships occur in the third year, and the fourth year is devoted to electives.

USMLE

Step 1: Required. Students must record a passing score for promotion.
Step 2: Clinical Skills (CS): Required. Students must only record a score.
Step 2: Clinical Knowledge (CK): Required. Students must only record a score.

Selection Factors

Admission is based upon character, motivation, intellectual ability, and achievement as judged by recommendations of premedical advisors, personal interviews with members of the faculty at the School of Medicine, college grades, and MCAT scores. In recent years, the number of applications filed by well-qualified residents of Louisiana has exceeded the number of places available. For this reason, places have not been offered to nonresidents. Determination of state residence is determined by LSU system regulations. Thirty colleges are represented in the 2008 entering class. The School of Medicine in Shreveport does not discriminate in applicant selection on the basis of race, sex, creed, national origin, age, or handicap.

Financial Aid

Scholarships and long-term, low-interest loan funds are available to students with financial need. In the past, no accepted students have been unable to meet their financial needs. Scholarships and loans are available to students in all four years and are based on applicants' showing verified need. Certain awards are given in recognition primarily of academic accomplishment and promise. The school offers summer employment to many students, but does not advise employment during school sessions, which would interfere with academic performance. Financial need has no bearing on an applicant's acceptance. Applications for financial assistance are furnished by the Financial Aid Office after applicants have been accepted.

Information about Diversity Programs

Applications from students from groups underrepresented in medicine are encouraged and will be given every consideration. All students are encouraged to take advantage of the services provided by the Office of Multicultural Affairs. They include a pre-matriculation program, an MCAT preparation course, and a summer research program for high school students, as well as informal counseling for medical students and applicants.

Campus Information

Setting

The medical school is located near the intersection of I-49 and I-20, in a peaceful neighborhood near the geographic center of Shreveport. Thus, affordable housing is available within a short commute.

Enrollment

For 2008, total enrollment was: 556

Special Features

The hospital includes an ACS-verified Adult Level-One Trauma Center, a Level-One Pediatric Trauma Center and a Pediatric ICU, as well as all features of a tertiary care hospital.

Housing

On-campus housing is not offered; however, safe affordable housing is abundantly available within a short commuting distance.

Satellite Campuses/Facilities

The school is affiliated with other local and regional hospitals.

Application Process and Requirements 2010–2011

Primary Application Service: AMCAS
Earliest filing date: June 1, 2009
Latest filing date: November 1, 2009

Secondary Application Required?: Yes
Sent to: All Louisiana applicants
URL: Provided by school
Student Admissions, (318) 675-5190,
shvadm@lsuhsc.edu
Fee: Yes, $50
Fee waiver available: Yes
Earliest filing date: June 1, 2009
Latest filing date: December 15, 2009

MCAT® required?: Yes
Latest MCAT® considered: September 2009
Oldest MCAT® considered: August 2006

Early Decision Program: School does have EDP
Applicants notified: October 1, 2009
EDP available for: Residents only

Regular Acceptance Notice
Earliest date: October 17, 2009
Latest date: Until class is full
Applicant's Response to Acceptance
Offer – Maximum Time: Two weeks

Requests for Deferred
Entrance Considered: Yes

Deposit to Hold Place in Class: Yes
Deposit (Resident): $250
Deposit (Non-resident): $250
Deposit due: May 15, 2010
Applied to tuition: Yes
Deposit refundable: Yes
Refundable by: May 15, 2010

Estimated number of new entrants: 118
EDP: 12, special program: n/a

Start Month/Year: July 30, 2010

Interview Format: Two closed file and one open file, non-stress interviews. Regional interviews are not available.

Other Programs

PREPARATORY PROGRAMS
Postbaccalaureate Program: No
Summer Program: Yes, www.sh.lsuhsc.edu/multicultural/front.htm
Shirley Roberson, (318) 675-5049,
srober1@lsuhsc.edu

COMBINED DEGREE PROGRAMS
Baccalaureate/M.D.: No
M.D./M.P.H.: No
M.D./M.B.A.: No
M.D./J.D.: No
M.D./Ph.D.: Yes, www.admissions.lsuhsc.edu

Premedical Coursework

Course	Req.	Rec.	Lab.	Hrs.
Inorganic Chemistry	•		•	8
Behavioral Sciences				
Biochemistry		•		6
Biology				
Biology/Zoology	•		•	8
Calculus				
College English	•			6
College Mathematics				

Course	Req.	Rec.	Lab.	Hrs.
Computer Science				
Genetics		•		6
Humanities				
Organic Chemistry	•		•	8
Physics	•		•	8
Psychology				
Social Sciences				
Other Science			•	6

Selection Factors: 2008 Accepted Applicants

Proportion of Accepted Applicants with Relevant Experience (Data Self-Reported to AMCAS®)		
Community Service/Volunteer		68%
Medically-Related Work		80%
Research		63%

Shaded bar represents school's accepted scores ranging from the 10th percentile to the 90th percentile   School Median ●   National Median ●

Overall GPA	2.0	2.1	2.2	2.3	2.4	2.5	2.6	2.7	2.8	2.9	3.0	3.1	3.2	3.3	3.4	3.5	3.6	3.7	(3.8)	3.9	4.0
Science GPA	2.0	2.1	2.2	2.3	2.4	2.5	2.6	2.7	2.8	2.9	3.0	3.1	3.2	3.3	3.4	3.5	3.6	3.7	(3.8)	3.9	4.0

MCAT® Total Numeric Score 9 10 11 12 13 14 15 16 17 18 19 20 21 22 23 24 25 26 27 28 (29) 30 31 (32) 33 34 35 36 37 38 39 40 41 42 43

Writing Sample				J	K	L	M	N	(O)	P	(Q)	R	S	T
Verbal Reasoning	3	4	5	6	7	8	(9)	(10)	11	12	13	14	15
Biological Sciences	3	4	5	6	7	8	9	(10)	(11)	12	13	14	15
Physical Sciences	3	4	5	6	7	8	9	(10)	(11)	12	13	14	15

Acceptance & Matriculation Data for 2008–2009 First Year Class

	Resident	Non-resident	International	Total
Applications	570	132	1	703
Interviewed	234	1	0	235
Deferred	1	0	0	1
Matriculants				
Early Assurance Program	n/a	n/a	n/a	n/a
Early Decision Program	16	0	0	16
Baccalaureate/M.D.	n/a	n/a	n/a	n/a
M.D./Ph.D.	0	0	0	0
Matriculated	116	0	0	**116**

Applications accepted from International Applicants: No

Specialty Choice

2004, 2005, 2006 Graduates, Specialty Choice (As reported by program directors to GME Track™)	
Anesthesiology	4%
Emergency Medicine	7%
Family Practice	11%
Internal Medicine	13%
Obstetrics/Gynecology	7%
Orthopaedic Surgery	3%
Pediatrics	7%
Psychiatry	2%
Radiology	5%
Surgery	10%

Matriculant Demographics: 2008–2009 First Year Class

Men: 61   **Women:** 55

Matriculants' Self-Reported Race/Ethnicity

Mexican American	1	Korean	0
Cuban	1	Vietnamese	1
Puerto Rican	0	Other Asian	1
Other Hispanic	0	Total Asian	8
Total Hispanic	2	Native American	2
Chinese	1	Black	3
Asian Indian	4	Native Hawaiian	0
Pakistani	0	White	102
Filipino	1	Unduplicated Number	
Japanese	0	of Matriculants	116

Science and Math Majors: 88%
Matriculants with:
Baccalaureate degree: 99%
Graduate degree(s): 6%

Financial Information

Source: 2007–2008 LCME I-B survey and 2008–2009 AAMC TSF questionnaire

	Residents	Non-residents
Total Cost of Attendance	$35,107	$49,255
Tuition and Fees	$10,461	$24,609
Other (includes living expenses)	$23,064	$23,064
Health Insurance (can be waived)	$1,582	$1,582

Average 2008 Graduate Indebtedness: $119,207
% of Enrolled Students Receiving Aid: 87%

Criminal Background Check

This medical school requires a criminal background check prior to matriculation.

Tulane University School of Medicine

New Orleans, Louisiana

Office of Admissions and Student Affairs
Tulane University School of Medicine
1430 Tulane Avenue, SL67
New Orleans, Louisiana 70112-2699
T 504 988 5187 **F** 504 988 6462

Admissions www.mcl.tulane.edu/admissions
Main www.mcl.tulane.edu
Financial www.finaidhsc.tulane.edu
E-mail medsch@tulane.edu

Private Institution

Dr. Benjamin Sachs, Dean

Dr. Marc J. Kahn, Senior Associate Dean for Admissions and Student Affairs

Dr. Ernest Steed, Assistant Dean for Student Affairs

Dr. Barbara S. Beckman, Associate Dean for Admissions

Michael T. Goodman, Director of Financial Aid

General Information

Tulane University School of Medicine, a private, nonsectarian institution, was founded in 1834. Today it is one of the eleven colleges comprising Tulane University and is the 15th oldest medical school in the United States.

Mission Statement

Tulane has a rich tradition of education characterized by an environment that is both supportive and enriching in every sense. It strives to present the ideal environment for preparing students to be expert and compassionate clinicians.

Curricular Highlights

Community Service Requirement: Required.
Research/Thesis Requirement: Optional.

Tulane School of Medicine offers a four-year program leading to the M.D. degree. While the emphasis in the first two years is on the principles of the basic medical sciences, the goal of the first two years is helping students develop clinical problem-solving skills instead of emphasizing the transmission of facts devoid of clinical context. The program in Foundations in Medicine, which spans the first two years, is responsible for instructing students in the complex art and science of the patient-doctor interaction. This objective is accomplished through lectures, small-group discussions, clinical demonstrations, visits to community health facilities, and interactions with both real patients and individuals trained as patient instructors. The third and fourth years provide experience in clinical settings where the emphasis is on patient care and community health. Flexibility is attained throughout the four years by designating approximately one-

third of scheduled curriculum time for elective courses and selected advanced studies. The curriculum is under constant review by faculty and students. Tulane offers a wide variety of support systems for medical students, including test-taking skills workshops.

USMLE

Step 1: Required. Students must only record a score.
Step 2: Clinical Skills (CS): Required. Students must record a passing total score to graduate.
Step 2: Clinical Knowledge (CK): Required. Students must record a passing total score to graduate.

Selection Factors

In evaluating applicants, the Committee on Admissions relies on such criteria as grade point averages, MCAT scores, faculty appraisals from the applicant's college, special accomplishments and talents, and the substance and level of courses taken in a particular college. Tulane has not established mandatory minimal MCAT or GPA scores, as all components of the application, cognitive and non-cognitive, are taken into account.

Financial Aid

Scholarships and loans (federal, private, and Tulane programs) are available to students based on an analysis of the individual's financial needs. Additionally, each year approximately 25 students are awarded scholarships, which are based exclusively upon academic merit.

Information about Diversity Programs

Tulane encourages qualified disadvantaged students and students from groups underrepresented in medicine to apply. Special activities available for, but not limited to, students from groups underrepresented in medicine include tutorial and counseling services for students in medical school. The diversity in composition of the members of the Committee on Admissions is reflected in the composition of the medical student body.

Campus Information

Setting
Tulane University School of Medicine is located in downtown New Orleans, a few blocks from the New Orleans Superdome and the French Quarter.

Enrollment
For 2008, total enrollment was: 661

Special Features
The School of Medicine and the Tulane University Hospital and Clinic are two components of the Tulane University Health Sciences Center. Other components of the Center include: the School of Public Health and Tropical Medicine, the Tulane/Xavier Center for Bioenvironmental Research, the Tulane National Primate Research Center, and the F. Edward Hebert Research Center. Twelve Centers of Excellence include the Depaul-Tulane Behavioral Health Center, Tulane Cancer Center, Tulane Center for Abdominal Transplant, Tulane Institute of Sports Medicine, Tulane-Xavier National Women's Center, Tulane Center for Gene Therapy, and Tulane Cardio-Vascular Center of Excellence.

Housing
Reasonably priced housing of all kinds is widely available, including the Deming Pavilion student residence, which is adjacent to the Tulane University Hospital and Clinic and across the street from the medical school.

Satellite Campuses/Facilities
Tulane School of Medicine has affiliation agreements with more than 10 hospitals and clinics in New Orleans and other communities; four of its principal clinical teaching facilities are in close proximity to the School of Medicine: the Medical Center of Louisiana in New Orleans (Charity Hospitals), University Hospital (a Charity Hospital), Veterans Affairs Medical Center, and the Tulane University Hospital and Clinic.

Application Process and Requirements 2010–2011

Primary Application Service: AMCAS
Earliest filing date: June 1, 2009
Latest filing date: December 15, 2009

Secondary Application Required?: Yes
Sent to: All applicants
URL: www.som.tulane.edu/departments/admissions/ Secondary_App/Tulane_Secondary_App.pdf
Fee: Yes, $100
Fee waiver available: No
Earliest filing date: June 1, 2009
Latest filing date: January 15, 2010

MCAT® required?: Yes
Latest MCAT® considered: August 2009
Oldest MCAT® considered: 2004

Early Decision Program: School does have EDP
Applicants notified: October 15, 2009
EDP available for: Both Residents and Non-residents

Regular Acceptance Notice
Earliest date: October 16, 2009
Latest date: Until class is full
Applicant's Response to Acceptance Offer – Maximum Time: Two weeks

Requests for Deferred Entrance Considered: Yes

Deposit to Hold Place in Class: Yes
Deposit (Resident): $500
Deposit (Non-resident): $500
Deposit due: May 15, 2009
Applied to tuition: Yes
Deposit refundable: Yes
Refundable by: May 15, 2010

Estimated number of new entrants: 177
EDP: 10, special program: n/a

Start Month/Year: August 2010

Interview Format: Selected applicants are invited for interviews. Regional interviews are not available.

Other Programs

PREPARATORY PROGRAMS
Postbaccalaureate Program: Yes, www.som.tulane.edu/anatomy/scb/acpinfo.htm
Summer Program: No
Master of Science in Pharmacology: www.pharmacology.tulane.edu
Master of Science in Genetics: www.som.tulane.edu/human_genetics/masters.html

COMBINED DEGREE PROGRAMS
Baccalaureate/M.D.: No
M.D./M.P.H.: Yes, www.mdmph.tulane.edu
M.D./M.B.A.: Yes, Marc Kahn, M.D., (504) 988-6735, mkahn@tulane.edu
M.D./J.D.: No
M.D./Ph.D.: Yes, www.som.tulane.edu/psp
James E. Robinson, M.D., (504) 988-5422, jrobinso@tulane.edu

Premedical Coursework

Course	Req.	Rec.	Lab.	Hrs.
Inorganic Chemistry	•		•	6
Behavioral Sciences				
Biochemistry				
Biology				
Biology/Zoology	•		•	6
Calculus				
College English	•			6
College Mathematics				

Course	Req.	Rec.	Lab.	Hrs.
Computer Science				
Genetics				
Humanities				
Organic Chemistry	•		•	6
Physics	•		•	6
Psychology				
Social Sciences				
Other				

Selection Factors: 2008 Accepted Applicants

Proportion of Accepted Applicants with Relevant Experience (Data Self-Reported to AMCAS®)		
Community Service/Volunteer		75%
Medically-Related Work		86%
Research		77%

Shaded bar represents school's accepted scores ranging from the 10th percentile to the 90th percentile   **School Median** ○   **National Median** ○

Overall GPA	2.0	2.1	2.2	2.3	2.4	2.5	2.6	2.7	2.8	2.9	3.0	3.1	3.2	3.3	3.4	3.5	③.6	3.7	3.8	3.9	4.0
Science GPA	2.0	2.1	2.2	2.3	2.4	2.5	2.6	2.7	2.8	2.9	3.0	3.1	3.2	3.3	3.4	③.5	3.6	3.7	3.8	3.9	4.0

MCAT® Total Numeric Score 9 10 11 12 13 14 15 16 17 18 19 20 21 22 23 24 25 26 27 28 29 30 ㉛ ㉜ 33 34 35 36 37 38 39 40 41 42 43

Writing Sample			J	K	L	M	N	O	P	Ⓠ	R	S	T
Verbal Reasoning	3	4	5	6	7	8	9	⑩	11	12	13	14	15
Biological Sciences	3	4	5	6	7	8	9	10	⑪	12	13	14	15
Physical Sciences	3	4	5	6	7	8	9	⑩	⑪	12	13	14	15

Acceptance & Matriculation Data for 2008–2009 First Year Class

	Resident	Non-resident	International	Total
Applications	437	7564	306	8307
Interviewed	63	553	5	621
Deferred	2	4	0	6
Matriculants				
Early Assurance Program	7	0	0	7
Early Decision Program	2	15	0	17
Baccalaureate/M.D.	n/a	n/a	n/a	n/a
M.D./Ph.D.	3	19	0	22
Matriculated	27	150	1	**178**

Applications accepted from International Applicants: Yes

Specialty Choice

2004, 2005, 2006 Graduates, Specialty Choice (As reported by program directors to GME Track™)

Anesthesiology	4%
Emergency Medicine	7%
Family Practice	8%
Internal Medicine	17%
Obstetrics/Gynecology	5%
Orthopaedic Surgery	5%
Pediatrics	8%
Psychiatry	5%
Radiology	5%
Surgery	6%

Matriculant Demographics: 2008–2009 First Year Class

Men: 97   **Women:** 81

Matriculants' Self-Reported Race/Ethnicity

Mexican American	0	Korean	3
Cuban	1	Vietnamese	1
Puerto Rican	0	Other Asian	4
Other Hispanic	2	Total Asian	34
Total Hispanic	3	Native American	0
Chinese	9	Black	2
Asian Indian	10	Native Hawaiian	0
Pakistani	1	White	141
Filipino	7	Unduplicated Number	
Japanese	1	of Matriculants	178

Science and Math Majors: 62%
Matriculants with:
Baccalaureate degree: 100%
Graduate degree(s): 30%

Financial Information

Source: 2007–2008 LCME I-B survey and 2008–2009 AAMC TSF questionnaire

	Residents	Non-residents
Total Cost of Attendance	$70,535	$70,535
Tuition and Fees	$47,234	$47,234
Other (includes living expenses)	$21,408	$21,408
Health Insurance (can be waived)	$1,893	$1,893

Average 2008 Graduate Indebtedness: $180,712
% of Enrolled Students Receiving Aid: 84%

Criminal Background Check

This medical school does not require a criminal background check prior to matriculation.

Johns Hopkins University School of Medicine

Baltimore, Maryland

Committee on Admissions
Johns Hopkins University School of Medicine
733 North Broadway, Suite G-49
Baltimore, Maryland 21205
T 410 955 3182   **F** 410 955 7494

Admissions www.hopkinsmedicine.org/admissions
Main www.hopkinsmedicine.org/som
Financial www.hopkinsmedicine.org/ admissions/afford.html
E-mail somadmiss@jhmi.edu

Private Institution

Dr. Edward D. Miller, Dean and Chief Executive Officer

Dr. James L. Weiss, Associate Dean for Admissions

Dr. Thomas Koenig, Associate Dean for Student Affairs

Dr. Daniel H. Teraguchi, Assistant Dean for Student Affairs

Hermione M. Hicks, Assistant Dean for Admissions

Terra Jones, Director, Financial Aid

General Information

Johns Hopkins University School of Medicine, founded in 1893, is a private, nondenominational institution which fosters the training of medical practitioners, teachers, and biomedical scientists. The medical center provides library facilities, the Reed Residence Hall, off-campus housing assistance, cafeterias, recreational sports in the Cooley Center, and performing arts programs. Preclinical courses are given in the adjacent basic science complex. Medical care facilities such as the Johns Hopkins Hospital and the Outpatient Center provide an extensive and diverse patient base for the teaching of all clinical subjects. Students also attend educational programs conducted at community hospitals in Baltimore and pursue elective experiences at other medical schools in the U.S. and foreign countries.

Mission Statement

The Johns Hopkins University School of Medicine is dedicated to preparing students to practice compassionate medicine of the highest standards and to contributing to the advancement of medical knowledge.

Curricular Highlights

Community Service Requirement: Optional.
Research/Thesis Requirement: Encouraged. Exceptional research opportunities are available.

The curriculum provides sound foundations in basic sciences and clinical medicine while retaining the flexibility required for students to identify and develop diverse career interests. All students receive honors, high pass, pass or fail grades in lieu of letter grades. The M.D.

program includes the integration of basic sciences and clinical experiences and the expanded use of case-based, small-group learning sessions. Students learn the medical interview and basic physical examination in the first months of medical school, and working with community physicians practices through years 1 and 2. For more information, see *www.hopkinsmedicine.org*. First-year includes integrated coverage of introductory basic sciences, neuroscience, epidemiology, and introduction to clinical medicine. Second-year includes the study of advanced basic sciences, behavioral sciences, clinical skills, and beginning clerkships. In the third and fourth-years, with the assistance of faculty advisors, students develop individualized programs incorporating required clerkships in major clinical areas and electives. Students may use electives for specialized clerkships, research, and public health experiences.

USMLE

Step 1: Required. Students must only record a score.
Step 2: Clinical Skills (CS): Required. Students must only record a score.
Step 2: Clinical Knowledge (CK): Required. Students must only record a score.

Selection Factors

A Bachelor's degree is required in addition to proven academic competence, previous achievements and activities help the Committee on Admissions to evaluate applicants' suitability for medicine. Applicants who have unusual talents, strong humanistic qualities, demonstrated leadership, and creative abilities are sought. There are no residency requirements for U.S. citizens. Applications are encouraged from international students. Students matriculating at Hopkins are required to undergo a criminal background check. Due to space limitations, Hopkins does not admit transfer students. JHU complies with federal and state laws prohibiting discrimination.

Financial Aid

Financial aid in the form of federal and institutional grants and loans is awarded solely on the basis of need. Financial considerations do not influence admission decisions. Parents' financial information is required of all students

requesting institutional aid. Students' awards fully meet their demonstrated financial need. The cost for living expenses is based on a 12-month budget. Student fellowship stipends are frequently available for projects carried out in summers. Non-U.S. citizens without permanent resident or immigrant visa status are not eligible to receive financial aid. International students must establish an escrow account currently in the amount of $270,000 and subject to change.

Information about Diversity Programs

Johns Hopkins is committed to enrolling a diverse student population with a passion for improving health locally and on a global scale. Hopkins' priorities include enhancing the cultural competencies of all its medical students to reduce health disparities. Hopkins has an excellent record of enrolling high quality students from disadvantaged backgrounds and who are underrepresented in medicine. Contact the Assistant Dean for Student Affairs for more information.

Campus Information

Setting

The School of Medicine is located in east Baltimore, 20 minutes by car from the undergraduate campus and a short walk from the Inner Harbor. The medical campus includes the Schools of Public Health, Nursing, and Johns Hopkins Hospital. The 44-acre campus is accessible by subway and a free Hopkins'shuttle provided to students and faculty.

Enrollment

For 2008, total enrollment was: 460

Housing

Students may live in Reed Hall, the primary residence for the School of Medicine. Students also live throughout Baltimore, where rental costs can be relatively low.

Regional/Satellite Campuses

In addition to the Johns Hopkins Hospital, students may also serve their clinical rotations at the Bayview Medical Center, located three miles from the main medical campus.

Application Process and Requirements 2010–2011

Primary Application Service: AMCAS
Earliest filing date: June 1, 2009
Latest filing date: October 15, 2009

Secondary Application Required?: Yes
Sent to: All applicants
URL: www.hopkinsmedicine.org/admissions
Fee: Yes, $80
Fee waiver available: Yes
Earliest filing date: June 1, 2009
Latest filing date: December 1, 2009

MCAT® required?: Yes
Latest MCAT® considered: September 2009
Oldest MCAT® considered: 2006

Early Decision Program: School does have EDP
Applicants notified: October 1, 2009
EDP available for: Both Residents
and Non-residents

Regular Acceptance Notice
Earliest date: October 15, 2009
Latest date: Varies
Applicant's Response to Acceptance
Offer – Maximum Time: Three weeks

Requests for Deferred
Entrance Considered: Yes

Deposit to Hold Place in Class: No
Deposit (Resident): n/a
Deposit (Non-resident): n/a
Deposit due: n/a
Applied to tuition: n/a
Deposit refundable: n/a
Refundable by: n/a

Estimated number of new entrants: 120
EDP: 0, special program: n/a

Start Month/Year: August 2010

Interview Format: Interviews are one-one-one.
Regional interview available in limited areas.

Other Programs

PREPARATORY PROGRAMS
Postbaccalaureate Program: Yes,
www.jhu.edu/postbac/
Summer Program: No

COMBINED DEGREE PROGRAMS
Baccalaureate/M.D.: No
M.D./M.P.H.: No
M.D./M.B.A.: No
M.D./J.D.: No
M.D./Ph.D.: Yes, www.hopkinsmedicine.org/
admissions/dualdegree.html, Sharon Welling,
(410) 955-8543, swellin1@jhmi.edu

Premedical Coursework

Course	Req.	Rec.	Lab.	Qtrs.
Inorganic Chemistry	•		•	8
Behavioral Sciences				
Biochemistry				
Biology	•		•	8
Biology/Zoology				
Calculus	•			6
College English				
College Mathematics				

Course	Req.	Rec.	Lab.	Qtrs.
Computer Science		•		
Genetics				
Humanities				
Organic Chemistry	•		•	8
Physics	•		•	8
Psychology				
Social Sciences				
Humanities or Social & Behavioral Sciences	•			24

Selection Factors: 2008 Accepted Applicants

Proportion of Accepted Applicants with Relevant Experience (Data Self-Reported to AMCAS®)		
Community Service/Volunteer		75%
Medically-Related Work		88%
Research		95%

Shaded bar represents school's accepted scores ranging from the 10th percentile to the 90th percentile. School Median ● National Median ●

Overall GPA	2.0	2.1	2.2	2.3	2.4	2.5	2.6	2.7	2.8	2.9	3.0	3.1	3.2	3.3	3.4	3.5	3.6	3.7	3.8	(3.9)	4.0
Science GPA	2.0	2.1	2.2	2.3	2.4	2.5	2.6	2.7	2.8	2.9	3.0	3.1	3.2	3.3	3.4	3.5	3.6	3.7	3.8	(3.9)	4.0

MCAT® Total Numeric Score 9 10 11 12 13 14 15 16 17 18 19 20 21 22 23 24 25 26 27 28 29 30 31 (32) 33 34 35 (36) 37 38 39 40 41 42 43

Writing Sample				J	K	L	M	N	O	P	(Q)	(R)	S	T
Verbal Reasoning	3	4	5	6	7	8	9	(10)	(11)	12	13	14	15
Biological Sciences	3	4	5	6	7	8	9	10	(11)	(12)	13	14	15
Physical Sciences	3	4	5	6	7	8	9	10	(11)	12	(13)	14	15

Acceptance & Matriculation Data for 2008–2009 First Year Class

	Resident	Non-resident	International	Total
Applications	372	5374	343	6089
Interviewed	80	625	53	758
Deferred	3	8	0	11
Matriculants				
Early Assurance Program	n/a	n/a	n/a	n/a
Early Decision Program	0	0	0	0
Baccalaureate/M.D.	n/a	n/a	n/a	n/a
M.D./Ph.D.	0	8	0	8
Matriculated	18	93	7	**118**

Applications accepted from International Applicants: Yes

Specialty Choice

2004, 2005, 2006 Graduates, Specialty Choice (As reported by program directors to GME Track™)	
Anesthesiology	3%
Emergency Medicine	6%
Family Practice	2%
Internal Medicine	20%
Obstetrics/Gynecology	1%
Orthopaedic Surgery	5%
Pediatrics	11%
Psychiatry	2%
Radiology	7%
Surgery	6%

Matriculant Demographics: 2008–2009 First Year Class

Men: 59 **Women:** 59

Matriculants' Self-Reported Race/Ethnicity

Mexican American	1	Korean	3
Cuban	0	Vietnamese	2
Puerto Rican	1	Other Asian	2
Other Hispanic	4	Total Asian	31
Total Hispanic	5	Native American	1
Chinese	14	Black	7
Asian Indian	10	Native Hawaiian	1
Pakistani	1	White	70
Filipino	0	Unduplicated Number	
Japanese	0	of Matriculants	118

Science and Math Majors: 67%
Matriculants with:
 Baccalaureate degree: 100%
 Graduate degree(s): 10%

Financial Information

Source: 2007–2008 LCME I-B survey
and 2008–2009 AAMC TSF questionnaire

	Residents	Non-residents
Total Cost of Attendance	$57,911	$57,911
Tuition and Fees	$39,108	$39,108
Other (includes living expenses)	$16,151	$16,151
Health Insurance (cannot be waived)	$2,652	$2,652

Average 2008 Graduate Indebtedness: $96,614
% of Enrolled Students Receiving Aid: 88%

Criminal Background Check

This medical school requires a criminal background check prior to matriculation.

Uniformed Services University of the Health Sciences F. Edward Hébert School of Medicine

Bethesda, Maryland

Admissions Office, Room A-1041
Uniformed Services University of the Health
Sciences F. Edward Hébert School of Medicine
4301 Jones Bridge Road
Bethesda, Maryland 20814-4799
T 301 295 3101   **F** 301 295 3545

Admissions www.usuhs.mil/admissions.html
Main www.usuhs.mil
Financial n/a
E-mail admissions@usuhs.mil

Public Institution

Dr. Larry W. Laughlin, M.D., Ph.D., Dean

Dr. Margaret Calloway, M.D., CDR, MC, USN, Associate Dean for Recruitment and Admissions

Dr. Cynthia I. Macri, M.D., CAPT, MC, USN, Vice President for Recruitment and Diversity

Joan C. Stearman, M.S.W., Director, Office of Admissions

General Information

Created by public law in 1972, the Uniformed Services University of the Health Sciences (USUHS) was founded to prepare young men and women for careers as health care professionals in the uniformed services. The school's charter is to provide a comprehensive education in medicine and to select individuals who demonstrate potential for and commitment to careers as medical officers in the uniformed services.

Mission Statement

USUHS is the nation's federal health sciences university and is committed to excellence in military medicine and public health during peace and war. Our mission is to provide the nation with health professionals dedicated to career service in the Department of Defense and the United States Public Health Service and with scientists who serve the common good.

Curricular Highlights

Community Service Requirement: Optional.
Research/Thesis Requirement: Optional.

The school has a four-year program culminating in the doctor of medicine degree. Basic science instruction predominates in the initial two academic years, with the final two years devoted to clinical education. Basic science instruction is correlated both interdisciplinarily and clinically. The integration between the clinical and basic sciences is progressive and proceeds with involvement in patient care activities early in the curriculum, starting with the first semester of the first year. The overall program is designed to educate students to serve as providers of primary health care. The curriculum also includes basic military orientation and concentration on unique aspects of military medicine. A conventional letter grading system is used.

USMLE

Step 1: Required. Students must record a passing score for graduation, but not promotion.
Step 2: Clinical Skills (CS): Required. Students must record a passing total score to graduate.
Step 2: Clinical Knowledge (CK): Required. Students must record a passing total score to graduate.

Selection Factors

The school employs a three-stage, progressive screening process for selecting entrants. The first stage consists of the submission of an AMCAS application; the second, the submission of supplementary materials; and the third, personal interviews, which are conducted at the campus. Advancement in the process is competitive, based on candidates' personal and intellectual characteristics. The Committee on Admissions does not discriminate on the basis of sex, race, religion, marital status, or national origin.

Financial Aid

Upon entering the first-year class of the School of Medicine, a student will be commissioned and serve on active duty in the grade of Second Lieutenant in either the Army or Air Force or an Ensign in the Navy or Public Health Service, receiving the pay and benefits of that grade. The time spent in medical school is not creditable toward retirement until retirement eligibility has been established. At graduation, students are promoted to Captain in the Air Force or Army or Lieutenant in the Navy and PHS upon receipt of the M.D. degree. Graduates are obligated to serve on active duty as medical officers for not less than seven years, as well as six years inactive ready reserve. The period of time spent in internship or residency training is not acceptable toward satisfying this seven-year obligation. A student who is dropped from the program for any reason may be required to perform active duty for a period of time equal to the time spent in the program. A disenrolled student may also be required to reimburse the government for tuition and fees. However, one year will be the minimum required active duty for persons separated from the school, regardless of the time spent in the program.

Information about Diversity Programs

The Office of Recruitment and Diversity provides a welcoming environment to all students by promoting and encouraging expression of their diverse ethnic, cultural, economic, and experiential backgrounds. Competitive applicants from groups underrepresented in medicine are actively encouraged to apply. The application and admissions processes are the same for all students. The staff supports all students throughout the four years of medical school, recognizing that each individual's unique circumstances may require various levels of support and encouragement. The learning environment is enhanced by the four major student-sponsored groups: Women in Medicine and Science, the Asian Pacific American Medical Student Association, the Latino Medical Student Association, and the Student National Medical Association. Faculty support is provided by the Office of Recruitment and Diversity to advance the community outreach efforts of these student groups.

Campus Information

Setting
Our university is located just outside the nation's capital, within walking distance of the NIH and the National Library of Medicine. We are located near public transportation, shopping, dining, national parks and recreational facilities.

Enrollment
For 2008, total enrollment was: 672

Special Features
The University's nationally ranked military and civilian faculty conduct cutting edge research in the biomedical sciences, combat casualty care and infectious diseases.

Housing
As on-campus housing is not available, students are provided a non-taxable housing allowance.

Application Process and Requirements 2010–2011

Primary Application Service: AMCAS
Earliest filing date: June 1, 2009
Latest filing date: November 15, 2009

Secondary Application Required?: Yes
Sent to: All applicants
Contact: (301) 295-3101, admissions@usuhs.mil
Fee: No
Fee waiver available: n/a
Earliest filing date: June 1, 2009
Latest filing date: December 15, 2009

MCAT® required?: Yes
Latest MCAT® considered: September 2009
Oldest MCAT® considered: April 2007

Early Decision Program: School does not have EDP

COMBINED DEGREE PROGRAMS
Baccalaureate/M.D.: No
M.D./M.P.H.: No
M.D./M.B.A.: No
M.D./J.D.: No
M.D./Ph.D.: Yes,
http://cim.usuhs.mil/geo/mdphd.htm

Premedical Coursework

Course	Req.	Rec.	Lab.	Hrs.
Inorganic Chemistry	•		•	8
Behavioral Sciences				
Biochemistry				
Biology	•		•	8
Biology/Zoology				
Calculus	•			3
College English	•			6
College Mathematics				

Course	Req.	Rec.	Lab.	Hrs.
Computer Science				
Genetics				
Humanities				
Organic Chemistry	•		•	8
Physics	•		•	8
Psychology				
Social Sciences				
Other				

Selection Factors: 2008 Accepted Applicants

Proportion of Accepted Applicants with Relevant Experience (Data Self-Reported to AMCAS)	
Community Service/Volunteer	66%
Medically-Related Work	79%
Research	62%

Shaded bar represents school's accepted scores ranging from the tile to the 90th percentile. School Median ● National Median ●

GPA 2.0 2.1 2.2 2.3 2.4 2.5 2.6 2.7 2.8 2.9 3.0 3.1 **3.2 3.3 3.4 3.5 (3.6)** 3.7 3.8 3.9 4.0
PA 2.0 2.1 2.2 2.3 2.4 2.5 2.6 2.7 2.8 2.9 3.0 **3.1 3.2 3.3 3.4 (3.5)** 3.6 3.7 3.8 3.9 4.0

Total Numeric Score 9 10 11 12 13 14 15 16 17 18 19 20 21 22 23 24 25 26 **27 28 29 (30) 31 (32) 33** 34 35 36 37 38 39 40 41 42 43

				J	K	L	M	N	O	(P)	(Q)	R	S	T
ample														
asoning	3	4	5	6	7	**8**	**9**	**(10)**	11	12	13	14	15
Sciences	3	4	5	6	7	8	**9**	**(10)**	**(11)**	12	13	14	15
ciences	3	4	5	6	7	8	**9**	**(10)**	**(11)**	12	13	14	15

tance & Matriculation or 2008–2009 ear Class

	Resident	Non-resident	International	Total
ons	115	1827	8	1950
ed	35	535	0	570
	0	3	0	3
ants				
surance Program	n/a	n/a	n/a	n/a
cision Program	0	0	0	0
reate/M.D.	n/a	n/a	n/a	n/a
.D.	0	1	0	1
lated	6	165	0	**171**

ions accepted from International Applicants: No

culant Demographics: –2009 First Year Class

..... .21   **Women:** 50

Matriculants' Self-Reported Race/Ethnicity

Mexican American	2	**Korean**	6
Cuban	2	**Vietnamese**	2
Puerto Rican	3	**Other Asian**	3
Other Hispanic	6	**Total Asian**	22
Total Hispanic	13	**Native American**	1
Chinese	7	**Black**	3
Asian Indian	1	**Native Hawaiian**	1
Pakistani	0	**White**	144
Filipino	6	**Unduplicated Number**	
Japanese	1	**of Matriculants**	171

Science and Math Majors: 68%
Matriculants with:
  Baccalaureate degree: 100%
  Graduate degree(s): 12%

Specialty Choice

2004, 2005, 2006 Graduates, Specialty Choice (As reported by program directors to GME Track™)	
Anesthesiology	3%
Emergency Medicine	4%
Family Practice	10%
Internal Medicine	6%
Obstetrics/Gynecology	4%
Orthopaedic Surgery	2%
Pediatrics	8%
Psychiatry	4%
Radiology	2%
Surgery	5%

Financial Information

Source: 2007–2008 LCME I-B survey and 2008–2009 AAMC TSF questionnaire

	Residents	Non-residents
Total Cost of Attendance	n/a	n/a
Tuition and Fees	n/a	n/a
Other (includes living expenses)	n/a	n/a
Health Insurance	n/a	n/a

Average 2008 Graduate Indebtedness: n/a
% of Enrolled Students Receiving Aid: n/a

Criminal Background Check

This medical school requires a criminal background check prior to matriculation.

University of Maryland School of Medicine

Baltimore, Maryland

Committee on Admissions, Suite 190
University of Maryland School of Medicine
685 West Baltimore Street
Baltimore, Maryland 21201-1559
T 410 706 7478   **F** 410 706 0467

Admissions www.medschool.umaryland.edu/
admissions
Main www.medschool.umaryland.edu
Financial www.umaryland.edu/fin
E-mail admissions@som.umaryland.edu

Public Institution

Dr. E. Albert Reece, Dean

*Dr. Milford M. Foxwell Jr.,
Associate Dean for Admissions*

Patricia Scott, Director of Financial Aid

*Dr. Donna L. Parker, Associate Dean
for Student Affairs*

General Information

Organized in 1807, The University of Maryland School of Medicine is the nation's oldest public medical college. The first class was graduated in 1810. Among the first to erect its own hospital for clinical instruction, the university also established the first intramural residency for senior students.

Mission Statement

The University of Maryland School of Medicine is dedicated to providing excellence in biomedical education, basic and clinical research, quality patient care, and service to improve the health of the citizens of Maryland and beyond. The School is committed to the education and training of M.D., M.D./M.P.H., M.D./Ph.D., M.D./M.S. in BioEngineering, graduate, physical therapy, and medical research technology students. The school will recruit and develop faculty to serve as exemplary role models for our students.

Curricular Highlights

Community Service Requirement: Optional.
Research/Thesis Requirement: Optional.

During the first two years of medical school the basic sciences are integrated and taught as systems, using interdisciplinary teaching by both basic and clinical science faculty. Mornings include lecture and small group sessions; afternoons are devoted to independent study. Curricular materials are available online and laptop computers are required. "Introduction to Clinical Medicine" begins early in the first year and continues through year two, offering instruction in clinical diagnosis, intimate human behavior, problem-based learning, biomedical ethics and dynamics of ambulatory care. Clinical clerkships during the last two years include a month in family medicine and an

emphasis on ambulatory teaching in other disciplines and two months of subinternship.

USMLE

Step 1: Required. Students must record a passing score for promotion.
Step 2: Clinical Skills (CS): Required. Students must only record a score.
Step 2: Clinical Knowledge (CK): Required. Students must only record a score.

Selection Factors

Applications are accepted from citizens and permanent residents of the U.S. and citizens of Canada. All AMCAS applicants are invited to submit a Stage II application. Selection of students is based on careful appraisal of character, motivation for medicine, academic achievement, MCAT scores, letters of reference, extracurricular activities and interviews. The University does not discriminate on the basis of race, creed, sex, national origin, age or handicap.

Financial Aid

Scholarships and loans are available for students with demonstrable need. The amount of the award may vary according to need and the level of funding available.

Information about Diversity Programs

The School of Medicine values diversity very highly in the educational process and is committed to the recruitment and retention of talented students from underrepresented and disadvantaged backgrounds. A major focus of our recruitment efforts is to provide information on admissions requirements and preparation for medical school, the selection process, and educational and research opportunities at the School of Medicine. There are no fixed quotas for any group and the admissions procedures are the same for all applicants. The Office of Admissions will make a special effort to provide information that is relevant to prospective applicants in these groups. Information can be obtained from Ms. Raushanah Kareem, in the Office of Admissions.

Campus Information

Setting

The professional campus is located in downtown Baltimore within easy walking distance of the

new Hippodrome Theatre, Inner Harbor, Maryland Science Center, National Aquarium and Pier 6 Pavilion. Oriole Park at Camden Yards and M&T Bank Stadium sit adjacent to campus.

Enrollment

For 2008, total enrollment was: 616

Special Features

Built in 1812, the meticulously restored Davidge Hall is the oldest building in North America in continuous use for medical education. The Health Sciences and Human Services Library is the second largest medical library building on the East Coast. Adjacent to the medical center's new Weinberg and Gudelsky clinical towers are the world-renowned Shock Trauma Center, the Baltimore Veterans Administration Medical Center, the University of Maryland Biotechnology Institute and the new UMB Biopark.

Housing

On-campus housing is available at a cost of about $700-1600/month. The new University Suites features furnished apartments plus study lounges, 24-hour security and on-site garage parking. The surrounding neighborhood provides even more choices for students, with both apartments and individual homes (townhomes) available for rent (average $800-1200/month) or purchase. The majority of our students live within walking distance of the campus, particularly during the first two years of medical school.

Satellite Campuses/Facilities

Students complete most of their junior year clinical clerkships at the University of Maryland Medical System and Baltimore Veterans Affairs Medical Center, but do rotate through several of our affiliated community hospitals for selected rotations. During the fourth year of medical school our students will see patients during their ambulatory months at physician's offices in underserved areas of Baltimore City, Western and Southern Maryland and the Eastern Shore.

Application Process and Requirements 2010–2011

Primary Application Service: AMCAS
Earliest filing date: June 1, 2009
Latest filing date: November 1, 2009

Secondary Application Required?: Yes
Sent to: All applicants
Contact: Ms. Tawanda Sykes, (410) 706-7478, tsykes@som.umaryland.edu
Fee: Yes, $70
Fee waiver available: No
Earliest filing date: July 15, 2009
Latest filing date: December 15, 2009

MCAT® required?: Yes
Latest MCAT® considered: September 2009
Oldest MCAT® considered: January 2006

Early Decision Program: School does have EDP
Applicants notified: October 1, 2009
EDP available for: Both Residents and Non-residents

Regular Acceptance Notice
Earliest date: October 15, 2009
Latest date: Until class is full
Applicant's Response to Acceptance Offer – Maximum Time: Three weeks

Requests for Deferred Entrance Considered: Yes

Deposit to Hold Place in Class: No
Deposit (Resident): n/a
Deposit (Non-resident): n/a
Deposit due: n/a
Applied to tuition: n/a
Deposit refundable: n/a
Refundable by: n/a

Estimated number of new entrants: 160
EDP: 5, special program: n/a

Start Month/Year: August 2010

Interview Format: Two, one-on-one interviews with faculty or student. Regional interviews are not available.

Other Programs

PREPARATORY PROGRAMS
Postbaccalaureate Program: No
Summer Program: Yes, Dr. Sandra Dolan, (410) 706-7669, sdolan@clc.umaryland.edu

COMBINED DEGREE PROGRAMS
Baccalaureate/M.D.: No
M.D./M.P.H.: Yes, www.medschool.umaryland.edu/MD_MPH/
Dr. Jordan Warnick, (410) 706-3026, jwarnick@som.umaryland.edu
M.D./M.B.A.: No
M.D./J.D.: No
M.D./Ph.D.: Yes, Nancy Malson, (410) 706-3990, nmalson@som.umaryland.edu
MD/MS BioEngineering and M.D./M.P.P: Yes, Dr. Jordan Warnick, (410) 706-3026, jwarnick@som.umaryland.edu

Premedical Coursework

Course	Req.	Rec.	Lab.	Hrs.
Inorganic Chemistry	•		•	8
Behavioral Sciences				
Biochemistry		•		
Biology				
Biology/Zoology	•		•	8
Calculus				
College English	•			6
College Mathematics				

Course	Req.	Rec.	Lab.	Hrs.
Computer Science		•		
Genetics		•		
Humanities		•		
Organic Chemistry	•		•	8
Physics	•		•	8
Psychology				
Social Sciences				
Other				

Selection Factors: 2008 Accepted Applicants

Proportion of Accepted Applicants with Relevant Experience (Data Self-Reported to AMCAS®)		
Community Service/Volunteer		69%
Medically-Related Work		91%
Research		86%

Shaded bar represents school's accepted scores ranging from the 10th percentile to the 90th percentile. School Median ● National Median ●

Overall GPA 2.0 2.1 2.2 2.3 2.4 2.5 2.6 2.7 2.8 2.9 3.0 3.1 3.2 3.3 3.4 **3.5 3.6 (3.7) 3.8 3.9 4.0**
Science GPA 2.0 2.1 2.2 2.3 2.4 2.5 2.6 2.7 2.8 2.9 3.0 3.1 3.2 **3.3 3.4 3.5 3.6 (3.7) 3.8 3.9 4.0**

MCAT® Total Numeric Score 9 10 11 12 13 14 15 16 17 18 19 20 21 22 23 24 25 26 27 28 29 30 **31 (32) 33 34 35 36 37** 38 39 40 41 42 43

Writing Sample			J	K	L	M	**N O P (Q) R S**			T
Verbal Reasoning	3	4	5	6	7	8	**9 (10) 11 12**	13	14	15
Biological Sciences	3	4	5	6	7	8	**9 10 (11) 12 13**		14	15
Physical Sciences	3	4	5	6	7	8	**9 10 (11) 12 13**		14	15

Acceptance & Matriculation Data for 2008–2009 First Year Class

	Resident	Non-resident	International	Total
Applications	790	3607	187	4584
Interviewed	291	264	7	562
Deferred	5	2	0	7
Matriculants				
Early Assurance Program	0	0	0	0
Early Decision Program	3	0	0	3
Baccalaureate/M.D.	n/a	n/a	n/a	n/a
M.D./Ph.D.	3	3	0	6
Matriculated	117	43	0	**160**

Applications accepted from International Applicants: Only Canadian

Matriculant Demographics: 2008–2009 First Year Class

Men: 70   **Women:** 90

Matriculants' Self-Reported Race/Ethnicity

Mexican American	1	Korean	4
Cuban	1	Vietnamese	1
Puerto Rican	1	Other Asian	5
Other Hispanic	2	Total Asian	35
Total Hispanic	4	Native American	0
Chinese	10	Black	17
Asian Indian	12	Native Hawaiian	0
Pakistani	1	White	102
Filipino	2	Unduplicated Number	
Japanese	1	of Matriculants	160

Science and Math Majors: 68%
Matriculants with:
    Baccalaureate degree: 100%
    Graduate degree(s): 6%

Specialty Choice

2004, 2005, 2006 Graduates Specialty Choices (As reported by program directors to GME Track™)

Anesthesiology	4%
Emergency Medicine	8%
Family Practice	8%
Internal Medicine	23%
Obstetrics/Gynecology	4%
Orthopaedic Surgery	3%
Pediatrics	10%
Psychiatry	3%
Radiology	2%
Surgery	8%

Financial Information

Source: 2007–2008 LCME I-B survey and 2008–2009 AAMC TSF questionnaire

	Residents	Non-residents
Total Cost of Attendance	$53,157	$72,027
Tuition and Fees	$24,249	$43,119
Other (includes living expenses)	$26,736	$26,736
Health Insurance (can be waived)	$2,172	$2,172

Average 2008 Graduate Indebtedness: $138,252
% of Enrolled Students Receiving Aid: 84%

Criminal Background Check

This medical school does not require a criminal background check prior to matriculation.

Boston University School of Medicine

Boston, Massachusetts

Admissions Office, Building L, Rm. 124
Boston University School of Medicine
72 East Concord Street
Boston, Massachusetts 02118
T 617 638 4630 **F** 617 638 4718

Admissions www.bumc.bu.edu/admissions/
Main www.bumc.bu.edu/busm/
Financial www.bumc.bu.edu/osfs
E-mail medadms@bu.edu

Private Institution

Dr. Karen Antman, Dean

Dr. Robert A. Witzburg, Associate Dean and Director of Admissions

Dr. Jonathan Woodson, Associate Dean for Diversity and Multicultural Affairs

Kathy Stavropoulos, Executive Director for Student Financial Services

Dr. Phyllis L. Carr, Associate Dean for Student Affairs

Ellen Difiore, Registrar

General Information

The New England Female Medical College, founded in 1848, was the first medical college for women in the world. In 1873 the college became the Boston University School of Medicine, the first coeducational medical school in the U.S. The current health sciences campus includes the Schools of Medicine, Dental Medicine, and Public Health, as well as the hospital, Boston Medical Center, the Division of Graduate Medical Sciences, and extensive research facilities.

Mission Statement

To educate and train students, physicians, and scientists who will be committed to excellence in the practice of medicine, in biomedical research, and in public health, and who will be prepared for careers in a changing and increasingly diverse society.

Curricular Highlights

Community Service Requirement: Optional. Many students and faculty participate.
Research/Thesis Requirement: Optional. Thesis may be required for dual degree programs.

BUSM offers a flexible program of critical inquiry and rigorous study in the biological, social, and behavioral sciences. The first-year focus is on normal structure and function, unified by Integrated Problems, a problem-based, clinically focused seminar. Introduction to Clinical Medicine has students interviewing and evaluating patients beginning in the first week of school. The basic sciences are linked with applications in clinical practice, emphasizing

multidisciplinary, team-based learning. The second-year focus is on pathophysiology, with an integrated, multidisciplinary format led by basic science and clinical faculty. The core clinical training of the third year includes clerkships in all the major disciplines, with ambulatory and inpatient experience in generalist and subspecialty venues. There is also opportunity for clinical electives. The fourth year includes advanced clerkships and is largely elective. Research opportunities are available in basic science and clinical disciplines, and students may pursue electives in international health. Any academic year may be spread over two calendar years and students may pursue any of several dual degree programs.

USMLE

Step 1: Required. Students must record a passing score for promotion.
Step 2: Clinical Skills (CS): Required. Students must only record a score.
Step 2: Clinical Knowledge (CK): Required. Students must only record a score.

Selection Factors

Applicants are selected not only on the basis of academic record, recommendations, research experience, and involvement in community activities and service, but also by qualities of personality, character, and resilience. A personal interview is an integral part of the admissions process. All interviews are granted at the discretion of the Committee on Admissions.

Financial Aid

BUSM is committed to ensuring that all accepted students can secure the necessary financial resources; need-based aid is available to students in all years. The Office of Student Financial Services administers its portfolio of scholarships and loans, assists students in securing aid from outside sources, conducts debt management seminars, offers entrance and exit counseling, and provides student financial management information. Financial need is not considered in the admissions process. There are no special institutional financial funds disbursed for international students. Unless an international student has an I-551 or I-151 resident alien card, federally insured loans are not available. Students may secure private educational

loans with a co-applicant who is a creditworthy U.S. citizen or resident alien.

Information about Diversity Programs

BUSM is committed to diversity in the faculty and student body. Programs for the recruitment and support of students from groups underrepresented in medicine are managed by the Office of Admissions and the Office of Diversity and Multicultural Affairs. All applications are processed through the Office of Admissions.

Campus Information

Setting

BU Medical Center is a beautiful urban campus, shared by clinical, educational, and research institutions. The four-square-block campus, located in the heart of Boston, is accessible by public transportation and is within walking distance of residential areas, shops, and cultural institutions.

Enrollment

For 2008, total enrollment was: 695

Special Features

Students complete most of their clinical training at Boston Medical Center Hospital (BMC), a very diverse institution with the busiest emergency department in New England and large programs in both ambulatory and inpatient care. BMC hosts residency training programs in all disciplines. BUSM graduates pursue careers in primary care and in the subspecialties, in full-time clinical practice and in academic centers, in rural and urban settings, in all parts of the U.S., and in international health.

Housing

Limited on-campus housing is available; most students choose to live off-campus. Rents vary, ranging from $650 and up, depending on student choice regarding location and number of roommates.

Satellite Campuses/Facilities

Basic science programs are on-campus. Clinical training is largely on-campus, but each student has some off-campus rotations, ensuring that all students experience different venues and styles of practice. All experience are supervised by full-time BUSM faculty.

Application Process and Requirements 2010–2011

Primary Application Service: AMCAS
Earliest filing date: June 1, 2009
Latest filing date: November 2, 2009

Secondary Application Required?: Yes
Sent to: All applicants
URL: Provided after receipt of initial application
Contact: Office of Admissions, (617) 638-4630, medadms@bu.edu
Fee: Yes, $100
Fee waiver available: Yes
Earliest filing date: June 1, 2009
Latest filing date: January 4, 2010

MCAT® required?: Yes
Latest MCAT® considered: Any scores available through AMCAS prior to January 2, 2010
Oldest MCAT® considered: 2006

Early Decision Program: School does have EDP
Applicants notified: October 1, 2009
EDP available for: Both Residents and Non-residents

Regular Acceptance Notice
Earliest date: Early January 2010
Latest date: Until class is full
Applicant's Response to Acceptance Offer – Maximum Time: Two weeks

Requests for Deferred Entrance Considered: No

Deposit to Hold Place in Class: Yes
Deposit (Resident): $500
Deposit (Non-resident): $500
Deposit due: May 15, 2010
Applied to tuition: Yes
Deposit refundable: Yes
Refundable prior to: May 15, 2010

Estimated number of new entrants: 132
EDP: 3, special program: 40

Start Month/Year: August 2010

Interview Format: On-campus interview required. Regional interviews are not available.

Other Programs

PREPARATORY PROGRAMS
Postbaccalaureate Program: Yes, www.bu.edu/met/adult_college_programs/boston_university_metropol itan_college_undergraduate_programs/college_certificate_program/postbaccalaureate_certificate/index.html
Summer Program: No
Early Medical School Selection Program: www.bumc.bu.edu/Dept/Content.aspx?DepartmentID=45&PageID=1295, Jonathan Woodson, M.D., (617) 638-4163, Jonathan.Woodson@bmc.org
Master of Arts in Medical Sciences: Yes, http://cobalt.bumc.bu.edu/current/Catalog/medsci/intro.htm

COMBINED DEGREE PROGRAMS
Baccalaureate/M.D.: Yes, www.bu.edu/cas/forms/accelerated.pdf
M.D./M.P.H.: Yes, www.bumc.bu.edu/sph
M.D./M.B.A.: Yes, http://management.bu.edu/gpo/dual/mdmba/index.html
M.D./Ph.D.: Yes, www.bumc.bu.edu/gms

Premedical Coursework

Course	Req.	Rec.	Lab.	Sems.
Inorganic Chemistry	•		•	2
Behavioral Sciences		•		2
Biochemistry		•		1
Biology	•		•	2
Biology/Zoology				
Calculus				
College English	•			2
College Mathematics		•		2
Computer Science				

Course	Req.	Rec.	Lab.	Sems.
Genetics		•		1
Humanities	•			2
Organic Chemistry	•		•	2
Physics	•			2
Psychology				
Social Sciences		•		2
Molecular Biology		•		1
Biostatistics & Epidemiology		•		1

Selection Factors: 2008 Accepted Applicants

Proportion of Accepted Applicants with Relevant Experience (Data Self-Reported to AMCAS®)		
Community Service/Volunteer		71%
Medically-Related Work		90%
Research		88%

Shaded bar represents school's accepted scores ranging from the 10th percentile to the 90th percentile   School Median ●   National Median ●

Overall GPA 2.0 2.1 2.2 2.3 2.4 2.5 2.6 2.7 2.8 2.9 3.0 3.1 3.2 3.3 3.4 3.5 3.6 3.7 (3.8) 3.9 4.0
Science GPA 2.0 2.1 2.2 2.3 2.4 2.5 2.6 2.7 2.8 2.9 3.0 3.1 3.2 3.3 3.4 3.5 3.6 (3.7) 3.8 3.9 4.0

MCAT® Total Numeric Score 9 10 11 12 13 14 15 16 17 18 19 20 21 22 23 24 25 26 27 28 29 30 31 (32 33) 34 35 36 37 38 39 40 41 42 43

Writing Sample			J	K	L	M	N	O	P	(Q)	R	S	T
Verbal Reasoning	3	4	5	6	7	8	9	(10)	11	12	13	14	15
Biological Sciences	3	4	5	6	7	8	9	10	(11)	12	13	14	15
Physical Sciences	3	4	5	6	7	8	9	10	(11)	12	13	14	15

Acceptance & Matriculation Data for 2008–2009 First Year Class

	Resident	Non-resident	International	Total
Applications	696	9383	659	10738
Interviewed	124	862	48	1034
Deferred	1	3	0	4
Matriculants				
Early Assurance Program	2	17	0	19
Early Decision Program	0	0	0	0
Baccalaureate/M.D.	2	15	1	18
M.D./Ph.D.	1	4	1	6
Matriculated	25	144	9	**178**

Applications accepted from International Applicants: Yes

Specialty Choice

2004, 2005, 2006 Graduates, Specialty Choice (As reported by program directors to GME Track™)

Anesthesiology	3%
Emergency Medicine	4%
Family Practice	5%
Internal Medicine	22%
Obstetrics/Gynecology	6%
Orthopaedic Surgery	4%
Pediatrics	8%
Psychiatry	3%
Radiology	7%
Surgery	7%

Matriculant Demographics: 2008–2009 First Year Class

Men: 87   **Women:** 91

Matriculants' Self-Reported Race/Ethnicity

Mexican American	8	Korean	4
Cuban	2	Vietnamese	4
Puerto Rican	1	Other Asian	4
Other Hispanic	8	Total Asian	56
Total Hispanic	18	Native American	0
Chinese	21	Black	16
Asian Indian	20	Native Hawaiian	0
Pakistani	0	White	96
Filipino	2	Unduplicated Number	
Japanese	1	of Matriculants	178

Science and Math Majors: 62%
Matriculants with:
   Baccalaureate degree: 99%
   Graduate degree(s): 24%

Financial Information

Source: 2007–2008 LCME I-B survey and 2008–2009 AAMC TSF questionnaire

	Residents	Non-residents
Total Cost of Attendance	$67,741	$67,741
Tuition and Fees	$45,286	$45,286
Other (includes living expenses)	$20,337	$20,337
Health Insurance (can be waived)	$2,118	$2,118

Average 2008 Graduate Indebtedness: $170,059
% of Enrolled Students Receiving Aid: 81%

Criminal Background Check

This medical school requires a criminal background check prior to matriculation.

Harvard Medical School
Boston, Massachusetts

Office of the Committee on Admissions
Harvard Medical School
25 Shattuck Street
306 Gordon Hall
Boston, Massachusetts 02115-6092
T 617 432 1550   **F** 617 432 3307

Admissions http://hms.harvard.edu/admissions/
Main http://hms.harvard.edu
Financial www.hms.harvard.edu/finaid/
E-mail admissions_office@hms.harvard.edu

Private Institution

*Dr. Jeffrey S. Flier, Dean
of the Faculty of Medicine*

*Dr. Robert J. Mayer, Faculty Associate
Dean for Admissions*

*Dr. Darrell N. Smith, Faculty Assistant
Dean for Admissions*

*Dr. Alvin F. Poussaint, Associate Dean
for Student Affairs*

Robert D. Coughlin, Director of Financial Aid

Joanne M. McEvoy, Director of Admissions

General Information

A leader in medical education since its inception in 1782, the Harvard Medical School forms the center of one of the nation's premier locations for medical training, research and practice. Clinical teaching is carried out in several hospitals, including Massachusetts General, Brigham and Women's, Children's Boston, Beth Israel Deaconess, Mount Auburn, and Cambridge Hospitals. The Massachusetts Mental Health Center and the McLean Hospital are psychiatric facilities. Massachusetts Eye and Ear Infirmary, the Schepens Eye Institute, and several community-based health centers provide additional opportunities for patient care, teaching, and research. Other affiliated institutions include the West Roxbury and Brockton VA Medical Centers, the Forsythe Institute, and the Spaulding Rehabilitation Hospital. The school has seven basic and two social science departments and over 10,000 affiliated faculty, including more than 6,000 full and part-time faculty instructors. Harvard Medical School has been home to 12 Nobel Laureates and many nationally and internationally recognized researchers and medical scholars.

Mission Statement

The mission of Harvard Medical School is to create and nurture a diverse community of the best people committed to leadership in alleviating human suffering caused by disease.

Curricular Highlights

Community Service Requirement: Optional.
Research/Thesis Requirement: Encouraged for NP; required for HST.

The New Pathway Program (NP) is a problem-based curriculum that emphasizes small-group tutorials and self-directed learning, complemented by laboratories and lectures. Students are expected to analyze problems, locate relevant material in library and computer-based resources, and develop habits of lifelong learning and independent study. The NP Program enrolls 135 students each year. A second M.D. pathway is the Harvard-M.I.T. Division of Health Sciences and Technology Program (HST). This collaboration between the Harvard Medical School and the Massachusetts Institute of Technology is designed for students with a strong interest and background in quantitative science. Courses in the first two years are taught at both HMS and MIT by faculty drawn from both institutions. HST students are expected to become conversant with the underlying quantitative and molecular aspects of medicine and biomedical science, achieved through a deep understanding of the physical and biological sciences, complemented with hands-on experience in the clinic. HST enrolls 30 students per year. Basic science and clinical content are interwoven throughout the four years in both programs.

USMLE

Step 1: Required. Students must record a passing score for graduation, but not promotion.
Step 2: Clinical Skills (CS): Required. Students must record a passing total score to graduate.
Step 2: Clinical Knowledge (CK): Required. Students must record a passing total score to graduate.

Selection Factors

Academic excellence is expected. Committee members consider the entire application, including the essay, extracurricular activities, life experiences, research, community work, and the comments contained in letters of recommendation. Harvard Medical School looks for evidence of integrity, maturity, humanitarian concerns, leadership potential, and an aptitude for working with people. The 2008 entering class came from 64 different undergraduate institutions, including representatives from 34 U.S. States and 12 foreign countries. The Harvard Medical School does not accept applications for advanced standing or transfer.

Financial Aid

All financial aid is awarded on the basis of need. A vigorous effort is made to assist accepted applicants in meeting their medical education costs through loans, medically related employment, and scholarships. Foreign students are eligible to be considered for need-based institutional scholarships and loans.

Information about Diversity Programs

Harvard Medical School is committed to the enrollment of a diverse body of talented students who will reflect the character of the people whose health needs the medical profession must serve. HMS's commitment to a diverse student population is reflected not only in the variety of institutions from which students are accepted, but also in the ethnic and economic backgrounds of the student body. For over 30 years, HMS has had one of the highest minority student enrollment and graduation rates of any United States medical school. The HMS Office of Recruitment and Multicultural Affairs provides support services to individuals from groups under-represented in medicine.

Campus Information

Setting

The Harvard Medical School campus is an integral part of the Longwood Medical and Academic Area (LMA), a community of health and educational institutions located adjacent to Fenway Park in the city of Boston, Massachusetts. Adjoining the medical school are the Harvard School of Public Health, the Harvard School of Dental Medicine, and the Francis A. Countway Library.

Enrollment

For 2008, total enrollment was: 728

Housing

On-campus housing for single students is available in Vanderbilt Hall, a residence complex next to the Harvard Medical School. Students may choose to live in one of the residential communities neighboring the Longwood Medical Area.

Application Process and Requirements 2010–2011

Primary Application Service: AMCAS
Earliest filing date: June 1, 2009
Latest filing date: October 15, 2009

Secondary Application Required?: Yes
Sent to: All applicants
URL: Sent via e-mail after verification of AMCAS application.
Contact: Admissions Office, (617) 432-1550, admissions_office@hms.harvard.edu
Fee: Yes, $85
Fee waiver available: Yes
Earliest filing date: July 1, 2009
Latest filing date: November 1, 2009

MCAT® required?: Yes
Latest MCAT® considered: September 2009
Oldest MCAT® considered: 2006

Early Decision Program: School does not have EDP
Applicants notified: n/a
EDP available for: n/a

Regular Acceptance Notice
Earliest date: March 1, 2010
Latest date: Varies
Applicant's Response to Acceptance Offer – Maximum Time: Three weeks

Requests for Deferred Entrance Considered: Yes

Deposit to Hold Place in Class: No
Deposit (Resident): n/a
Deposit (Non-resident): n/a
Deposit due: n/a
Applied to tuition: n/a
Deposit refundable: n/a
Refundable by: n/a

Estimated number of new entrants: 165
EDP: n/a, special program: n/a

Start Month/Year: August 2010

Interview Format: On-campus only; scheduled selectively. Regional interviews are not available.

Other Programs

PREPARATORY PROGRAMS
Postbaccalaureate Program: No
Summer Program: No

COMBINED DEGREE PROGRAMS
Baccalaureate/M.D.: No
M.D./M.P.H.: Yes, www.hms.harvard.edu/dualdegrees/index.html, Admissions Office, (617) 432-1550, admissions_office@hms.harvard.edu
M.D./M.B.A.: Yes www.hbs.edu/mba/academics/mdmba.html
(617) 432-1550, admissions_office@hms.harvard.edu
M.D./J.D.: No
M.D./Ph.D.: Yes, www.hms.harvard.edu/md_phd/
(617) 432-0991, mdphd@hms.harvard.edu
Additional Program: Yes, www.hms.harvard.edu/dualdegrees/index.html
(617) 432-1550, admissions_office@hms.harvard.edu

Premedical Coursework

Course	Req.	Rec.	Lab.	Sems.
Inorganic Chemistry	•		•	2
Behavioral Sciences				
Biochemistry		•		1
Biology	•		•	2
Biology/Zoology				
Calculus	•			2
College English				
College Mathematics				

Course	Req.	Rec.	Lab.	Sems.
Computer Science				
Genetics				
Humanities				
Organic Chemistry	•		•	2
Physics	•			2
Psychology				
Social Sciences				
Writing				2

Selection Factors: 2008 Accepted Applicants

Proportion of Accepted Applicants with Relevant Experience (Data Self-Reported to AMCAS®)			Community Service/Volunteer	75%
			Medically-Related Work	93%
			Research	95%

Shaded bar represents school's accepted scores ranging from the 10th percentile to the 90th percentile. School Median ● National Median ●

Overall GPA 2.0 2.1 2.2 2.3 2.4 2.5 2.6 2.7 2.8 2.9 3.0 3.1 3.2 3.3 3.4 3.5 3.6 3.7 3.8 (3.9) 4.0
Science GPA 2.0 2.1 2.2 2.3 2.4 2.5 2.6 2.7 2.8 2.9 3.0 3.1 3.2 3.3 3.4 3.5 3.6 3.7 3.8 (3.9) 4.0

MCAT® Total Numeric Score 9 10 11 12 13 14 15 16 17 18 19 20 21 22 23 24 25 26 27 28 29 30 31 (32) 33 34 35 (36) 37 38 39 40 41 42 43

Writing Sample			J	K	L	M	N	O	P	(Q)	(R)	S	T
Verbal Reasoning	3	4	5	6	7	8	9	(10)	(11)	12	13	14	15
Biological Sciences	3	4	5	6	7	8	9	10	(11)	12	(13)	14	15
Physical Sciences	3	4	5	6	7	8	9	10	(11)	12	(13)	14	15

Acceptance & Matriculation Data for 2008–2009 First Year Class

	Resident	Non-resident	International	Total
Applications	411	5598	453	6462
Interviewed	104	955	112	1171
Deferred	1	9	0	10
Matriculants				
Early Assurance Program	n/a	n/a	n/a	n/a
Early Decision Program	0	0	0	0
Baccalaureate/M.D.	n/a	n/a	n/a	n/a
M.D./Ph.D.	2	8	1	11
Matriculated	24	133	8	**165**

Applications accepted from International Applicants: Yes

Specialty Choice

2004, 2005, 2006 Graduates, Specialty Choice (As reported by program directors to GME Track™)	
Anesthesiology	2%
Emergency Medicine	7%
Family Practice	2%
Internal Medicine	19%
Obstetrics/Gynecology	3%
Orthopaedic Surgery	4%
Pediatrics	9%
Psychiatry	5%
Radiology	6%
Surgery	5%

Matriculant Demographics: 2008–2009 First Year Class

Men: 85   **Women:** 80

Matriculants' Self-Reported Race/Ethnicity

Mexican American	5	**Korean**	3
Cuban	1	**Vietnamese**	1
Puerto Rican	2	**Other Asian**	8
Other Hispanic	6	**Total Asian**	57
Total Hispanic	14	**Native American**	3
Chinese	24	**Black**	16
Asian Indian	16	**Native Hawaiian**	0
Pakistani	1	**White**	81
Filipino	3	**Unduplicated Number**	
Japanese	2	**of Matriculants**	165

Science and Math Majors: 60%
Matriculants with:
  Baccalaureate degree: 100%
  Graduate degree(s): 15%

Financial Information
Source: 2007–2008 LCME I-B survey and 2008–2009 AAMC TSF questionnaire

	Residents	Non-residents
Total Cost of Attendance	$62,900	$62,900
Tuition and Fees	$41,819	$41,819
Other (includes living expenses)	$19,677	$19,677
Health Insurance (can be waived)	$1,404	$1,404

Average 2008 Graduate Indebtedness: $107,750
% of Enrolled Students Receiving Aid: 83%

Criminal Background Check

This medical school does not require a criminal background check prior to matriculation.

Tufts University School of Medicine

Boston, Massachusetts

Office of Admissions
Tufts University School of Medicine
136 Harrison Avenue
Boston, Massachusetts 02111
T 617 636 6571 **F** unpublished

Admissions www.tufts.edu/med/admissions
Main www.tufts.edu/med
Financial www.tufts.edu/med/about/offices/
finaid/index.html
E-mail med-admissions@tufts.edu

Private Institution

Dr. Michael Rosenblatt, Dean

Dr. David Neumeyer, Dean for Admissions

Colleen Romain, Director of Minority Affairs

Tara Olsen, Director of Financial Aid

Thomas M. Slavin, Director of Admissions

John Matias, Associate Dean of Admissions

General Information

Tufts University was founded in 1852 in Medford, Massachusetts; the School of Medicine was established in Boston in 1893. Close association of the School of Medicine with 30-plus hospitals currently affords ample facilities for clinical experience.

Mission Statement

To produce a competent, compassionate physician who is skilled and well-educated in a core of general knowledge; one who is capable of building on this core to achieve educational and career goals and to maintain the task of lifelong learning.

Curricular Highlights

Community Service Requirement: Required.
Research/Thesis Requirement: Optional.

Students experience a progressive development of clinical knowledge, skills, and attitudes required as a professional in medicine today. The curriculum emphasizes the basic skills needed by a generalist physician and includes newly expanded topics such as information management, computer literacy, and negotiation/management/team building skills, in addition to integrated topics such as nutrition, gerontology, health care economics, and ethics. Community and ambulatory-based learning experiences are incorporated throughout to reflect the changing environment of health care. In the third year, students develop their clinical skills and learn to take responsibility for patient care under close preceptor supervision at a number of affiliated sites representing a wide variety of clinical settings. The goal of the fourth year of the curriculum is to expand the basic clinical knowledge and skills acquired

in the first three years, enabling the student to manage clinical problems with the degree of independence required of the first-year postgraduate level of medical training.

USMLE

Step 1: Required. Students must record a passing score for promotion.
Step 2: Clinical Skills (CS): Required. Students must only record a score.
Step 2: Clinical Knowledge (CK): Required. Students must only record a score.

Selection Factors

The selection of candidates for admission to the first year is based not only on performance in the required premedical courses, but also on the applicant's entire academic record and extracurricular experiences. Letters of recommendation and additional information supplied by the applicant are reviewed for indications of promise and fitness for a medical career. Personal interviews are a prerequisite for admission and are granted only by invitation of the Admissions Committee. Preference is given to U.S. citizens and permanent residents who will receive a bachelor's degree from an U.S. college or university prior to matriculation. Tufts accepts transfers from other U.S. LCME-accredited medical schools into the second- and third-year classes in years when vacancies have been created by attrition. The number of seats available has traditionally been extremely limited. In some years, no transfer openings are available.

Financial Aid

Up to 75 percent of students participate in the federal government's student loan programs at some time during their four years of study. Additionally, limited scholarship and loan assistance is available directly from Tufts for students who qualify on the basis of need. Approximately 33 percent of students receive financial aid directly from Tufts at some time during their four years of study.

Information about Diversity Programs

Tufts has a strong commitment to affirmative action and seeks to provide an atmosphere of nondiscrimination for members of groups underrepresented in medicine as well as an

accessible campus and support services for persons with disabilities.

Campus Information

Setting

The School of Medicine is located within a health sciences campus that includes the School of Dental Medicine, the Sackler School of Graduate Biomedical Sciences, the Friedman School of Nutrition Science and Policy, the Sackler Center for Health Communications, the Jaharis Center for Biomedical and Nutrition Sciences, the Jean Mayer Nutrition Research Center, and the New England Medical Center.

Enrollment

For 2008, total enrollment was: 705

Special Features

TUSM has created a unique cadre of combined-degree programs by which students can attain an M.D./Ph.D., an M.D./M.P.H, or an M.D./M.B.A. in Health Management. TUSM also offers a Maine Track, with clinical training focused at Maine Medical Center and other sites in Maine.

Housing

A limited amount of on-campus housing is available in Posner Hall, the Health Sciences Campus dormitory. Most TUSM students live off-campus. In the late spring of each year, the Student Affairs Office hires a seasonal off-campus housing coordinator to assist students at the Boston Health Sciences Campus in finding off-campus housing. The coordinator typically distributes general information about the Greater Boston housing market and maintains listings of available housing opportunities.

Satellite Campuses/Facilities

Most of the school's clinical affiliates are located in the metropolitan Boston area. Nevertheless, students should expect to participate in rotations that are located outside of Boston, including some at the Baystate Medical Center (the western campus of TUSM) in Springfield, Massachusetts, and Eastern Maine Medial Center in Bangor, Maine.

Application Process and Requirements 2010–2011

Primary Application Service: AMCAS
Earliest filing date: June 1, 2009
Latest filing date: November 1, 2009

Secondary Application Required?: Yes
Sent to: All applicants
URL: www.tufts.edu/med/admissions/md/howtoapply/secondary.html
Fee: Yes, $105
Fee waiver available: Yes
Earliest filing date: June 1, 2009
Latest filing date: January 15, 2010

MCAT® required?: Yes
Latest MCAT® considered: September 2009
Oldest MCAT® considered: January 2005

Early Decision Program: School does have EDP
Applicants notified: October 1, 2009
EDP available for: Both Residents and Non-residents

Regular Acceptance Notice
Earliest date: October 15, 2009
Latest date: Until class is full
Applicant's Response to Acceptance Offer – Maximum Time: Two weeks

Requests for Deferred Entrance Considered: Yes

Deposit to Hold Place in Class: Yes
Deposit (Resident): $100
Deposit (Non-resident): $100
Deposit due: With response to acceptance offer
Applied to tuition: Yes
Deposit refundable: Yes
Refundable by: May 15, 2010

Estimated number of new entrants: 178
EDP: 2, special program: 20

Start Month/Year: August 2010

Interview Format: On-campus interviews conducted September–March. Regional interviews are not available.

Other Programs

PREPARATORY PROGRAMS
Postbaccalaureate Program: No
Summer Program: Yes, Colleen Romain, (617) 636-6534, colleen.romain@tufts.edu

COMBINED DEGREE PROGRAMS
Baccalaureate/M.D.: No
M.D./M.P.H.: Yes, www.tufts.edu/med/education/phpd/mph/pathways/mdmph_dvmmph/index.html
M.D./M.B.A.: Yes, www.tufts.edu/med/education/combinedmd/mdmba/index.html
M.D./J.D.: No
M.D./Ph.D.: Yes, www.tufts.edu/sackler/programs/combined.html

Premedical Coursework

Course	Req.	Rec.	Lab.	Sems.
Inorganic Chemistry	•		•	2
Behavioral Sciences				
Biochemistry				
Biology	•		•	2
Biology/Zoology				
Calculus				
College English				
College Mathematics				

Course	Req.	Rec.	Lab.	Sems.
Computer Science				
Genetics				
Humanities				
Organic Chemistry	•		•	2
Physics	•		•	2
Psychology				
Social Sciences				
Other				

Selection Factors: 2008 Accepted Applicants

Proportion of Accepted Applicants with Relevant Experience (Data Self-Reported to AMCAS®)		
Community Service/Volunteer	70%
Medically-Related Work	84%
Research	84%

Shaded bar represents school's accepted scores ranging from the 10th percentile to the 90th percentile   School Median ●   National Median ●

Overall GPA 2.0 2.1 2.2 2.3 2.4 2.5 2.6 2.7 2.8 2.9 3.0 3.1 3.2 3.3 3.4 3.5 3.6 3.7 (3.8) 3.9 4.0
Science GPA 2.0 2.1 2.2 2.3 2.4 2.5 2.6 2.7 2.8 2.9 3.0 3.1 3.2 3.3 3.4 3.5 3.6 (3.7) 3.8 3.9 4.0

MCAT® Total Numeric Score 9 10 11 12 13 14 15 16 17 18 19 20 21 22 23 24 25 26 27 28 29 30 31 (32) 33 34 (35) 36 37 38 39 40 41 42 43

	J	K	L	M	N	O	P	Q	R	S	T
Writing Sample								(Q)			

Verbal Reasoning	3	4	5	6	7	8	9	(10)	(11)	12	13	14	15
Biological Sciences	3	4	5	6	7	8	9	10	(11)	(12)	13	14	15
Physical Sciences	3	4	5	6	7	8	9	10	(11)	(12)	13	14	15

Acceptance & Matriculation Data for 2008–2009 First Year Class

	Resident	Non-resident	International	Total
Applications	698	8004	401	9103
Interviewed	166	705	3	874
Deferred	3	4	0	7
Matriculants				
Early Assurance Program	8	13	2	23
Early Decision Program	0	1	0	1
Baccalaureate/M.D.	n/a	n/a	n/a	n/a
M.D./Ph.D.	1	3	0	4
Matriculated	52	125	1	**178**

Applications accepted from International Applicants: Yes

Specialty Choice

2004, 2005, 2006 Graduates, Specialty Choice (As reported by program directors to GME Track™)	
Anesthesiology	7%
Emergency Medicine	8%
Family Practice	7%
Internal Medicine	23%
Obstetrics/Gynecology	2%
Orthopaedic Surgery	4%
Pediatrics	11%
Psychiatry	2%
Radiology	6%
Surgery	10%

Matriculant Demographics: 2008–2009 First Year Class

Men: 97   **Women:** 81

Matriculants' Self-Reported Race/Ethnicity

Mexican American	5	**Korean**	5
Cuban	2	**Vietnamese**	0
Puerto Rican	0	**Other Asian**	1
Other Hispanic	4	**Total Asian**	43
Total Hispanic	11	**Native American**	0
Chinese	22	**Black**	10
Asian Indian	12	**Native Hawaiian**	1
Pakistani	3	**White**	124
Filipino	0	**Unduplicated Number**	
Japanese	1	**of Matriculants**	178

Science and Math Majors: 62%
Matriculants with:
      Baccalaureate degree: 98%
      Graduate degree(s): 10%

Financial Information

Source: 2007–2008 LCME I-B survey and 2008–2009 AAMC TSF questionnaire

	Residents	Non-residents
Total Cost of Attendance	$70,533	$70,533
Tuition and Fees	$48,992	$48,992
Other (includes living expenses)	$18,565	$18,565
Health Insurance (can be waived)	$2,976	$2,976

Average 2008 Graduate Indebtedness: $192,162
% of Enrolled Students Receiving Aid: 80%

Criminal Background Check

This medical school does not require a criminal background check prior to matriculation.

University of Massachusetts Medical School
Worcester, Massachusetts

University of Massachusetts Medical School
Office of Admissions
55 Lake Avenue, North, Room S1-112
Worcester, Massachusetts 01655
T 508 856 2323 **F** 508 856 3629

Admissions www.umassmed.edu/som/admissions
Main www.umassmed.edu/education
Financial www.umass.edu/financialaid/index.aspx
E-mail admissions@umassmed.edu

Public Institution

Dr. Terence Flotte, Dean

Dr. John Paraskos,
Associate Dean for Admissions

Dr. Danna B. Peterson, Assistant Dean of
Student Affairs/Diversity and Minority Affairs

Betsy Groves, Director of Financial Aid

General Information
Established in 1962, the University of Massachusetts Medical School accepted its first class in 1970. UMMS is committed to training physicians in a wide range of medical disciplines and emphasizes training for practice in general medicine and the primary care specialties in the public sector and in underserved areas of Massachusetts. This mission has since been expanded to include graduate education in the biomedical sciences and nursing, graduate medical education, and continuing medical education for health professionals. The school's clinical partner is UMass Memorial Medical Center, consisting of two acute care hospitals with a total of 761 beds. Clinical education is also conducted at a number of affiliated community hospitals and health centers in the region. UMMS Worcester is adjacent to the Massachusetts Biotechnology Research Park, which houses a number of UMass research programs including the Program in Molecular Medicine, the Cancer Center, and the Worcester Foundation for Biomedical Research.

Mission Statement
The mission of the University of Massachusetts Medical School is to serve the people of the Commonwealth through excellence in health sciences education, clinical care, research, and public service.

Curricular Highlights
Community Service Requirement: Optional.
Research/Thesis Requirement: Optional.

The UMMS curriculum encourages interdisciplinary learning and integration of the basic and clinical sciences, with special attention to clinical correlation of subject matter in the preclinical years. Emphasis in the first year is on normal structure and function with a bal-

ance of small-group learning and large-group function. Emphasis in the second year is on the etiology of disease, pathophysiology, pharmacology, and clinical diagnosis. The third and fourth years are a continuum of required clerkships and both clinical and research electives with emphasis on integration. UMMS encourages students to participate in research programs in advanced biomedical studies.

USMLE
Step 1: Required. Students must record a passing score for graduation, but not promotion.
Step 2: Clinical Skills (CS): Required. Students must only record a score.
Step 2: Clinical Knowledge (CK): Required. Students must only record a score.

Selection Factors
Current policy limits admission to the M.D. program to students who are Massachusetts residents. Residents and non-residents of Massachusetts are eligible for admission to the joint M.D./Ph.D. program through the Graduate School of Biomedical Sciences and the Medical School. All applicants must be U.S. citizens or have permanent resident status. The admissions committee bases its evaluation of applicants on academic ability and achievement, MCAT scores, and such factors as extracurricular achievement, maturity, motivation, and character as these are reflected in letters of recommendation from preprofessional advisory committees and other persons. Interviews are arranged by invitation only. Applicants are selected on the basis of their individual merits without regard to race, sex, creed, national origin, age, or disability. UMMS has a set of technical standards for admission and promotion, which are available upon request. Two semesters of biology or zoology are required.

Financial Aid
Please refer to the UMMS Financial Aid Web page.

Information about Diversity Programs
For additional information, please contact the Associate Vice Chancellor for School Services at 508-856-2444.

Campus Information

Setting
UMMS is in Worcester, MA and thus conveniently located in central Massachusetts. UMass Memorial Health Care is the clinical partner of UMMS and the largest health care system serving central and western Massachusetts. The medical school and clinical affiliate share adjoining buildings. There are numerous institutions of higher learning in the area offering culturally diverse activities. The campus is accessible by local bus and taxicab services.

Enrollment
For 2008, total enrollment was: 445

Special Features
The UMMS clinical affiliate, UMass Memorial Health Care, houses a regional trauma center and provides specialized education in primary, secondary, tertiary, and quaternary health care. A recently expanded research facility in close proximity to the biotech park has made the campus a focus for biotechnology research in Massachusetts. Students are given the opportunity for international rotations.

Housing
On-campus housing is not available. There are many affordable apartments within fifteen minutes of the medical school. Rents average $800-$1,000 per month.

Satellite Campuses/Facilities
Student rotations are divided among multiple campuses of UMass Memorial Health Care: University, Memorial, and Hahnemann Campuses and Clinton, Marlborough, Wing Memorial, and HealthAlliance Hospitals. The school is also affiliated with other suburban medical centers, such as the Berkshire Medical Center, Milford-Whitinsville Regional Hospital, St. Elizabeth's Hospital in Brighton, St. Vincent Hospital at Worcester Medical Center, and the Day Kimball Hospital in Connecticut. Students are required to have their own transportation.

Application Process and Requirements 2010–2011

Primary Application Service: AMCAS
Earliest filing date: June 1, 2009
Latest filing date: November 1, 2009

Secondary Application Required?: Yes
Sent to: All verified applicants
Contact: Admissions Office, 508-856-2323, admissions@umassmed.edu
Fee: Yes, $75
Fee waiver available: Yes
Earliest filing date: After verified application received
Latest filing date: Must be completed by December 15, 2009

MCAT® required?: Yes
Latest MCAT® considered: September 2009
Oldest MCAT® considered: 2006

Early Decision Program: School does have EDP
Applicants notified: October 1, 2009
EDP available for: Residents only

Regular Acceptance Notice
Earliest date: October 15, 2009
Latest date: Until Class is Full
Applicant's Response to Acceptance
Offer – Maximum Time: Two weeks

Requests for Deferred
Entrance Considered: Yes

Deposit to Hold Place in Class: Yes
Deposit (Resident): $100
Deposit (Non-resident): $100
Deposit due: With response to acceptance offer
Applied to tuition: Yes
Deposit refundable: Yes
Refundable by: May 15, 2010

Estimated number of new entrants: 125
EDP: 10, special program: n/a

Start Month/Year: August 2010

Interview Format: Students meet one-on-one with two interviewers. Off campus interviews are available.

Other Programs

PREPARATORY PROGRAMS
Postbaccalaureate Program: No
Summer Program: Yes, www.umassmed.edu/summer
Summer Enrichment Program: www.umassmed.edu/outreach/sep.aspx

COMBINED DEGREE PROGRAMS
Baccalaureate/M.D.: No
M.D./M.P.H.: No
M.D./M.B.A.: No
M.D./J.D.: No
M.D./Ph.D.: Yes, www.umassmed.edu/MDPhD/index.aspx

Premedical Coursework

Course	Req.	Rec.	Lab.	Sems.	Course	Req.	Rec.	Lab.	Sems.
Inorganic Chemistry	•		•	2	Computer Science		•		2
Behavioral Sciences					Genetics				
Biochemistry		•			Organic Chemistry	•		•	2
Biology	•		•	2	Physics	•		•	2
Biology/Zoology	•		•	2	Psychology				
Calculus					Social Sciences				
College English	•			2	Statistics		•		2
College Mathematics					Other				

Selection Factors: 2008 Accepted Applicants

Proportion of Accepted Applicants with Relevant Experience (Data Self-Reported to AMCAS®)		
Community Service/Volunteer		70%
Medically-Related Work		83%
Research		84%

Shaded bar represents school's accepted scores ranging from the 10th percentile to the 90th percentile. **School Median ●** **National Median ●**

Overall GPA	2.0	2.1	2.2	2.3	2.4	2.5	2.6	2.7	2.8	2.9	3.0	3.1	3.2	3.3	3.4	3.5	3.6	(3.7)	3.8	3.9	4.0
Science GPA	2.0	2.1	2.2	2.3	2.4	2.5	2.6	2.7	2.8	2.9	3.0	3.1	3.2	3.3	3.4	3.5	3.6	(3.7)	3.8	3.9	4.0

MCAT® Total Numeric Score 9 10 11 12 13 14 15 16 17 18 19 20 21 22 23 24 25 26 27 28 29 30 31 32 (33) 34 35 36 37 38 39 40 41 42 43

Writing Sample			J	K	L	M	N	O	P	(Q)	R	S	T
Verbal Reasoning	3	4	5	6	7	8	9	(10)	(11)	12	13	14	15
Biological Sciences	3	4	5	6	7	8	9	10	(11)	12	13	14	15
Physical Sciences	3	4	5	6	7	8	9	10	(11)	12	13	14	15

Acceptance & Matriculation Data for 2008–2009 First Year Class

	Resident	Non-resident	International	Total
Applications	726	85	3	814
Interviewed	437	23	0	460
Deferred	3	0	0	3
Matriculants				
Early Assurance Program	n/a	n/a	n/a	n/a
Early Decision Program	2	0	0	2
Baccalaureate/M.D.	n/a	n/a	n/a	n/a
M.D./Ph.D.	4	3	0	7
Matriculated	111	3	0	**114**

Applications accepted from International Applicants: No

Specialty Choice

2004, 2005, 2006 Graduates, Specialty Choice (As reported by program directors to GME Track™)	
Anesthesiology	5%
Emergency Medicine	13%
Family Practice	12%
Internal Medicine	20%
Obstetrics/Gynecology	6%
Orthopaedic Surgery	3%
Pediatrics	13%
Psychiatry	4%
Radiology	5%
Surgery	5%

Matriculant Demographics: 2008–2009 First Year Class

Men: 55   **Women:** 59

Matriculants' Self-Reported Race/Ethnicity

Mexican American	1	Korean	2
Cuban	1	Vietnamese	0
Puerto Rican	2	Other Asian	3
Other Hispanic	2	Total Asian	10
Total Hispanic	5	Native American	0
Chinese	1	Black	6
Asian Indian	4	Native Hawaiian	0
Pakistani	1	White	99
Filipino	0	**Unduplicated Number**	
Japanese	0	**of Matriculants**	114

Science and Math Majors: 61%
Matriculants with:
Baccalaureate degree: 100%
Graduate degree(s): 13%

Financial Information

Source: 2007–2008 LCME I-B survey and 2008–2009 AAMC TSF questionnaire

	Residents	Non-residents
Total Cost of Attendance	$41,118	$41,118
Tuition and Fees	$14,238	$14,238
Other (includes living expenses)	$23,668	$23,668
Health Insurance (can be waived)	$3,212	$3,212

Average 2008 Graduate Indebtedness: $117,332
% of Enrolled Students Receiving Aid: 97%

Criminal Background Check

This medical school requires a criminal background check prior to matriculation.

Michigan State University
College of Human Medicine

East Lansing, Michigan

College of Human Medicine, Office of Admissions
A239 Life Science
Michigan State University
East Lansing, Michigan 48824-1317
T 517 353 9620 **F** 517 432 0021

Admissions http://MDadmissions.msu.edu
Main http://humanmedicine.msu.edu
Financial http://finaid.msu.edu/med
E-mail MDadmissions@msu.edu

Public Institution

Dr. Marsha Rappley, Dean

Dr. Wanda Lipscomb, Associate Dean for Student Affairs, Diversity and Outreach

Dr. Christine Shafer, Assistant Dean for Admissions

Jay Bryde, Admissions Officer

Letitia Fowler, Admissions Senior Counselor

Diane Batten, Coordinator of Medical Student Financial Aid

General Information

The College of Human Medicine (CHM), founded in response to Michigan's need for primary care physicians, has expanded to meet growing needs. Students begin at either the MSU campus in East Lansing or at the new Grand Rapids location. After two preclinical years of basic science and clinical skills, students enter clinical years at a community campus.

Mission Statement

The College of Human Medicine at Michigan State University is committed to educating exemplary physicians and scholars, discovering and disseminating new knowledge, and providing service at home and abroad. We enhance our communities by providing outstanding primary and specialty care, promoting the dignity and inclusion of all people, and responding to the needs of the medically underserved.

Curricular Highlights

Community Service Requirement: Required.
Community Service: Students enjoy meaningful service.
Research/Thesis Requirement: Optional.
Research Thesis: Research available.

The curriculum integrates basic biological, behavioral, and social sciences, using a developmental approach to learning; early teaching of clinical skills, and clinical training utilizing a community-integrated approach. Grading is on a modified pass/no pass system; clinical honors performance is recognized. Block I is a 2½ semester experience in which fundamental medical science is presented in a structured,

discipline-based format. It also comprises basic clinical skills, mentor group, longitudinal patient exposure, opportunities for independent as well as supplementary learning experiences, and a clinical correlations course that integrates basic science and medicine. Block II presents a clinical problem-based format with emphasis on small-group learning and use of a clinical context for basic science concepts, clinical skills training, and special topics seminars over two semesters. Block III includes 60 weeks of required clerkships and 20 weeks of elective clerkships. Family medicine is a required clerkship. Students may complete elective clerkships in other locations, including third world countries. A Rural Physician Program and the Leadership in Medicine for the Underserved/ Vulnerable Program, with an international component, are offered.

USMLE

Step 1: Required. Students must record a passing score for promotion.
Step 2: Clinical Skills (CS): Required. Students must record a passing total score to graduate.
Step 2: Clinical Knowledge (CK): Required. Students must record a passing total score to graduate.

Selection Factors

CHM seeks a class that is academically competent, reflective of the rural and urban character of Michigan, and representative of a wide spectrum of personalities, backgrounds, and talents. Disadvantaged and minority students are encouraged to apply. Ability to pay is not a factor. Selection criteria is multifactorial and includes year-to-year and cumulative GPA (including postbac and graduate); best MCAT performance; fit with the school's mission; relevant clinical and community service; assessments of motivation, ability to communicate, and problem-solve; maturity and suitability for the MSU program; state of residence, and potential to contribute to the overall quality of the entering class. CHM considers U.S. and Canadian residents and applicants with U.S. permanent resident status.

Financial Aid

Information about specific scholarships and financial aid can be obtained from the Office of Financial Aid at *http://finaid.msu.edu/med.*

Information about Diversity Programs

The Advanced Baccalaureate Learning Experience (ABLE) is a 13-month, enriched academic experience offered to an invited group of disadvantaged students who have applied for admission to CHM. Students who successfully complete the ABLE program are offered regular admission to CHM's entering class.

Campus Information

Setting

One preclinical setting, the MSU Big Ten 5,200-acre, park-like campus in East Lansing, embraces 9,428 graduate and professional students, including law, osteopathic medicine, and veterinary students. The new preclinical campus is in the rapidly expanding "Medical Mile" area of downtown Grand Rapids. Clinical training occurs in one of the seven fully supported community campuses in Michigan: Flint, Grand Rapids, Kalamazoo, Lansing, Saginaw, Traverse City, and the Upper Peninsula (Marquette).

Enrollment

For 2008, total enrollment was: 550

Special Features

Students enjoy a cooperative experience where interests and needs are supported by the ABLE program, an extended curriculum option, research opportunities, the Rural Physician Program, and the Leadership in Medicine for the Underserved/ Vulnerable Program, international opportunities, the resources of MSU and seven communities in Michigan.

Housing

Affordable housing is readily available at all sites. Additionally, MSU operates three large on-campus apartment complexes and accommodations for graduate and professional students on campus.

Satellite Campuses/Facilities

Clinical campuses (Flint, Grand Rapids, Kalamazoo, Lansing, Saginaw, Traverse City and the Upper Peninsula) comprise full-time, part-time, and volunteer faculty in the clinical disciplines. Students are connected to an array of health care resources in the community that allow for hands-on learning, exposure to diverse patient problems, research, and experience in varied medical practice settings.

Application Process and Requirements 2010–2011

Primary Application Service: AMCAS
Earliest filing date: June 1, 2009
Latest filing date: November 15, 2009

Secondary Application Required?: Yes
Sent to: All applicants with fee paid.
URL: URL provided upon receipt of $60 Secondary Application fee.
Fee: Yes, $60
Fee waiver available: Yes
Earliest filing date: August 2009
Latest filing date: February 2010

MCAT® required?: Yes
Latest MCAT® considered: September 2009
Oldest MCAT® considered: April 2006

Early Decision Program: School does have EDP
Applicants notified: October 1, 2009
EDP available for: Both Residents and Non-residents

Regular Acceptance Notice
Earliest date: October 15, 2009
Latest date: Varies
Applicant's Response to Acceptance Offer – Maximum Time: Two weeks

Requests for Deferred Entrance Considered: Yes

Deposit to Hold Place in Class: Yes
Deposit (Resident): $100
Deposit (Non-resident): $100
Deposit due: With response to acceptance offer
Applied to tuition: Yes
Deposit refundable: Yes
Refundable by: May 15, 2010

Estimated number of new entrants: 200
EDP: 5, special program: 25

Start Month/Year: August 2010

Interview Format: Individual 30 minute student and faculty interviews. Regional interviews are being considered.

Other Programs

PREPARATORY PROGRAMS
Postbaccalaureate Program: Yes,
http://MDadmissions.msu.edu/main/able.htm
Summer Program: No

COMBINED DEGREE PROGRAMS
Baccalaureate/M.D.: No
M.D./M.P.H.: Yes, http://publichealth.msu.edu
M.D./M.B.A.: No
M.D./J.D.: No
M.D./Ph.D.: Yes,
http://MDadmissions.msu.edu/main/mdphd.htm

Premedical Coursework

Course	Req.	Rec.	Lab.	Sems.	Course	Req.	Rec.	Lab.	Sems.
Inorganic Chemistry	•		•	2	Computer Science		•		
Behavioral Sciences		•			Genetics		•		
Biochemistry		•			Humanities	•			2
Biology	•		•	2	Organic Chemistry	•		•	2
Biology/Zoology					Physics		•		
Calculus					Psychology		•		
College English	•			2	Social Sciences		•		
College Mathematics				1	2 Upper-Level Biology	•			2

Selection Factors: 2008 Accepted Applicants

Proportion of Accepted Applicants with Relevant Experience (Data Self-Reported to AMCAS®)		
Community Service/Volunteer		80%
Medically-Related Work		93%
Research		85%

Shaded bar represents school's accepted scores ranging from the 10th percentile to the 90th percentile ▮   School Median ● National Median ●

Overall GPA 2.0 2.1 2.2 2.3 2.4 2.5 2.6 2.7 2.8 2.9 3.0 3.1 **3.2 3.3 3.4 3.5 (3.6) 3.7 3.8 3.9** 4.0
Science GPA 2.0 2.1 2.2 2.3 2.4 2.5 2.6 2.7 2.8 2.9 3.0 **3.1 3.2 3.3 3.4 (3.5) 3.6 3.7 3.8 3.9** 4.0

MCAT® Total Numeric Score 9 10 11 12 13 14 15 16 17 18 19 20 21 22 23 24 25 **26 27 28 29(30)31(32)33** 34 35 36 37 38 39 40 41 42 43

Writing Sample			J	K	L	**M N O (P) (Q) R**	S	T
Verbal Reasoning	3	4	5	6	**7 8 9 (10) 11**	12	13	14	15
Biological Sciences	3	4	5	6	7	**8 9 (10) (11) 12**	13	14	15
Physical Sciences	3	4	5	6	7	**8 9 (10) (11) 12**	13	14	15

Acceptance & Matriculation Data for 2008–2009 First Year Class

	Resident	Non-resident	International	Total
Applications	1283	3272	303	4858
Interviewed	323	167	20	510
Deferred	7	2	0	9
Matriculants				
Early Assurance Program	0	0	0	0
Early Decision Program	4	0	0	4
Baccalaureate/M.D.	10	0	0	10
M.D./Ph.D.	2	0	0	2
Matriculated	115	36	5	**156**

Applications accepted from International Applicants: Canadian only

Specialty Choice

2004, 2005, 2006 Graduates, Specialty Choice (As reported by program directors to GME Track™)	
Anesthesiology	6%
Emergency Medicine	9%
Family Practice	16%
Internal Medicine	15%
Obstetrics/Gynecology	6%
Orthopaedic Surgery	2%
Pediatrics	11%
Psychiatry	5%
Radiology	5%
Surgery	7%

Matriculant Demographics: 2008–2009 First Year Class

Men: 79   **Women:** 77

Matriculants' Self-Reported Race/Ethnicity

Mexican American	2	Korean	2
Cuban	0	Vietnamese	4
Puerto Rican	1	Other Asian	3
Other Hispanic	5	Total Asian	23
Total Hispanic	8	Native American	2
Chinese	3	Black	8
Asian Indian	14	Native Hawaiian	0
Pakistani	0	White	114
Filipino	0	Unduplicated Number	
Japanese	0	of Matriculants	156

Science and Math Majors: 67%
Matriculants with:
    Baccalaureate degree: 100%
    Graduate degree(s): 17%

Financial Information
Source: 2007–2008 LCME I-B survey and 2008–2009 AAMC TSF questionnaire

	Residents	Non-residents
Total Cost of Attendance	$57,580	$92,794
Tuition and Fees	$30,459	$65,673
Other (includes living expenses)	$25,731	$25,731
Health Insurance (can be waived)	$1,390	$1,390

Average 2008 Graduate Indebtedness: $160,937
% of Enrolled Students Receiving Aid: 95%

Criminal Background Check

This medical school does not require a criminal background check prior to matriculation.

University of Michigan Medical School

Ann Arbor, Michigan

Admissions Office
4303 Medical Science I Building
University of Michigan Medical School
Ann Arbor, Michigan 48109-0624
T 734 764 6317   **F** 734 763 0453

Admissions www.med.umich.edu/medschool/admissions
Main www.med.umich.edu/medschool
Financial www.med.umich.edu/medschool/financialaid
E-mail umichmedadmiss@umich.edu

Public Institution

Dr. James Woolliscroft, Dean

Dr. Steven Gay, Assistant Dean of Admissions

Dr. David Gordon, Assistant Dean for Diversity and Career Development

Robert F. Ruiz, Director of Admissions

Carmen Colby, Director of Financial Aid

General Information

The University of Michigan Medical School was founded in 1850. This school was the first to establish a university-owned hospital. Today, the medical center occupies more than 30 buildings, the world's largest one-site complex devoted to health care, education, and research. The Health System consistently ranks as one of the top ten in the nation.

Mission Statement

The University of Michigan Medical School seeks to graduate a diverse cohort of physicians who are dedicated to life-long learning. Our goals include educating individuals committed to achieving the highest standards of competency required to provide exemplary patient care. We seek to graduate culturally competent physicians who will assume leadership roles in the areas of clinical medicine, research, and teaching. Physicians who graduate from the University of Michigan will demonstrate a strong foundation in biomedical sciences; empathetic interpersonal skills; an ability to identify and reduce health risk factors; an ability to obtain and interpret relevant patient information and to make effective clinical decisions; a commitment to achieving personal and professional excellence; and the critical attributes of compassion, honesty, and integrity.

Curricular Highlights

Community Service Requirement: Optional.
Research/Thesis Requirement: Optional.

In the first year, the introductory Patients and Populations course acquaints medical students with genetics, principles of disease, epidemiology, and evidence-based medicine. After that, most of the material is structured within Normal Organ Systems sequences and a Microbiology and Infectious Disease course. Clinical skills are taught in focused one- and two-week modules throughout the first and second years, beginning with the medical interview and history-taking skills and moving to physical examination practice. In the two-year Family Centered Experience, pairs of first-year students are assigned to a family in the community. These families will serve as resources to help medical students understand how health changes, chronic conditions, and serious illnesses affect patients and those close to them. The second year curriculum features Abnormal Organ Systems sequences. It includes additional patient cases and continuing reinforcement of information gathering and critical appraisal skills. Clinical skills modules will continue with expectations for mastery of more advanced physical examination, history-taking, and communication skills. Clinical training in the third year includes required rotations, and opportunities for career exploratory electives. Fourth-year requirements include a subinternship and an ICU experience, as well as a course in Advanced Medical Therapeutics. In the subinternship, students are assigned their own patient caseload and they perform with almost the same level of responsibility as a resident. The fourth year includes eight weeks of vacation and interviewing time, as well as 12 weeks of electives, with opportunities for off-campus and international rotations. All courses in the first year are graded pass/fail. In the subsequent years, faculty assign students grades of honors, high pass, pass, or fail.

USMLE

Step 1: Required. Students must record a passing score for promotion.
Step 2: Clinical Skills (CS): Required. Students must record a passing total score to graduate.
Step 2: Clinical Knowledge (CK): Required. Students must record a passing total score to graduate.

Selection Factors

The Admissions Committee is dedicated to matriculating those individuals with the skills, intelligence, and personal attributes to become leaders in medicine. Although admitted students all have demonstrated the ability to succeed academically, other attributes such as compassion, empathy, altruism, leadership, honesty, and communication and interpersonal skills are viewed as being critical to future excellence. The committee considers that all information pertaining to the ability, personality, and character of the applicant is relevant. Although a solid background in science is required, students with expertise in a wide variety of fields, including the humanities, arts, and engineering, are encouraged to apply.

Financial Aid

Application for financial aid may be initiated following acceptance to the medical school.

Information about Diversity Programs

The University of Michigan is committed to training a diverse cohort of physicians who are capable of caring for an increasingly diverse patient population. Medical students of color are very active in organizations such as LANAMA (Latino/a American/Native American Medical Association) and BMA (Black Medical Association). These students are also actively involved in setting the agenda for diversity and cultural competency programs, and participate in the Health System's Multi-cultural Community Health Alliance.

Campus Information

Setting

The University of Michigan Medical School is nestled in a large medical center surrounded by tree-lined streets, city parks and bike paths.

Enrollment

For 2008, total enrollment was: 678

Housing

While some students choose campus housing, most students opt to live in apartments near the medical center.

Application Process and Requirements 2010–2011

Primary Application Service: AMCAS
Earliest filing date: June 1, 2009
Latest filing date: October 15, 2009

Secondary Application Required?: Yes
Sent to: All applicants
URL: n/a
Fee: Yes, $85
Fee waiver available: Yes
Earliest filing date: July 1, 2009
Latest filing date: November 31, 2009

MCAT® required?: Yes
Latest MCAT® considered: September 2009
Oldest MCAT® considered: 2006

Early Decision Program: School does not have EDP
Applicants notified: n/a
EDP available for: n/a

Regular Acceptance Notice
Earliest date: October 15, 2009
Latest date: Until class is full
Applicant's Response to Acceptance Offer – Maximum Time: May 15, 2010

Requests for Deferred Entrance Considered: Yes

Deposit to Hold Place in Class: No
Deposit (Resident): n/a
Deposit (Non-resident): n/a
Deposit due: n/a
Applied to tuition: n/a
Deposit refundable: n/a
Refundable by: n/a

Estimated number of new entrants: 170
EDP: n/a, special program: n/a

Start Month/Year: August 2010

Interview Format: Regional interviews are not available.

Other Programs

PREPARATORY PROGRAMS
Postbaccalaureate Program: No
Summer Program: Yes

COMBINED DEGREE PROGRAMS
Baccalaureate/M.D.: No
M.D./M.P.H.: Yes, www.sph.umich.edu/academics/degrees.html
M.D./M.B.A.: Yes, http://med.umich.edu/med students/curRes/dualDegree/mdMBA/index.html
M.D./J.D.: Yes
M.D./Ph.D.: Yes, www.med.umich.edu/medschool/mstp/

Premedical Coursework

Course	Req.	Rec.	Lab.	Hrs.
Inorganic Chemistry	•		•	4
Behavioral Sciences				
Biochemistry	•			3
Biology	•		•	6
Biology/Zoology				
Calculus				
College English	•			6
College Mathematics				

Course	Req.	Rec.	Lab.	Hrs.
Computer Science				
Genetics				
Humanities				18
Organic Chemistry	•		•	4
Physics	•		•	6
Psychology				
Social Sciences				
Other				

Selection Factors: 2008 Accepted Applicants

Proportion of Accepted Applicants with Relevant Experience (Data Self-Reported to AMCAS®)		
Community Service/Volunteer		72%
Medically-Related Work		87%
Research		93%

Shaded bar represents school's accepted scores ranging from the 10th percentile to the 90th percentile.   School Median ●   National Median ●

Overall GPA	2.0	2.1	2.2	2.3	2.4	2.5	2.6	2.7	2.8	2.9	3.0	3.1	3.2	3.3	3.4	3.5	3.6	3.7	(3.8)	3.9	4.0
Science GPA	2.0	2.1	2.2	2.3	2.4	2.5	2.6	2.7	2.8	2.9	3.0	3.1	3.2	3.3	3.4	3.5	3.6	3.7	(3.8)	3.9	4.0

MCAT® Total Numeric Score 9 10 11 12 13 14 15 16 17 18 19 20 21 22 23 24 25 26 27 28 29 30 31 (32) 33 34 35 (36) 37 38 39 40 41 42 43

Writing Sample			J	K	L	M	N	O	P	(Q)	R	S	T
Verbal Reasoning	3	4	5	6	7	8	9	(10)	(11)	12	13	14	15
Biological Sciences	3	4	5	6	7	8	9	10	(11)	12	(13)	14	15
Physical Sciences	3	4	5	6	7	8	9	10	(11)	12	(13)	14	15

Acceptance & Matriculation Data for 2008–2009 First Year Class

	Resident	Non-resident	International	Total
Applications	1048	4675	83	5806
Interviewed	181	620	0	801
Deferred	7	10	0	17
Matriculants				
Early Assurance Program	0	0	0	0
Early Decision Program	0	0	0	0
Baccalaureate/M.D.	0	0	0	0
M.D./Ph.D.	3	7	0	10
Matriculated	79	90	1	**170**

Applications accepted from International Applicants: No

Specialty Choice

2004, 2005, 2006 Graduates, Specialty Choice (As reported by program directors to GME Track™)	
Anesthesiology	8%
Emergency Medicine	8%
Family Practice	5%
Internal Medicine	14%
Obstetrics/Gynecology	4%
Orthopaedic Surgery	3%
Pediatrics	8%
Psychiatry	2%
Radiology	6%
Surgery	8%

Matriculant Demographics: 2008–2009 First Year Class

Men: 81   **Women:** 89

Matriculants' Self-Reported Race/Ethnicity

Mexican American	1	Korean	6
Cuban	1	Vietnamese	1
Puerto Rican	1	Other Asian	5
Other Hispanic	6	Total Asian	44
Total Hispanic	9	Native American	2
Chinese	13	Black	5
Asian Indian	12	Native Hawaiian	1
Pakistani	3	White	110
Filipino	3	Unduplicated Number	
Japanese	1	of Matriculants	170

Science and Math Majors: 64%
Matriculants with:
Baccalaureate degree: 98%
Graduate degree(s): 9%

Financial Information

Source: 2007–2008 LCME I-B survey and 2008–2009 AAMC TSF questionnaire

	Residents	Non-residents
Total Cost of Attendance	$48,057	$64,277
Tuition and Fees	$26,005	$41,485
Other (includes living expenses)	$20,052	$20,792
Health Insurance (can be waived)	$2,000	$2,000

Average 2008 Graduate Indebtedness: $111,139
% of Enrolled Students Receiving Aid: 92%

Criminal Background Check

This medical school requires a criminal background check prior to matriculation.

Wayne State University School of Medicine

Detroit, Michigan

Office of Admissions
320 East Canfield, Suite 322
Detroit, Michigan 48201
T 313 577 1466   **F** 313 577 9420

Admissions www.med.wayne.edu/admissions
Main www.med.wayne.edu
Financial www.med.wayne.edu/student_affairs/
financial_aid
E-mail admissions@med.wayne.edu

Public Institution

Dr. Robert M. Mentzer Jr., Dean

*Dr. Silas Norman Jr., Assistant Dean
for Admissions*

*Julia Simmons, Director, Diversity and
Integrated Student Services Office*

Deirdre Moore, Assistant Director, Financial Aid

Dr. Robert R. Frank, Executive Vice Dean

General Information
The School of Medicine, which originated in 1868, is the oldest component of Wayne State University.

Mission Statement
The mission of the Wayne State University School of Medicine is to provide the Michigan community with medical and biotechnical resources, in the form of scientific knowledge and trained professionals, so as to improve the overall health of the community.

Curricular Highlights
Community Service Requirement: Optional. A co-curricular program is available.
Research/Thesis Requirement: Optional.

The curriculum employs a combination of traditional and newer approaches to the teaching of medical students. Year 1 begins with an introductory Clinical Medicine course which runs through all four years including: human sexuality, medical interviewing, physical diagnosis, public health and prevention, and evidence-based medicine. Year 1 is organized around the disciplines of structure (anatomy, histology, and embryology) and function (biochemistry, physiology, genetics, and nutrition), and ends with an integrated neuroscience course. Second year is a completely integrated year focusing on pathophysiology, including immunology/microbiology and pharmacology. Year 3 is a series of clinical clerkships including medicine, surgery, pediatrics, family medicine, psychiatry, neurology, and obstetrics/gynecology. During Year 3 all students have a six-month Continuity clerkship. Year 4 is predominately an elective year with only three required one month rotations: emergency medicine, a sub-internship, and an ambulatory

block month. The School of Medicine uses traditional lectures, small-group and panel discussions, computer-assisted instruction, and multimedia in its teaching program. Standardized patients are used for student practice and assessment in the new Richard J. Mazurek, M.D. Medical Education Commons.

USMLE
Step 1: Required. Students must record a passing score for promotion.
Step 2: Clinical Skills (CS): Required. Students must only record a score.
Step 2: Clinical Knowledge (CK): Required. Students must record a passing total score to graduate.

Selection Factors
Consideration is given to the entire record, GPA, MCAT scores, recommendations, and interview results, as these reflect the applicant's personality, maturity, character, and suitability for medicine. Additionally, the committee regards health care experience as desirable. Following an initial screening process, individuals with competitive applications are selected to complete a secondary application. As a state-supported school, the institution must give preference to Michigan residents; however, out-of-state applicants are encouraged to apply. Applicants whose educational backgrounds include academic work outside the United States must have completed two years of coursework at a U.S. or Canadian college, including the prerequisite courses. Interviews are required, but scheduled only with those applicants who are given serious consideration. Students are urged to apply by November 1.

Financial Aid
Financial aid awards administered by the School of Medicine are made by the financial aid officer based on federal guidelines and those established by the Committee on Financial Aid and Scholarships, which includes student representation. The College Work-Study Program and other medically oriented jobs are generally available to eligible students for the summer break. Financial aid seminars are held for incoming students and their families. Additional information is available by calling the Office of Financial Aid at (313) 577-1039 or visiting its Web site.

Information about Diversity Programs
The school supports a one-year postbaccalaureate program for disadvantaged medical school applicants from Michigan who have been denied admission, but who appear to have the potential for academic success. The program consists of pre-medical science courses, academic skills training, personal adjustment counseling, and academic tutoring. Successful students are guaranteed admission to the School of Medicine. For information, write Julia Simmons, Director, Office of Diversity and Integrated Student Services.

Campus Information
Setting
WSUSOM is located in the 236 acre Detroit Medical Center in Detroit, and consists of Scott Hall; Richard J. Mazurek, M.D. Medical Education Commons; Shiffman Medical Library; Lande Medical Research Building; Elliman Clinical Research Building; and the C.S. Mott Building.

Enrollment
For 2008, total enrollment was: 1172

Special Features
Harper University Hospital, Hutzel Women's Hospital, the Children's Hospital of Michigan, Detroit Receiving Hospital, University Health Center, the Rehabilitation Institute of Michigan, and the John Dingell V.A. Medical Center make up the Detroit Medical Center (DMC). In addition, the SEMCME (SE Michigan Center for Medical Education) brings together Wayne State University, the DMC, and community-based teaching hospitals in the Southeastern Michigan metropolitan area.

Housing
On-campus resident housing is available on the main campus located near the medical center. The Office of Student Organizations maintains a list of affordable apartments located near the medical school.

Application Process and Requirements 2010–2011

Primary Application Service: AMCAS
Earliest filing date: June 1, 2009
Latest filing date: December 15, 2009

Secondary Application Required?: Yes
Sent to: Screened applicants
Contact: Dawn Yargeau
(313) 577-1466, admissions@med.wayne.edu
Fee: Yes, $50
Fee waiver available: Yes
Earliest filing date: July 15, 2009
Latest filing date: March 1, 2010

MCAT® required?: Yes
Latest MCAT® considered: September 2009
Oldest MCAT® considered: September 2006

Early Decision Program: School does have EDP
Applicants notified: October 1, 2009
EDP available for: Both Residents
and Non-residents

Regular Acceptance Notice
Earliest date: October 18, 2009
Latest date: Varies
Applicant's Response to Acceptance
Offer – Maximum Time: Three weeks

**Requests for Deferred
Entrance Considered:** Yes

Deposit to Hold Place in Class: Yes
Deposit (Resident): $50
Deposit (Non-resident): $50
Deposit due: With response to acceptance offer
Applied to tuition: Yes
Deposit refundable: No
Refundable by: n/a

Estimated number of new entrants: 290
EDP: 5, special program: 17

Start Month/Year: August 2010

Interview Format: One-on-one with an
Admission Committee member. Regional
interviews are not available.

Other Programs

PREPARATORY PROGRAMS
Postbaccalaureate Program: Yes,
Julia Simmons, (313) 577-1598
jsimmons@med.wayne.edu
Summer Program: Yes, Julia Simmons,
(313) 577-1598, jsimmons@med.wayne.edu

COMBINED DEGREE PROGRAMS
Baccalaureate/M.D.: Yes, http://honors.wayne.
edu/medstart.php
Nancy Galster, (313) 577-3030, ad4469@wayne.edu
M.D./M.P.H.: No
M.D./M.B.A.: No
M.D./J.D.: No
M.D./Ph.D.: Yes, www.mdphdprogram.med.
wayne.edu/
Ambika Mathur, Ph.D., (313) 577-1455
amathur@med.wayne.edu

Premedical Coursework

Course	Req.	Rec.	Lab.	Qtrs.
Inorganic Chemistry	•		•	2
Behavioral Sciences				
Biochemistry		•		1
Biology				
Biology/Zoology	•		•	2
Calculus				
College English	•			2
College Mathematics				

Course	Req.	Rec.	Lab.	Qtrs.
Computer Science				
Genetics				
Humanities				
Organic Chemistry	•		•	2
Physics	•		•	2
Psychology				
Social Sciences				
Other				

Selection Factors: 2008 Accepted Applicants

Proportion of Accepted Applicants with Relevant Experience (Data Self-Reported to AMCAS)		Community Service/Volunteer	71%
		Medically-Related Work	90%
		Research	81%

Shaded bar represents school's accepted scores ranging from the 10th percentile to the 90th percentile   School Median ● National Median ●

Overall GPA	2.0	2.1	2.2	2.3	2.4	2.5	2.6	2.7	2.8	2.9	3.0	3.1	3.2	3.3	3.4	3.5	3.6	(3.7)	3.8	3.9	4.0
Science GPA	2.0	2.1	2.2	2.3	2.4	2.5	2.6	2.7	2.8	2.9	3.0	3.1	3.2	3.3	3.4	3.5	3.6	(3.7)	3.8	3.9	4.0

MCAT® Total Numeric Score 9 10 11 12 13 14 15 16 17 18 19 20 21 22 23 24 25 26 27 28 29 30 31 (32) 33 34 35 36 37 38 39 40 41 42 43

Writing Sample			J	K	L	M	N	O	(P)	(Q)	R	S	T	
Verbal Reasoning	3	4	5	6	7	8	9	(10)	11	12	13	14	15	
Biological Sciences	3	4	5	6	7	8	9	10	(11)	12	13	14	15	
Physical Sciences	3	4	5	6	7	8	9	10	(11)	12	13	14	15	

Acceptance & Matriculation Data for 2008–2009 First Year Class

	Resident	Non-resident	International	Total
Applications	1396	2411	452	4259
Interviewed	505	161	73	739
Deferred	1	3	1	5
Matriculants				
Early Assurance Program	0	0	0	0
Early Decision Program	4	0	0	4
Baccalaureate/M.D.	11	0	0	11
M.D./Ph.D.	3	0	0	3
Matriculated	246	27	17	**290**

Applications accepted from International Applicants: Canadian Only

Matriculant Demographics: 2008–2009 First Year Class

Men: 156   **Women:** 134

Matriculants' Self-Reported Race/Ethnicity

Mexican American	1	Korean	5
Cuban	1	Vietnamese	1
Puerto Rican	0	Other Asian	6
Other Hispanic	1	Total Asian	64
Total Hispanic	3	Native American	4
Chinese	9	Black	14
Asian Indian	36	Native Hawaiian	1
Pakistani	6	White	184
Filipino	3	**Unduplicated Number**	
Japanese	1	**of Matriculants**	290

Science and Math Majors: 66%
Matriculants with:
    Baccalaureate degree: 99%
    Graduate degree(s): 15%

Specialty Choice

2004, 2005, 2006 Graduates, Specialty Choice (As reported by program directors to GME Track™)	
Anesthesiology	5%
Emergency Medicine	14%
Family Practice	7%
Internal Medicine	18%
Obstetrics/Gynecology	6%
Orthopaedic Surgery	4%
Pediatrics	7%
Psychiatry	3%
Radiology	8%
Surgery	6%

Financial Information

Source: 2007–2008 LCME I-B survey
and 2008–2009 AAMC TSF questionnaire

	Residents	Non-residents
Total Cost of Attendance	$52,159	$81,549
Tuition and Fees	$28,425	$57,515
Other (includes living expenses)	$21,548	$21,848
Health Insurance (can be waived)	$2,186	$2,186

Average 2008 Graduate Indebtedness: $143,203
% of Enrolled Students Receiving Aid: 90%

Criminal Background Check

This medical school does not require a criminal
background check prior to matriculation.

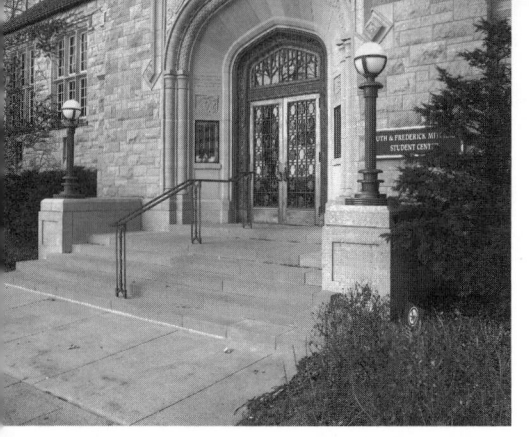

Mayo Clinic College of Medicine
Mayo Medical School
Rochester, Minnesota

Mayo Medical School
200 First Street, SW
Rochester, Minnesota 55905
T 507 284 2316   **F** 507 284 2634

Admissions www.mayo.edu/mms/md-admissions.html
Main www.mayo.edu/mms
Financial www.mayo.edu/mms/md-tuition.html
E-mail medschoolAdmissions@mayo.edu

Private Institution

Dr. Keith D. Lindor, Dean

Dr. Patricia A. Barrier, Associate Dean for Student Affairs

Dr. Eddie L. Greene, Director for Diversity

Barbara L. Porter, Assistant Dean for Student Affairs

David L. Dahlen, Director of Financial Aid and Registrar

General Information

Mayo Medical School is an integral part of Mayo Clinic, the world's largest group practice of medicine. Resources of MMS include a diverse patient population of more than 500,000 registrants annually, four affiliated hospitals with facilities for clinical and basic research, primary care facilities including several rural health centers, and affiliations with physicians who practice in surrounding communities and states.

Mission Statement

Mayo Medical School will use the patient-centered focus and strengths of Mayo Clinic to educate physicians to serve society by assuming leadership roles in medical practice, education, and research.

Curricular Highlights

Community Service Requirement: Optional.
Research/Thesis Requirement: Required.

The innovative patient-based curriculum is characterized by extensive early patient interaction and creative integration of sciences in all segments of the curriculum. In the first two years, courses occur in integrated blocks and contain a clinical component with experiences related to topics covered in the classroom. Themes of basic science, clinical experiences, leadership, physician and society, principles of pharmacology, and basic and advanced doctoring are represented throughout the curriculum. First and second year selectives engage students in career exploration, shadowing, and volunteer work. Year three is devoted to developing skills in all of the basic clinical clerkships, moving beyond acquiring information to the level of synthesis and diagnosis. One

quarter of the third year is an opportunity to explore the realm of scientific investigation, as every student completes a research endeavor under the mentorship of an experienced Mayo investigator. Over 80 percent of students publish and/or present their research while in medical school. Year four requirements include a sub-internship and rotations in family medicine, pediatrics, surgery, and emergency medicine. A social medicine rotation is offered to understand the role of community in the mission of medicine. Integrated into the fourth-year curriculum is a three week didactic experience in which students explore preventive medicine, biomedical ethics, palliative medicine and clinical pharmacology. The remainder of the fourth year is fully elective which allows students to customize their learning.

USMLE

Step 1: Required. Students must record a passing score for promotion.
Step 2: Clinical Skills (CS): Required. Students must record a passing total score to graduate.
Step 2: Clinical Knowledge (CK): Required. Students must record a passing total score to graduate.

Selection Factors

Mayo Medical School is dedicated to enrolling students with superior academic credentials who possess leadership characteristics and have a profound desire to commit their lives to service. An evaluation of the entire AMCAS application, including the academic record, MCAT scores, research, healthcare exploration, and service experiences, is considered in the initial review. For selected candidates three letters of recommendation will be requested. If the applicant qualifies, an onsite interview is granted. Appointment notification occurs approximately every four weeks throughout the admissions cycle. Appointments continue to be offered to fill the class up to the time of matriculation. All matriculates must have completed prerequisite courses and must possess a baccalaureate degree granted from an accredited United States or Canadian college or university; the final two years of coursework must be completed at this school. Mayo does not discriminate on the basis of race, sex, creed,

national origin, age, or disability in its educational programs or activities. Mayo Medical School does not accept transfer students.

Financial Aid

A generous scholarship program provides every student significant financial support. Financial aid in the form of loans and need-based grants are also available.

Information about Diversity Programs

Mayo Medical School actively seeks to recruit and matriculate a diverse class of students.

Campus Information

Setting

Mayo Medical School is located in Rochester, Minnesota, a vibrant, friendly city that provides a highly livable environment for more than 32,000 Mayo Clinic staff and students.

Enrollment

For 2008, total enrollment was: 172

Special Features

Mayo Clinic's three practices and regional health system comprise the largest integrated private group practice in the world. Thus, the clinical resources experienced as a Mayo medical student are unparalleled.

Housing

On-campus housing is not available. A list of affordable housing options in areas adjacent to the campus can be provided to new students.

Satellite Campuses/Facilities

In addition to the Mayo Clinic in Rochester, Minnesota, rotations can be completed at Mayo Clinic's group practice sites in Arizona and Florida.

Application Process and Requirements 2010–2011

Primary Application Service: AMCAS
Earliest filing date: June 1, 2009
Latest filing date: October 15, 2009

Secondary Application Required?: No
Sent to: n/a
URL: n/a
Fee: Yes, $100
Fee waiver available: Yes
Earliest filing date: n/a
Latest filing date: n/a

MCAT® required?: Yes
Latest MCAT® considered: September 2009
Oldest MCAT® considered: 2007

Early Decision Program: School does not have EDP
Applicants notified: n/a
EDP available for: n/a

Regular Acceptance Notice
Earliest date: October 15, 2009
Latest date: Until class is full
Applicant's Response to Acceptance Offer – Maximum Time: Two weeks

Requests for Deferred Entrance Considered: Yes

Deposit to Hold Place in Class: Yes

Deposit (Resident): $100
Deposit (Non-resident): $100
Deposit due: With response to acceptance offer
Applied to tuition: No
Deposit refundable: Yes, Refundable upon matriculation

Estimated number of new entrants: 50
EDP: n/a, special program: n/a

Start Month/Year: July 2010

Interview Format: Two one-on-one interviews with Admissions Committee members. Regional interviews are not available.

Other Programs

PREPARATORY PROGRAMS
Postbaccalaureate Program: No
Summer Program: Yes, www.mayo.edu/mms/prospective-students.html, Marcy Landswerk, (507) 284-2316, landswerk.marcy@mayo.edu

COMBINED DEGREE PROGRAMS
Baccalaureate/M.D.: No
M.D./M.P.H.: Yes, www.mayo.edu/mms/academic-enrichment.html
M.D./M.B.A.: No
M.D./J.D.: Yes, www.mayo.edu/mms/academic-enrichment.html
M.D./Ph.D.: Yes, www.mayo.edu/mms/md-phd.html

Premedical Coursework

Course	Req.	Rec.	Lab.	Sems.	Course	Req.	Rec.	Lab.	Sems.
Inorganic Chemistry	•		•	2	Computer Science				
Behavioral Sciences					Genetics				
Biochemistry	•			1	Humanities				
Biology	•		•	2	Organic Chemistry	•		•	2
Biology/Zoology					Physics	•		•	2
Calculus					Psychology				
College English					Social Sciences				
College Mathematics					Other				

Selection Factors: 2008 Accepted Applicants

Proportion of Accepted Applicants with Relevant Experience (Data Self-Reported to AMCAS®)		
Community Service/Volunteer		83%
Medically-Related Work		87%
Research		92%

Shaded bar represents school's accepted scores ranging from the 10th percentile to the 90th percentile. School Median ● National Median ●

Overall GPA	2.0	2.1	2.2	2.3	2.4	2.5	2.6	2.7	2.8	2.9	3.0	3.1	3.2	3.3	3.4	3.5	3.6	3.7	3.8	(3.9)	4.0	
Science GPA	2.0	2.1	2.2	2.3	2.4	2.5	2.6	2.7	2.8	2.9	3.0	3.1	3.2	3.3	3.4	3.5	3.6	3.7	(3.8)	3.9	4.0	

MCAT® Total Numeric Score 9 10 11 12 13 14 15 16 17 18 19 20 21 22 23 24 25 26 27 28 29 30 31 (32) 33 34 (35) 36 37 38 39 40 41 42 43

Writing Sample			J	K	L	M	N	O	P	(Q)	R	S	T
Verbal Reasoning	3	4	5	6	7	8	9	(10)	(11)	12	13	14	15
Biological Sciences	3	4	5	6	7	8	9	10	(11)	(12)	13	14	15
Physical Sciences	3	4	5	6	7	8	9	10	(11)	(12)	13	14	15

Acceptance & Matriculation Data for 2008–2009 First Year Class

	Resident	Non-resident	International	Total
Applications	404	3160	175	3739
Interviewed	43	255	13	311
Deferred	1	0	0	1
Matriculant				
Early Assurance Program	n/a	n/a	n/a	n/a
Early Decision Program	n/a	n/a	n/a	n/a
Baccalaureate/M.D.	n/a	n/a	n/a	n/a
M.D./Ph.D.	1	5	0	6
Matriculated	11	37	2	**50**

Applications accepted from International Applicants: Yes

Matriculant Demographics: 2008–2009 First Year Class

Men: 24 **Women:** 26

Matriculants' Self-Reported Race/Ethnicity

Mexican American	2	Korean	0
Cuban	0	Vietnamese	0
Puerto Rican	0	Other Asian	0
Other Hispanic	0	Total Asian	13
Total Hispanic	2	Native American	2
Chinese	5	Black	1
Asian Indian	5	Native Hawaiian	3
Pakistani	1	White	32
Filipino	1	Unduplicated Number	
Japanese	1	of Matriculants	50

Science and Math Majors: 58%
Matriculants with:
Baccalaureate degree: 100%
Graduate degree(s): 10%

Specialty Choice

2004, 2005, 2006 Graduates, Specialty Choice (As reported by program directors to GME Track™)	
Anesthesiology	9%
Emergency Medicine	6%
Family Practice	8%
Internal Medicine	15%
Obstetrics/Gynecology	4%
Orthopaedic Surgery	2%
Pediatrics	13%
Psychiatry	3%
Radiology	13%
Surgery	3%

Financial Information

Source: 2007–2008 LCME I-B survey and 2008–2009 AAMC TSF questionnaire

	Residents	Non-residents
Total Cost of Attendance	$59.698	$59,698
Tuition and Fees	$29,800	$29,800
Other (includes living expenses)	$29,898	$29,898
Health Insurance (can be waived)	$0	$0

Average 2008 Graduate Indebtedness: $74,181
% of Enrolled Students Receiving Aid: 100%

Criminal Background Check

This medical school requires a criminal background check prior to matriculation.

University of Minnesota Medical School
Minneapolis, Minnesota

University of Minnesota
Medical School – Twin Cities
MMC 293, 420 Delaware St SE
Minneapolis, Minnesota 55455
T 612 625 7977   **F** 612 625 8228

Admissions www.meded.umn.edu/admissions (TC),
www.med.umn.edu/duluth/admissions (DU)
Main www.med.umn.edu/
Financial www.meded.umn.edu/financial (TC),
www.med.umn.edu/duluth/admissions/tuition/home.
html (DU)
E-mail meded@umn.edu (Twin Cities),
medadmis@d.umn.edu (Duluth)

Public Institution

Dr. Deborah Powell, Dean

Dr. Gary L. Davis, Senior Associate Dean, Duluth Campus

Dr. Lillian A. Repesh, Associate Dean for Admissions and Student Affairs, Duluth

Paul T. White, J.D., Associate Dean of Admissions, Twin Cities

Dr. Joycelyn Dorscher, Director of Center of American Indian and Minority Health

Mary Tate, Director of Minority Affairs and Diversity, Twin Cities

General Information

Founded in 1888, the University of Minnesota Medical School is located on the Twin Cities campus of the University. A two-year basic science regional campus is located in Duluth. The medical school is a unit of the U of M Academic Health Center.

Mission Statement

Committed to innovation and diversity, the Medical School educates physicians, scientists, and health professionals; generates knowledge and treatments; and cares for patients and communities with compassion and respect. We value excellence, inclusiveness, collaboration and discovery.

Curricular Highlights

Community Service Requirement: Optional.
Research/Thesis Requirement: Optional.

In the Medical School curriculum, progress is based on competency achievement, not time. This innovative program offers integrated instruction in scientific foundations of medicine and clinical sciences. An emphasis on critical thinking and self-directed learning is built into courses, reinforced by Foundations of Critical Thinking cases that span the curriculum. Early clinical exposure includes direct patient care focusing on understanding health care processes. Significant flexibility in the structure and scheduling of the 3rd year and beyond allows students to pursue a wide range of clinical/academic interests. Each student has an advisor throughout medical school to ensure mastery

of required competencies. The Twin Cities campus offers a Medical Scientist Training Program and other combined degrees, while Duluth has a mission focused on preparing students for family practice in rural Minnesota and Native American communities.

USMLE

Step 1: Required. Students must record a passing score for promotion.
Step 2: Clinical Skills (CS): Required. Students must record a passing total score to graduate.
Step 2: Clinical Knowledge (CK): Required. Students must record a passing total score to graduate.

Selection Factors

Legal residents of Minnesota are given preference for admission, but qualified out-of-state applicants are also encouraged to apply. Commitment to improving the human condition, unassailable professional conduct, outstanding interpersonal skills, dedication to lifelong learning and cultural sensitivity are evaluated. The medical school seeks to matriculate a diverse student body *(www.meded.umn.edu/admissions/index.cfm).* Applicant qualifications are evaluated through recommendation letters, post-secondary experiences, undergraduate education, responses to the supplemental application, and on-site interviews. In addition, the medical school's Duluth campus seeks persons with traits that indicate a high potential for becoming a family physician in rural Minnesota or American Indian communities. Duluth applicants must be U.S. citizens or have permanent resident status. Transfer students are rarely accepted into Year 3 on the Twin Cities campus. Students accepted to the Twin Cities and Duluth campuses enter a class of 170 and 60 students, respectively. The University of Minnesota Medical School does not discriminate on the basis of race, gender, creed, sexual orientation, disability, or national origin.

Financial Aid

Financial aid applicants must file the FAFSA. Loans and scholarship aid are available. Tuition rates for new matriculates are fixed through a cost-of-degree tuition policy. For information, contact B.J. Gibson *[TC]*(612/625-4998,

www. meded.umn.edu/financial) or Dina Flaherty *[DU]* (218/726-6548, *www.med.umn.edu/duluth/admissions/tuition/home.html).*

Information about Diversity Programs

Minnesota is committed to the recruitment and education of students from groups underrepresented in medicine. For more information, contact the Office of Minority Affairs and Diversity (Twin Cities, 612/625-1494), or the Center of American Indian and Minority Health. CAIMH is headquartered in Duluth (218/726-7235) and also has a Twin Cities office (612/624-0465).

Campus Information

Setting
The Twin Cities campus is located on the second largest university campus in the United States. Most major hospitals in the Minneapolis-St. Paul area are affiliated with the Medical School. The Duluth program is located on the U of MN Duluth campus in northeastern Minnesota and has affiliations with Duluth hospitals.

Enrollment
For 2008, total enrollment was: 945

Special Features
The Medical School provides a wide range of clinical and research opportunities *(www.meded.umn.edu/clerkships/index.cfm; www.med.umn.edu/RPAP/; www.med.umn.edu/imer/; www.ahc.umn.edu/; www.meded.umn.edu/resopps/).*

Housing
Medical student fraternities *[TC]* and private housing are available in the campus neighborhoods; both campuses maintain a list of resources for affordable off-campus housing.

Satellite Campuses/Facilities
The two-year program at the Medical School's Duluth campus was established to increase the number of family practice physicians with a commitment to serve in rural Minnesota or American Indian communities. Students transition to the Twin Cities for years 3 and 4 with the opportunity to complete some rotations in Duluth as well as participate in RPAP. For more information: Susan Christensen (218/726-8511; medadmis@d.umn.edu).

Application Process and Requirements 2010–2011

Primary Application Service: AMCAS
Earliest filing date: June 1, 2009
Latest filing date: November 15, 2009

Secondary Application Required?: Yes
Sent to: All
URL: n/a
Fee: Yes, $75
Fee waiver available: Yes
Earliest filing date: 2009
Latest filing date: January 31, 2010

MCAT® required?: Yes
Latest MCAT® considered: September 2009
Oldest MCAT® considered: 2006

Early Decision Program: School does have EDP
Applicants notified: October 1, 2009
EDP available for: Both Residents and Non-residents

Regular Acceptance Notice
Earliest date: October 15, 2009
Latest date: Until class is full
Applicant's Response to Acceptance Offer – Maximum Time: Two weeks

Requests for Deferred Entrance Considered: Yes

Deposit to Hold Place in Class: Yes
Deposit (Resident): $100
Deposit (Non-resident): $100
Deposit due: With response to acceptance offer
Applied to tuition: Yes
Deposit refundable: Yes
Refundable by: May 15, 2010

Estimated number of new entrants: 230
EDP: 20, special program: 5

Start Month/Year: August 2010

Interview Format: Individual interviews are conducted. Regional interviews are not available.

Other Programs

PREPARATORY PROGRAMS
Postbaccalaureate Program: No
Summer Program: Yes, www.caimh.org
Pre-matriculation Program: Yes, www.caimh.org

COMBINED DEGREE PROGRAMS
Baccalaureate/M.D.: Yes, www.med.umn.edu/duluth/admissions/home.html, Susan Christensen (218) 726-8511, medadmis@d.umn.edu
M.D./M.P.H.: Yes, www.sph.umn.edu/education/degrees/home.html, Sarah Harper, (612) 626-3740; (800) 774-8636, harpe014@umn.edu
M.D./M.B.A.: Yes, www.meded.umn.edu/admissions/MD-MBA.cfm, Tracy Keeling, (612) 625-5555, tkeeling@umn.edu
M.D./J.D.: Yes, www.meded.umn.edu/admissions/JD-MD.cfm, Carol Rachac, (612) 625-3356, crachac@umn.edu
M.D./Ph.D.: Yes, www.med.umn.edu/mdphd/home.html Susan Shurson, (612) 625-3680, shurs002@umn.edu
Additional: Yes, M.D./M.H.I., www.hinfgrad.umn.edu/mhi/MD-MHI.html Stewart Speedie, (612) 624-4657, speed002@umn.edu

Premedical Coursework

Course	Req.	Rec.	Lab.	Qtrs.
Inorganic Chemistry	•		•	1
Behavioral Sciences				
Biochemistry		•		1
Biology	•		•	1
Biology/Zoology				
Calculus				
College English				
College Mathematics				
Computer Science				

Course	Req.	Rec.	Lab.	Qtrs.
Genetics		•		
Humanities	•			1
Organic Chemistry	•		•	2
Physics	•		•	2
Psychology		•		1
Social Sciences	•			1
Statistics		•		
Ethics		•		
Foreign Language		•		

Selection Factors: 2008 Accepted Applicants

Proportion of Accepted Applicants with Relevant Experience (Data Self-Reported to AMCAS)	
Community Service/Volunteer	77%
Medically-Related Work	86%
Research	79%

Shaded bar represents school's accepted scores ranging from the 10th percentile to the 90th percentile   School Median ●   National Median ●

Overall GPA	2.0	2.1	2.2	2.3	2.4	2.5	2.6	2.7	2.8	2.9	3.0	3.1	3.2	3.3	3.4	3.5	3.6	3.7	(3.8)	3.9	4.0
Science GPA	2.0	2.1	2.2	2.3	2.4	2.5	2.6	2.7	2.8	2.9	3.0	3.1	3.2	3.3	3.4	3.5	3.6	(3.7)	3.8	3.9	4.0

MCAT® Total Numeric Score 9 10 11 12 13 14 15 16 17 18 19 20 21 22 23 24 25 26 27 28 29 30 31 (32) 33 34 35 36 37 38 39 40 41 42 43

Writing Sample			J	K	L	M	N	O	(P)	(Q)	R	S	T
Verbal Reasoning	3	4	5	6	7	8	9	(10)	11	12	13	14	15
Biological Sciences	3	4	5	6	7	8	9	10	(11)	12	13	14	15
Physical Sciences	3	4	5	6	7	8	9	10	(11)	12	13	14	15

Acceptance & Matriculation Data for 2008–2009 First Year Class

	Resident	Non-resident	International	Total
Applications	1226	3116	222	4564
Interviewed	389	220	12	621
Deferred	4	0	0	4
Matriculants				
Early Assurance Program	0	0	0	0
Early Decision Program	14	1	0	15
Baccalaureate/M.D.	2	0	0	2
M.D./Ph.D.	3	3	0	6
Matriculated	193	34	3	**230**

Applications accepted from International Applicants: Yes

Matriculant Demographics: 2008–2009 First Year Class

Men: 118   **Women:** 112

Matriculants' Self-Reported Race/Ethnicity

Mexican American	4	**Korean**	2
Cuban	0	**Vietnamese**	1
Puerto Rican	3	**Other Asian**	4
Other Hispanic	1	**Total Asian**	25
Total Hispanic	7	**Native American**	7
Chinese	9	**Black**	9
Asian Indian	5	**Native Hawaiian**	0
Pakistani	1	**White**	184
Filipino	2	**Unduplicated Number**	
Japanese	1	**of Matriculants**	230

Science and Math Majors: 67%
Matriculants with:
   Baccalaureate degree: 100%
   Graduate degree(s): 6%

Specialty Choice

2004, 2005, 2006 Graduates, Specialty Choice (As reported by program directors to GME Track™)	
Anesthesiology	6%
Emergency Medicine	7%
Family Practice	17%
Internal Medicine	18%
Obstetrics/Gynecology	5%
Orthopaedic Surgery	4%
Pediatrics	9%
Psychiatry	3%
Radiology	4%
Surgery	7%

Financial Information

Source: 2007–2008 LCME I-B survey and 2008–2009 AAMC TSF questionnaire

	Residents	Non-residents
Total Cost of Attendance	$55,418	$62,951
Tuition and Fees	$32,427	$39,960
Other (includes living expenses)	$20,795	$20,795
Health Insurance (can be waived)	$2,196	$2,196

Average 2008 Graduate Indebtedness: $176,561
% of Enrolled Students Receiving Aid: 95%

Criminal Background Check

This medical school requires a criminal background check prior to matriculation.

University of Mississippi School of Medicine

Jackson, Mississippi

Associate Dean for Admissions
University of Mississippi School of Medicine
2500 North State Street
Jackson, Mississippi 39216-4505
T 601 984 5010   **F** 601 984 5008

Admissions http://som.umc.edu/admissions.html
Main http://som.umc.edu
Financial http://som.umc.edu/
acceptedAppl.html#FinanAssist
E-mail AdmitMD@som.umsmed.edu

Public Institution

Dr. Daniel W. Jones, Dean

Dr. Steven T. Case, Associate Dean for Admissions

Dr. Jasmine P. Taylor, Associate Dean for Multicultural Affairs

Stacey Mathews, Director of Student Financial Aid

Dr. Peggy M. Davis, Director of Admissions

Barbara M. Westerfield, Registrar

General Information

The School of Medicine, created by a special act of the Board of Trustees in June 1903, operated as a two-year school in Oxford until 1955, when it expanded to four years and moved to the new University of Mississippi Medical Center in Jackson. The Medical Center now houses the Schools of Medicine, Nursing, Health Related Professions, Dentistry, Graduate Studies in Health Sciences, and the 722-bed University Hospitals and Health System.

Mission Statement

The primary mission of the University of Mississippi School of Medicine is to offer an accredited program of medical education that will provide well-trained physicians and certain supporting health care professionals, in numbers consistent with the health care needs of the state, who are responsive to the health problems of the people and committed to medical education as a continuum, which must prevail throughout professional life.

Curricular Highlights

Community Service Requirement: Optional. Medical students staff the Jackson Free Clinic
Research/Thesis Requirement: Optional.

During the two preclinical years, students learn the sciences basic to the study of medicine and participate in laboratory exercises, small-group discussion, computer-assisted learning, and independent study. The preclinical curriculum was revised to increase integration and improve the sequencing of course content and provide earlier clinical experience for students.

The third year involves full-time clinical study as students rotate through the major clinical disciplines and participate in the team care of patients in the University Hospitals and Clinics, Veterans Affairs Medical Center, and various community settings. The fourth year consists of eight required calendar month blocks that may be taken at any time during the eleven months available from July through May. Fourth-year clinical clerkships provide greater depth of study in core areas of medicine, as well as in a student's anticipated medical specialty. Opportunities exist for advanced study and research in basic science departments and for electives at other institutions in this country or abroad.

USMLE

Step 1: Required. Students must record a passing score for promotion.
Step 2: Clinical Skills (CS): Required. Students must record a passing total score to graduate.
Step 2: Clinical Knowledge (CK): Required. Students must record a passing total score to graduate.

Selection Factors

The Admissions Committee selects applicants on a competitive basis without regard to age, sex, sexual orientation, race, creed, national origin, marital status, handicap, or veteran status. Strong preference is given to legal residents of Mississippi; in recent years, non-residents have not been admitted. Interviews are arranged at the discretion of the Admissions Committee; major considerations are undergraduate BCPM GPA and MCAT scores. Interviews are used to assess non-cognitive variables and communication skills. Experiences listed on an AMCAS application document nonacademic and professional attributes, and premedical faculty evaluations reveal an applicant's approach to academic study and professionalism. For details, see *http://som.umc.edu/admissions.html#EvalApps*. Mississippi residents enrolled in other medical schools accredited by the Liaison Committee on Medical Education may be considered for advanced standing transfer.

Financial Aid

Accepted students may apply for financial aid. The school participates in federal scholarship and loan programs (such as Perkins and Stafford) and state-funded Mississippi Rural Physician Scholarship and State Medical Education Loan/Scholarship programs. Eligible students may qualify for limited scholarship funds provided by private donors. For details, see *http://som.umc.edu/acceptedappl.html# FinanAssist.*

Information about Diversity Programs

The Admissions Committee encourages students from groups underrepresented in medicine to apply for admission. Information about pipeline programs and support provided by the Division of Multicultural Affairs can be obtained at: *http://mca.umc.edu/.*

Campus Information

Setting

The Medical Center is located on a 164 acre campus in Jackson. The state capital and Mississippi's largest city, Jackson offers a wide array of professional arts attractions. Recreational facilities include a 30,000-acre reservoir, just 15 minutes from the campus.

Enrollment

For 2008, total enrollment was: 430

Special Features

The opening of a new adult medical and surgical hospital in 2006 marked the completion of a project to replace the original teaching hospital with four new state-of-the-art hospitals. The Medical Center opened a 57,000 square foot student union – with a state-of-the-art fitness center and gymnasium – in 1999. Medical students sponsor the Jackson Free Clinic that provides medical care to homeless and uninsured patients on Saturdays.

Housing

Rent averages from $450-$750 a month for area apartments.

Satellite Campuses/Facilities

The Jackson Medical Mall, one mile from the campus, houses the hospital's clinics, offices for the Jackson Heart Study and the Medical Center's new Cancer Institute. Originally the city's first shopping mall, the Jackson Medical Mall is recognized as a national model of urban revitalization.

Application Process and Requirements 2010–2011

Primary Application Service: AMCAS
Earliest filing date: June 1, 2009
Latest filing date: October 15, 2009

Secondary Application Required?: Yes
Sent to: URL and password provided after receipt of AMCAS application.
URL: http://som.umc.edu/docs/SecondaryApplication.pdf
Fee: Yes, $50
Fee waiver available: Yes
Earliest filing date: June 1, 2009
Latest filing date: December 1, 2009

MCAT® required?: Yes
Latest MCAT® considered: September 2009
Oldest MCAT® considered: April 2006

Early Decision Program: School does have EDP
Applicants notified: Not later than October 1, 2009
EDP available for: Residents only

Regular Acceptance Notice
Earliest date: October 16, 2009
Latest date: Until class is full
Applicant's Response to Acceptance Offer – Maximum Time: Two weeks

Requests for Deferred Entrance Considered: Yes

Deposit to Hold Place in Class: Yes
Deposit (Resident): $50
Deposit (Non-resident): $100
Deposit due: Deposit must accompany response to acceptance offer
Applied to tuition: Yes
Deposit refundable: Yes
Refundable by: May 15, 2010

Estimated number of new entrants: 120
EDP: 10, special program: n/a

Start Month/Year: August 3, 2010

Interview Format: Three semi-structured, one-on-one interviews. Regional interviews are not available.

Other Programs

PREPARATORY PROGRAMS
Postbaccalaureate Program: Yes, http://som.umc.edu/admissions.html#PPT
Summer Program: Yes, http://mca.umc.edu/
Pre-matriculation Program: Yes, http://mca.umc.edu/programs/pre_mat.html
MedCorp Program: Yes, http://mca.umc.edu/programs/medcorp.html

COMBINED DEGREE PROGRAMS
Baccalaureate/M.D.: No
M.D./M.P.H.: No
M.D./M.B.A.: No
M.D./J.D.: No
M.D./Ph.D.: Yes, http://som.umc.edu/admissions.html#MDPhD

Premedical Coursework

Course	Req.	Rec.	Lab.	Hrs.
Inorganic Chemistry	•		•	8
Behavioral Sciences		•		
Biochemistry		•		
Biology				
Biology/Zoology	•		•	8
Calculus		•		3
College English	•			6
College Mathematics	•			6
Computer Science				

Course	Req.	Rec.	Lab.	Hrs.
Genetics		•		3
Humanities		•		
Organic Chemistry	•		•	8
Physics	•		•	8
Psychology		•		
Social Sciences		•		
Vertebrate Anatomy		•		3
Histology		•		3
Physiology		•		3

Selection Factors: 2008 Accepted Applicants

Proportion of Accepted Applicants with Relevant Experience (Data Self-Reported to AMCAS®)		
Community Service/Volunteer	83%
Medically-Related Work	72%
Research	55%

Shaded bar represents school's accepted scores ranging from the 10th percentile to the 90th percentile. School Median ● National Median ●

Overall GPA 2.0 2.1 2.2 2.3 2.4 2.5 2.6 2.7 2.8 2.9 3.0 3.1 3.2 3.3 **3.4 3.5 3.6 3.7 (3.8)** 3.9 4.0

Science GPA 2.0 2.1 2.2 2.3 2.4 2.5 2.6 2.7 2.8 2.9 3.0 3.1 **3.2 3.3 3.4 3.5 3.6 (3.7)** 3.8 3.9 4.0

MCAT® Total Numeric Score 9 10 11 12 13 14 15 16 17 18 19 20 21 22 **23 24 25 26 (27) 28 29 30 31 (32) 33** 34 35 36 37 38 39 40 41 42 43

Writing Sample			J	K	**L**	**M**	**(N)**	**O**	**P**	**(Q)**	R	S	T
Verbal Reasoning	3	4	5	6	**7**	**8**	**(9)**	**(10)**	**11**	12	13	14	15
Biological Sciences	3	4	5	6	7	8	**(9)**	**10**	**(11)**	**12**	13	14	15
Physical Sciences	3	4	5	6	**7**	**8**	**(9)**	**10**	**(11)**	12	13	14	15

Acceptance & Matriculation Data for 2008–2009 First Year Class

	Resident	Non-resident	International	Total
Applications	265	0	1	266
Interviewed	193	0	0	193
Deferred	0	0	0	0
Matriculants				
Early Assurance Program	0	0	0	0
Early Decision Program	9	0	0	9
Baccalaureate/M.D.	n/a	n/a	n/a	n/a
M.D./Ph.D.	3	0	0	3
Matriculated	110	0	0	**110**

Applications accepted from International Applicants: No

Matriculant Demographics: 2008–2009 First Year Class

Men: 55   **Women:** 55

Matriculants' Self-Reported Race/Ethnicity

Mexican American	0	Korean	1
Cuban	1	Vietnamese	1
Puerto Rican	0	Other Asian	2
Other Hispanic	0	Total Asian	9
Total Hispanic	1	Native American	1
Chinese	1	Black	10
Asian Indian	3	Native Hawaiian	0
Pakistani	1	White	91
Filipino	0	Unduplicated Number	
Japanese	0	of Matriculants	110

Science and Math Majors: 77%
Matriculants with:
     Baccalaureate degree: 100%
     Graduate degree(s): 12%

Specialty Choice

2004, 2005, 2006 Graduates, Specialty Choice (As reported by program directors to GME Track™)	
Anesthesiology	6%
Emergency Medicine	8%
Family Practice	10%
Internal Medicine	22%
Obstetrics/Gynecology	6%
Orthopaedic Surgery	6%
Pediatrics	12%
Psychiatry	3%
Radiology	4%
Surgery	5%

Financial Information

Source: 2007–2008 LCME I-B survey and 2008–2009 AAMC TSF questionnaire

	Residents	Non-residents
Total Cost of Attendance	$38,377	$53,870
Tuition and Fees	$11,649	$27,142
Other (includes living expenses)	$24,731	$24,731
Health Insurance (can be waived)	$1,997	$1,997

Average 2008 Graduate Indebtedness: $105,536
% of Enrolled Students Receiving Aid: 92%

Criminal Background Check

This medical school requires a criminal background check prior to matriculation.

Saint Louis University School of Medicine

St. Louis, Missouri

Saint Louis University School of Medicine
Office of Admissions
1402 S. Grand Blvd. M226
St. Louis, Missouri 63104
T 314 977 9870   **F** 314 977 9825

Admissions http://medschool.slu.edu/admissions
Main www.slu.edu
Financial http://medschool.slu.edu/sfp
E-mail slumd@slu.edu

Private Institution

Dr. Philip Alderson, Dean

*Dr. L. James Willmore,
Associate Dean, Admissions*

Sandra Pritt, Student Financial Services

General Information

Established in 1836, Saint Louis University School of Medicine has the distinction of awarding the first M.D. degree west of the Mississippi River. The school is recognized as a pioneer in geriatric medicine, organ transplantation, chronic disease prevention, cardiovascular disease, neurosciences, and vaccine research, among others. The School of Medicine trains physicians and biomedical scientists, conducts medical research, and provides health services on a local, national, and international level.

Mission Statement

Beyond the important objective of training physicians who are scholars of human biology, the School of Medicine strives to graduate physicians who manifest in their personal and professional lives an appreciation of humanistic medicine. We regard humanistic medicine as a constellation of ethical and professional attitudes, which affect the physician's interactions with patients, colleagues, and society. Among these attitudes are concern for the sanctity of human life; commitment to dignity and respect in the provision of medical care to all patients; devotion to social justice, especially regarding inequities in the availability of health care; humility and awareness of medicine's limitations in the care of the sick; appreciation of the role of non-medical factors in a patient's state of well-being or illness; and mature, well-balanced professional behavior that derives from comfortable relationships with members of the human family and one's Creator.

Curricular Highlights

Community Service Requirement: Optional. Distinction in Community Service
Research/Thesis Requirement: Optional. Distinction of Research

The M.D. curriculum provides coordination and integration of the basic and clinical sciences across all four years. Additionally, it follows established principles of adult learning, and so is a hybrid of lectures, small-group activities, early clinical activities, self-directed learning, and problem-solving exercises. The first two years of the curriculum are devoted to the study of the fundamental sciences basic to medicine. In year two, a series of integrated modules that are organ-based are coupled with the acquisition of fundamental clinical skills required to begin the clinical clerkships that are taught in the Applied Clinical Skills and Patient, Physician, and Society and Bedside Diagnosis course series. The last two years concentrate on the further development and refinement of essential clinical skills, while also providing ongoing integration of the basic sciences into clinical practice. The grading system consists of the following levels: honors, pass, and fail.

USMLE

Step 1: Required. Students must record a passing score for promotion.
Step 2: Clinical Skills (CS): Required. Students must record a passing total score to graduate.
Step 2: Clinical Knowledge (CK): Required. Students must record a passing total score to graduate.

Selection Factors

Saint Louis University School of Medicine encourages applications from persons who have demonstrated a high level of academic achievement and who manifest in their personal lives those human qualities that are required for a career of service to society.

Financial Aid

Our mission is to assist you in identifying and providing resources to meet the costs associated with our standard student budget. Qualified students may be able to receive scholarship and/or loan funds from federal, state, and University programs. Funds based on financial need require the annual filing of the Free Application for Federal Student Aid (FAFSA). Parental financial information is required on the FAFSA to be considered for University need-based scholarships and loan programs.

Information about Diversity Programs

The School of Medicine is committed to promoting diversity in the classroom and in the clinics so that all students understand and learn from each other about the practice of medicine in a diverse environment. The Office of Multicultural Affairs (OMA) assists students from diverse backgrounds to be successful as they pursue a career as a physician.

Campus Information

Setting

The medical school is located in the city's arts district five minutes from the Gateway Arch on the Mississippi Riverfront.

Enrollment

For 2008, total enrollment was: 711

Special Features

A Simulation Laboratory and a Clinical Skills Center provide the latest methodology for instruction and evaluation using standardized patients and high end devices to learn clinical skills, in addition to the regular training sites. The new research building provides state-of-the-art facilities for health sciences research that touches lives and provides service to the community.

Housing

St. Louis and the surrounding area offer plenty of affordable housing.

Satellite Campuses/Facilities

Major teaching affiliations include The University Hospital, Cardinal Glennon Children's Medical Center, St. Elizabeth's Hospital, St. John's Mercy Medical Center, St. Mary's Hospital, DesPeres Hospital, Forrest Park Hospital, and St. Louis Veterans Affairs Hospitals.

Application Process and Requirements 2010–2011

Primary Application Service: AMCAS
Earliest filing date: June 1, 2009
Latest filing date: December 15, 2009

Secondary Application Required?: Yes
Sent to: All applicants
URL: www.oasprod3.com/schools/slusom
Fee: Yes, $100
Fee waiver available: Yes
Earliest filing date: June 1, 2009
Latest filing date: February 15, 2010

MCAT® required?: Yes
Latest MCAT® considered: September 2009
Oldest MCAT® considered: April 2006

Early Decision Program: School does have EDP
Applicants notified: October 1, 2009
EDP available for: Both Residents
and Non-residents

Regular Acceptance Notice
Earliest date: October 15, 2009
Latest date: Until class is full
**Applicant's Response to Acceptance
Offer – Maximum Time:** Two weeks

**Requests for Deferred
Entrance Considered:** Yes

Deposit to Hold Place in Class: Yes
Deposit (Resident): $100
Deposit (Non-resident): $100
Deposit due: With response to acceptance offer
Applied to tuition: Yes
Deposit refundable: Yes
Refundable by: May 15, 2010

Estimated number of new entrants: 175
EDP: 3, special program: 30

Start Month/Year: August 2010

Interview Format: A single one-on-one interview. Some regional interviews may be offered.

Other Programs

PREPARATORY PROGRAMS
Postbaccalaureate Program: No
Summer Program: No

COMBINED DEGREE PROGRAMS
Baccalaureate/M.D.: Yes,
www.slu.edu/colleges/AS/phs/medScholars.html
M.D./M.P.H.: Yes, http://publichealth.slu.edu/
programs/mph/mdmph.html, Bernard Backer,
(314) 977-8144, backerb@slu.edu
M.D./M.B.A.: Yes, www.slu.edu/x16691.xml
M.D./J.D.: No
M.D./Ph.D.: Yes, http://medschool.slu.edu/
admissions/index.php?page=mdphd-program,
Andrew Lechner, Ph.D., (314) 977-9877,
lechnera@slu.edu

Premedical Coursework

Course	Req.	Rec.	Lab.	Hrs.	Course	Req.	Rec.	Lab.	Hrs.
Inorganic Chemistry	•		•	8	Computer Science				
Behavioral Sciences					Genetics				
Biochemistry		•			Humanities		•		12
Biology					Organic Chemistry	•		•	8
Biology/Zoology	•		•	8	Physics	•		•	8
Calculus					Psychology				
College English	•			6	Social Sciences				
College Mathematics					Other				

Selection Factors: 2008 Accepted Applicants

Proportion of Accepted Applicants with Relevant Experience (Data Self-Reported to AMCAS*)		
Community Service/Volunteer		71%
Medically-Related Work		86%
Research		82%

Shaded bar represents school's accepted scores ranging from the 10th percentile to the 90th percentile. School Median ● National Median

Overall GPA	2.0 2.1 2.2 2.3 2.4 2.5 2.6 2.7 2.8 2.9 3.0 3.1 3.2 3.3 3.4 **3.5 3.6 3.7 (3.8) 3.9** 4.0
Science GPA	2.0 2.1 2.2 2.3 2.4 2.5 2.6 2.7 2.8 2.9 3.0 3.1 3.2 3.3 **3.4 3.5 3.6 (3.7) 3.8 3.9** 4.0

MCAT® Total Numeric Score	9 10 11 12 13 14 15 16 17 18 19 20 21 22 23 24 25 26 27 28 **29 30 31 (32) 33 34 35 36** 37 38 39 40 41 42 43
Writing Sample	J K L **M N O P (Q) R** S T
Verbal Reasoning	3 4 5 6 7 8 **9 (10) 11 12 13** 14 15
Biological Sciences	3 4 5 6 7 8 **9 10 (11) 12 13** 14 15
Physical Sciences	3 4 5 6 7 8 **9 10 (11) 12 13** 14 15

Acceptance & Matriculation Data for 2008–2009 First Year Class

	Resident	Non-resident	International	Total
Applications	371	5729	257	6357
Interviewed	110	788	39	937
Deferred	2	6	1	9
Matriculants				
Early Assurance Program	0	0	0	0
Early Decision Program	0	0	0	0
Baccalaureate/M.D.	9	20	0	29
M.D./Ph.D.	1	3	0	4
Matriculated	43	128	5	**176**

Applications accepted from International Applicants: Yes

Matriculant Demographics: 2008–2009 First Year Class

Men: 98   **Women:** 78

Matriculants' Self-Reported Race/Ethnicity

Mexican American	1	Korean	7
Cuban	1	Vietnamese	5
Puerto Rican	1	Other Asian	5
Other Hispanic	2	Total Asian	54
Total Hispanic	5	Native American	0
Chinese	11	Black	10
Asian Indian	17	Native Hawaiian	0
Pakistani	2	White	111
Filipino	6	Unduplicated Number	
Japanese	3	of Matriculants	176

Science and Math Majors: 73%
Matriculants with:
Baccalaureate degree: 99%
Graduate degree(s): 7%

Specialty Choice

2004, 2005, 2006 Graduates, Specialty Choice (As reported by program directors to GME Track™)	
Anesthesiology	6%
Emergency Medicine	5%
Family Practice	8%
Internal Medicine	17%
Obstetrics/Gynecology	6%
Orthopaedic Surgery	4%
Pediatrics	14%
Psychiatry	6%
Radiology	6%
Surgery	5%

Financial Information

Source: 2007–2008 LCME I-B survey and 2008–2009 AAMC TSF questionnaire

	Residents	Non-residents
Total Cost of Attendance	$66,253	$66,253
Tuition and Fees	$44,435	$44,435
Other (includes living expenses)	$19,682	$19,682
Health Insurance (can be waived)	$2,136	$2,136

Average 2008 Graduate Indebtedness: $173,346
% of Enrolled Students Receiving Aid: 87%

Criminal Background Check

This medical school requires a criminal background check after matriculation.

University of Missouri School of Medicine

Columbia, Missouri

Marivern Easton, Director of Admissions & Records
Office of Med. Education, MA215 Med. Sci. Bldg
Univ. of Missouri School of Medicine
One Hospital Drive, Columbia, Missouri 65212
T 573 882 9219   **F** 573 884 2988

Admissions http://som.missouri.edu/admit.shtml/
Main http://som.missouri.edu/
Financial http://som.missouri.edu/financial/
E-mail MizzouMed@missouri.edu

Public Institution

Dr. Robert Churchill, Sr. Interim Dean

Dr. Linda Headrick, Senior Associate Dean for Education & Faculty Development

Cheri Marks, Coordinator of Financial Aid

Dr. Rachel Brown, Associate Dean for Student Programs

Dr. Michael Hosokawa, Associate Dean for Curriculum

General Information

The University of Missouri School of Medicine was established in 1872. The MU Health Sciences Center includes the University Hospital, and multiple specialized and community clinics, both inpatient and outpatient. The MU School of Medicine has additional affiliations with other hospitals and clinics across the state.

Mission Statement

The mission of MU School of Medicine is to educate physicians to provide effective patient-centered care for the people of Missouri and beyond. Patient-centered care reflects a respect for individual patient's values, preferences, and expressed needs. This care is grounded in the best available evidence and conserves limited resources, and it depends on shared decision-making and active patient participation. Our graduates' care will be marked by compassion, empathy, and patient advocacy. Our graduates also will be: honest, with high ethical standards; knowledgeable in biomedical sciences, evidence-based practice, and societal and cultural issues; critical-thinkers and problem-solvers; able to communicate with patients and other health-care team members; committed to improving quality and safety; and committed to lifelong learning and mastering information.

Curricular Highlights

Community Service Requirement: Optional.
Research/Thesis Requirement: Optional.

USMLE

Step 1: Required. Students must record a passing score for promotion.
Step 2: Clinical Skills (CS): Required. Students must record a passing total score to graduate.
Step 2: Clinical Knowledge (CK): Required. Students must record a passing total score to graduate.

Selection Factors

The Admissions Committee conducts required on-campus personal interviews. Strong preference is given to Missouri residents. Exceptional residents of other states may also be admitted. Non-Missouri residents are evaluated on an individual basis, and may be asked to provide evidence of Missouri ties, diversity, and/or exceptional academics. Selection for interview is based upon academic performance; personal qualities such as motivation, social concern, and integrity; and tested motivation for medicine. Early Decision Program applicants must be Missouri residents with 3.75 cum GPA and MCAT sum of 30 with no individual section score below 9. The School of Medicine does not discriminate on the basis of race, sex, creed, national origin, age, handicap, religion, or status as a Vietnam-era veteran in admission or access to or treatment or employment in its programs and activities.

Financial Aid

Students are admitted to the School of Medicine without regard to financial circumstances. MU participates in federal scholarship and loan programs. The institutional scholarship program is primarily need-based. Institutional long-term loans are available and MU also operates an emergency short-term loan program.

Information about Diversity Programs

The University of Missouri is committed to the recruitment and education of disadvantaged and nontraditional applicants and applicants from groups underrepresented in medicine. The School of Medicine sponsors summer programs targeting rural and disadvantaged high school students, although students from across Missouri may participate.

Campus Information

Setting

The University of Missouri School of Medicine is located in the heart of the University of Missouri's main campus, allowing students to use its programs and facilities. MU has affiliations with all five hospitals in the city and a number of satellite and specialty clinics in the mid-Missouri area.

Enrollment

For 2008, total enrollment was: 387

Housing

Most medical students live in privately-owned apartments, condominiums, and townhouses; some purchase their own homes.

Satellite Campuses/Facilities

Students may choose to complete all elective clinical rotations in and around Columbia, or off-site in Missouri or across the country. Students may participate in the Rural Track Program, which offers rural sites for both clerkship and elective experiences.

Application Process and Requirements 2010–2011

Primary Application Service: AMCAS
Earliest filing date: June 1, 2009
Latest filing date: November 1, 2009

Secondary Application Required?: Yes
Sent to: All Missouri residents
and screened out-of-state applicants
Marivern Easton, (573) 882-9219
eastonm@health.missouri.edu
URL: n/a
Fee: Yes, $75
Fee waiver available: Yes
Earliest filing date: July 1, 2009
Latest filing date: January 15, 2010

MCAT® required?: Yes
Latest MCAT® considered: September 2009
Oldest MCAT® considered: 2006

Early Decision Program: School does have EDP
Applicants notified: October 1, 2009
EDP available for: Residents only

Regular Acceptance Notice
Earliest date: October 15, 2009
Latest date: Until class is full
**Applicant's Response to Acceptance
Offer – Maximum Time:** 30 days

**Requests for Deferred
Entrance Considered:** Yes

Deposit to Hold Place in Class: Yes
Deposit (Resident): $100
Deposit (Non-resident): $100
Deposit due: Within 30 days of acceptance offer
until July, after which less time is given.
Applied to tuition: Yes
Deposit refundable: Yes
Refundable by: May 15, 2010

Estimated number of new entrants: 96
EDP: 4, special program: 23

Start Month/Year: July 2010

Interview Format: Two open file, one-on-one
interviews by Admissions Committee members are
required. Regional interviews are not available.

Other Programs

PREPARATORY PROGRAMS
Postbaccalaureate Program: No
Summer Program: No

COMBINED DEGREE PROGRAMS
Baccalaureate/M.D.: No
M.D./M.P.H.: No
M.D./M.B.A.: No
M.D./J.D.: No
M.D./Ph.D.: Yes, Douglas Anthony, M.D., Ph.D.,
(573) 884-4079, mdphd@missouri.edu

Premedical Coursework

Course	Req.	Rec.	Lab.	Hrs.
Inorganic Chemistry	•		•	8
Behavioral Sciences				
Biochemistry		•		
Biology	•		•	8
Biology/Zoology				
Calculus				
College English				
College Mathematics	•			3

Course	Req.	Rec.	Lab.	Hrs.
Computer Science				
Genetics				
Humanities		•		
Organic Chemistry	•		•	8
Physics	•		•	8
Psychology				
Social Sciences		•		
English Composition		•		6

Selection Factors: 2008 Accepted Applicants

Proportion of Accepted Applicants with Relevant Experience (Data Self-Reported to AMCAS®)		
Community Service/Volunteer		65%
Medically-Related Work		68%
Research		67%

Shaded bar represents school's accepted scores ranging from the 10th percentile to the 90th percentile — School Median ● National Median ●

Overall GPA	2.0	2.1	2.2	2.3	2.4	2.5	2.6	2.7	2.8	2.9	3.0	3.1	3.2	3.3	3.4	3.5	3.6	3.7	(3.8)	3.9	4.0
Science GPA	2.0	2.1	2.2	2.3	2.4	2.5	2.6	2.7	2.8	2.9	3.0	3.1	3.2	3.3	3.4	3.5	3.6	3.7	(3.8)	3.9	4.0

MCAT® Total Numeric Score 9 10 11 12 13 14 15 16 17 18 19 20 21 22 23 24 25 26 27 28 29 30 (31) 32 33 34 35 36 37 38 39 40 41 42 43

Writing Sample		J	K	L	M	N	O	(P)	(Q)	R	S	T
Verbal Reasoning	3	4	5	6	7	8	9	(10)	11	12	13	14	15
Biological Sciences	3	4	5	6	7	8	9	10	(11)	12	13	14	15
Physical Sciences	3	4	5	6	7	8	9	(10)	(11)	12	13	14	15

Acceptance & Matriculation Data for 2008–2009 First Year Class

	Resident	Non-resident	International	Total
Applications	447	882	15	1344
Interviewed	215	91	0	306
Deferred	2	0	0	2
Matriculants				
Early Assurance Program	23	0	0	23
Early Decision Program	3	0	0	3
Baccalaureate/M.D.	n/a	n/a	n/a	n/a
M.D./Ph.D.	0	0	0	0
Matriculated	80	15	0	**95**

Applications accepted from International Applicants: No

Specialty Choice

2004, 2005, 2006 Graduates, Specialty Choice (As reported by program directors to GME Track™)	
Anesthesiology	5%
Emergency Medicine	6%
Family Practice	15%
Internal Medicine	11%
Obstetrics/Gynecology	6%
Orthopaedic Surgery	3%
Pediatrics	15%
Psychiatry	3%
Radiology	6%
Surgery	6%

Matriculant Demographics: 2008–2009 First Year Class

Men: 50   **Women:** 45

Matriculants' Self-Reported Race/Ethnicity

Mexican American	0	Korean	1
Cuban	0	Vietnamese	0
Puerto Rican	0	Other Asian	3
Other Hispanic	1	Total Asian	12
Total Hispanic	1	Native American	4
Chinese	2	Black	6
Asian Indian	5	Native Hawaiian	0
Pakistani	0	White	75
Filipino	1	Unduplicated Number	
Japanese	0	of Matriculants	95

Science and Math Majors: 75%
Matriculants with:
Baccalaureate degree: 100%
Graduate degree(s): 15%

Financial Information

Source: 2007–2008 LCME I-B survey
and 2008–2009 AAMC TSF questionnaire

	Residents	Non-residents
Total Cost of Attendance	$43,036	$66,548
Tuition and Fees	$24,856	$48,368
Other (includes living expenses)	$16,304	$16,304
Health Insurance (can be waived)	$1,876	$1,876

Average 2008 Graduate Indebtedness: $131,948
% of Enrolled Students Receiving Aid: 96%

Criminal Background Check

This medical school does not require a criminal background check prior to matriculation.

University of Missouri — Kansas City
School of Medicine

Kansas City, Missouri

Council on Selection
University of Missouri — Kansas City
School of Medicine
2411 Holmes
Kansas City, Missouri 64108-2792
T 816 235 1870   **F** 816 235 6579

Admissions www.umkc.edu/admissions
Main www.med.umkc.edu
Financial www.sfa.umkc.edu
E-mail medicine@umkc.edu

Public Institution

Dr. Betty M. Drees, Dean

*Dr. R. Stephen Griffith, Chair,
Council on Selection*

*Dr. Susan B. Wilson, Associate Dean,
Cultural Enhancement and Diversity*

Jan Brandow, Director of Student Financial Aid

*Alice Arredondo, Assistant Dean for
Admissions & Recruitment*

General Information

The Board of Curators of the University of
Missouri authorized the establishment of a
medical school at the University of Missouri-
Kansas City in 1969. Located on a 135-acre
Hospital Hill campus, the medical school is
near both the schools and colleges of the university and affiliated community hospitals.

Mission Statement

The mission of the University of Missouri-Kansas
City School of Medicine is to prepare graduates
so that they are able to enter and complete
graduate programs in medical education, qualify
for medical licensure, provide competent medical
care, and have the educational background
necessary for lifelong learning in order to address
the health care needs of our state and nation.

Curricular Highlights

Community Service Requirement: Optional.
Research/Thesis Requirement: Optional.

The School of Medicine, with the College of
Arts and Sciences and the School of Biological
Sciences, offers a year-round program leading
to baccalaureate and M.D. degrees in six calendar years. The student is required to complete
both degrees and has the freedom to major in
any department of the School of Biological
Sciences or the College of Arts and Sciences.
The program is designed primarily for high
school seniors entering college. To receive the
baccalaureate degree, the student must complete 120 semester hours of credit. Under the
guidance of a clinician-scholar, called a docent,
small groups of first and second-year students
are introduced to medicine in community hospitals where they can observe patients and

their problems. During the first two years of
the program, the student is occupied predominantly with arts and sciences coursework, with
about one-fourth of the time being devoted to
introduction to medicine courses. After these
two years the student advances, with the
approval of the Council on Evaluation, to Year
3 of the six-year program. During the last four
years of the curriculum, the student, with
guidance from a docent and education team
coordinator, plans a program for meeting the
curricular requirements. Two months of Years
4 through 6 are spent with the docent on an
inpatient internal medicine rotation. The
remaining months of each year are spent in a
number of other required and elective course
offerings in the basic and clinical sciences and
the humanities and social sciences. Students
spend two academic terms in arts and sciences
coursework during the last four years of the
program. Basic, clinical, and behavioral science
information is presented and emphasized
throughout the program. Each student is
expected to acquire a firm, broad base of information in each of these major content areas.
The academic program provides the medical
student with a realistic working knowledge of
community health problems and resources.
There is a strong student support system. An
alternative path is available for extended study.

USMLE

Step 1: Required. Students must record a passing
score for promotion.
Step 2: Clinical Skills (CS): Required. Students
must record a passing total score to graduate.
Step 2: Clinical Knowledge (CK): Required.
Students must record a passing total score to
graduate.

Selection Factors

Selection criteria are: (1) the applicant's academic potential as judged by quality of high
school courses, rank in high school class, and
scores on the ACT In the 2008-2009 entering
class, the average ACT score fell at the 95th
percentile, and the average rank-in-class was at
the 94th percentile; (2) personal qualities,
including maturity, leadership, reliability, motivation for medicine, range of interests, interpersonal skills, compassion, and job/volunteer
experience. After the Council on Selection

carefully reviews all applicants, those who
appear to be well qualified are invited for
interviews. If invited, the applicant is notified
by e-mail or phone and is required to be present at the scheduled date and time of the interview. Students are considered on the basis of
their individual qualifications without regard
to race, creed, sex, or national origin. Interview
statistics* for B.A./M.D. are reflected in the
Acceptance & Matriculation Chart. The program also accepts a small number of students
with at least a Bachelor's degree. Called M.D.-
Only, they are required to take the MCAT and,
if admitted, pursue the last four years of the
program. Promoting third-year B.A./M.D. students and M.D.O. students are listed in
Acceptance & Matriculation Chart as
"Matriculants." The school also accepts transfers. The admissions deadline for M.D.-Only
and transfer students can be found on the
school Web site.

Financial Aid

A variety of financial assistance is available to
all medical students. Additional information
and applications for financial aid may be
obtained from: Student Financial Aid Office,
UMKC, 5115 Oak, Kansas City, Missouri
64110. Priority financial aid application date is
March 1.

Information about Diversity Programs

Information for students from groups under-
represented in medicine is available from Dr.
Susan B. Wilson, Associate Dean for Cultural
Enhancement and Diversity, or Mary Anne
Morgenegg, Coordinator, Council on Selection
at the School of Medicine.

Campus Information

Enrollment

For 2008, total enrollment was: 623

Application Process and Requirements 2010–2011

Primary Application Service: School Specific
Earliest filing date: August 1, 2009
Latest filing date: November 1, 2009

Secondary Application Required?: Yes
Sent to: All applicants
URL: n/a
Fee: No
Fee waiver available: n/a
Earliest filing date: n/a
Latest filing date: n/a

MCAT® required?: Yes for M.D. - only
Latest MCAT® considered: June 2009
Oldest MCAT® considered: 2006

Early Decision Program: School does not have EDP
Applicants notified: n/a
EDP available for: n/a

Regular Acceptance Notice
Earliest date: April 1, 2010
Latest date: Varies
Applicant's Response to Acceptance Offer – Maximum Time: 30 days

Requests for Deferred Entrance Considered: No

Deposit to Hold Place in Class: Yes
Deposit (Resident): $100
Deposit (Non-resident): $100
Deposit due: With response to acceptance offer
Applied to tuition: Yes
Deposit refundable: Yes
Refundable by: 15 days

Estimated number of new entrants: 100
EDP: n/a, **special program:** 100

Start Month/Year: August 2010

Interview Format: Two thirty-minute interviews. Regional interviews are not available.

Other Programs

PREPARATORY PROGRAMS
Postbaccalaureate Program: No
Summer Program: No

COMBINED DEGREE PROGRAMS
Baccalaureate/M.D.: Yes, www.med.umkc.edu
M.D./M.P.H.: No
M.D./M.B.A.: No
M.D./J.D.: No
M.D./Ph.D.: No

Premedical Coursework

Course	Req.	Rec.	Lab.	Hrs.	Course	Req.	Rec.	Lab.	Hrs.
Inorganic Chemistry					Computer Science				
Behavioral Sciences					Genetics				
Biochemistry					Humanities				
Biology					Organic Chemistry				
Biology/Zoology					Physics				
Calculus					Psychology				
College English					Social Sciences				
College Mathematics					Other				

Selection Factors: 2008 Accepted Applicants

Proportion of Accepted Applicants with Relevant Experience (Data Self-Reported to AMCAS®)		
Community Service/Volunteer		63%
Medically-Related Work		88%
Research		75%

Shaded bar represents school's accepted scores ranging from the 10th percentile to the 90th percentile. School Median ● National Median ●

Overall GPA 2.0 2.1 2.2 2.3 2.4 2.5 2.6 2.7 **2.8 2.9 3.0 3.1 3.2 3.3 (3.4) 3.5 3.6 3.7 3.8 3.9 4.0**

Science GPA 2.0 2.1 2.2 2.3 2.4 2.5 2.6 **2.7 2.8 2.9 3.0 3.1 (3.2) 3.3 3.4 3.5 3.6 3.7 3.8 3.9 4.0**

MCAT® Total Numeric Score 9 10 11 12 13 14 15 16 17 18 19 20 **21 22 23 24 25 26 27 28 (29) 30 31 (32) 33 34** 35 36 37 38 39 40 41 42 43

Writing Sample			J	K	L	**M**	**N**	**O**	**(P)**	**(Q)**	R	S	T
Verbal Reasoning	3	4	**5**	**6**	**7**	**(8)**	**9**	**(10)**	**11**	**12**	13	14	15
Biological Sciences	3	4	5	6	**7**	**8**	**9**	**(10)**	**(11)**	**12**	**13**	14	15
Physical Sciences	3	4	5	6	**7**	**8**	**9**	**(10)**	**(11)**	**12**	13	14	15

Acceptance & Matriculation Data for 2008–2009 First Year Class

	Resident	Non-resident	International	Total
Applications	43	43	0	86
Interviewed	141*	142*	0	283
Deferred	0	0	0	0
Matriculants				
Early Assurance Program	n/a	n/a	n/a	n/a
Early Decision Program	0	0	0	0
Baccalaureate/M.D.	53	47	0	100
M.D./Ph.D.	n/a	n/a	n/a	n/a
Matriculated	43	43	0	**86**

Applications accepted from International Applicants: No

Specialty Choice

2004, 2005, 2006 Graduates, Specialty Choice (As reported by program directors to GME Track™)	
Anesthesiology	9%
Emergency Medicine	5%
Family Practice	9%
Internal Medicine	20%
Obstetrics/Gynecology	6%
Orthopaedic Surgery	2%
Pediatrics	12%
Psychiatry	2%
Radiology	4%
Surgery	7%

Matriculant Demographics: 2008–2009 First Year Class

Men: 40   **Women:** 46

Matriculants' Self-Reported Race/Ethnicity

Mexican American	0	Korean	0
Cuban	0	Vietnamese	0
Puerto Rican	0	Other Asian	38
Other Hispanic	2	Total Asian	40
Total Hispanic	2	Native American	1
Chinese	1	Black	2
Asian Indian	2	Native Hawaiian	0
Pakistani	0	White	39
Filipino	0	Unduplicated Number	
Japanese	0	of Matriculants	86

Science and Math Majors: 7%
Matriculants with:
      Baccalaureate degree: 9%
      Graduate degree(s): 5%

Financial Information

Source: 2007–2008 LCME I-B survey and 2008–2009 AAMC TSF questionnaire

	Residents	Non-residents
Total Cost of Attendance	$54,430	$81,899
Tuition and Fees	$28,810	$56,279
Other (includes living expenses)	$25,620	$25,620
Health Insurance (cannot be waived)	$0	$0

Average 2008 Graduate Indebtedness: $141,135
% of Enrolled Students Receiving Aid: 85%

Criminal Background Check

This medical school requires a criminal background check prior to matriculation.

Washington University School of Medicine

St. Louis, Missouri

Office of Admissions
Washington University in St. Louis School of Medicine
660 South Euclid Avenue, #8107
St. Louis, Missouri 63110
T 314 362 6858 **F** 314 362 4658

Admissions medschool.wustl.edu/admissions
Main medschool.wustl.edu
Financial www.wusmfinaid.wustl.edu
E-mail wumscoa@wustl.edu

Private Institution

Dr. Larry J. Shapiro, Dean and Executive Vice Chancellor for Medical Affairs

Dr. W. Edwin Dodson, Associate Vice Chancellor and Associate Dean for Admissions

Dr. Will Ross, Associate Dean, Diversity Programs

Robert McCormack, Assistant Dean and Director of Financial Aid

General Information

Dedicated solely to medical education and located at the heart of the 230-acre Washington University Medical Center, the Farrell Learning and Teaching Center provides a state-of-the-art facility in which to learn the compassionate delivery of scientific medicine. This facility complements the outstanding clinical resources at Barnes-Jewish Hospital, and at St. Louis Children's Hospital, two of the top academic hospitals in the country. Learning among the most talented classmates in the country and in world class facilities, medical students at Washington University enjoy a supportive and non-competitive environment where opportunities for discovery, learning and self-fulfillment abound.

Mission Statement

The mission of Washington University is the promotion of learning by students and by faculty. Teaching, the transmission of knowledge, is central to our mission, as is research, the creation of new knowledge. Our goals are: to foster excellence in our teaching, research, scholarship, and service; to prepare students with attitudes, skills, and habits of lifelong learning and with leadership skills, enabling them to be useful members of a global society; and to be an exemplary institution in our home community, St. Louis, as well as in the nation and the world.

Curricular Highlights

Community Service Requirement: Optional.
Research/Thesis Requirement: Optional.

The curriculum provides a state-of-the-art foundation in the science and the art of medicine. Instruction is by lecture and small-group interactive sessions, and includes problem-based exercises and self-directed learning using computers and other resources led by faculty facilitators. Medical humanities and ethics are integrated into the four years of medical training, with emphasis given to the sociological and cultural concerns of patients and to the adaptation of medical care to their needs. Patient contact begins in the first semester of the first year and the fourth year is all electives. There are abundant opportunities in basic and clinical research. A five-year M.A. and M.D. degree program is available for students desiring one or two years of research training, while a Medical Scientist Training Program leads to both M.D. and Ph.D. degrees. A pass/fail grading system is used in the first year.

USMLE

Step 1: Optional.
Step 2: Clinical Skills (CS): Optional.
Step 2: Clinical Knowledge (CK): Optional.

Selection Factors

A good doctor must be compassionate and understanding, as well as a good scientist. To this end, the School of Medicine selects students who, in addition to possessing keen minds, demonstrate sensitivity and a commitment to serve others. Hence, students are selected on the basis of character, attitude, interest, intellectual ability, motivation, maturity, and achievement as indicated by superior academic and extracurricular accomplishments. Policies and programs are nondiscriminatory, and full consideration is given to all applicants without regard to sex, age, race, handicap, sexual preference, creed, or national or ethnic origin. Students from groups underrepresented in medicine are encouraged to apply. Selected applicants are invited to interview, which is required for acceptance.

Financial Aid

The financial resources of an applicant do not enter into the selection process. Tuition is set at entry and does not increase during the four years of medical school. Students who document finanical need can receive need-based financial aid comprised of both scholarships and loans with need-based medical student borrowing currently capped at $20,000 per year ($80,000 over four years). Merit-based full-tuition scholarships are awarded to selected students in each entering class and are renewable.

Information about Diversity Programs

Washington University is strongly committed to the recruitment, selection, education, and graduation of an increased number of students from groups underrepresented in medicine. Students are supported by an active chapter of the Student National Medical Association and a network of faculty from diverse groups.

Campus Information

Setting

The Washington University Medical Center extends over 12 city blocks and is adjacent to the 1,371 acre Forest Park.

Enrollment

For 2008, total enrollment was: 591

Special Features

An education from Washington University School of Medicine prepares graduates for leadership and readies them for rigorous postgraduate clinical training, leading edge research, and rewarding medical careers. Learning takes place at the edge of what is known alongside exceptional colleagues and in state-of-the-art facilities. There are abundant clinical and research opportunities, including one of the largest genome sequencing facilities in the world. Generous need-based financial aid helps limit indebtedness.

Housing

St. Louis is nationally recognized for its abundant, convenient, safe, and affordable housing. The bus and light rail system are free to students. The on-campus Spencer T. Olin Residence Hall is connected to the medical school buildings.

Application Process and Requirements 2010–2011

Primary Application Service: AMCAS
Earliest filing date: June 1, 2009
Latest filing date: December 1, 2009

Secondary Application Required?: Yes
Sent to: All applicants
URL: http://wumsapply.wustl.edu
Fee: Yes, $50
Fee waiver available: Yes
Earliest filing date: July 1, 2009
Latest filing date: December 31, 2009

MCAT® required?: Yes
Latest MCAT® considered: September 2009
Oldest MCAT® considered: September 2006

Early Decision Program: School does not have EDP
Applicants notified: n/a
EDP available for: n/a

Regular Acceptance Notice
Earliest date: November 1, 2009
Latest date: Until class is full
Applicant's Response to Acceptance Offer – Maximum Time: Two weeks

Requests for Deferred Entrance Considered: Yes

Deposit to Hold Place in Class: Yes
Deposit (Resident): $100
Deposit (Non-resident): $100
Deposit due: With response to acceptance offer
Applied to tuition: Yes
Deposit refundable: Yes
Refundable by: May 15, 2010

Estimated number of new entrants: 120
EDP: n/a, special program: 20

Start Month/Year: August 2010

Interview Format: Open, unstructured, one-on-one. Regional interviews are not available.

Other Programs

Preparatory Programs
Postbaccalaureate Program: Yes, http://ucollege.wustl.edu/programs/special-programs
Elizabeth Fogt, Director of Advising and Student Services, (314) 935-6778, efogt@artsci.wustl.edu
Summer Program: No

Combined Degree Programs
Baccalaureate/M.D.: Yes, http://uscholars.wustl.edu
M.D./M.P.H.: No
M.D./M.B.A.: No
M.D./J.D.: No
M.D./Ph.D.: Yes, http://mstp.wustl.edu

Premedical Coursework

Course	Req.	Rec.	Lab.	Sems.
Inorganic Chemistry	•			2
Behavioral Sciences				
Biochemistry				
Biology	•			2
Biology/Zoology				
Calculus	•			2
College English				
College Mathematics				

Course	Req.	Rec.	Lab.	Sems.
Computer Science				
Genetics				
Humanities				
Organic Chemistry	•			2
Physics	•			2
Psychology				
Social Sciences				
Other				

Selection Factors: 2008 Accepted Applicants

Proportion of Accepted Applicants with Relevant Experience (Data Self-Reported to AMCAS®)		
Community Service/Volunteer		73%
Medically-Related Work		82%
Research		94%

Shaded bar represents school's accepted scores ranging from the 10th percentile to the 90th percentile.
School Median ● National Median ●

Overall GPA	2.0	2.1	2.2	2.3	2.4	2.5	2.6	2.7	2.8	2.9	3.0	3.1	3.2	3.3	3.4	3.5	3.6	3.7	3.8	(3.9)	4.0
Science GPA	2.0	2.1	2.2	2.3	2.4	2.5	2.6	2.7	2.8	2.9	3.0	3.1	3.2	3.3	3.4	3.5	3.6	3.7	3.8	(3.9)	4.0

MCAT® Total Numeric Score 9 10 11 12 13 14 15 16 17 18 19 20 21 22 23 24 25 26 27 28 29 30 31 (32) 33 34 35 36 37 (38) 39 40 41 42 43

Writing Sample			J	K	L	M	N	O	P	(Q)	R	S		T
Verbal Reasoning	3	4	5	6	7	8	9	(10)	11	(12)	13	14		15
Biological Sciences	3	4	5	6	7	8	9	10	(11)	12	(13)	14		15
Physical Sciences	3	4	5	6	7	8	9	10	(11)	12	(13)	14		15

Acceptance & Matriculation Data for 2008–2009 First Year Class

	Resident	Non-resident	International	Total
Applications	176	3584	262	4022
Interviewed	61	1037	58	1156
Deferred	2	9	0	11
Matriculants				
Early Assurance Program	n/a	n/a	n/a	n/a
Early Decision Program	0	0	0	0
Baccalaureate/M.D.	7	86	5	98
M.D./Ph.D.	2	20	2	24
Matriculated	9	106	7	**122**

Applications accepted from International Applicants: Yes

Specialty Choice

2004, 2005, 2006 Graduates, Specialty Choice (As reported by program directors to GME Track™)	
Anesthesiology	7%
Emergency Medicine	5%
Family Practice	0%
Internal Medicine	18%
Obstetrics/Gynecology	3%
Orthopaedic Surgery	7%
Pediatrics	19%
Psychiatry	4%
Radiology Diagnostic	5%
Surgery General	6%

Matriculant Demographics: 2008–2009 First Year Class

Men: 63   **Women:** 59

Matriculants' Self-Reported Race/Ethnicity

Mexican American	6	**Korean**	4
Cuban	0	**Vietnamese**	0
Puerto Rican	0	**Other Asian**	1
Other Hispanic	2	**Total Asian**	31
Total Hispanic	7	**Native American**	1
Chinese	16	**Black**	8
Asian Indian	9	**Native Hawaiian**	0
Pakistani	0	**White**	70
Filipino	1	**Unduplicated Number**	
Japanese	0	**of Matriculants**	122

Science and Math Majors: 78%
Matriculants with:
    Baccalaureate degree: 100%
    Graduate degree(s): 7%

Financial Information

Source: 2007–2008 LCME I-B survey and 2008–2009 AAMC TSF questionnaire

	Residents	Non-residents
Total Cost of Attendance	$61,222	$61,222
Tuition and Fees	$45,550	$45,550
Other (includes living expenses)	$15,672	$15,672
Health Insurance (can not be waived)	$0	$0

Average 2008 Graduate Indebtedness: $101,191
% of Enrolled Students Receiving Aid: 87%

Criminal Background Check

This medical school requires a criminal background check prior to matriculation.

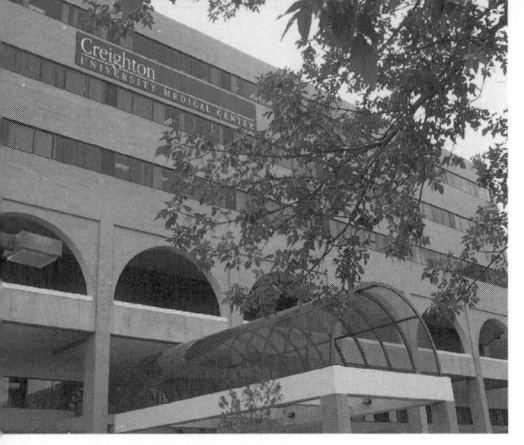

Creighton University School of Medicine
Omaha, Nebraska

Creighton University School of Medicine
Office of Medical Admissions
2500 California Plaza
Omaha, Nebraska 68178
T 402 280 2799   **F** 402 280 1241

Admissions http://www2.creighton.edu/medschool/medicine.oma/index.php
Main http://www2.creighton.edu/medschool/
Financial http://www2.creighton.edu/financialaid/
E-mail medschadm@creighton.edu

Private Institution

Dr. Rowen K. Zetterman, Dean

*Dr. Henry C. Nipper,
Assistant Dean for Admissions*

*Dr. Sade Kosoko-Lasaki, Associate Vice President
for Multicultural and Community Affairs*

Karen Malloy, Financial Aid Coordinator

Garland Jarmon, Jr., Director of Admissions

General Information

Creighton University School of Medicine opened in 1892, 14 years after the opening of the parent university, a Jesuit, Catholic institution. The Criss Complex houses the School of Medicine and its Medical Education Center offering wireless small-group rooms, student lounges, Wellness Center and lecture halls. In the anatomy suites, students use CT scans as instructional aides. We podcast all M1 & M2 lectures and administer all exams in our 72-seat computer classroom. Clinical instruction is carried out at Creighton University Medical Center (where medical students access patient labs via their PDAs) as well as in other affiliated hospitals and clinics.

Mission Statement

In the Catholic, Jesuit tradition of Creighton University, the mission of the School of Medicine is to improve the human condition through excellence in educating students, physicians and the public, advancing knowledge, and providing comprehensive patient care. Vision Statement: We will be a School of Medicine respected by our peers for excellence in teaching, research, and clinical care. We will be distinguished for preparing graduates who achieve excellence in their chosen fields and who demonstrate extraordinary compassion and commitment to the service of others.

Curricular Highlights

Community Service Requirement: Optional.
Opportunities: ILAC, Magis Clinic, Project CURA
Research/Thesis Requirement: Optional.

The curriculum integrates basic and clinical science in all four years. Year one combines strong basic science content with the fundamentals of physical diagnosis and interviewing techniques. Year two is organized around a series of organ system-based courses and clinical skills training, including longitudinal clinics. Year three is comprised of core clerkships in a variety of inpatient and ambulatory settings. In year four students continue clinical training in critical care, surgery, and primary care and explore their interests through electives. Clinical experiences, and ethical and societal issues, are prominent in the curriculum in each year. Instructional methodology uses case-based small-group sessions and computer-assisted instruction. Close faculty/student relationships provide for mentoring and advising of students. Students are graded against curriculum standards on an honors/satisfactory/unsatisfactory system in order to encourage a sense of community in each class.

USMLE

Step 1: Required. Students must record a passing score for promotion.
Step 2: Clinical Skills (CS): Required. Students must only record a score.
Step 2: Clinical Knowledge (CK): Required. Students must only record a score.

Selection Factors

The qualities of intellectual ability and curiosity, emotional maturity, honesty, proper motivation, proven scholastic ability, significant service to humanity, and documented medical experience are of highest importance. A formal interview on campus is required prior to acceptance. No restrictions are placed on applicants due to race, religion, sex, national or ethnic origin, age, disability, veteran status, or state of residence. Creighton values diversity in its medical classes. Advantage is given to applicants who complete their pre-professional education at Creighton. Both the AMCAS and Creighton's secondary applications are required of all applicants.

Financial Aid

In addition to student loans and other government programs, a limited number of scholarships are available for those who are academically well qualified and have strong records of service to others.

Information about Diversity Programs

Qualified candidates from groups who are underrepresented in medicine are encouraged to apply. Creighton's Office of Health Sciences Multicultural and Community Affairs has several active programs to increase diversity and provide appropriate support services. The office administers several diversity programs, including pipeline and premedical postbaccalaureate programs.

Campus Information

Setting

Creighton's 100-acre campus and medical center are near Omaha's revitalized downtown and new arena. All of Creighton's schools and colleges are located on one campus.

Enrollment

For 2008, total enrollment was: 501

Special Features

"…service is a primary goal of education…our graduates and their mentors should be advocates of justice and crafters of a social order." – Fr. John Schlegel, S.J., President. Student life at the School of Medicine is personified by "balance" between academics and service to others. Activities include the Institute for Latin American Concern in the Dominican Republic, Project CURA, and the student-operated Magis Clinic. Although not required, all students do community service. The school also supports a student Wellness Council that organizes such events as picnics, movie nights, and stress management sessions; a Wellness Center; and the Wellness Chronicle. A variety of sports, music, and recreational activities is available on campus or nearby.

Housing

Safe, affordable housing is available on campus or nearby. Creighton offers two student parking garages which ease parking.

Satellite Campuses/Facilities

Satellite Campuses/Facilities: Opportunities for off-campus experiences exist in Phoenix, San Francisco, Indian Health Service, and the Dominican Republic.

Application Process and Requirements 2010–2011

Primary Application Service: AMCAS
Earliest filing date: July 1, 2009
Latest filing date: November 1, 2009

Secondary Application Required?: Yes
Sent to: All applicants
URL: www.oasprod3.com/Schools/
CreightonSOM/Login.aspx
Fee: Yes, $95
Fee waiver available: Yes
Earliest filing date: July 1, 2009
Latest filing date: January 15, 2010

MCAT® required?: Yes
Latest MCAT® considered: September 2009
Oldest MCAT® considered: January 2007

Early Decision Program: School does have EDP
Applicants notified: October 1, 2009
EDP available for: Both Residents and Non-residents

Regular Acceptance Notice
Earliest date: October 16, 2009
Latest date: Until class is full
Applicant's Response to Acceptance Offer – Maximum Time: 14 days

Requests for Deferred Entrance Considered: Yes

Deposit to Hold Place in Class: Yes
Deposit (Resident): $100
Deposit (Non-resident): $100
Deposit due: With response to acceptance offer
Applied to tuition: Yes
Deposit refundable: Yes
Refundable by: May 15, 2010

Estimated number of new entrants: 126
EDP: 1, special program: 7

Start Month/Year: August 2010

Interview Format: Two open-file one-on-one interviews with a faculty representative and a medical student. Regional interviews are not available.

Other Programs

PREPARATORY PROGRAMS
Postbaccalaureate Program: Yes,
http://www2.creighton.edu/health/hsmaca/
premedicalpost-bacprogram/index.php,
(402) 280-2799, postbac.appl@creighton.edu
Summer Program: No
Summer Research Institute:
http://medicine.creighton.edu/research/
student_research_opportunities.htm

COMBINED DEGREE PROGRAMS
Baccalaureate/M.D.: No
M.D./M.P.H.: No
M.D./M.B.A.: No
M.D./J.D.: No
M.D./Ph.D.: Yes, www2.creighton.edu/fileadmin/
user/Registrar/docs/archive/MD_06-08.pdf

Premedical Coursework

Course	Req.	Rec.	Lab.	Hrs.
Inorganic Chemistry	•	•		8
Behavioral Sciences				
Biochemistry		•		
Biology	•	•		8
Biology/Zoology				
Calculus				
College English	•			6
College Mathematics				
Computer Science				

Course	Req.	Rec.	Lab.	Hrs.
Genetics		•		
Humanities		•		
Organic Chemistry	•		•	8
Physics	•		•	8
Psychology				
Social Sciences				
Spanish		•		
Molecular Biology		•		
Physiology		•		

Selection Factors: 2008 Accepted Applicants

Proportion of Accepted Applicants with Relevant Experience (Data Self-Reported to AMCAS®)		Community Service/Volunteer	77%
		Medically-Related Work	86%
		Research	73%

Shaded bar represents school's accepted scores ranging from the 10th percentile to the 90th percentile   School Median ●   National Median ●

Overall GPA	2.0 2.1 2.2 2.3 2.4 2.5 2.6 2.7 2.8 2.9 3.0 3.1 3.2 3.3 3.4 3.5 3.6 3.7 (3.8) 3.9 4.0
Science GPA	2.0 2.1 2.2 2.3 2.4 2.5 2.6 2.7 2.8 2.9 3.0 3.1 3.2 3.3 3.4 3.5 3.6 (3.7) 3.8 3.9 4.0

MCAT® Total Numeric Score 9 10 11 12 13 14 15 16 17 18 19 20 21 22 23 24 25 26 27 28 29 30 (31) 32 33 34 35 36 37 38 39 40 41 42 43

Writing Sample			J	K	L	M	N	O	(P)	(Q) R S T
Verbal Reasoning	3	4	5	6	7	8	9	(10)	11	12 13 14 15
Biological Sciences	3	4	5	6	7	8	9	(10)	(11)	12 13 14 15
Physical Sciences	3	4	5	6	7	8	9	(10)	(11)	12 13 14 15

Acceptance & Matriculation Data for 2008–2009 First Year Class

	Resident	Non-resident	International	Total
Applications	183	5319	153	5655
Interviewed	55	528	3	586
Deferred	0	4	0	4
Matriculants				
Early Assurance Program	0	5	0	5
Early Decision Program	0	0	0	0
Baccalaureate/M.D.	n/a	n/a	n/a	n/a
M.D./Ph.D.	0	0	0	0
Matriculated	16	109	1	**126**

Applications accepted from International Applicants: Yes

Matriculant Demographics: 2008–2009 First Year Class

Men: 63   **Women:** 63

Matriculants' Self-Reported Race/Ethnicity

Mexican American	3	Korean	3
Cuban	2	Vietnamese	3
Puerto Rican	0	Other Asian	0
Other Hispanic	0	Total Asian	15
Total Hispanic	5	Native American	1
Chinese	2	Black	4
Asian Indian	5	Native Hawaiian	1
Pakistani	1	White	103
Filipino	1	Unduplicated Number	
Japanese	3	of Matriculants	126

Science and Math Majors: 75%
Matriculants with:
Baccalaureate degree: 100%
Graduate degree(s): 10%

Specialty Choice

2004, 2005, 2006 Graduates, Specialty Choice (As reported by program directors to GME Track™)	
Anesthesiology	10%
Emergency Medicine	4%
Family Practice	7%
Internal Medicine	21%
Obstetrics/Gynecology	11%
Orthopaedic Surgery	6%
Pediatrics	10%
Psychiatry	5%
Radiology Diagnostic	8%
Surgery General	6%

Financial Information

Source: 2007–2008 LCME I-B survey and 2008–2009 AAMC TSF questionnaire

	Residents	Non-residents
Total Cost of Attendance	$64,497	$64,497
Tuition and Fees	$43,496	$43,496
Other (includes living expenses)	$19,181	$19,181
Health Insurance (can not be waived)	$1,820	$1,820

Average 2008 Graduate Indebtedness: $192,296
% of Enrolled Students Receiving Aid: 95%

Criminal Background Check

This medical school requires a criminal background check prior to matriculation.

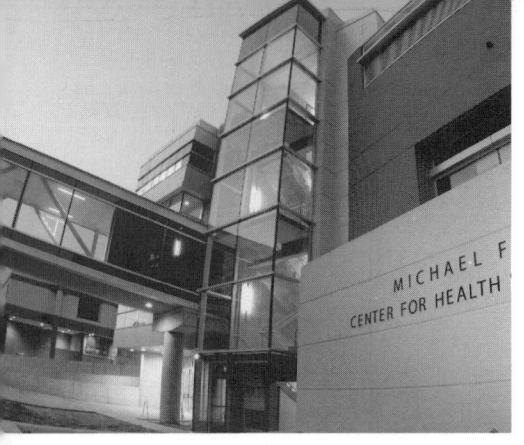

University of Nebraska College of Medicine

Omaha, Nebraska

Office of Admissions and Students
University of Nebraska Medical Center
College of Medicine
985527 Nebraska Medical Center
Omaha, Nebraska 68198-5527
T 402 559 2259   F 402 559 6840

Admissions www.unmc.edu/dept/uncom
Main www.unmc.edu/dept/com
Financial www.unmc.edu/student/
studentservices/financialaid
E-mail grrogers@unmc.edu

Public Institution

Dr. John L. Gollan, Dean

*Dr. Jeffrey W. Hill, Associate Dean,
Office of Admissions and Students*

*Judith Walker, Assistant Director
of Financial Aid*

Gigi Rogers, Administrative Coordinator

General Information

Medical education has been continuous in Omaha since students first entered the Omaha Medical College in the fall of 1881. This modern medical center is a major health resource for the State of Nebraska and the surrounding areas. Several integrated units fulfill the mission of the University of Nebraska Medical Center: The Colleges of Medicine, Nursing, Pharmacy, and Dentistry, the Office of Graduate Studies and Research, the Meyer Rehabilitation Institute, the Eppley Institute for Research in Cancer and Allied Diseases, Nebraska Medical Center (Clarkson and University Hospital), and UNMC Physicians. The School of Allied Health Professions is part of the College of Medicine. These facilities are supplemented by direct teaching affiliations with the Veterans Affairs Medical Center and eight community hospitals.

Mission Statement

The mission of the University of Nebraska Medical Center is to improve the health of Nebraska through premier educational programs, innovative research, the highest quality patient care, and outreach to underserved populations.

Curricular Highlights

Community Service Requirement: Required.
Research/Thesis Requirement: Optional.

The College of Medicine enjoys a distinguished record of excellence in medical education. Our goal is for students to acquire the knowledge, skills, experience, and new pattern of behavior that is required in today's rapidly changing health care system, which emphasizes customer satisfaction, practice efficiency, cost management, preventive medicine, teamwork and a spirit of collaboration between health professionals.

USMLE

Step 1: Required. Students must record a passing score for promotion.
Step 2: Clinical Skills (CS): Required. Students must only record a score.
Step 2: Clinical Knowledge (CK): Required. Students must only record a score.

Selection Factors

Selection is based on a total assessment of each candidate's motivation, interests, character, demonstrated intellectual ability, previous academic record and its trends, personal interview, scores on the MCAT, and general fitness and promise for a career in medicine. Admission is based on individual qualifications without regard to age, sex, sexual preference, race, national origin, handicap, or religious or political beliefs. Strong preference is given to residents of Nebraska, but a small number of students from other states may be accepted. The potential for service to underserved communities is taken into consideration during the preadmission evaluation.

Financial Aid

Some scholarships are available each year. Several fellowships and assistantships are available to students who desire to take one or two years of graduate study or research in the basic sciences.

Information about Diversity Programs

The University of Nebraska College of Medicine is committed to increasing the number of physicians from groups currently underrepresented in the medical profession. Information is available through the Office of Student Equity and Multicultural Affairs at (402) 559-4437.

Campus Information

Setting

The University of Nebraska College of Medicine is located in the heart of Omaha. Recreational and cultural activities include the Omaha Symphony Orchestra, the Old Market, the Joslyn Art Museum, the Omaha Community Playhouse, and the nationally recognized Opera Omaha. The Henry Doorly Zoo contains the world's largest indoor tropical rain forest and an IMAX theater. Spectator sports in Omaha include a full range of high school and collegiate sports and minor league teams. Omaha is the home of the College Baseball World Series.

Enrollment

For 2008, total enrollment was: 481

Special Features

The University of Nebraska College of Medicine strives to be a regional and national leader in the education of primary care health professionals, in the application of information technology to health care, and in research and clinical services related to cancer, transplantation, neurosciences, cardiovascular disease, genetics, rural health, and other major areas of healthcare need. UNMC is world-renowned in the treatment of lymphoma and leukemia, and has one of the two most active bone marrow transplant programs in the country. The LifeNet helicopter transport service transfers acutely ill patients from distances up to 200 miles from Omaha to the teaching services of the Nebraska Medical Center. The Clinical Skills Laboratory in the Michael F. Sorrell Center has a 40-seat instructional/preparatory room, 10 large exam rooms, six smaller exam rooms, a hospital suite and two simulation suites. Additionally, the CSL is equipped with high-tech simulation models for interactive instruction.

Housing

Campus housing is available and many affordable apartments are within walking distance.

Satellite Campuses/Facilities

The clinical facilities at the University of Nebraska Medical Center include the Nebraska Medical Center, University Medical Associates, and the Meyer Rehabilitation Institute. The Nebraska Medical Center is the primary teaching hospital for the College of Medicine. The College has affiliations with community hospitals throughout the state. The Omaha Veterans Affairs Medical Center is fully integrated into the educational programs of the College of Medicine.

Application Process and Requirements 2010–2011

Primary Application Service: AMCAS
Earliest filing date: June 1, 2009
Latest filing date: November 1, 2009

Secondary Application Required?: Yes
Sent to: All applicants
URL: http://net.unmc.edu/apply
Contact: Jackie O'Hara, (402) 559-2259
johara@unmc.edu
Fee: Yes, $70
Fee waiver available: Yes
Earliest filing date: n/a
Latest filing date: January 15, 2010

MCAT® required?: Yes
Latest MCAT® considered: September 2009
Oldest MCAT® considered: January 2007

Early Decision Program: School does have EDP
Applicants notified: October 1, 2009
EDP available for: Both Residents and Non-residents

Regular Acceptance Notice
Earliest date: December 2009
Latest date: Until class is full
Applicant's Response to Acceptance Offer – Maximum Time: Two weeks

Requests for Deferred Entrance Considered: No

Deposit to Hold Place in Class: Yes
Deposit (Resident): $100
Deposit (Non-resident): $100
Deposit due: With response to acceptance offer
Applied to tuition: Yes
Deposit refundable: Yes
Refundable by: May 15, 2010

Estimated number of new entrants: 130
EDP: 35, special program: n/a

Start Month/Year: August 2010

Interview Format: By invitation only. Regional interviews are not available.

Other Programs

PREPARATORY PROGRAMS
Postbaccalaureate Program: No
Summer Program: Yes, www.unmc.edu/dept/cce/smdep, (800) 701-9665, smdep@unmc.edu
Summer Undergraduate Research: Yes, www.unmc.edu/dept/summerresearch, Jeanne Ferbrache, (402) 559-3937, jferbrache@unmc.edu

COMBINED DEGREE PROGRAMS
Baccalaureate/M.D.: No
M.D./M.P.H.: Yes, Jessica B. Tschirren, MPA, (402) 561-7586, jtschirren@unmc.edu
M.D./M.B.A.: No
M.D./J.D.: No
M.D./Ph.D.: Yes, www.unmc.edu/mdphd
Sonja Cox, (402) 559-8242, sacox@unmc.edu

Premedical Coursework

Course	Req.	Rec.	Lab.	Qtrs.	Course	Req.	Rec.	Lab.	Qtrs.
Inorganic Chemistry	•		•	8	Computer Science				
Behavioral Sciences					Genetics		•		3
Biochemistry	•			3	Humanities		•		12
Biology	•		•	8	Organic Chemistry	•		•	8
Biology/Zoology					Physics	•			8
Calculus	•			3	Psychology				
College English	•			3	Social Sciences				
College Mathematics					Other				

Selection Factors: 2008 Accepted Applicants

Proportion of Accepted Applicants with Relevant Experience (Data Self-Reported to AMCAS)	
Community Service/Volunteer	73%
Medically-Related Work	75%
Research	70%

Shaded bar represents school's accepted scores ranging from the 10th percentile to the 90th percentile. School Median ● National Median ●

Overall GPA 2.0 2.1 2.2 2.3 2.4 2.5 2.6 2.7 2.8 2.9 3.0 3.1 3.2 3.3 3.4 3.5 3.6 3.7 **(3.8)** 3.9 4.0
Science GPA 2.0 2.1 2.2 2.3 2.4 2.5 2.6 2.7 2.8 2.9 3.0 3.1 3.2 3.3 3.4 3.5 3.6 **(3.7)** 3.8 3.9 4.0

MCAT® Total Numeric Score 9 10 11 12 13 14 15 16 17 18 19 20 21 22 23 24 25 26 27 28 29 **(30)** 31 **32** 33 34 35 36 37 38 39 40 41 42 43

Writing Sample			J	K	L	M	N	O	**(P)**	**(Q)**	R	S	T	
Verbal Reasoning	3	4	5	6	7	8	9	**(10)**	11	12	13	14	15	
Biological Sciences	3	4	5	6	7	8	9	10	**(11)**	12	13	14	15	
Physical Sciences	3	4	5	6	7	8	9	**(10)**	**(11)**	12	13	14	15	

Acceptance & Matriculation Data for 2008–2009 First Year Class

	Resident	Non-resident	International	Total
Applications	294	1105	13	1412
Interviewed	213	179	0	392
Deferred	3	0	0	3
Matriculants				
Early Assurance Program	n/a	n/a	n/a	n/a
Early Decision Program	44	2	0	46
Baccalaureate/M.D.	n/a	n/a	n/a	n/a
M.D./Ph.D.	2	1	0	3
Matriculated	110	14	0	**124**

Applications accepted from International Applicants: No

Specialty Choice

2004, 2005, 2006 Graduates, Specialty Choice (As reported by program directors to GME Track™)	
Anesthesiology	8%
Emergency Medicine	7%
Family Practice	12%
Internal Medicine	17%
Obstetrics/Gynecology	4%
Orthopaedic Surgery	3%
Pediatrics	10%
Psychiatry	5%
Radiology	4%
Surgery	5%

Matriculant Demographics: 2008–2009 First Year Class

Men: 73   **Women:** 51

Matriculants' Self-Reported Race/Ethnicity

Mexican American	3	Korean	3
Cuban	0	Vietnamese	1
Puerto Rican	0	Other Asian	1
Other Hispanic	0	Total Asian	5
Total Hispanic	3	Native American	2
Chinese	0	Black	4
Asian Indian	0	Native Hawaiian	0
Pakistani	0	White	114
Filipino	0	Unduplicated Number	
Japanese	0	of Matriculants	124

Science and Math Majors: 60%
Matriculants with:
Baccalaureate degree: 99%
Graduate degree(s): 5%

Financial Information

Source: 2007–2008 LCME I-B survey and 2008–2009 AAMC TSF questionnaire

	Residents	Non-residents
Total Cost of Attendance	$40,833	$72,179
Tuition and Fees	$23,845	$55,191
Other (includes living expenses)	$16,024	$16,024
Health Insurance (can be waived)	$964	$964

Average 2008 Graduate Indebtedness: $129,504
% of Enrolled Students Receiving Aid: 96%

Criminal Background Check

This medical school requires a criminal background check prior to matriculation.

University of Nevada School of Medicine

Reno, Nevada

Office of Admissions and Student Affairs
University of Nevada School of Medicine
Mail Stop 0357
Reno, Nevada 89557-0357
T 775 784 6063   **F** 775 784 6194

Admissions www.medicine.nevada.edu/dept/asa/
default.asp
Main www.medicine.nevada.edu/
Financial www.medicine.nevada.edu/dept/asa/
students/financial_assistance_home.htm
E-mail asa@med.unr.edu

Public Institution

Dr. Ole Theinhaus, Dean

Dr. Peggy Dupey, Interim Assistant Dean for Admissions and Student Affairs

Ann Diggins, Director of Recruitment and Student Services

General Information

The University of Nevada School of Medicine is a state-supported, community-based, university-integrated school which relies heavily on community physicians as teachers and community health facilities as sites for the majority of its clinical education. The school is dedicated to selecting individuals with diverse backgrounds who will learn to be compassionate and competent physicians. Students study comprehensive health care delivery considering the needs of the individual, the family, and the community.

Mission Statement

To provide educational opportunities for Nevadans, to improve the quality of healthcare for citizens of Nevada, to create new biomedical knowledge through education, research, patient care and community service, and to provide continuing medical education.

Curricular Highlights

Community Service Requirement: Optional.
Research/Thesis Requirement: Optional.

The first two years of the program are concentrated in classrooms and laboratories on the Reno campus. The curriculum emphasizes the biomedical and behavioral sciences basic to medicine. Basic science disciplines are integrated with each other and with clinical problems to promote the learning of problem-solving skills. A clinical correlation course, which explores the basics of biomedical ethics, is taught. Early clinical training is provided for students to learn patient interviewing and doctor-patient relationship skills and the basics of physical examination and diagnosis. Throughout the first and second years, students spend time with a physician to observe medical practice in the office setting and clinic settings. There are also opportunities to participate in basic and clinical science research

throughout the curriculum. The third and fourth years emphasize a balance of ambulatory and inpatient medical education designed to better prepare students for residency. Third and fourth year students study clinical medicine in Reno, Las Vegas, and rural Nevada.

USMLE

Step 1: Required. Students must record a passing score for promotion.
Step 2: Clinical Skills (CS): Required. Students must record a passing total score to graduate.
Step 2: Clinical Knowledge (CK): Required. Students must record a passing total score to graduate.

Selection Factors

Candidates are evaluated on the basis of academic performance; results of the MCAT; the nature and depth of scholarly, extracurricular, and health care-related activities during college years (excellence and balance of the natural sciences, social sciences, and humanities); academic letters of evaluation; and the personal interview. A small number of non-resident applicants from Alaska, Idaho, Montana, or Wyoming or residents of northern California counties bordering Nevada (medical catchment area) are considered. Applicants from other western states should contact the office of admissions for updated eligibility information. Applicants are required to be U.S. citizens or have a permanent resident visa. Only those students who are currently enrolled and in good academic standing at LCME-accredited medical schools and have a strong residential tie to Nevada are considered for transfer to the second and third years. The number of positions available for transfer is strictly limited by attrition and compatibility to the school's curriculum. Only U.S. citizens are considered. Transfer applications from students attending foreign medical schools are not considered. Completion of a criminal background check is required of all accepted applicants. The fee for this background check is $51.25.

Financial Aid

Every attempt is made to assist students and their families in meeting both their financial obligations to the School of Medicine and the student's essential personal needs. Financial

status is not a determinant in selecting qualified applicants. A limited number of loans and scholarships are available on the basis of need and merit. Determination of financial aid awards is made after acceptance.

Information about Diversity Programs

The School of Medicine is committed to the recruitment, selection, and retention of individuals who are members of groups traditionally underrepresented in American medicine. Residents of the state of Nevada and individuals who meet the non-resident criteria and who are from such backgrounds are encouraged to apply. The University of Nevada, Reno, does not discriminate on the basis of race, color, religion, sex, age, creed, national origin, veteran status, physical or mental disability, and in accordance with university policy, sexual orientation, in any program or activity it operates.

Campus Information

Enrollment

For 2008, total enrollment was: 237

Special Features

The Reno campus features state-of-the art research facilities, a new medical education building with the latest wireless technology, and a Human Patient Simulator (S.T.A.N.). Students have opportunities to work in several clinical facilities. The Las Vegas campus features a Level I trauma center.

Housing

Housing is available within short distances of campuses.

Satellite Campuses/Facilities

The University of Nevada School of Medicine is a state-wide institution with varied clinical sites including a Level I trauma center and numerous research and rural clinical opportunities.

Application Process and Requirements 2010–2011

Primary Application Service: AMCAS
Earliest filing date: June 1, 2009
Latest filing date: November 1, 2009

Secondary Application Required?: Yes
Sent to: Screened applicants
Contact: Patricia Romney, (775) 784-6063, promney@medicine.nevada.edu
Fee: Yes, $45
Fee waiver available: Yes
Earliest filing date: August 1, 2009
Latest filing date: December 1, 2009

MCAT® required?: Yes
Latest MCAT® considered: September 2009
Oldest MCAT® considered: 2006

Early Decision Program: School does have EDP
Applicants notified: October 1, 2009
EDP available for: Both Residents and Non-residents

Regular Acceptance Notice
Earliest date: January 15, 2010
Latest date: Varies
Applicant's Response to Acceptance Offer – Maximum Time: Two weeks

Requests for Deferred Entrance Considered: Yes

Deposit to Hold Place in Class: No
Deposit (Resident): n/a
Deposit (Non-resident): n/a
Deposit due: n/a
Applied to tuition: n/a
Deposit refundable: n/a
Refundable by: n/a

Estimated number of new entrants: 62
EDP: 5, special program: n/a

Start Month/Year: August 2010

Interview Format: Interviews are blind and semi-structured. Applicants are interviewed in Reno and Las Vegas.

Other Programs

PREPARATORY PROGRAMS
Postbaccalaureate Program: No
Summer Program: No

COMBINED DEGREE PROGRAMS
Baccalaureate/M.D.: Yes, www.medicine.nevada.edu/dept/asa/prospective_applicants/programs_md.htm, Gina Sella, (775) 682-8354, gsella@medicine.nevada.edu
M.D./M.P.H.: Yes, www.medicine.nevada.edu/dept/asa/prospective_applicants.programs_home.htm
M.D./M.B.A.: Yes, www.medicine.nevada.edu/dept/asa/prospective_applicants/programs_home.htm
M.D./J.D.: No
M.D./Ph.D.: Yes, www.medicine.nevada.edu/dept/asa/prospective_applicants/programs_graduate.htm, David Lupan, Ph.D., (775) 784-4908, asa@med.unr.edu

Premedical Coursework

Course	Req.	Rec.	Lab.	Hrs.
Inorganic Chemistry	•		•	8
Behavioral Sciences	•			6
Biochemistry		•		
Biology	•		•	12
Biology/Zoology				
Calculus		•		
College English		•		
College Mathematics		•		

Course	Req.	Rec.	Lab.	Hrs.
Computer Science		•		
Genetics		•		
Humanities		•		
Organic Chemistry	•		•	8
Physics	•		•	8
Psychology		•		
Social Sciences		•		
Microbiology/Immunology		•		

Selection Factors: 2008 Accepted Applicants

Proportion of Accepted Applicants with Relevant Experience (Data Self-Reported to AMCAS')	
Community Service/Volunteer	74%
Medically-Related Work	89%
Research	79%

Shaded bar represents school's accepted scores ranging from the 10th percentile to the 90th percentile. School Median ● National Median ●

Overall GPA	2.0	2.1	2.2	2.3	2.4	2.5	2.6	2.7	2.8	2.9	3.0	3.1	3.2	3.3	3.4	3.5	3.6	(3.7)	3.8	3.9	4.0
Science GPA	2.0	2.1	2.2	2.3	2.4	2.5	2.6	2.7	2.8	2.9	3.0	3.1	3.2	3.3	3.4	3.5	3.6	(3.7)	3.8	3.9	4.0

MCAT® Total Numeric Score 9 10 11 12 13 14 15 16 17 18 19 20 21 22 23 24 25 26 27 28 29 30 (31) 32 33 34 35 36 37 38 39 40 41 42 43

Writing Sample			J	K	L	M	N	O	(P)	(Q)	R	S	T
Verbal Reasoning	3	4	5	6	7	8	9	(10)	11	12	13	14	15
Biological Sciences	3	4	5	6	7	8	9	10	(11)	12	13	14	15
Physical Sciences	3	4	5	6	7	8	9	(10)	(11)	12	13	14	15

Acceptance & Matriculation Data for 2008–2009 First Year Class

	Resident	Non-resident	International	Total
Applications	145	1061	15	1221
Interviewed	134	43	0	177
Deferred	0	1	0	1
Matriculants				
Early Assurance Program	n/a	n/a	n/a	n/a
Early Decision Program	1	0	0	1
Baccalaureate/M.D.	n/a	n/a	n/a	n/a
M.D./Ph.D.	n/a	n/a	n/a	n/a
Matriculated	51	11	0	**62**

Applications accepted from International Applicants: No

Matriculant Demographics: 2008–2009 First Year Class

Men: 29 **Women:** 33

Matriculants' Self-Reported Race/Ethnicity

Mexican American	0	Korean	1
Cuban	1	Vietnamese	0
Puerto Rican	0	Other Asian	1
Other Hispanic	0	Total Asian	15
Total Hispanic	1	Native American	0
Chinese	2	Black	1
Asian Indian	7	Native Hawaiian	0
Pakistani	1	White	44
Filipino	2	Unduplicated Number	
Japanese	1	of Matriculants	62

Science and Math Majors: 77%
Matriculants with:
Baccalaureate degree: 100%
Graduate degree(s): 15%

Specialty Choice

2004, 2005, 2006 Graduates, Specialty Choice (As reported by program directors to GME Track™)	
Anesthesiology	7%
Emergency Medicine	10%
Family Practice	14%
Internal Medicine	17%
Obstetrics/Gynecology	6%
Orthopaedic Surgery	4%
Pediatrics	12%
Psychiatry	5%
Radiology	5%
Surgery	4%

Financial Information

Source: 2007–2008 LCME I-B survey and 2008–2009 AAMC TSF questionnaire

	Residents	Non-residents
Total Cost of Attendance	$38,825	$59,190
Tuition and Fees	$14,303	$34,668
Other (includes living expenses)	$22,520	$22,520
Health Insurance (can be waived)	$2,002	$2,002

Average 2008 Graduate Indebtedness: $108,224
% of Enrolled Students Receiving Aid: 89%

Criminal Background Check

This medical school requires a criminal background check prior to matriculation.

Dartmouth Medical School
Hanover, New Hampshire

Dartmouth Medical School
Office of Admissions
3 Rope Ferry Road
Hanover, New Hampshire 03755-1404
T 603 650 1505   **F** 603 650 1560

Admissions http://dms.dartmouth.edu/admissions/
Main http://dms.dartmouth.edu/
Financial http://dms.dartmouth.edu admissions/financial_aid/
E-mail dms.admissions@dartmouth.edu

Private Institution

Dr. William Green, Dean

Andrew G. Welch, Director of Admissions

Dr. Lori Alvord, Associate Dean of Student and Multicultural Affairs

G. Dino Koff, Director of Financial Aid

General Information

Dartmouth Medical School, the fourth oldest U.S. medical school, is a partner of Dartmouth-Hitchcock Medical Center (DHMC). DHMC serves a patient population of 1.6 million and includes Mary Hitchcock Memorial Hospital, Dartmouth-Hitchcock Clinic, and the Veterans Affairs Hospital in White River Junction, Vermont. Other facilities contributing to the integration of advanced research and quality care within DHMC include the Norris Cotton Cancer Center, Children's Hospital at Dartmouth, and the Borwell Research Building; DHMC is a major force for medical treatment and discovery and is the site of numerous clinical trials. Additional teaching sites span nationally and internationally from the New England states to California to Tanzania. A faculty of approximately 2,000 affords ample opportunity for individual instruction.

Mission Statement

Dartmouth Medical School educates outstanding leaders prepared to transform medicine and science. The school aspires to be the best in the world at expanding knowledge and using it wisely to improve health, all done in the context of the tradition of collegiality of Dartmouth and the values its community honors. We are committed to the challenges of discovery and innovation and to their application to health care that meets the needs and wants of patients and society.

Curricular Highlights

Community Service Requirement: Optional.
Research/Thesis Requirement: Optional.

The DMS curriculum integrates basic and clinical sciences throughout medical school. Its hallmarks are longitudinal experiences in the basic and clinical sciences, early introduction to patient care, small-group instruction, close relationships with faculty, and opportunities for independent learning. DMS uses various pedagogies, including problem-based learning, lectures, and small elective courses. Year One includes On Doctoring, a course that pairs students with faculty practitioners in the clinical environment. The Scientific Basis of Medicine, an interdisciplinary pathophysiology course combined with an introduction to the mechanisms of disease and the principles of clinical medicine, is a feature of Year Two. Six seven-week clerkships, elective time, and opportunities to practice in diverse settings shape the third year. The fourth year includes two required clerkships, a sub-internship, and four short courses, but students largely spend this year refining their interests through electives.

USMLE

Step 1: Required. Students must only record a score.
Step 2: Clinical Skills (CS): Required. Students must only record a score.
Step 2: Clinical Knowledge (CK): Required. Students must only record a score.

Selection Factors

The admissions committee carefully reviews the entire application with attention to personal, scholastic, and scientific qualifications. DMS does not employ numeric cutoffs or inflexible criteria. Selected applicants interview in Hanover from September to March. DMS supports equal opportunity for all persons and does not discriminate on the basis of race, color, religion, national or ethnic origin, sex, age, sexual orientation, gender identity or expression, disability, or military or veteran status in admission or access to, or treatment or employment in, its programs and practices.

Financial Aid

DMS practices need-blind admissions. Application fee waivers are granted to individuals who have received an AMCAS fee waiver. All accepted U.S. citizens and permanent residents with documented need are offered financial aid packages. DMS awards scholarships and loans on the basis of need as indicated by the FAFSA, the Need Access form, the DMS financial aid application, and supporting documentation. Financial support for foreign students is limited.

Information about Diversity Programs

DMS seeks to enroll a talented and diverse class of students from various racial, ethnic, cultural, religious, and socio-economic backgrounds. Lori Alvord, M.D. is Associate Dean of Student and Multicultural Affairs.

Campus Information

Setting

DMS is located in the classic New England town of Hanover, NH, on the campus of Dartmouth College. DMS and the surrounding communities provide abundant cultural and recreational opportunities. A sample of venues includes the Hopkins Center, with frequent concerts, films, lectures, and artistic performances, and the Hood Museum, which boasts impressive permanent and temporary exhibits.

Enrollment

For 2008, total enrollment was: 319

Special Features

DMS offers both small classes and one of the nation's top 16 major teaching hospitals. With a patient population of nearly 1.6 million people, Dartmouth medical students gain exposure to a broad spectrum of patients and treatments and are well-prepared for residency training.

Housing

Housing is available on and off-campus.

Satellite Campuses/Facilities

DMS provides a variety of clinical training opportunities; students gain exposure to various patient populations, healthcare delivery systems, and management models. Locations such as Tuba City, AZ; Orange County, CA; San Francisco, CA; Bethel, AK; the Florida Keys, Dar es Salaam, Tanzania; and every New England state (except Massachusetts) are only some of the possibilities. Students may also study at the internationally known Dartmouth Institute for Health Policy and Clinical Practice.

Application Process and Requirements 2010–2011

Primary Application Service: AMCAS
Earliest filing date: June 1, 2009
Latest filing date: November 1, 2009

Secondary Application Required?: Yes
Sent to: All applicants
URL: http://dms.dartmouth.edu/admissions/instrs_to_applicants.shtml
Contact: Office of Admissions, (603) 650-1505, dms.admissions@dartmouth.edu
Fee: Yes, $85
Fee waiver available: Yes
Earliest filing date: June 1, 2009
Latest filing date: January 4, 2010

MCAT® required?: No
Latest MCAT® considered: September 2009
Oldest MCAT® considered: 2007

Early Decision Program: School does not have EDP
Applicants notified: n/a
EDP available for: n/a

Regular Acceptance Notice
Earliest date: October 15, 2009
Latest date: Until class is full
Applicant's Response to Acceptance Offer – Maximum Time: Two weeks

Requests for Deferred Entrance Considered: Yes

Deposit to Hold Place in Class: No
Deposit (Resident): n/a
Deposit (Non-resident): n/a
Deposit due: n/a
Applied to tuition: n/a
Deposit refundable: n/a
Refundable by: n/a

Estimated number of new entrants: 83
EDP: 0, special program: n/a

Start Month/Year: August 2010

Interview Format: Two half-hour interviews. Regional interviews are not available.

Other Programs

PREPARATORY PROGRAMS
Postbaccalaureate Program: No
Summer Program: Yes,
Kalindi Trietley, (603) 650-6535
Kalindi.E.Trietley@Dartmouth.edu

Combined Degree Programs
Baccalaureate/M.D.: No
M.D./M.P.H.: Yes, http://dms.dartmouth.edu/admissions/admission/
M.D./M.B.A.: Yes, http://tuck.dartmouth.edu/
M.D./J.D.: No
M.D./Ph.D.: Yes, http://dms.dartmouth.edu/admissions/curriculum/mdphd/

Premedical Coursework

Course	Req.	Rec.	Lab.	Hrs.	Course	Req.	Rec.	Lab.	Hrs.
Inorganic Chemistry	•			8	Computer Science				
Behavioral Sciences					Genetics				
Biochemistry		•		3	Humanities				
Biology	•			8	Organic Chemistry	•			8
Biology/Zoology					Physics	•			8
Calculus	•			3	Psychology				
College English					Social Sciences				
College Mathematics					Other				

Selection Factors: 2008 Accepted Applicants

Proportion of Accepted Applicants with Relevant Experience (Data Self-Reported to AMCAS®)		
Community Service/Volunteer		77%
Medically-Related Work		91%
Research		93%

Shaded bar represents school's accepted scores ranging from the 10th percentile to the 90th percentile. School Median ● National Median ●

Overall GPA	2.0	2.1	2.2	2.3	2.4	2.5	2.6	2.7	2.8	2.9	3.0	3.1	3.2	3.3	3.4	3.5	3.6	3.7	(3.8)	3.9	4.0
Science GPA	2.0	2.1	2.2	2.3	2.4	2.5	2.6	2.7	2.8	2.9	3.0	3.1	3.2	3.3	3.4	3.5	3.6	3.7	(3.8)	3.9	4.0

MCAT® Total Numeric Score 9 10 11 12 13 14 15 16 17 18 19 20 21 22 23 24 25 26 27 28 29 30 31 (32) 33 (34) 35 36 37 38 39 40 41 42 43

Writing Sample			J	K	L	M	N	O	P	(Q)	R	S	T
Verbal Reasoning	3	4	5	6	7	8	9	(10)	(11)	12	13	14	15
Biological Sciences	3	4	5	6	7	8	9	10	(11)	(12)	13	14	15
Physical Sciences	3	4	5	6	7	8	9	10	(11)	12	13	14	15

Acceptance & Matriculation Data for 2008–2009 First Year Class

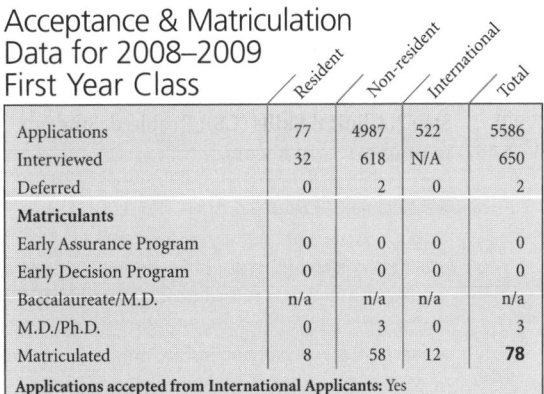

	Resident	Non-resident	International	Total
Applications	77	4987	522	5586
Interviewed	32	618	N/A	650
Deferred	0	2	0	2
Matriculants				
Early Assurance Program	0	0	0	0
Early Decision Program	0	0	0	0
Baccalaureate/M.D.	n/a	n/a	n/a	n/a
M.D./Ph.D.	0	3	0	3
Matriculated	8	58	12	**78**

Applications accepted from International Applicants: Yes

Matriculant Demographics: 2008–2009 First Year Class

Men: 44   **Women:** 34

Matriculants' Self-Reported Race/Ethnicity

Mexican American	1	**Korean**	1
Cuban	0	**Vietnamese**	0
Puerto Rican	0	**Other Asian**	0
Other Hispanic	4	**Total Asian**	11
Total Hispanic	5	**Native American**	1
Chinese	5	**Black**	1
Asian Indian	2	**Native Hawaiian**	0
Pakistani	1	**White**	47
Filipino	2	**Unduplicated Number**	
Japanese	0	**of Matriculants**	78

Science and Math Majors: 68%
Matriculants with:
Baccalaureate degree: 100%
Graduate degree(s): 5%

Specialty Choice

2004, 2005, 2006 Graduates, Specialty Choice (As reported by program directors to GME Track™)	
Anesthesiology	6%
Emergency Medicine	7%
Family Practice	10%
Internal Medicine	14%
Obstetrics/Gynecology	4%
Orthopaedic Surgery	4%
Pediatrics	8%
Psychiatry	6%
Radiology	7%
Surgery	11%

Financial Information

Source: 2007–2008 LCME I-B survey and 2008–2009 AAMC TSF questionnaire

	Residents	Non-residents
Total Cost of Attendance	$58,410	$58,410
Tuition and Fees	$40,900	$40,900
Other (includes living expenses)	$15,450	$15,450
Health Insurance (can be waived)	$2,060	$2,060

Average 2008 Graduate Indebtedness: $120,930
% of Enrolled Students Receiving Aid: 87%

Criminal Background Check

Please see School's Web site.

University of Medicine and Dentistry of New Jersey — New Jersey Medical School

Newark, New Jersey

Director of Admissions
UMDNJ — New Jersey Medical School
185 South Orange Avenue C-653
Newark, New Jersey 07103
T 973 972 4631   **F** 973 972 7986

Admissions http://njms.umdnj.edu/education/
admissions
Main http://njms.umdnj.edu
Financial www.umdnj.edu/studentfinancialaid
E-mail njmsadmiss@umdnj.edu

Public Institution

Dr. Robert L. Johnson, Interim Dean

Dr. Maria Soto-Greene, Vice Dean

Dr. George F. Heinrich, Associate Dean for Admissions and Special Programs

Elaine Varas, University Director of Student Financial Aid

Mercedes M. Rivero, Director of Admissions

General Information

New Jersey Medical School (NJMS), formerly Seton Hall College of Medicine and Dentistry, is the state's oldest academic medical institution. More than 600 faculty and 1,300 volunteer faculty in our 20 academic departments play a critical role in transforming our students into qualified clinicians who will meet and exceed the healthcare needs of New Jersey and the nation. Clinical instruction is carried out at the University Hospital, Hackensack University Medical Center, Veterans Affairs Medical Center, St. Barnabus Medical Center, Newark Beth Israel Medical Center, Morristown Memorial Hospital, Overlook Hospital, Mountainside Hospital and Kessler Institute for Rehabilitation.

Mission Statement

To educate students, physicians, and scientists to meet society's current and future healthcare needs through patient-centered education; pioneering research; innovative clinical, rehabilitative and preventive care; and collaborative community outreach.

Curricular Highlights

Community Service Requirement: Optional.
Research/Thesis Requirement: Optional.

Years 1 and 2 are devoted to providing an understanding of the basic sciences integrated with early clinical exposure and a comprehensive introduction to the field of medicine through a course called the "Physician's Core." The basic sciences are taught utilizing a variety of teaching modalities, including lectures, laboratories and small-group sessions. Students receive components of their clinical training in the Clinical Skills Training Center, which fea-

tures 12 simulated patient examination rooms equipped to monitor mock patient encounters with standardized patients. Years 3 and 4 are devoted to providing in-depth exposure to clinical medicine. In Year 3, students rotate through the major disciplines in medicine (internal medicine, surgery, family medicine, pediatrics, psychiatry and obstetrics-gynecology) and in Year 4, students will assume a higher degree of autonomy and responsibility as they rotate through acting internships and an emergency medicine rotation, and select from a wide range of electives, both at NJMS and throughout the country.

USMLE

Step 1: Required. Students must record a passing score for promotion.
Step 2: Clinical Skills (CS): Required. Students must record a passing total score to graduate.
Step 2: Clinical Knowledge (CK): Required. Students must record a passing total score to graduate.

Selection Factors

Applicants are selected on the basis of academic excellence, leadership qualities, demonstrated compassion for others and broad extracurricular experiences. Related factors such as passion, perseverance, special aptitudes and stamina are also considered. Intense competition tends to favor those with stronger credentials. Although some preference is given to residents of NJ, out-of-state residents are encouraged to apply.

Financial Aid

The student financial aid programs are a centrally managed operation at UMDNJ and not considered in the admissions process. Financial Aid Professionals meet and advise accepted students regarding the financial aspects of their medical education.

Information about Diversity Programs

NJMS is committed to the recruitment of a diverse student body as well as enhancing the cultural competency of all its medical students in order to improve access to care for underserved populations. Several programs have been established to support these goals. Information may be obtained by contacting the Office of Special Programs at (973) 972-3762.

Campus Information

Setting

Located in Newark's University Heights, NJMS is minutes from the Prudential Sports Arena, the Newark Bears Riverfront Stadium, NJ Performing Arts Center, Ironbound district, Weequahic Golf Course and Branch Brook Park. Manhattan is just a 15-minute train ride away. Many buildings on the 65-acre campus are connected, making it convenient to travel from classrooms and labs to the library, University Hospital and student apartments.

Enrollment

For 2008, total enrollment was: 708

Special Features

In recent years, NJMS has received over $104 million in extramural grants supporting basic, clinical and translational research. NJMS is also home to the Global Tuberculosis Institute, The Institute for Ophthalmology and Visual Science, and the Center for Emerging and Reemerging Pathogens. NJMS is a charter member of the New Jersey Stem Cell Research and Education Foundation. Designated Areas of Excellence include: Brain Injury and Stroke, Cancer/Oncology, Cardiovascular Biology, Cellular Signal Transduction, Immunology, Infectious Diseases, Neurosciences, Psychiatry/Behavioral Sciences. NJMS faculty contributions include: the development of the worldwide standard in knee replacement, the New Jersey Knee; a patented method for the early detection of Lyme disease; the identification of pediatric AIDS and the development of drug-therapy to reduce the likelihood of pre-natal transmission; and proof of the connection between smoking and cancer resulting in the warning message printed on cigarette packages.

Housing

There is an on-campus student apartment building that houses 465 students in 234 residential apartments. The 14-story building includes a private exterior courtyard and a parking garage.

Application Process and Requirements 2010–2011

Primary Application Service: AMCAS
Earliest filing date: June 1, 2009
Latest filing date: December 1, 2009

Secondary Application Required?: Yes
Sent to: All applicants
Contact: njmsadmiss@umdnj.edu
Fee: Yes, $80
Fee waiver available: Yes
Earliest filing date: July 1, 2009
Latest filing date: December 15, 2009

MCAT® required?: Yes
Latest MCAT® considered: September 2009
Oldest MCAT® considered: 1999

Early Decision Program: School does have EDP
Applicants notified: October 1, 2009
EDP available for: Both Residents
and Non-residents

Regular Acceptance Notice
Earliest date: October 15, 2009
Latest date: Varies
Applicant's Response to Acceptance
Offer – Maximum Time: Two weeks

Requests for Deferred
Entrance Considered: Yes

Deposit to Hold Place in Class: Yes
Deposit (Resident): $100
Deposit (Non-resident): $100
Deposit due: Within two weeks of acceptance
Applied to tuition: Yes
Deposit refundable: Yes
Refundable by: May 15, 2010

Estimated number of new entrants: 170
EDP: 20, special program: 25

Start Month/Year: August 2010

Interview Format: One-to-one,
non-stress interview with faculty.

Other Programs

PREPARATORY PROGRAMS
Postbaccalaureate Program: No
Summer Program: Yes
Dolores Anthony, (973) 972-3762
anthondd@umdnj.edu

Combined Degree Programs
Baccalaureate/M.D.: Yes, http://njms.umdnj.edu/
education/admissions/seven_year_ba_md.cfm,
Lisa Houston, (973) 972-4631,
njmadmiss@umdnj.edu
M.D./M.P.H.: Yes, http://sph.umdnj.edu
M.D./M.B.A.: Yes,
http://njms.umdnj.edu/education/
admissions/md_mba.cfm
M.D./J.D.: No
M.D./Ph.D.: Yes, http://njms.umdnj.edu/
education/admissions/md_phd.cfm

Premedical Coursework

Course	Req.	Rec.	Lab.	Hrs.
Inorganic Chemistry	•		•	8
Behavioral Sciences				
Biochemistry		•		
Biology		•		
Biology/Zoology	•		•	8
Calculus				
College English	•			6
College Mathematics		•		3

Course	Req.	Rec.	Lab.	Hrs.
Computer Science				
Genetics		•		
Humanities				
Organic Chemistry	•		•	8
Physics	•		•	8
Psychology				
Social Sciences				
Other				

Selection Factors: 2008 Accepted Applicants

Proportion of Accepted Applicants with Relevant Experience (Data Self-Reported to AMCAS®)		
Community Service/Volunteer		64%
Medically-Related Work		84%
Research		78%

Shaded bar represents school's accepted scores ranging from the 10th percentile to the 90th percentile. School Median ● National Median ●

Overall GPA	2.0	2.1	2.2	2.3	2.4	2.5	2.6	2.7	2.8	2.9	3.0	3.1	3.2	3.3	3.4	3.5	3.6	(3.7)	3.8	3.9	4.0
Science GPA	2.0	2.1	2.2	2.3	2.4	2.5	2.6	2.7	2.8	2.9	3.0	3.1	3.2	3.3	3.4	3.5	(3.6)	3.7	3.8	3.9	4.0

MCAT® Total Numeric Score 9 10 11 12 13 14 15 16 17 18 19 20 21 22 23 24 25 26 27 28 29 30 31 (32) 33 34 35 36 37 38 39 40 41 42 43

Writing Sample			J	K	L	M	N	O	(P)	(Q)	R	S	T
Verbal Reasoning	3	4	5	6	7	8	9	(10)	11	12	13	14	15
Biological Sciences	3	4	5	6	7	8	9	10	(11)	12	13	14	15
Physical Sciences	3	4	5	6	7	8	9	10	(11)	12	13	14	15

Acceptance & Matriculation Data for 2008–2009 First Year Class

	Resident	Non-resident	International	Total
Applications	1159	3032	52	4243
Interviewed	632	23	0	665
Deferred	1	0	0	1
Matriculants				
Early Assurance Program	1	0	0	1
Early Decision Program	22	0	0	22
Baccalaureate/M.D.	19	1	0	20
M.D./Ph.D.	5	0	0	5
Matriculated	185	9	0	**194**

Applications accepted from International Applicants: No

Matriculant Demographics: 2008–2009 First Year Class

Men: 121   **Women:** 73

Matriculants' Self-Reported Race/Ethnicity

Mexican American	0	Korean	15
Cuban	3	Vietnamese	1
Puerto Rican	5	Other Asian	2
Other Hispanic	12	Total Asian	73
Total Hispanic	20	Native American	0
Chinese	18	Black	17
Asian Indian	33	Native Hawaiian	0
Pakistani	4	White	94
Filipino	0	Unduplicated Number	
Japanese	0	of Matriculants	194

Science and Math Majors: 66%
Matriculants with:
    Baccalaureate degree: 98%
    Graduate degree(s): 14%

Specialty Choice

2004, 2005, 2006 Graduates, Specialty Choice (As reported by program directors to GME Track™)	
Anesthesiology	7%
Emergency Medicine	8%
Family Practice	5%
Internal Medicine	17%
Obstetrics/Gynecology	5%
Orthopaedic Surgery	5%
Pediatrics	12%
Psychiatry	5%
Radiology	6%
Surgery	7%

Financial Information

Source: 2007–2008 LCME I-B survey
and 2008–2009 AAMC TSF questionnaire

	Residents	Non-residents
Total Cost of Attendance	$49,839	$64,082
Tuition and Fees	$26,113	$40,356
Other (includes living expenses)	$21,905	$21,905
Health Insurance (can be waived)	$1,821	$1,821

Average 2008 Graduate Indebtedness: $132,677
% of Enrolled Students Receiving Aid: 83%

Criminal Background Check

This medical school requires a criminal background check prior to matriculation.

University of Medicine and Dentistry of New Jersey — Robert Wood Johnson Medical School

Piscataway, New Jersey

Associate Dean for Admissions
University of Medicine and Dentistry of New Jersey
Robert Wood Johnson Medical School
675 Hoes Lane
Piscataway, New Jersey 08854-5635
T 732 235 4576 **F** 732 235 5078

Admissions http://rwjms.umdnj.edu/admissions
Main http://rwjms.umdnj.edu
Financial www.umdnj.edu/studentfinancialaid
E-mail rwjapadm@umdnj.edu

Public Institution

Dr. Peter S. Amenta, Dean

Dr. Carol A. Terregino, Associate Dean for Admissions

Dr. Cheryl Dickson, Assistant Dean for Multicultural Affairs

Marshall Anthony, Associate Director of Financial Aid

Meryle Kramer, Admissions Officer

General Information

Robert Wood Johnson Medical School, formerly Rutgers Medical School, has campuses in Piscataway, New Brunswick and Camden. A full complement of clinical training facilities including Robert Wood Johnson University Hospital, Bristol Myers Squibb Children's Hospital, Cooper University Hospital and numerous ambulatory sites provide outstanding educational experiences. The medical school encompasses 22 basic science and clinical departments and more than 2,500 full-time and volunteer faculty members.

Mission Statement

The medical school is dedicated to the pursuit of excellence in education, research, health care delivery and the promotion of community health. Excellence is achieved through the work of a scholarly and creative faculty and a high-achieving and diverse student body.

Curricular Highlights

Community Service Requirement: Optional. Distinction in Service to the Community
Research/Thesis Requirement: Optional. Distinction in Research or Distinction in Medical Education.

The preclerkship pass/fail curriculum provides for early introduction to patient care via the Patient Centered Medicine course, integration of clinical skills into the basic sciences, and opportunity for self-directed learning. There is ample elective time in the third year. In the fourth year students rotate in emergency medicine and critical care, a sub-internship, outpatient subspecialties and 20 weeks of electives. A longitudinal primary care experience and an independent project round out the clinical curriculum. The Clinical Skills Center runs a summative clinical assessment. Each clerkship has an OSCE, and grading is on a 5-point scale. There are a number of dual degree options including a program in Clinical and Translational research. The M.D./Ph.D. is a tri-institutional program with Princeton University and Rutgers University.

USMLE

Step 1: Required. Students must record a passing score for promotion.
Step 2: Clinical Skills (CS): Required. Students must record a passing total score to graduate.
Step 2: Clinical Knowledge (CK): Required. Students must record a passing total score to graduate.

Selection Factors

Preference is given to New Jersey residents. Out-of-state applicants are encouraged to apply. Admission is determined on the basis of academics, MCAT, preprofessional evaluations, character, motivation, and interview. We believe that a diverse student body contributes to the educational program of all students. Selection and recruitment is based on a holistic review of each applicant's experiences, personal qualities and potential to enhance the learning environment. Applications from members of groups underrepresented in medicine are encouraged. Interviews are by invitation. Matriculants must submit to a criminal background check.

Financial Aid

Financial aid is awarded on the basis of evaluated need. All awards consist of a package of loans and grants when funds are available. New funds have been allocated for scholarships. Counseling services are available.

Information about Diversity Programs

Robert Wood Johnson Medical School is committed to the education of physicians from groups underrepresented in medicine. Applications from in-state and out-of-state candidates are welcome. Numerous support services are available for disadvantaged students, including a pre-matriculation summer program.

Campus Information

Setting

The facilities of the Piscataway campus include the Kessler Teaching Labs/Clinical Skills Center and the Research Tower, University Behavioral Health Care Center, the Center for Advanced Biotechnology and Medicine and the Environmental and Occupational Health Sciences Institute, UMDNJ School of Public Health and the Robert Wood Johnson Medical School Research Building, the current site for the Stem Cell Institute. The New Brunswick campus includes the Cancer Hospital, BMS Children's Hospital, Children's Specialized Hospital, the Child Health Institute, the Cancer Institute of New Jersey. The Camden Regional Campus is close to the historic river front, and across the river from Philadelphia. The medical school and Cooper University Hospital facilities are adjacent to each other.

Enrollment

For 2008, total enrollment was: 680

Special Features

The medical school hosts 85 centers and institutes including the Cancer Institute of New Jersey, the Cardiovascular Institute, the Child Health Institute of New Jersey, the Center for Advanced Biotechnology and Medicine, and the Environmental and Occupational Health Sciences Institute. Students provide continuity care to the community in Urban Health Initiatives, the Promise Clinic and the Homeless and Indigent Population Health Outreach Project. They tailor their medical school experiences as Student Scholars, researchers, leaders of organizations and non-credit electives and as international travelers. Scholarly and social lives are rich.

Housing

On-campus housing is currently not available. Students are assisted in finding affordable housing.

Satellite Campuses/Facilities

Camden is a regional campus. One third of the class completes clinical training at this single-hospital site. Students in the New Brunswick program rotate among three hospital sites.

Application Process and Requirements 2010–2011

Primary Application Service: AMCAS
Earliest filing date: June 1, 2009
Latest filing date: December 1, 2009

Secondary Application Required?: No
Sent to: n/a
URL: n/a
Fee: Yes, $75
Fee waiver available: Yes
Earliest filing date: n/a
Latest filing date: n/a

MCAT® required?: Yes
Latest MCAT® considered: September 2009
Oldest MCAT® considered: September 2006

Early Decision Program: School does have EDP
Applicants notified: October 1, 2009
EDP available for: Both Residents and Non-residents

Regular Acceptance Notice
Earliest date: October 16, 2009
Latest date: Until class is full
Applicant's Response to Acceptance Offer – Maximum Time: Two weeks

Requests for Deferred Entrance Considered: Yes

Deposit to Hold Place in Class: Yes
Deposit (Resident): $50
Deposit (Non-resident): $50
Deposit due: With response to acceptance offer
Applied to tuition: Yes
Deposit refundable: Yes
Refundable by: May 15, 2010

Estimated number of new entrants: 156
EDP: 5, special program: 10

Start Month/Year: August 2010

Interview Format: One (faculty) or two (faculty and student) interviews. Applicants can interview on any of the campuses.

Other Programs

PREPARATORY PROGRAMS
Postbaccalaureate Program: No
Summer Program: Yes, Cheryl Dickson, M.D. (732) 235-2144, dicksoca@umdnj.edu

COMBINED DEGREE PROGRAMS
Baccalaureate/M.D.: Yes, http://lifesci.rutgers.edu/~hpo/
M.D./M.P.H.: Yes, http://sph.umdnj.edu Tina Greco, (732) 235-4017, grecotm@umdnj.edu
M.D./M.B.A.: Yes, David Seiden, Ph.D. (732) 235-4577, seiden@umdnj.edu
M.D./J.D.: Yes, Carol A. Terregino, M.D. (732) 235-4577, terregca@umdnj.edu
M.D./Ph.D.: Yes, http://rwjms.umdnj.edu/research/scientist_training/ Terri Kinzy, Ph.D., (732) 235-5450, kinzytg@umdnj.edu

Premedical Coursework

Course	Req.	Rec.	Lab.	Sems.
Inorganic Chemistry	•		•	2
Behavioral Sciences		•		
Biochemistry		•		
Biology				
Biology/Zoology	•		•	2
Calculus				
College English	•			2
College Mathematics	•			1
Computer Science				

Course	Req.	Rec.	Lab.	Sems.
Genetics		•		
Humanities		•		
Organic Chemistry	•		•	2
Physics	•		•	2
Psychology		•		
Social Sciences		•		
Molecular Biology		•		
Statistics		•		
Cell Biology		•		

Selection Factors: 2008 Accepted Applicants

Proportion of Accepted Applicants with Relevant Experience (Data Self-Reported to AMCAS®)		
Community Service/Volunteer		66%
Medically-Related Work		90%
Research		81%

Shaded bar represents school's accepted scores ranging from the 10th percentile to the 90th percentile. School Median ● National Median ●

Overall GPA 2.0 2.1 2.2 2.3 2.4 2.5 2.6 2.7 2.8 2.9 3.0 3.1 3.2 3.3 3.4 3.5 3.6 (3.7) 3.8 3.9 4.0

Science GPA 2.0 2.1 2.2 2.3 2.4 2.5 2.6 2.7 2.8 2.9 3.0 3.1 3.2 3.3 3.4 3.5 3.6 (3.7) 3.8 3.9 4.0

MCAT® Total Numeric Score 9 10 11 12 13 14 15 16 17 18 19 20 21 22 23 24 25 26 27 28 29 30 31 (32) 33 34 35 36 37 38 39 40 41 42 43

Writing Sample			J	K	L	M	N	O	P	(Q)	R	S	T
Verbal Reasoning	3	4	5	6	7	8	9	(10)	11	12	13	14	15
Biological Sciences	3	4	5	6	7	8	9	10	(11)	12	13	14	15
Physical Sciences	3	4	5	6	7	8	9	10	(11)	12	13	14	15

Acceptance & Matriculation Data for 2008–2009 First Year Class

	Resident	Non-resident	International	Total
Applications	1159	2187	32	3378
Interviewed	418	97	0	515
Deferred	5	1	0	6
Matriculants				
Early Assurance Program	0	0	0	0
Early Decision Program	6	0	0	6
Baccalaureate/M.D.	10	0	0	10
M.D./Ph.D.	3	3	0	6
Matriculated	140	26	0	**166**

Applications accepted from International Applicants: No

Matriculant Demographics: 2008–2009 First Year Class

Men: 74 **Women:** 92

Matriculants' Self-Reported Race/Ethnicity

Mexican American	2	**Korean**	7
Cuban	2	**Vietnamese**	0
Puerto Rican	2	**Other Asian**	1
Other Hispanic	5	**Total Asian**	46
Total Hispanic	10	**Native American**	0
Chinese	11	**Black**	15
Asian Indian	21	**Native Hawaiian**	0
Pakistani	3	**White**	97
Filipino	2	**Unduplicated Number**	
Japanese	2	**of Matriculants**	166

Science and Math Majors: 59%
Matriculants with:
    Baccalaureate degree: 100%
    Graduate degree(s): 6%

Specialty Choice

2004, 2005, 2006 Graduates, Specialty Choice (As reported by program directors to GME Track™)	
Anesthesiology	4%
Emergency Medicine	5%
Family Practice	7%
Internal Medicine	22%
Obstetrics/Gynecology	4%
Orthopaedic Surgery	4%
Pediatrics	12%
Psychiatry	6%
Radiology	8%
Surgery	6%

Financial Information

Source: 2007–2008 LCME I-B survey and 2008–2009 AAMC TSF questionnaire

	Residents	Non-residents
Total Cost of Attendance	$55,174	$69,417
Tuition and Fees	$26,452	$40,695
Other (includes living expenses)	$26,755	$26,755
Health Insurance (can be waived)	$1,967	$1,967

Average 2008 Graduate Indebtedness: $132,911
% of Enrolled Students Receiving Aid: 81%

Criminal Background Check

This medical school requires a criminal background check prior to matriculation.

University of New Mexico School of Medicine

Albuquerque, New Mexico

University of New Mexico Health Sciences Center School of Medicine, Office of Admissions, MSC09 5085, Health Sciences Library and Informatics Center, Room 125
Albuquerque, New Mexico 87131-0001
T 505 272 4766   F 505 925 6031

Admissions http://hsc.unm.edu/som/admissions
Main http://hsc.unm.edu/som
Financial http://hsc.unm.edu/som/admissions/aid.shtml
E-mail somadmissions@salud.unm.edu

Public Institution

Dr. Paul B. Roth, Dean

Dr. David G. Bear, Assistant Dean for Admissions

Dr. Valerie Romero-Leggott, Vice President of Diversity

Janell Valdez, Financial Aid Supervisor

Marlene Ballejos, Admissions Director

General Information

This internationlly renowned program was established in 1961, and The University of New Mexico enrolled its first 24 medical students in September of 1964. The School of Medicine is both a professional and graduate school where students may earn an M.D. degree, a Ph.D. degree, a combined M.D./Ph.D. degree, a combined M.D./M.P.H., or B.S. or M.S. degrees in several allied health science fields. Medical education at the resident and postgraduate levels is offered through the University's teaching hospital and various state-of-the-art facilities.

Mission Statement

The mission of the University of New Mexico is to educate students, scientists, physicians and other health professionals in the art and science of medicine through the transmission of biomedical knowledge acquired from research and patient care. We aspire to improve the health of all New Mexicans by being a model of excellence in education while working to reduce disparities among medically underrepresented populations and communities.

Curricular Highlights

Community Service Requirement: Required. A community research project is required.
Research/Thesis Requirement: Required. A research project and report is required.

The School of Medicine utilizes a hybrid curriculum, which incorporates the integration of basic sciences and clinical medicine with problem-based and student-centered learning techniques. Early clinical skills are coupled with medical education taught from three perspectives: biologic, population, and behavioral, and these perspectives are continued throughout the

clinical years. Medical students are exposed to patient care during the first year of education, and finish that year with a 9-week, in-depth Practical Immersion Experience (PIE) in a professional setting in one of New Mexico's communities. The goals of the curriculum are to graduate physicians who are enthusiastic and responsible for their continued learning; have the ability to define problems, formulate questions, and carry out scholarly inquiry; are skilled in self and peer assessment; and have a broad perspective on the importance of human biology, behavior, environment, culture, and social setting in the health of individuals and populations. Student assessment is competency-based and values mastery of knowledge, critical appraisal, interpersonal and clinical skills, and peer and self-assessment.

USMLE

Step 1: Required. Students must record a passing score for promotion.
Step 2: Clinical Skills (CS): Required. Students must record a passing total score to graduate.
Step 2: Clinical Knowledge (CK): Required. Students must only record a score.

Selection Factors

Upon receipt of the AMCAS application, applicants who pass initial screening will be sent a supplemental application and an invitation to interview. In general, only those applicants with ties to the state of New Mexico or residents of WICHE states (Montana and Wyoming) will receive consideration for admission. Selection is based upon scholastic achievement, performance on the MCAT, personal interviews with members of the Admissions Committee, and recommendations.

Financial Aid

The school makes accessible federal, state and institutional aid in the form of scholarships, grants, and loans. Both need-based and merit-based funding are available to students. The amount of an award varies according to the student's need and the level of funding available. The Office of Financial Aid assists all students in locating necessary funds to support their medical education.

Information about Diversity Programs

The mission of the Office of Diversity is to

promote racial, ethnic, socio-economic, and geographic diversity in the UNM Health Sciences Center and to develop a variety of opportunities addressing key issues in diversity. Strategies to achieve this mission include creating college awareness and identifying, recruiting, and supporting students, residents, and faculty from these diverse backgrounds.

Campus Information

Setting
Albuquerque is home to a unique blend of culture and cuisine, styles and stories, peoples, pursuits, and panoramas.

Enrollment
For 2008, total enrollment was: 299

Special Features
The School of Medicine facilities include a Basic Medical Sciences Building, a Biomedical Research Facility, the Health Sciences Library and Informatics Center, the Mental Health Center, the UNM Children's Hospital, the Children's Psychiatric Center, the Family Practice Center, the Mind Imaging Center, Clinical and Translational Science Center, and the Cancer Research and Treatment Center. Other components include: Addiction and Substance Abuse Programs, Brain Imaging Center, Center for Disease Medicine, Center for Environmental Health Sciences, Center for Telehealth, Center on Aging, Children's Hospital Heart Center, Clinical Trials Center, General Clinical Research Center, Geriatric Education Center, HSC Institute for Ethics, New Mexico AIDS Education and Training Center, New Mexico Immunization Coalition, New Mexico Poison Control Center, Sleep Disorders Center, School of Medicine Center for Community Partnerships and Speech/Language/Swallow Center.

Housing
On-campus housing is not available.

Satellite Campuses/Facilities
Student clinical rotations are divided among University Hospital and several other locations in the Albuquerque area.

Application Process and Requirements 2010–2011

Primary Application Service: AMCAS
Earliest filing date: June 1, 2009
Latest filing date: November 15, 2009

Secondary Application Required?: Yes
Sent to: Screened applicants
URL: http://hsc.unm.edu/som/admissions
Fee: Yes, $75
Fee waiver available: Yes
Earliest filing date: August 1, 2009
Latest filing date: February 1, 2010

MCAT® required?: Yes
Latest MCAT® considered: September 2009
Oldest MCAT® considered: 2005

Early Decision Program: School does have EDP
Applicants notified: October 1, 2009
EDP available for: Both Residents and Non-residents

Regular Acceptance Notice
Earliest date: March 15, 2010
Latest date: Until class is full
Applicant's Response to Acceptance Offer – Maximum Time: Two weeks

Requests for Deferred Entrance Considered: Yes

Deposit to Hold Place in Class: Yes
Deposit (Resident): $100
Deposit (Non-resident): $100
Deposit due: May 15, 2010
Applied to tuition: Yes
Deposit refundable: Yes
Refundable by: May 15, 2010

Estimated number of new entrants: 75
EDP: 6, special program: 7

Start Month/Year: July 2010

Interview Format: Two one-on-one interviews by committee members.

Other Programs

PREPARATORY PROGRAMS
Postbaccalaureate Program: Yes,
http://hsc.unm.edu/som/asc/
Steven Mitchell, (505) 925-4441,
oasis@salud.unm.edu
Summer Program: No

COMBINED DEGREE PROGRAMS
Baccalaureate/M.D.: Yes,
http://hsc.unm.edu/som/combinedbamd
Kathy Kersting, (505) 925-4500
combinedbamd@salud.unm.edu
M.D./M.P.H.: Yes, http://hsc.unm.edu/som/
admissions/programs_restore.shtml, Gaylea Garcia,
(505) 272-4173, garciag@salud.unm.edu
M.D./M.B.A.: No
M.D./J.D.: No
M.D./Ph.D.: Yes, http://hsc.unm.edu/som/
programs/mdphd, Fernando Valenzuela,
(505) 272-1887, bsgp@salud.unm.edu

Premedical Coursework

Course	Req.	Rec.	Lab.	Hrs.
Inorganic Chemistry	•		•	8
Behavioral Sciences				
Biochemistry	•			3
Biology				
Biology/Zoology	•		•	8
Calculus				
College English				
College Mathematics				

Course	Req.	Rec.	Lab.	Hrs.
Computer Science				
Genetics				
Humanities				
Organic Chemistry	•		•	8
Physics	•			6
Psychology				
Anatomy & Physiology		•	•	
Microbiology		•		
Immunology		•		

Selection Factors: 2008 Accepted Applicants

Proportion of Accepted Applicants with Relevant Experience (Data Self-Reported to AMCAS*)		
Community Service/Volunteer		77%
Medically-Related Work		90%
Research		72%

Shaded bar represents school's accepted scores ranging from the 10th percentile to the 90th percentile. School Median ● National Median ●

Overall GPA 2.0 2.1 2.2 2.3 2.4 2.5 2.6 2.7 2.8 2.9 3.0 3.1 3.2 3.3 3.4 3.5 3.6 ⦿3.7 3.8 3.9 4.0
Science GPA 2.0 2.1 2.2 2.3 2.4 2.5 2.6 2.7 2.8 2.9 3.0 3.1 3.2 3.3 3.4 3.5 ⦿3.6 3.7 3.8 3.9 4.0

MCAT® Total Numeric Score 9 10 11 12 13 14 15 16 17 18 19 20 21 22 23 24 25 26 27 ⦿28 29 30 31 ◉32 33 34 35 36 37 38 39 40 41 42 43

Writing Sample			J	K	L	M	N	O	Ⓟ	Ⓠ	R	S	T
Verbal Reasoning	3	4	5	6	7	8	Ⓨ9	◉10	11	12	13	14	15
Biological Sciences	3	4	5	6	7	8	9	Ⓨ10	◉11	12	13	14	15
Physical Sciences	3	4	5	6	7	8	Ⓨ9	10	◉11	12	13	14	15

Acceptance & Matriculation Data for 2008–2009 First Year Class

	Resident	Non-resident	International	Total
Applications	207	364	5	576
Interviewed	183	36	0	219
Deferred	6	0	0	6
Matriculants				
Early Assurance Program	n/a	n/a	n/a	n/a
Early Decision Program	0	0	0	0
Baccalaureate/M.D.	n/a	n/a	n/a	n/a
M.D./Ph.D.	1	0	0	1
Matriculated	73	2	0	**75**

Applications accepted from International Applicants: No

Matriculant Demographics: 2008–2009 First Year Class

Men: 33 **Women:** 42

Matriculants' Self-Reported Race/Ethnicity

Mexican American	17	**Korean**	0
Cuban	1	**Vietnamese**	0
Puerto Rican	0	**Other Asian**	1
Other Hispanic	9	**Total Asian**	5
Total Hispanic	25	**Native American**	5
Chinese	4	**Black**	1
Asian Indian	0	**Native Hawaiian**	0
Pakistani	0	**White**	60
Filipino	0	**Unduplicated Number**	
Japanese	1	**of Matriculants**	75

Science and Math Majors: 72%
Matriculants with:
Baccalaureate degree: 100%
Graduate degree(s): 15%

Specialty Choice

2004, 2005, 2006 Graduates, Specialty Choice (As reported by program directors to GME Track™)	
Anesthesiology	5%
Emergency Medicine	6%
Family Practice	12%
Internal Medicine	21%
Obstetrics/Gynecology	11%
Orthopaedic Surgery	2%
Pediatrics	13%
Psychiatry	1%
Radiology	5%
Surgery	4%

Financial Information
Source: 2007–2008 LCME I-B survey and 2008–2009 AAMC TSF questionnaire

	Residents	Non-residents
Total Cost of Attendance	$38,173	$65,545
Tuition and Fees	$17,621	$44,993
Other (includes living expenses)	$20,410	$20,410
Health Insurance (cannot be waived)	$142	$142

Average 2008 Graduate Indebtedness: $119,564
% of Enrolled Students Receiving Aid: 88%

Criminal Background Check

This medical school requires a criminal background check prior to matriculation.

Albany Medical College
Albany, New York

Office of Admissions, Mail Code 3
Albany Medical College
47 New Scotland Avenue
Albany, New York 12208
T 518 262 5521   **F** 518 262 5887

Admissions www.amc.edu/academic/Undergraduate
_Admissions/
Main www.amc.edu/Academic/
Financial www.amc.edu/academic/
Undergraduate/FinancialAid.html
E-mail admissions@mail.amc.edu

Private Institution

Dr. Vincent Verdile, Dean

*Joanne H. Nanos, Director, Admissions
and Student Records*

Ann Loughman, Director of Financial Aid

*Dr. Henry Pohl, Vice Dean for
Academic Administration*

General Information
Founded in 1839, Albany Medical College is
one of the oldest medical schools in the country and one of the largest teaching hospitals in
New York State. The college is coeducational,
nondenominational, and privately supported.
The college and the 650-bed Albany Medical
Center Hospital comprise Albany Medical
Center. Patient care, from primary to tertiary,
is provided for over 2.5 million residents of
eastern New York and western New England.

Mission Statement
The mission of the Albany Medical College is
to: (1) educate medical students, all physicians,
bio-medical scientists, and other health professionals to meet future primary and specialty
health care needs, (2) foster biomedical
research that leads to scientific advances and
improvement of public health, and (3) provide
a broad range of patient services.

Curricular Highlights
Community Service Requirement: Optional.
M.D. with Distinction in Service
Research/Thesis Requirement: Optional.
M.D. with Distinction in Research

Basic and clinical sciences are integrated into
themes stressing normal function in Year 1 and
pathological processes in Year 2. There are also
five longitudinal themes integrated throughout
the curriculum: clinical skills, ethical and
health systems issues, evidence-based medicine, nutrition, and informatics. In every
theme, learning focuses on clinical presentations. Beginning in Year 1, students learn to
interview and examine both real and standardized patients. Clinical skills competence is
highlighted throughout the four years. Basic
science knowledge is reinforced during years 3
and 4. Primary care is emphasized throughout

the four years. Year 3 clerkships focus on care
in ambulatory settings. Year 4 required rotations concentrate on care in hospital-based settings, preparing students for residency and
practice. The remainder of fourth year includes
electives chosen by the students and a required
course in learning how to teach.

USMLE
Step 1: Required. Students must record a passing
score for graduation, but not promotion.
Step 2: Clinical Skills (CS): Required. Students
must record a passing total score to graduate.
Step 2: Clinical Knowledge (CK): Required.
Students must record a passing total score to
graduate.

Selection Factors
In selecting students, emphasis is placed upon
integrity, character, academic achievement,
motivation, emotional stability, and social and
intellectual suitability. The college is committed to the belief that educational opportunities
should be available to all eligible persons without regard to race, creed, age, gender, religion,
marital status, handicap, national origin, or
sexual orientation. Admission is not restricted
to state residents. The committee evaluates
applications based on a number of factors in
addition to MCAT scores and GPAs.
Invitations for interview are made at the discretion of the committee. Preapplication
inquiries or questions concerning the status of
applications are always welcome.

Financial Aid
The mission of the Financial Aid Office is to be
the primary source of information and education about financing a degree. Outreach events
and media are provided to guide the development of students' immediate and long-range
spending plans that secure their financial
future. The office awards and certifies need-
based aid for 88% of enrolled students and
provides lifetime service to graduated students.

Information about Diversity Programs
We believe that Albany Medical College's mission is enriched by a community of people
with diverse backgrounds. Recognition and
respect of all differences that exist is crucial to
the development of core professional attributes

in our students, to the continued nurturing of
such attributes among our faculty, staff and
workforce. To that end we seek to recruit students who will bring a diversity of thought,
experience and backgrounds to our community. Please call the Office of Student Affairs at
(518) 262-5634 for more information.

Campus Information

Setting
Albany is the capital of New York and a part of
the tri-city area which includes Schenectady
and Troy. Rich in history, Albany has diverse
cultural and recreational opportunities. Fifteen
area colleges and universities add to the
region's eclectic appeal.

Enrollment
For 2008, total enrollment was: 572

Special Features
Albany Medical Center Hospital provides
sophisticated health care to more than 2 million
people in 24 counties. A recently completed
renovation invested approximately $15 million
and added 45,000 square feet of new construction. The new addition permitted several outpatient services and all physician offices to move
to one location and opened space within the
hospital to add 25 additional inpatient beds.

Housing
On-campus housing is not available. The college maintains a list of affordable apartments
within a 5-mile radius. Rents average $500–
$900 per month.

Satellite Campuses/Facilities
The medical college is affiliated with other
hospitals in New York State. Clinical departments utilize a network of community physicians to serve the ambulatory care educational
needs of students. The college, which is combined with Albany Medical Center Hospital on
its campus, is also affiliated with the Veterans
Administration Hospital, community hospitals, and private and community clinics in surrounding counties.

Application Process and Requirements 2010–2011

Primary Application Service: AMCAS
Earliest filing date: June 1, 2009
Latest filing date: November 15, 2009

Secondary Application Required?: Yes
Sent to: All applicants
Contact: Admissions Staff
(518) 262-5521, admissions@mail.amc.edu
Fee: Yes, $105
Fee waiver available: Yes
Earliest filing date: June 2009
Latest filing date: January 15, 2010

MCAT® required?: Yes
Latest MCAT® considered: September 2009
Oldest MCAT® considered: 2006

Early Decision Program: School does not have EDP
Applicants notified: n/a
EDP available for: n/a

Regular Acceptance Notice
Earliest date: November 1, 2009
Latest date: Until class is full
Applicant's Response to Acceptance Offer – Maximum Time: Two weeks

Requests for Deferred Entrance Considered: Yes

Deposit to Hold Place in Class: Yes
Deposit (Resident): $100
Deposit (Non-resident): $100
Deposit due: With response to acceptance offer
Applied to tuition: Yes
Deposit refundable: Yes
Refundable by: May 15, 2010

Estimated number of new entrants: 138
EDP: n/a, special program: n/a

Start Month/Year: August 2010

Interview Format: Individual interviews by Admissions Committee. Regional interviews are not available.

Other Programs

PREPARATORY PROGRAMS
Postbaccalaureate Program: No
Summer Program: No

COMBINED DEGREE PROGRAMS
Baccalaureate/M.D.: Yes,
Johanna Comanzo, (518) 262-5529
combineddegreeprograms@mail.amc.edu
M.D./M.P.H.: No
M.D./M.B.A.: No
M.D./J.D.: No
M.D./Ph.D.: No
Additional Program: No

Premedical Coursework

Course	Req.	Rec.	Lab.	Hrs.	Course	Req.	Rec.	Lab.	Hrs.
Inorganic Chemistry	•		•	6	Computer Science				
Behavioral Sciences					Genetics				
Biochemistry					Humanities				
Biology	•		•	6	Organic Chemistry	•		•	6
Biology/Zoology	•		•	6	Physics	•		•	6
Calculus					Psychology				
College English					Social Sciences				
College Mathematics					Other				

Selection Factors: 2008 Accepted Applicants

Proportion of Accepted Applicants with Relevant Experience (Data Self-Reported to AMCAS®)		
Community Service/Volunteer		66%
Medically-Related Work		85%
Research		78%

Shaded bar represents school's accepted scores ranging from the 10th percentile to the 90th percentile.   School Median ●   National Median ●

Overall GPA	2.0	2.1	2.2	2.3	2.4	2.5	2.6	2.7	2.8	2.9	3.0	3.1	3.2	3.3	3.4	3.5	(3.6)	3.7	3.8	3.9	4.0
Science GPA	2.0	2.1	2.2	2.3	2.4	2.5	2.6	2.7	2.8	2.9	3.0	3.1	3.2	3.3	3.4	3.5	(3.6)	3.7	3.8	3.9	4.0

MCAT® Total Numeric Score 9 10 11 12 13 14 15 16 17 18 19 20 21 22 23 24 25 26 27 28 29 30 31 32 (33) 34 35 36 37 38 39 40 41 42 43

Writing Sample			J	K	L	M	N	O	P	(Q)	R	S	T
Verbal Reasoning	3	4	5	6	7	8	9	(10)	11	12	13	14	15
Biological Sciences	3	4	5	6	7	8	9	10	(11)	12	13	14	15
Physical Sciences	3	4	5	6	7	8	9	10	(11)	12	13	14	15

Acceptance & Matriculation Data for 2008–2009 First Year Class

	Resident	Non-resident	International	Total
Applications	1590	6684	610	8884
Interviewed	153	382	30	565
Deferred	0	3	0	3
Matriculants				
Early Assurance Program	0	0	0	0
Early Decision Program	0	0	0	0
Baccalaureate/M.D.	26	18	0	44
M.D./Ph.D.	n/a	n/a	n/a	n/a
Matriculated	58	82	3	**143**

Applications accepted from International Applicants: Yes

Specialty Choice

2004, 2005, 2006 Graduates, Specialty Choice (As reported by program directors to GME Track™)	
Anesthesiology	5%
Emergency Medicine	11%
Family Practice	8%
Internal Medicine	11%
Obstetrics/Gynecology	4%
Orthopaedic Surgery	4%
Pediatrics	14%
Psychiatry	5%
Radiology	2%
Surgery	8%

Matriculant Demographics: 2008–2009 First Year Class

Men: 75   **Women:** 68

Matriculants' Self-Reported Race/Ethnicity

Mexican American	2	Korean	3
Cuban	1	Vietnamese	4
Puerto Rican	1	Other Asian	3
Other Hispanic	1	Total Asian	49
Total Hispanic	4	Native American	2
Chinese	12	Black	2
Asian Indian	25	Native Hawaiian	0
Pakistani	2	White	86
Filipino	1	Unduplicated Number	
Japanese	2	of Matriculants	143

Science and Math Majors: 65%
Matriculants with:
Baccalaureate degree: 93%
Graduate degree(s): 28%

Financial Information

Source: 2007–2008 LCME I-B survey and 2008–2009 AAMC TSF questionnaire

	Residents	Non-residents
Total Cost of Attendance	$66,123	$66,813
Tuition and Fees	$44,623	$44,623
Other (includes living expenses)	$18,980	$19,670
Health Insurance (can be waived)	$2,520	$2,520

Average 2008 Graduate Indebtedness: $161,316
% of Enrolled Students Receiving Aid: 82%

Criminal Background Check

This medical school requires a criminal background check prior to matriculation.

Albert Einstein College of Medicine of Yeshiva University

Bronx, New York

Office of Admissions, Albert Einstein College of
Medicine of Yeshiva U Jack and Pearl Resnick Campus
1300 Morris Park Avenue
Bronx, New York 10461
T 718 430 2106   F 718 430 8840

Admissions www.aecom.yu.edu/home/admissions/
Main www.aecom.yu.edu/home/overview.asp
Financial www.aecom.yu.edu/admissions/stafford.asp
E-mail admissions@aecom.yu.edu

Private Institution

Dr. Allen M. Spiegel, Dean

Noreen Kerrigan, Assistant Dean for Student Admissions

Dr. Milton A. Gumbs, Associate Dean for Diversity Enhancement

Charles DeRubeis, Financial Aid Director

Dr. Albert Kuperman, Associate Dean for Educational Affairs

Dr. Paul Marantz, Associate Dean for Clinical Research Education

General Information

Clinical education takes place in acute care hospitals, long-term care and skilled nursing facilities, hospices, and neighborhood health centers that serve a diverse population of patients in and around the NY metropolitan area. There are many facilities devoted to biomedical research and teaching, and a new building for genetic and translational research.

Mission Statement

Einstein combines scientific excellence with the social mission to improve human health through engagement in our local, national, and global communities. Einstein's dynamic curriculum unites the biomedical sciences and hands-on clinical training with the flexibility to pursue research and meet the healthcare needs of underserved populations in the Bronx, the greater New York metropolitan area, and beyond. Einstein attracts a diverse student body and provides a collegial and collaborative environment that fosters our students' growth as future clinicians, educators, physician scientists, and leaders in the field.

Curricular Highlights

Community Service Requirement: Optional.
Research/Thesis Requirement: Required.

Years 1 and 2 are interdisciplinary courses with self-directed case-based learning in small groups, and the "Introduction to Clinical Medicine" in which students see patients three weeks after matriculation. Year 3 consists of clerkship rotations. Year 4 provides experience in ambulatory care, Neurology and a hospital-based subin-

ternship. Fourth year electives include overseas exchange programs, global health fellowships, and research. Many students do a tuition-free/fellowship supported fifth year, to conduct year-long projects, or to study for the MPH Degree. Performance is Pass/Fail in Years 1 and 2, supplemented by Honors and detailed narrative reports in Years 3 and 4.

USMLE

Step 1: Required. Students must record a passing score for promotion.
Step 2: Clinical Skills (CS): Required. Students must record a passing total score to graduate.
Step 2: Clinical Knowledge (CK): Required. Students must record a passing total score to graduate.

Selection Factors

In addition to the usual selection factors, attention is paid to community service, potential for professional achievement, motivation, and evidence of other personal qualities deemed essential for the study and practice of medicine. Einstein seeks traditional and non-traditional applicants who add diversity to the class and bring various perspectives to the study and practice of medicine. (Non-discrimination statement at: *www.aecom.yu.edu/admissions/page.aspx?id=568.*)

Financial Aid

Every attempt is made to assist students in meeting their financial obligations to the college and their essential personal needs. About 50% of students receive institutional loans and/or scholarships; about 80% qualify for outside loans and/or grants.

Information about Diversity Programs

The College of Medicine welcomes applications from students who are from groups underrepresented in medicine and/or who are economically disadvantaged. The College's Office of Diversity Enhancement provides opportunities for students to participate in special programs for high school and college students. Individual counseling is provided to students in need of long-term assistance to assure retention. The Office offers a summer research program to college students. Information on a summer research program can be obtained at (718) 430-3091.

Campus Information

Setting

Located in a residential area of the northeast Bronx, surrounded by private homes and apartment buildings and near the Westchester County border, the area combines small-town living with easy access to Manhattan. Close by are the Bronx Zoo, Botanical Gardens, Yankee Stadium, City Island (a fishing and sailing community), Orchard Beach, and the sprawling Pelham Bay Park, where there is hiking, swimming, horseback riding, golfing, and bicycling.

Enrollment

For 2008, total enrollment was: 777

Special Features

There are fellowships for projects in basic and clinical research, global health, community and population health, and ethics and humanism. There is an Alternative Pathway to the M.D.-Ph.D. after Year 2, overseas exchange programs, a Clinical Research M.D./M.S. Program, a stipend for the M.P.H. Degree (anywhere in the world), a Medical Spanish Program, and a program for Personal Wellness.

Housing

Housing at Einstein is outstanding. Apartments are large. Rents are low. Security is excellent. There are studios, one- and two-bedroom apartments with a/c, fully equipped eat-in-kitchens, and ample closet space. Parking, laundry facilities, children's playground, and a large athletic facility are on the premises. Housing is available to all Einstein students and to their spouses or committed partners.

Satellite Campuses/Facilities

Facilities include: Beth Israel Medical Center, Bronx-Lebanon Hospital, Jacobi Medical Center, North Shore/Long Island Jewish Medical Center, Montefiore and the Jack D. Weiler Hospitals, Bronx Children's Psychiatric Center, Bronx Psychiatric Center, Four Winds Hospital, Beth Abraham Hospital, Hebrew Home for the Aged, Morningside House, the Parker Jewish Geriatric Institute, the Children's Evaluation and Rehabilitation Center, the Division of Substance Abuse, and the Sound View Throgs Neck Community Mental Health Center.

Application Process and Requirements 2010–2011

Primary Application Service: AMCAS
Earliest filing date: June 1, 2009
Latest filing date: November 1, 2009

Secondary Application Required?: Yes
Sent to: All applicants
URL: www.aecom.yu.edu/admissions/admissionApplication.asp
Fee: Yes, $115
Fee waiver available: Yes
Earliest filing date: July 1, 2009
Latest filing date: March 15, 2010

MCAT® required?: Yes
Latest MCAT® considered: September 2009
Oldest MCAT® considered: 2006

Early Decision Program: School does have EDP
Applicants notified: October 1, 2009
EDP available for: Both Residents and Non-residents

Regular Acceptance Notice
Earliest date: January 15, 2010
Latest date: Until class is full
Applicant's Response to Acceptance Offer
Maximum Time: Two weeks until May 1, 2010; one week thereafter

Requests for Deferred Entrance Considered: Yes

Deposit to Hold Place in Class: Yes
Deposit (Resident): $100
Deposit (Non-resident): $100
Deposit due: With response to acceptance offer
Applied to tuition: Yes
Deposit refundable: Yes
Refundable by: May 15, 2010

Estimated number of new entrants: 183
EDP: 2, special program: 5

Start Month/Year: August 2010

Interview Format: One interview with a faculty member only. Regional interviews are not available.

Other Programs

PREPARATORY PROGRAMS
Postbaccalaureate Program: No
Summer Program: Yes, www.aecom.yu.edu/phd/index.asp?surp
Minority Student Summer Research Opportunity Program: www.aecom.yu.edu/admissions/page.aspx?ID=9564, Ms. Nilda Soto, (718) 430-3091, soto@aecom.yu.edu
Hispanic Center of Excellence Summer Undergraduate Mentorship Program: www.aecom.yu.edu/hcoe/page.aspx?id=7512&efmensel=1970_submenu_2002_btnlink, Ms. Hope Spano, (718) 430-2792, hspano@aecom.yu.edu

COMBINED DEGREE PROGRAMS
Baccalaureate/M.D.: No
M.D./M.P.H.: Yes, www.aecom.yu.edu/uploadedFiles/IPHS/IPHS_MPH_Brochure.pdf, Dr. Albert Kuperman, (718) 430-3371, kuperman@aecom.yu.edu
M.D./M.B.A.: No
M.D./J.D.: No
M.D./Ph.D.: Yes, mstp.aecom.yu.edu/
Clinical Research Program: Yes, www.aecom.yu.edu/ooe/Special_Programs/clinical_research_md_ms_program.htm

Premedical Coursework

Course	Req.	Rec.	Lab.	Hrs.	Course	Req.	Rec.	Lab.	Hrs.
Inorganic Chemistry	•		•	8	Computer Science		•		3
Behavioral Sciences					Genetics		•		3
Biochemistry		•	•	4	Humanities				
Biology		•	•	8	Organic Chemistry	•		•	8
Biology/Zoology					Physics	•		•	8
Calculus					Psychology				
College English	•			6	Social Sciences				
College Mathematics	•			6	Other				

Selection Factors: 2008 Accepted Applicants

Proportion of Accepted Applicants with Relevant Experience (Data Self-Reported to AMCAS®)		
Community Service/Volunteer		68%
Medically-Related Work		86%
Research		89%

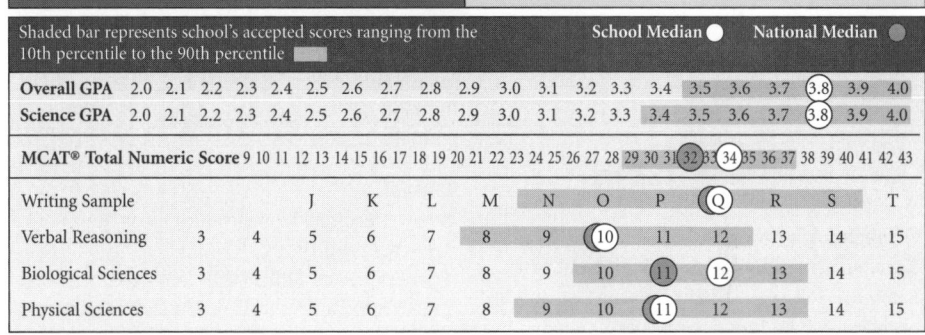

Shaded bar represents school's accepted scores ranging from the 10th percentile to the 90th percentile. School Median ● National Median ●

Overall GPA 2.0 2.1 2.2 2.3 2.4 2.5 2.6 2.7 2.8 2.9 3.0 3.1 3.2 3.3 3.4 3.5 3.6 3.7 (3.8) 3.9 4.0
Science GPA 2.0 2.1 2.2 2.3 2.4 2.5 2.6 2.7 2.8 2.9 3.0 3.1 3.2 3.3 3.4 3.5 3.6 3.7 (3.8) 3.9 4.0

MCAT® Total Numeric Score 9 10 11 12 13 14 15 16 17 18 19 20 21 22 23 24 25 26 27 28 29 30 31 (32) 33 (34) 35 36 37 38 39 40 41 42 43

Writing Sample			J	K	L	M	N	O	P	(Q)	R	S	T
Verbal Reasoning	3	4	5	6	7	8	9	(10)	11	12	13	14	15
Biological Sciences	3	4	5	6	7	8	9	10	(11)	(12)	13	14	15
Physical Sciences	3	4	5	6	7	8	9	10	(11)	12	13	14	15

Acceptance & Matriculation Data for 2008–2009 First Year Class

	Resident	Non-resident	International	Total
Applications	1518	5324	541	7883
Interviewed	360	831	45	1236
Deferred	1	0	0	1
Matriculants				
Early Assurance Program	0	0	0	0
Early Decision Program	1	1	0	2
Baccalaureate/M.D.	n/a	n/a	n/a	n/a
M.D./Ph.D.	5	10	1	16
Matriculated	77	101	4	**182**

Applications accepted from International Applicants: Yes

Specialty Choice

2004, 2005, 2006 Graduates, Specialty Choice (As reported by program directors to GME Track™)	
Anesthesiology	4%
Emergency Medicine	8%
Family Practice	2%
Internal Medicine	26%
Obstetrics/Gynecology	4%
Orthopaedic Surgery	4%
Pediatrics	18%
Psychiatry	5%
Radiology	7%
Surgery	4%

Matriculant Demographics: 2008–2009 First Year Class

Men: 85   **Women:** 97

Matriculants' Self-Reported Race/Ethnicity

Mexican American	2	Korean	10
Cuban	1	Vietnamese	1
Puerto Rican	4	Other Asian	4
Other Hispanic	9	Total Asian	45
Total Hispanic	14	Native American	2
Chinese	22	Black	11
Asian Indian	7	Native Hawaiian	0
Pakistani	1	White	113
Filipino	3	Unduplicated Number	
Japanese	1	of Matriculants	182

Science and Math Majors: 65%
Matriculants with:
Baccalaureate degree: 98%
Graduate degree(s): 9%

Financial Information
Source: 2007–2008 LCME I-B survey and 2008–2009 AAMC TSF questionnaire

	Residents	Non-residents
Total Cost of Attendance	$66,400	$66,400
Tuition and Fees	$44,780	$44,780
Other (includes living expenses)	$20,820	$20,820
Health Insurance (cannot be waived)	$0	$0

Average 2008 Graduate Indebtedness: $152,327
% of Enrolled Students Receiving Aid: 80%

Criminal Background Check

This medical school does not require a criminal background check prior to matriculation.

Columbia University
College of Physicians and Surgeons
New York, New York

Columbia University
College of Physicians and Surgeons
Admissions Office, Room 1-416
630 West 168th Street
New York, New York 10032
T 212 305 3595   F 212 305 3601

Admissions www.cumc.columbia.edu/dept/
ps/admissions
Main http://cumc.columbia.edu/dept/ps
Financial http://cumc.columbia.edu/student/finaid
E-mail psadmissions@columbia.edu

Private Institution

Dr. Lee Goldman, Dean, Executive Vice President for Health and Biomedical Sciences

Dr. Andrew G. Frantz, Associate Dean for Admissions

Dr. Hilda Y. Hutcherson, Associate Dean, Office of Diversity

Ellen Spilker, Executive Director, Office of Student Financial Planning

General Information

The College of Physicians and Surgeons originated in 1767 as the Medical Faculty of King's College and was the first school to award an earned doctor of medicine degree in the American colonies. The college is part of the Columbia University Medical Center. Clinical teaching is provided at CUMC; Roosevelt-St. Luke's Hospital Center and Harlem Hospital Center in Manhattan; Bassett Hospital in Cooperstown, NY; and Stamford Hospital in Connecticut.

Mission Statement

The mission of Columbia is to produce physicians who excel in both the science and art of medicine, and who will become leaders in their fields. It seeks to do this by providing an atmosphere that is collegial rather than competitive, and by offering students opportunities to express their interests in a wide variety of humanistic as well as scientific activities.

Curricular Highlights

Community Service Requirement: Optional.
Research/Thesis Requirement: Required.

Beginning in the fall of 2009, P&S will implement a new curriculum. Hallmarks of the new curriculum include: emphasis on collaboration and teamwork; cultivation of a commitment to life-long inquiry; a self-directed, faculty mentored, in-depth scholarly project in an area of special interest to the student; and a longitudinal approach to content that will teach basic science, professionalism, public health and clinical medicine throughout the four years. The preclinical component of the curriculum is now eighteen months long, integrating basic and clinical sciences with progressive clinical

skills building and patient responsibilities during the first semester. The major clinical year, divided into twelve week long blocks, will offer instruction in all areas of clinical medicine. Between blocks students will return to the campus for inter-sessions focused on topics relevant during clinical training. After the major clinical year students will have an additional fourteen months to explore their individual interests.

USMLE
Step 1: Required. Students must record a passing score for promotion.
Step 2: Clinical Skills (CS): Required. Students must record a passing score in each section to graduate.
Step 2: Clinical Knowledge (CK): Required. Students must record a passing score in each section to graduate.

Selection Factors
We seek applicants who have shown the greatest evidence of excellence and leadership potential in the science and art of medicine. Beyond academic ability, medicine also demands integrity, the ability to relate easily to others, and concern for their welfare. The school evaluates by several means: letters of recommendation, participation in extracurricular and summer activities, breadth of interests and undergraduate education, and the personal interview. Each year, some applicants are accepted who display extraordinary promise with regard to either the science or the art of medicine, even though they do not meet, in optimal measure, all of the criteria described above. CUMC seeks diversity of background among its applicants, geographical and otherwise; no preference is given to state of residence. Admission is possible for all qualified applicants regardless of sex, race, age, religion, sexual orientation, national origin, or handicap.

Financial Aid
Admission is not based on an applicant's ability to pay for medical school. The College makes every effort to help accepted students finance their medical education. More than $9 million in need-based grants/scholarships and low-cost loans have been awarded annually. To be considered for need-based funds, financial

data for student, spouse and parents must be provided. After "calculating" family resources, remaining need is met first with a package of low-cost loans, then with school grants and scholarships. Federal and private student loan programs are available to cover educational expenses that cannot be met by family resources. Students who do not qualify for need-based funds from the school can access Federal Stafford, Graduate PLUS, and private loans.

Information about Diversity Programs
The College has a strong commitment to increase the numbers of medical students from groups underrepresented in medicine. There is a highly diverse student body and faculty. For additional information, call (212) 305-4157.

Campus Information

Setting
Located on the Upper West Side of New York City, the CUMC is on a large multi-acre campus.

Enrollment
For 2008, total enrollment was: 651

Special Features
The New York State Psychiatric Institute building and Morgan Stanley Children's Hospital were recently opened. MS Children's Hospital is ranked among the top five pediatric hospitals in the nation. Faculty members Dr. Eric Kandel and Dr. Richard Axel are our most recent awarded Nobel Prizes in Neural Science.

Housing
On campus housing is available for single students, married couples, and domestic partnerships.

Satellite Campuses/Facilities
Students may train at some–or all–of P&S's affiliated hospitals in rural and urban settings. Columbia's Bassett track provides the first year and a half training in parallel with New York based students, and the next two and a half at a campus located in Cooperstown, NY. This program features education in an integrated health care system serving an extensive rural community.

Application Process and Requirements 2010–2011

Primary Application Service: AMCAS
Earliest filing date: June 1, 2009
Latest filing date: October 15, 2009

Secondary Application Required?: Yes
Sent to: All applicants
URL: https://app.applyyourself.com/?id=COL-MED
Fee: Yes, $85
Fee waiver available: Yes
Earliest filing date: June 1, 2009
Latest filing date: November 15, 2009

MCAT® required?: Yes
Latest MCAT® considered: September 2009
Oldest MCAT® considered: March 2007

Early Decision Program: School does not have EDP
Applicants notified: n/a
EDP available for: n/a

Regular Acceptance Notice
Earliest date: March 1, 2010
Latest date: Varies
**Applicant's Response to Acceptance
Offer – Maximum Time:** Three weeks

**Requests for Deferred
Entrance Considered:** Yes

Deposit to Hold Place in Class: No
Deposit (Resident): n/a
Deposit (Non-resident): n/a
Deposit due: n/a
Applied to tuition: n/a
Deposit refundable: n/a
Refundable by: n/a

Estimated number of new entrants: 153
EDP: n/a, special program: n/a

Start Month/Year: August 2010

Interview Format: Monday-Friday, September through February. Regional interviews are very rarely available.

Other Programs

PREPARATORY PROGRAMS
Postbaccalaureate Program: Yes,
www.columbia.edu/cu/gs/postbacc,
(212) 854-2881, pmaofficers@columbia.edu
Summer Program: Yes,
www.oda-ps.cumc.columbia.edu

COMBINED DEGREE PROGRAMS
Baccalaureate/M.D.: No
M.D./M.P.H.: Yes, www.mailman.hs.columbia.edu,
(212) 305-3927
M.D./M.P.H.: Yes, Betsy Asher, (202) 305-3927,
ba2239@columbia.edu
M.D./M.B.A.: Yes, http://www4.gsb.columbia.edu/mba,
Susan Sullivan, (212) 854-4557, sms12@columbia.edu
M.D./J.D.: No
M.D./Ph.D.: Yes, http://mdphd.columbia.edu,
Patrice Spitalnik, (212) 342-5653,
M.D.-Ph.D.@columbia.edu

Premedical Coursework

Course	Req.	Rec.	Lab.	Sems.
Inorganic Chemistry	•		•	2
Behavioral Sciences				
Biochemistry				
Biology	•		•	2
Biology/Zoology				
Calculus				
College English	•			2
College Mathematics				

Course	Req.	Rec.	Lab.	Sems.
Computer Science				
Genetics				
Humanities				
Organic Chemistry	•		•	2
Physics	•			2
Psychology				
Social Sciences				
Other				

Selection Factors: 2008 Accepted Applicants

Proportion of Accepted Applicants with Relevant Experience (Data Self-Reported to AMCAS®)		
Community Service/Volunteer		65%
Medically-Related Work		87%
Research		88%

Shaded bar represents school's accepted scores ranging from the 10th percentile to the 90th percentile ▬   School Median ⚪   National Median ⚪

Overall GPA	2.0	2.1	2.2	2.3	2.4	2.5	2.6	2.7	2.8	2.9	3.0	3.1	3.2	3.3	3.4	3.5	3.6	3.7	(3.8)	3.9	4.0
Science GPA	2.0	2.1	2.2	2.3	2.4	2.5	2.6	2.7	2.8	2.9	3.0	3.1	3.2	3.3	3.4	3.5	3.6	3.7	(3.8)	3.9	4.0

MCAT® Total Numeric Score	9	10	11	12	13	14	15	16	17	18	19	20	21	22	23	24	25	26	27	28	29	30	31	(32)	33	34	35	(36)	37	38	39	40	41	42	43

Writing Sample			J	K	L	M	N	O	P	(Q)	R	S	T
Verbal Reasoning	3	4	5	6	7	8	9	(10)	(11)	12	13	14	15
Biological Sciences	3	4	5	6	7	8	9	10	(11)	12	(13)	14	15
Physical Sciences	3	4	5	6	7	8	9	10	(11)	12	(13)	14	15

Acceptance & Matriculation Data for 2008–2009 First Year Class

	Resident	Non-resident	International	Total
Applications	1083	5390	453	6926
Interviewed	114	694	293	1101
Deferred	1	4	0	5
Matriculants				
Early Assurance Program	0	0	0	0
Early Decision Program	0	0	0	0
Baccalaureate/M.D.	n/a	n/a	n/a	n/a
M.D./Ph.D.	3	10	0	13
Matriculated	42	103	8	**153**

Applications accepted from International Applicants: Yes

Matriculant Demographics: 2008–2009 First Year Class

Men: 77   **Women:** 76

Matriculants' Self-Reported Race/Ethnicity

Mexican American	3	**Korean**	2
Cuban	1	**Vietnamese**	1
Puerto Rican	1	**Other Asian**	4
Other Hispanic	3	**Total Asian**	26
Total Hispanic	7	**Native American**	0
Chinese	14	**Black**	25
Asian Indian	5	**Native Hawaiian**	0
Pakistani	0	**White**	88
Filipino	1	**Unduplicated Number**	
Japanese	0	**of Matriculants**	153

Science and Math Majors: 65%
Matriculants with:
   Baccalaureate degree: 100%
   Graduate degree(s): 4%

Specialty Choice

2004, 2005, 2006 Graduates, Specialty Choice (As reported by program directors to GME Track™)	
Anesthesiology	6%
Emergency Medicine	6%
Family Practice	1%
Internal Medicine	19%
Obstetrics/Gynecology	4%
Orthopaedic Surgery	8%
Pediatrics	10%
Psychiatry	7%
Radiology	4%
Surgery	6%

Financial Information

Source: 2007–2008 LCME I-B survey and 2008–2009 AAMC TSF questionnaire

	Residents	Non-residents
Total Cost of Attendance	$64,290	$64,290
Tuition and Fees	$44,490	$44,490
Other (includes living expenses)	$17,198	$17,198
Health Insurance (can be waived)	$2,602	$2,602

Average 2008 Graduate Indebtedness: $113,146
% of Enrolled Students Receiving Aid: 83%

Criminal Background Check

This medical school does not require a criminal background check prior to matriculation.

Weill Cornell Medical College
New York, New York

Office of Admissions
Weill Cornell Medical College
445 East 69th Street
New York, New York 10021
T 212 746 1067   F 212 746 8052

Admissions www.med.cornell.edu/education/
admissions
Main www.med.cornell.edu
Financial www.med.cornell.edu/education/
admissions/app_fin_aid.html
E-mail wcmc-admissions@med.cornell.edu

Private Institution

Dr. Antonio M. Gotto, Jr., Dean

*Dr. Charles L. Bardes, Associate Dean
and Chair, Committee on Admissions*

*Dr. Carlyle H. Miller, Associate Dean
for Student Affairs*

Gladys Laden, Director of Financial Aid

Liliana Montano, Assistant Dean of Admissions

General Information
Founded in 1898 as Cornell University Medical College, the school's name was changed to the Joan and Sanford I. Weill Medical College of Cornell University in 1998. The medical school campus embraces the New York-Presbyterian Hospital, Memorial Sloan-Kettering Cancer Center, Rockefeller University, and the Hospital for Special Surgery. In addition, students train in clinical care throughout an affiliated network, including public, private, research, tertiary care, and community hospitals, as well as primary care sites.

Mission Statement
WMC is committed to excellence in research, teaching, patient care, and the advancement of the art and science of medicine. To this end, our mission is to provide the finest education possible for medical students, to provide superior continuing medical education for the life-long education of physicians throughout their careers, to conduct research at the cutting edge of knowledge, to improve the health care of the nation and world both now and for further generations, and to provide the highest level of clinical care for the communities we serve.

Curricular Highlights
Community Service Requirement: Optional.
Special degree program: M.D. with Honors in Service
Research/Thesis Requirement: Optional.
Special degree program: M.D. with Honors in Research

The first two years center on Problem-Based Learning (PBL), in which students learn by actively solving problems with the faculty in small group seminars. Lectures, anatomic dis-

section, experimental laboratories and journal clubs augment the learning experience. Basic science courses are integrated and multidisciplinary. Students begin to work with patients immediately during the three-year sequence of Medicine, Patients, and Society, which focuses on clinical skills, the doctor-patient relationship, health care systems, and ultimately ethics and end-of-life care. The core clinical clerkships include Medicine, Neurology, Obstetrics and Gynecology, Pediatrics, Primary Care, Psychiatry, Public Health, and Surgery. Year 4 provides the major time block for electives in clinical medicine, research, and international health experiences, as well as a return to advanced biomedical science.

USMLE
Step 1: Optional.
Step 2: Clinical Skills (CS): Optional.
Step 2: Clinical Knowledge (CK): Optional.

Selection Factors
WMC considers each applicant on an individual basis and welcomes those with backgrounds in the basic sciences, social sciences, and liberal arts. We encourage applicants to sample a broad range of academic disciplines and to explore one or more areas in depth. Participation in other activities should demonstrate commitment and initiative. We encourage applicants to explore medicine via research, clinical work, and volunteer service. We seek students who demonstrate emotional maturity, personal depth, commitment to others' well-being, and ethical and moral integrity. We seek to build a diverse class and emphasize diversity in all its dimensions, including race, ethnicity, educational background, personal experiences, and fields of interest. Typically a third of our entering students majored in liberal arts, and a quarter are 25 years of age or older.

Financial Aid
Admissions decisions are made without regard to applicants' financial status. All financial aid is based on need. Some 85% of the class receives financial aid, and about 50% receives grants from the College. Housing is guaranteed for all students and priced well below market rate. Financial support for community service, summer research, and international electives is

available for all students. The application fee will be waived if it represents a financial hardship to the applicant. Students who are not citizens or permanent residents of the United States are not eligible for Weill Cornell financial aid.

Information about Diversity Programs
Cornell University has been deeply committed to diversity from its very founding, and the Medical College upholds this principle. WMC's educational mission is dedicated to the inclusion of students from diverse ethnic, racial, social, economic, and educational backgrounds. Special summer research programs are available for college undergraduates who have a major interest in the medical problems of the underserved. Further information is available at *www.med. cornell.education/student/min_aff.html*.

Campus Information

Setting
Weill Cornell is located in the heart of New York City in the Upper East Side of Manhattan, a lovely residential neighborhood. Many of the city's cultural resources are a short walk away, including the Metropolitan Museum of Art, The Museum of Modern Art, Carnegie Hall, Central Park, among others.

Enrollment
For 2008, total enrollment was: 410

Special Features
World medicine is a major emphasis. Most students participate in international electives, spanning some eighty countries on six continents, with financial and logisitical support from the College.

Housing
Modern, reduced-cost on-campus housing is guaranteed for all students.

Satellite Campuses/Facilities
Students rotate throughout New York City at public, private, community, research, and tertiary care hospitals, as well as primary care sites.

Application Process and Requirements 2010–2011

Primary Application Service: AMCAS
Earliest filing date: June 2009
Latest filing date: October 15, 2009

Secondary Application Required?: Yes
Sent to: All applicants
URL: Sent to verified applicants only.
Contact: Office of Admissions
(212) 746-1067, wcmc-admissions@med.cornell.edu
Fee: Yes, $75
Fee waiver available: Yes
Earliest filing date: Depends on release of AMCAS application.
Latest filing date: November 15, 2009

MCAT® required?: Yes
Latest MCAT® considered: September 2009
Oldest MCAT® considered: September 2006

Early Decision Program: School does have EDP
Applicants notified: October 1, 2009
EDP available for: Both Residents and Non-residents

Regular Acceptance Notice
Earliest date: December 2009
Latest date: Until class is full
Applicant's Response to Acceptance Offer – Maximum Time: Two weeks

Requests for Deferred Entrance Considered: Yes

Deposit to Hold Place in Class: Yes
Deposit (Resident): $100
Deposit (Non-resident): $100
Deposit due: May 15, 2010
Applied to tuition: Yes
Deposit refundable: Yes
Refundable by: May 15, 2010

Estimated number of new entrants: 101
EDP: 1, special program: 3

Start Month/Year: August 2010

Interview Format: Two individual interviews with admissions committee members. No regional interviews.

Other Programs

PREPARATORY PROGRAMS
Postbaccalaureate Program: No
Summer Program: Yes,
www.med.cornell.edu/education/student/min_sum_pro.html, Elizabeth Wilson-Anstey, (212) 746-1058, eaanstey@med.cornell.edu

COMBINED DEGREE PROGRAMS
Baccalaureate/M.D.: No
M.D./M.P.H.: No
M.D./M.B.A.: Yes, www.med.cornell.edu/education
M.D./J.D.: No
M.D./Ph.D.: Yes, www.med.cornell.edu/mdphd, Ruth Gotian, (212) 746-6023, mdphd@med.cornell.edu

Premedical Coursework

Course	Req.	Rec.	Lab.	Sems.	Course	Req.	Rec.	Lab.	Sems.
Inorganic Chemistry	•		•	2	Genetics				
Behavioral Sciences					Humanities				
Biochemistry					Organic Chemistry	•		•	2
Biology	•		•	2	Physics	•		•	2
Biology/Zoology					Psychology				
Calculus		•		1	Social Sciences				
College English	•			2	Statistics		•		1
College Mathematics					Foreign Language		•		
Computer Science					Other				

Selection Factors: 2008 Accepted Applicants

Proportion of Accepted Applicants with Relevant Experience (Data Self-Reported to AMCAS)		
Community Service/Volunteer	70%
Medically-Related Work	87%
Research	94%

Shaded bar represents school's accepted scores ranging from the 10th percentile to the 90th percentile   School Median ●   National Median ●

Overall GPA	2.0	2.1	2.2	2.3	2.4	2.5	2.6	2.7	2.8	2.9	3.0	3.1	3.2	3.3	3.4	3.5	3.6	3.7	3.8	(3.9)	4.0
Science GPA	2.0	2.1	2.2	2.3	2.4	2.5	2.6	2.7	2.8	2.9	3.0	3.1	3.2	3.3	3.4	3.5	3.6	3.7	3.8	(3.9)	4.0

MCAT® Total Numeric Score 9 10 11 12 13 14 15 16 17 18 19 20 21 22 23 24 25 26 27 28 29 30 31 (32)33 34 35 (36)37 38 39 40 41 42 43

Writing Sample			J	K	L	M	N	O	P	(Q)	R	S	T
Verbal Reasoning	3	4	5	6	7	8	9	(10)	(11)	12	13	14	15
Biological Sciences	3	4	5	6	7	8	9	10	(11)	(12)	13	14	15
Physical Sciences	3	4	5	6	7	8	9	10	(11)	(12)	13	14	15

Acceptance & Matriculation Data for 2008–2009 First Year Class

	Resident	Non-resident	International	Total
Applications	1105	4383	339	5827
Interviewed	133	514	21	668
Deferred	2	7	1	10
Matriculants				
Early Assurance Program	n/a	n/a	n/a	n/a
Early Decision Program	0	1	0	1
Baccalaureate/M.D.	n/a	n/a	n/a	n/a
M.D./Ph.D.	2	10	0	12
Matriculated	31	69	1	**101**

Applications accepted from International Applicants: Yes

Specialty Choice

2004, 2005, 2006 Graduates, Specialty Choice (As reported by program directors to GME Track™)	
Anesthesiology	7%
Emergency Medicine	7%
Family Practice	1%
Internal Medicine	17%
Obstetrics/Gynecology	4%
Orthopaedic Surgery	2%
Pediatrics	12%
Psychiatry	8%
Radiology	5%
Surgery	10%

Matriculant Demographics: 2008–2009 First Year Class

Men: 54   **Women:** 47

Matriculants' Self-Reported Race/Ethnicity

Mexican American	3	**Korean**	5
Cuban	0	**Vietnamese**	2
Puerto Rican	1	**Other Asian**	1
Other Hispanic	9	**Total Asian**	15
Total Hispanic	12	**Native American**	1
Chinese	2	**Black**	8
Asian Indian	3	**Native Hawaiian**	0
Pakistani	0	**White**	72
Filipino	0	**Unduplicated Number**	
Japanese	2	**of Matriculants**	101

Science and Math Majors: 50%
Matriculants with:
Baccalaureate degree: 99%
Graduate degree(s): 11%

Financial Information

Source: 2007–2008 LCME I-B survey and 2008–2009 AAMC TSF questionnaire

	Residents	Non-residents
Total Cost of Attendance	$ 66,764	$ 66,764
Tuition and Fees	$ 44,465	$ 44,465
Other (includes living expenses)	$ 18,346	$ 18,346
Health Insurance (can be waived)	$ 3,953	$ 3,953

Average 2008 Graduate Indebtedness: $111,920
% of Enrolled Students Receiving Aid: 89%

Criminal Background Check

This medical school does not require a criminal background check prior to matriculation.

Mount Sinai School of Medicine of New York University

New York, New York

Office of Admissions,
Mount Sinai School of Medicine
Annenberg Building, Room 5-04
One Gustave L. Levy Place – Box 1002
New York, New York 10029-6574
T 212 241 6696   **F** 212 828 4135

Admissions www.mssm.edu/bulletin/admissions/
admissions.htm
Main www.mssm.edu
Financial www.mountsinai.org/Education/School
%20of%20Medicine/Degrees%20and%20Programs/
MD%20Program/Financial%20Aid
E-mail admissions@mssm.edu

Private Institution

Dr. Dennis Charney, Dean

Dr. Alan C. Carver, Assistant Dean for Admissions

Dr. Gary C. Butts, Associate Dean for Multicultural and Community Affairs

Dale Fuller, Director of Student Financial Services

General Information

Mount Sinai School of Medicine is privately endowed and affiliated with New York University. The medical center campus includes The Mount Sinai Hospital, research and service laboratories, teaching facilities, and the Graduate School of Biological Sciences. The school recently completed Phase II/IV of the total renovation of its educational space, and will soon start construction that will expand its research space by approximately thirty percent. Additional clinical training sites extend throughout New York City, New Jersey, Westchester County, and Long Island.

Mission Statement

The school is committed to serving science and society through outstanding research, education, patient care, and community service. We strive to develop new approaches to teaching, translate scientific discoveries into improvements in patient care, and identify new ways to enhance the health and educational opportunities of the communities we serve.

Curricular Highlights

Community Service Requirement: Optional.
Research/Thesis Requirement: Optional.

Mount Sinai School of Medicine's curriculum is designed to teach a core knowledge of the biological basis of health and disease, skills in critical thinking, life-long learning skills, professional and humanistic attitudes, a scientific approach to medicine, and an appreciation of the physician's obligations to society and the community. The curriculum emphasizes the interdisciplinary nature of the basic and clinical sciences; it utilizes lectures and small group, case-based seminars and laboratory exercises. Courses are graded pass/fail during the first two years, and honors/high pass/pass/fail in the last two years.

USMLE

Step 1: Required. Students must record a passing score for promotion.
Step 2: Clinical Skills (CS): Required. Students must record a passing total score to graduate.
Step 2: Clinical Knowledge (CK): Required. Students must record a passing total score to graduate.

Selection Factors

Excellence in scholarship, personal maturity, integrity, intellectual creativity, and motivation for medicine are important factors. The interview, recommendations, and MCAT scores are criteria for evaluation. All applicants are considered, regardless of race, sex, color, creed, age, national origin, handicap, veteran status, marital status, or sexual orientation.

Financial Aid

Applications for financial aid are treated confidentially, and awards are made by a faculty committee on financial aid. Each applicant is considered on an individual basis so that the school can provide maximal support for those who most need it. Financial aid may be offered in the form of a scholarship, a loan, or both, in accordance with the requirements of the individual situation and the availability of funds. Students who are not citizens or permanent residents of the United States are not eligible for financial assistance.

Information about Diversity Programs

Strongly motivated students from groups underrepresented in medicine are actively sought and encouraged to apply. A pre-entrance summer enrichment program is available for students who are accepted to the first-year class. Tutorial assistance is available for all students. The school's Center for Multicultural and Community Affairs provides leadership and coordination for minority affairs activities, multicultural diversity program activities, a variety of enrichment programs, and advisory and career counseling services.

Campus Information

Setting

The campus sits on the border between the Upper East Side of Manhattan and the thriving and vibrant community of East Harlem. Student housing is located across the street from the campus, as is Central Park. The Museum Mile, restaurants, shopping, and public transportation are all convenient to the campus.

Enrollment

For 2008, total enrollment was: 506

Special Features

The hospital and the school work together to remain at the cutting-edge of modern medicine, and to maintain regional and national leadership. Mount Sinai was the first U.S. medical school to establish academic Departments of Geriatrics and Environmental and Occupational Medicine, and is one of the few schools of medicine in the United States to have a Department of Health Policy. MD, M.D./Ph.D., M.D./M.P.H. and M.D./M.B.A. degrees are offered. There is extensive online support for the curriculum. Student feedback is highly valued. Special features include: a standardized patient facility, human simulator center, the Global Health Center, the Office of Research Opportunities, and the Center for Multicultural and Community Affairs.

Housing

Single students are guaranteed housing in Aron Hall, located across the street from the school. Couples housing is located within easy walking distance and is on a space available basis.

Satellite Campuses/Facilities

The main teaching site is the Mount Sinai Hospital, located on the main campus. Students also rotate to inpatient and ambulatory sites within a teaching consortium, among the largest in the country, which consists of outstanding public and private institutions in New York City and the suburbs of New Jersey.

Application Process and Requirements 2010–2011

Primary Application Service: AMCAS
Earliest filing date: June 1, 2009
Latest filing date: November 1, 2009

Secondary Application Required?: Yes
Sent to: All applicants
Contact: (212) 241-6996, admissions@mssm.edu
Fee: Yes, $105
Fee waiver available: Yes
Earliest filing date: July 15, 2009
Latest filing date: December 15, 2009

MCAT® required?: Yes
Latest MCAT® considered: September 2009
Oldest MCAT® considered: April 2007

Early Decision Program: School does have EDP
Applicants notified: October 1, 2009
EDP available for: Both Residents and Non-residents

Regular Acceptance Notice
Earliest date: November 1, 2009
Latest date: Until class is full
Applicant's Response to Acceptance Offer – Maximum Time: Two weeks

Requests for Deferred Entrance Considered: Yes

Deposit to Hold Place in Class: No
Deposit (Resident): n/a
Deposit (Non-resident): n/a
Deposit due: n/a
Applied to tuition: n/a
Deposit refundable: n/a
Refundable by: n/a

Estimated number of new entrants: 128
EDP: 1, special program: 12

Start Month/Year: August 12, 2010

Interview Format: Two thirty-minute interviews. Regional interviews are not available.

Other Programs

PREPARATORY PROGRAMS
Postbaccalaureate Program: Yes
(212) 241-6546, www.mountsinai.org/
Education/School%20of%20Medicine/Degrees%20
and%20Programs/Post-Baccalaureate%20Research
%20Education%20Program%20for%20Medicine
Summer Program: Yes
grads@mssm.edu, (212) 241-6546

COMBINED DEGREE PROGRAMS
Baccalaureate/M.D.: No
M.D./M.P.H.: Yes, (212) 241-7941
www.mssm.edu/cpm/mph/
M.D./M.B.A.: Yes, (212) 241-2260
www.mssm.edu/medschool/md_mba/
ray.cornbill@mssm.edu
M.D./J.D.: No
M.D./Ph.D.: Yes, mstp@mssm.edu
www.mssm.edu/gradschool/mstp/

Premedical Coursework

Course	Req.	Rec.	Lab.	Sems.
Inorganic Chemistry	•	•		2
Behavioral Sciences				
Biochemistry		•		
Biology	•		•	2
Biology/Zoology				
Calculus				
College English	•			2
College Mathematics	•			2

Course	Req.	Rec.	Lab.	Sems.
Computer Science				
Genetics		•		
Humanities				
Organic Chemistry	•		•	2
Physics	•			2
Psychology				
Social Sciences				
Other				

Selection Factors: 2008 Accepted Applicants

Proportion of Accepted Applicants with Relevant Experience (Data Self-Reported to AMCAS®)		
Community Service/Volunteer		71%
Medically-Related Work		85%
Research		85%

Shaded bar represents school's accepted scores ranging from the 10th percentile to the 90th percentile. School Median ● National Median ●

Overall GPA	2.0	2.1	2.2	2.3	2.4	2.5	2.6	2.7	2.8	2.9	3.0	3.1	3.2	3.3	3.4	3.5	3.6	3.7	(3.8)	3.9	4.0
Science GPA	2.0	2.1	2.2	2.3	2.4	2.5	2.6	2.7	2.8	2.9	3.0	3.1	3.2	3.3	3.4	3.5	3.6	(3.7)	3.8	3.9	4.0

MCAT® Total Numeric Score 9 10 11 12 13 14 15 16 17 18 19 20 21 22 23 24 25 26 27 28 29 30 31 (32) 33 34 35 (36) 37 38 39 40 41 42 43

Writing Sample				J	K	L	M	N	O	P	(Q)	R	S	T
Verbal Reasoning	3	4	5	6	7	8	9	(10)	(11)	12	13	14	15
Biological Sciences	3	4	5	6	7	8	9	10	(11)	(12)	13	14	15
Physical Sciences	3	4	5	6	7	8	9	10	(11)	(12)	13	14	15

Acceptance & Matriculation Data for 2008–2009 First Year Class

	Resident	Non-resident	International	Total
Applications	1467	4818	445	6730
Interviewed	257	563	27	847
Deferred	1	2	2	5
Matriculants				
Early Assurance Program	12	14	0	26
Early Decision Program	0	0	0	0
Baccalaureate/M.D.	n/a	n/a	n/a	n/a
M.D./Ph.D.	5	7	0	12
Matriculated	54	82	4	**140**

Applications accepted from International Applicants: Yes

Matriculant Demographics: 2008–2009 First Year Class

Men: 72   **Women:** 68

Matriculants' Self-Reported Race/Ethnicity

Mexican American	2	Korean	5
Cuban	5	Vietnamese	1
Puerto Rican	2	Other Asian	4
Other Hispanic	7	Total Asian	34
Total Hispanic	16	Native American	0
Chinese	15	Black	10
Asian Indian	9	Native Hawaiian	0
Pakistani	1	White	82
Filipino	0	Unduplicated Number	
Japanese	0	of Matriculants	140

Science and Math Majors: 45%
Matriculants with:
 Baccalaureate degree: 100%
 Graduate degree(s): 11%

Specialty Choice

2004, 2005, 2006 Graduates, Specialty Choice (As reported by program directors to GME Track™)	
Anesthesiology	7%
Emergency Medicine	4%
Family Practice	2%
Internal Medicine	25%
Obstetrics/Gynecology	3%
Orthopaedic Surgery	2%
Pediatrics	10%
Psychiatry	9%
Radiology	5%
Surgery	8%

Financial Information

Source: 2007–2008 LCME I-B survey and 2008–2009 AAMC TSF questionnaire

	Residents	Non-residents
Total Cost of Attendance	$57,990	$57,990
Tuition and Fees	$38,850	$38,850
Other (includes living expenses)	$18,380	$18,380
Health Insurance (can be waived)	$2,760	$2,760

Average 2008 Graduate Indebtedness: $133,186
% of Enrolled Students Receiving Aid: 71%

Criminal Background Check

This medical school requires a criminal background check prior to matriculation.

New York Medical College
Valhalla, New York

Office of Admissions
Administration Building
New York Medical College
Valhalla, New York 10595
T 914 594 4507 **F** 914 594 4976

Admissions www.nymc.edu/admit/medical/info/index.asp
Main www.nymc.edu
Financial www.nymc.edu/studentlife/sfs.htm
E-mail mdadmit@nymc.edu

Private Institution

Dr. Ralph A. O'Connell, Provost and Dean

Dr. Fern R. Juster, Associate Dean and Chair, Committee on Admissions

Dr. Gladys M. Ayala, Senior Associate Dean for Student Affairs

Anthony M. Sozzo IV, Associate Dean and Director of Student Financial Planning

Dr. Laurie Sullivan, Assistant Dean of Admissions

General Information
Founded in 1860, New York Medical College is located in suburban Westchester County, 25 miles from New York City. The university educates students for careers in medicine, biomedical science, and the health professions through its School of Medicine, Graduate School of Basic Medical Sciences, and School of Public Health.

Mission Statement
New York Medical College is a health sciences university whose purpose is to educate physicians, scientists, public health specialists, and other healthcare professionals, and to conduct biomedical and population-based research. Through its faculty and affiliated clinical partners, the College provides service to its community in an atmosphere of excellence, scholarship and professionalism. New York Medical College believes that the rich diversity of its student body and faculty is important to its mission of educating outstanding health care professionals for the multicultural world of the 21st century.

Curricular Highlights
Community Service Requirement: Optional.
Research/Thesis Requirement: Optional.

NYMC's goal is to provide a general professional education that prepares students for all career options in medicine. There is emphasis on critical thinking, evidence-based decision making, and cultural humility throughout the curriculum. Clinical exposure begins in the first year with a longitudinal assignment to a primary care physician where students focus on communication skills, history-taking, and preventive

medicine. In addition to traditional lectures and laboratory exercises, basic science courses utilize self directed study, small group discussion, computer assisted instruction, and problem-based learning. Clerkships in seven disciplines at a wide variety of hospitals and community-based clinical settings comprise the third year. In the required fourth year sub-internships, students are expected to function at the level of a beginning resident in required rotations and electives at medical institutions around the country and the world. Highlights of the curriculum include an optional Summer Research Fellowship Program between the first and second years; exposure to medical informatics; an integrated curriculum in biomedical ethics; rigorous sub-internships in Medicine or Pediatrics; palliative care components in the medicine clerkship; and a required fourth year rotation in Geriatric Medicine or Chronic Care Pediatrics.

USMLE
Step 1: Required. Students must record a passing score for promotion.
Step 2: Clinical Skills (CS): Required. Students must only record a score.
Step 2: Clinical Knowledge (CK): Required. Students must record a passing total score to graduate.

Selection Factors
The Admissions Committee selects students after considering factors of intellect, character, and personality pointing toward their ability to become informed and caring physicians. A history of academic excellence is essential. Undergraduate major is not a factor in selection. Clear evidence of a strong motivation toward medicine and a sense of dedication to the service of others is encouraged. Qualities of character and personality are evaluated from letters of evaluation, personal statements, and the interview. The school does not deny admission to any applicant on the basis of any legally prohibited discrimination involving, but not limited to, such factors as race, color, creed, religion, national or ethnic origin, age, sex, sexual orientation, or disability.

Financial Aid
Financial aid is awarded on the basis of need; scholarships, based on need, are available to

entering students. The college provides debt management and loan counseling services.

Information about Diversity Programs
New York Medical College seeks to admit a diverse class, including diversity of gender, race, ethnicity, cultural and economic background, and life experience. A diverse student body provides a valuable educational experience that prepares medical students for the real world of medical practice in a multicultural society.

Campus Information

Setting
NYMC, Westchester Medical Center, and Maria Fareri Children's Hospital/Regional Trauma Center are located on a 22-acre suburban campus. Affiliated hospitals and clinical sites are located in NYC and lower Hudson Valley.

Enrollment
For 2008, total enrollment was: 776

Special Features
New York Medical College is the only academic biomedical research institution between New York City and Albany, with $41 million in sponsored programs of research, training, and service.

Housing
On-campus housing is available on the main campus in Valhalla. Most first and second year students live on campus. Half of third and fourth year students live in Manhattan. The Housing Office maintains a list of off-campus housing opportunities.

Satellite Campuses/Facilities
New York Medical College's wide range of affiliated hospitals, including large urban medical centers, small suburban hospitals, and technologically advanced regional tertiary care facilities, provide extensive resources and educational opportunities.

Application Process and Requirements 2010–2011

Primary Application Service: AMCAS
Earliest filing date: June 1, 2009
Latest filing date: December 15, 2009

Secondary Application Required?: Yes
Sent to: All applicants
URL: www.nymc.edu/medadmission/Instructions.html
Fee: Yes, $100
Fee waiver available: Yes
Earliest filing date: July 1, 2009
Latest filing date: January 31, 2010

MCAT® required?: Yes
Latest MCAT® considered: September 2009
Oldest MCAT® considered: April 2007

Early Decision Program: School does have EDP
Applicants notified: October 1, 2009
EDP available for: Both Residents and Non-residents

Regular Acceptance Notice
Earliest date: December 7, 2009
Latest date: Until class is full
Applicant's Response to Acceptance Offer – Maximum Time: Two weeks

Requests for Deferred Entrance Considered: Yes

Deposit to Hold Place in Class: Yes
Deposit (Resident): $100
Deposit (Non-resident): $100
Deposit due: Within two weeks of acceptance
Applied to tuition: Yes
Deposit refundable: Yes
Refundable by: May 15, 2010

Estimated number of new entrants: 190
EDP: 2, special program: n/a

Start Month/Year: August 2010

Interview Format: One-on-one blind and minimally structured interviews. Regional interviews are not available.

Other Programs

PREPARATORY PROGRAMS
Postbaccalaureate Program: Yes, www.nymc.edu/gsbms/interdisciplinary.asp
Summer Program: No

COMBINED DEGREE PROGRAMS
Baccalaureate/M.D.: No
M.D./M.P.H.: Yes, www.nymc.edu/hs/department_programs.htm#M.D./M.P.H
M.D./M.B.A.: No
M.D./J.D.: No
M.D./Ph.D.: Yes, www.nymc.edu/gsbms/md-phd-program.asp

Premedical Coursework

Course	Req.	Rec.	Lab.	Sems.	Course	Req.	Rec.	Lab.	Sems.
Inorganic Chemistry	•		•	2	Computer Science				
Behavioral Sciences					Genetics				
Biochemistry		•			Humanities				
Biology	•		•	2	Organic Chemistry	•		•	2
Biology/Zoology					Physics	•		•	2
Calculus					Psychology				
College English	•			2	Social Sciences				
College Mathematics					Other				

Selection Factors: 2008 Accepted Applicants

Proportion of Accepted Applicants with Relevant Experience (Data Self-Reported to AMCAS)		
Community Service/Volunteer		66%
Medically-Related Work		92%
Research		86%

Shaded bar represents school's accepted scores ranging from the 10th percentile to the 90th percentile | School Median ● | National Median ●

| Overall GPA | 2.0 2.1 2.2 2.3 2.4 2.5 2.6 2.7 2.8 2.9 3.0 3.1 3.2 3.3 3.4 3.5 (3.6) 3.7 3.8 3.9 4.0 |
| Science GPA | 2.0 2.1 2.2 2.3 2.4 2.5 2.6 2.7 2.8 2.9 3.0 3.1 3.2 3.3 3.4 (3.5) 3.6 3.7 3.8 3.9 4.0 |

MCAT® Total Numeric Score 9 10 11 12 13 14 15 16 17 18 19 20 21 22 23 24 25 26 27 28 29 30 (31) 32 33 34 35 36 37 38 39 40 41 42 43

Writing Sample				J	K	L	M	N	O	P	(Q)	R	S	T
Verbal Reasoning	3	4	5	6	7	8	9	(10)	11	12	13	14	15
Biological Sciences	3	4	5	6	7	8	9	10	(11)	12	13	14	15
Physical Sciences	3	4	5	6	7	8	9	(10)	(11)	12	13	14	15

Acceptance & Matriculation Data for 2008–2009 First Year Class

	Resident	Non-resident	International	Total
Applications	1849	8697	549	11095
Interviewed	333	1029	20	1382
Deferred	3	6	0	9
Matriculants				
Early Assurance Program	n/a	n/a	n/a	0
Early Decision Program	0	1	0	1
Baccalaureate/M.D.	n/a	n/a	n/a	0
M.D./Ph.D.	n/a	n/a	n/a	0
Matriculated	48	137	2	**187**

Applications accepted from International Applicants: Yes

Matriculant Demographics: 2008–2009 First Year Class

Men: 92   **Women:** 95

Matriculants' Self-Reported Race/Ethnicity

Mexican American	1	Korean	8
Cuban	3	Vietnamese	4
Puerto Rican	4	Other Asian	7
Other Hispanic	2	Total Asian	57
Total Hispanic	9	Native American	0
Chinese	22	Black	10
Asian Indian	15	Native Hawaiian	2
Pakistani	2	White	110
Filipino	1	Unduplicated Number	
Japanese	1	of Matriculants	187

Science and Math Majors: 66%
Matriculants with:
     Baccalaureate degree: 99%
     Graduate degree(s): 12%

Specialty Choice

2004, 2005, 2006 Graduates, Specialty Choice (As reported by program directors to GME Track™)	
Anesthesiology	9%
Emergency Medicine	3%
Family Practice	3%
Internal Medicine	25%
Obstetrics/Gynecology	4%
Orthopaedic Surgery	4%
Pediatrics	13%
Psychiatry	3%
Radiology	10%
Surgery	7%

Financial Information

Source: 2007–2008 LCME I-B survey and 2008–2009 AAMC TSF questionnaire

	Residents	Non-residents
Total Cost of Attendance	$65,116	$69,980
Tuition and Fees	$42,536	$42,236
Other (includes living expenses)	$18,920	$24,084
Health Insurance (can be waived)	$3,660	$3,660

Average 2008 Graduate Indebtedness: $174,409
% of Enrolled Students Receiving Aid: 85%

Criminal Background Check

This medical school does not require a criminal background check prior to matriculation.

New York University School of Medicine
New York, New York

New York University School of Medicine
Office of Admissions
550 First Avenue
New York, New York 10016
T 212 263 5290   **F** 212 263 0720

Admissions www.med.nyu.edu/admissions
Main www.med.nyu.edu
Financial http://admissions.med.nyu.edu/financial-aid/
E-mail admissions@med.nyu.edu

Private Institution

Dr. Robert I. Grossman, Dean

Dr. Nancy B. Genieser,
Associate Dean of Admissions and Financial Aid

Mekbib Gemeda, Assistant Dean of Diversity Affairs

Joanne McGrath, Assistant Dean of Admissions

General Information

Founded in 1841, NYU School of Medicine is one of the nation's preeminent academic institutions. For over 150 years, NYU has trained thousands of physician-scientists who have enriched countless lives and helped shape medical history. Through scientific research, medical education, and patient care, NYU continues its deep, abiding commitment to improve the human condition. NYU is among the nation's leaders in consistently producing physician graduates who go on to become full-time members of medical school faculties. Students train at Bellevue, the nation's first hospital. NYU is a "private university in the public service." The School of Medicine combines the best of modern biomedical science with a rich tradition of caring for all populations at the highest level of human achievement.

Mission Statement

NYU has a threefold mission: the education and training of physicians and scientists, the search for new knowledge, and the care of the sick. The three are inseparable. Medicine can be handed on to succeeding generations only by long training in the scientific method of investigation and by the actual care of patients. Progress in medicine, which is medical research, must look constantly to the school for its investigators, and to the patient for its problems, whereas the whole future of medical care rests upon a continuing supply of physicians and upon the promise of new discovery. The purpose, then, can only be achieved by endeavor in all three directions — medical education, research, and patient care — and they must be carried on simultaneously, for they are wholly dependent upon each other, not only for inspiration, but also for their very means of success.

Curricular Highlights

Community Service Requirement: Optional. Most students participate in community service.
Research/Thesis Requirement: Optional. M.D. with honors given upon completion.

NYU's curriculum innovates basic science teaching and promotes independent, interdisciplinary learning through small-group seminars, problem-solving activities, and computer-assisted instruction. Interdepartmental faculty instruct students in thematic curricular modules during the first two years, providing students with the essential information base, concepts, and skills necessary to understand, apply, and continually build upon the foundation of clinical medicine. Clinical sciences study continues through the four years. Advanced biomedical concepts are brought forward during clerkships through palindromic case studies stressing the translation of molecular biological and molecular genetic knowledge into decision-making and clinical care. Required clerkships and electives throughout the third and fourth years allow students to design specific courses in line with their educational and career goals. Through the honors research program, independent study projects, and the Masters Scholars program, students forge mentored relationships and cultivate their interests including public health, bioethics, human rights, biomedical health sciences, and medical informatics.

USMLE

Step 1: Required. Students must only record a score.
Step 2: Clinical Skills (CS): Required. Students must only record a score.
Step 2: Clinical Knowledge (CK): Required. Students Must only record a score.

Selection Factors

Applicants are considered from several viewpoints: excellence in coursework, premedical committee evaluation, interview, trends in the student's college progress, and the MCAT. The committee does not rely solely on MCAT scores and GPAs. Volunteer activities, independent research, and accomplishments in the humanities and liberal arts fields are also strongly considered. Only international applicants who hold a permanent resident visa will be considered for admission.

Financial Aid

The Financial Aid Office reviews all applications for financial assistance. Enrolled students and new accepts are eligible to apply for assistance. For more information, see *http://admissions.med.nyu.edu/financial-aid/*.

Information about Diversity Programs

The School of Medicine is committed to admitting a diverse class. The Office of Diversity Affairs and Advisory Council has established programs and services to meet the academic, educational, personal, and cultural needs of students from groups underrepresented in medicine. See: *www.med.nyu.edu/diversity_affairs/index.html*.

Campus Information

Setting

NYUSOM lies at the heart of NYU Medical Center, which embraces NYU Hospitals Center (Tisch Hospital and the Rusk Institute for Rehabilitation Medicine,) and NYU's major hospital affiliates (Bellevue, Hospital for Joint Diseases, and the VA Hospital).

Enrollment

For 2008, total enrollment was: 737

Special Features

Bellevue is the primary location of clinical instruction and is also a significant research hub. Students complete much of their third-year clinical clerkships there, and many complete their fourth-year subinternships and clinical electives there, as well. Bellevue's Level I Treatment Center is an internationally recognized model for ER development.

Housing

There are three residence halls for students, ranging from single rooms to two bedroom apartments. All buildings are protected by security systems.

Application Process and Requirements 2010–2011

Primary Application Service: AMCAS
Earliest filing date: June 1, 2009
Latest filing date: October 15, 2009

Secondary Application Required?: Yes
Sent to: All applicants
URL: http://admissions.med.nyu.edu/how-apply
Fee: Yes, $100
Fee waiver available: Yes
Earliest filing date: July 1, 2009
Latest filing date: December 1, 2009

MCAT® required?: Yes
Latest MCAT® considered: September 2009
Oldest MCAT® considered: 2006

Early Decision Program: School does not have EDP
Applicants notified: n/a
EDP available for: n/a

Regular Acceptance Notice
Earliest date: December 15, 2009
Latest date: Until class is full
Applicant's Response to Acceptance Offer – Maximum Time: Two weeks

Requests for Deferred Entrance Considered: Yes

Deposit to Hold Place in Class: Yes
Deposit (Resident): $100
Deposit (Non-resident): $100
Deposit due: With response to acceptance offer
Applied to tuition: Yes
Deposit refundable: Yes
Refundable by: May 15, 2010

Estimated number of new entrants: 166
EDP: 0, special program: n/a

Start Month/Year: August 2010

Interview Format: One-on-one interview with a faculty member. Regional interviews are not available.

Other Programs

PREPARATORY PROGRAMS
Postbaccalaureate Program: Yes
www.nyu.edu/cas/prehealth/postbacc/index.html
Summer Program: Yes, www.med.nyu.edu/sackler/programs/summer.html

COMBINED DEGREE PROGRAMS
Baccalaureate/M.D.: No
M.D./M.P.H.: Yes, www.nyu.edu/mph
M.D./M.B.A.: No
M.D./J.D.: No
M.D./Ph.D.: Yes, http://mdphd.med.nyu.edu/
MD/MPA: Yes, http://wagner.nyu.edu/dualdegrees/dual3.php

Premedical Coursework

Course	Req.	Rec.	Lab.	Hrs.
Inorganic Chemistry	•	•		6
Behavioral Sciences				
Biochemistry		•		
Biology	•		•	6
Biology/Zoology				
Calculus				
College English	•			6
College Mathematics				

Course	Req.	Rec.	Lab.	Hrs.
Computer Science				
Genetics		•		
Humanities				
Organic Chemistry	•		•	6
Physics	•		•	6
Psychology				
Social Sciences				
Other				

Selection Factors: 2008 Accepted Applicants

Proportion of Accepted Applicants with Relevant Experience (Data Self-Reported to AMCAS°)		
Community Service/Volunteer		68%
Medically-Related Work		85%
Research		93%

Shaded bar represents school's accepted scores ranging from the 10th percentile to the 90th percentile   School Median ●   National Median ●

Overall GPA	2.0	2.1	2.2	2.3	2.4	2.5	2.6	2.7	2.8	2.9	3.0	3.1	3.2	3.3	3.4	3.5	3.6	3.7	(3.8)	3.9	4.0
Science GPA	2.0	2.1	2.2	2.3	2.4	2.5	2.6	2.7	2.8	2.9	3.0	3.1	3.2	3.3	3.4	3.5	3.6	3.7	(3.8)	3.9	4.0

MCAT® Total Numeric Score 9 10 11 12 13 14 15 16 17 18 19 20 21 22 23 24 25 26 27 28 29 30 31 (32) 33 34 (35) 36 37 38 39 40 41 42 43

Writing Sample				J		K		L		M	N	O	P	(Q)	R	S	T
Verbal Reasoning	3		4		5		6		7		8		9	(10)	(11)		12		13		14		15
Biological Sciences	3		4		5		6		7		8		9		10	(11)	(12)		13		14		15
Physical Sciences	3		4		5		6		7		8		9		10	(11)	(12)		13		14		15

Acceptance & Matriculation Data for 2008–2009 First Year Class

	Resident	Non-resident	International	Total
Applications	1378	5697	245	7320
Interviewed	246	694	14	954
Deferred	2	4	0	6
Matriculants				
Early Assurance Program	0	0	0	0
Early Decision Program	0	0	0	0
Baccalaureate/M.D.	n/a	n/a	n/a	n/a
M.D./Ph.D.	1	3	0	4
Matriculated	72	92	1	**165**

Applications accepted from International Applicants: Only Canadian

Matriculant Demographics: 2008–2009 First Year Class

Men: 87   **Women:** 78

Matriculants' Self-Reported Race/Ethnicity

Mexican American	1	**Korean**	7
Cuban	3	**Vietnamese**	1
Puerto Rican	2	**Other Asian**	4
Other Hispanic	3	**Total Asian**	52
Total Hispanic	8	**Native American**	1
Chinese	22	**Black**	5
Asian Indian	11	**Native Hawaiian**	0
Pakistani	1	**White**	100
Filipino	5	**Unduplicated Number**	
Japanese	3	**of Matriculants**	165

Science and Math Majors: 65%
Matriculants with:
    Baccalaureate degree: 99%
    Graduate degree(s): 3%

Specialty Choice

2004, 2005, 2006 Graduates, Specialty Choice (As reported by program directors to GME Track™)	
Anesthesiology	6%
Emergency Medicine	4%
Family Practice	0%
Internal Medicine	26%
Obstetrics/Gynecology	5%
Orthopaedic Surgery	6%
Pediatrics	9%
Psychiatry	4%
Radiology	8%
Surgery	6%

Financial Information

Source: 2007–2008 LCME I-B survey and 2008–2009 AAMC TSF questionnaire

	Residents	Non-residents
Total Cost of Attendance	$62,276	$62,276
Tuition and Fees	$43,976	$43,976
Other (includes living expenses)	$14,800	$14,800
Health Insurance (can be waived)	$3,500	$3,500

Average 2008 Graduate Indebtedness: $145,997
% of Enrolled Students Receiving Aid: 79%

Criminal Background Check

Please check the School Web site.

University at Buffalo School of Medicine & Biomedical Sciences

Buffalo, New York

Office of Medical Admissions
University at Buffalo
131 Biomedical Education Building
Buffalo, New York 14214-3013
T 716 829 3466   F 716 829 3849

Admissions www.smbs.buffalo.edu/ome/ome
_admission.htm
Main www.smbs.buffalo.edu
Financial src.buffalo.edu/financialaid
E-mail jjrosso@buffalo.edu

Public Institution

Dr. Michael Cain, Dean

Dr. Charles M. Severin, Associate Dean for Medical Education and Admissions

Dr. David A. Milling, Assistant Dean, Multicultural Affairs

Dr. Nancy Nielsen, Senior Associate Dean of Medical Education

General Information

The School of Medicine was founded in 1846 by Millard Fillmore and a group of physicians. In 1962, the University of Buffalo joined the State University of New York (SUNY) system. The University at Buffalo has the most comprehensive campus in the SUNY system and was honored in 1989 with election to the Association of American Universities. The clinical education program is conducted in cooperation with nine area hospitals.

Mission Statement

To provide well-trained physicians and other health care professionals who will attend to the health needs of citizens. To offer a source of continuing education to the community of health care providers. To provide a center of research and scholarship that will advance and promote health-related services. As a public institution, the mission places particular emphasis on diversity, inclusion, and the special needs of New York State, such as minority recruitment and retention, and the underserved urban and rural health populations.

Curricular Highlights

Community Service Requirement: Optional.
Research/Thesis Requirement: Optional.

The curriculum emphasizes the relevance of medical education to the practice of medicine and the relevance of basic science to clinical practice. It introduces patient contact and patient-centered learning in the first year of medical school, and it increases ambulatory care experiences in the clinical years. The first two years contain an integrated curriculum that includes the Introduction to Clinical Medicine course continuum, which prepares students in the knowledge, skills, and attitudes required for

third-year clinical clerkships and provides the foundation for a medical career. Ethics, the doctor-patient relationship, principles of health promotion, disease prevention, and promotion of self-learning and inquiry are emphasized, in addition to extensive education in the skills basic to medical practice and patient care. The clinical years include required clerkships and electives. There is ample time for additional electives during the senior year.

USMLE

Step 1: Required. Students must record a passing score for promotion.
Step 2: Clinical Skills (CS): Required. Students must only record a score.
Step 2: Clinical Knowledge (CK): Required. Students must only record a score.

Selection Factors

The Admissions Committee seeks to identify and select students who display favorable qualities deemed important for the pursuit of a career in medicine. In making its assessments and determinations, the committee relies on information contained in the application and in documents submitted in support of the applicant. Based on careful screening, applicants are invited to appear for an interview. Reapplications are treated no differently than initial applications. Rejected applicants should seek the advice and counsel of their premedical advisor. Students are accepted without regard to race, sex, creed, national origin, age, sexual preference, or handicap. All applicants will receive the "Technical Standards of the Medical School Curriculum" with the secondary application. Some preference is given to qualified residents of New York State. Competitive out-of-state applicants are encouraged to apply.

Financial Aid

The priority due date for receipt of the Free Application for Federal Student Aid (FAFSA) is March 1, 2010. Forms received after the deadline are subject to funds available. Financial aid requests are considered after admission. Awards are made based on need. In most requests, parental income information is required regardless of dependency status. A limited number of scholarships based on academic merit and financial need are provided each year.

Information about Diversity Programs

The Summer Enrichment and Support Program helps facilitate students' retention in medical school. It is designed for admitted first-year educationally and socioeconomically disadvantaged students. Tutorial and counseling services are available throughout the summer and academic year.

Campus Information

Setting

The medical school is located on a recently renovated 33-acre campus on Main Street, in the northeast corner of the city of Buffalo. The world-renowned Shock Trauma Center is located two miles from the main medical school building. There are several public parks, cultural institutions, and shopping areas located in the vicinity. The "Main Street Campus" is accessible by subway to downtown Buffalo and is within walking distance of the VA Medical Center.

Enrollment

For 2008, total enrollment was: 568

Special Features

Students receive training in world-renowned clinical centers, including the Children's Hospital Trauma Center and Roswell Park Memorial Cancer Institute. There are also numerous opportunities for clinical and basic science research and varied international clinical experiences.

Housing

While on-campus housing is not available, the University maintains a list of affordable apartments and homes within a 10-mile radius of the campus. Rents average $500–$700 per month.

Satellite Campuses/Facilities

Student rotations are divided among nine teaching hospitals and several clinics in the metro Buffalo area. The medical school is also affiliated with ambulatory care centers in outlying suburban areas.

Application Process and Requirements 2010–2011

Primary Application Service: AMCAS
Earliest filing date: June 1, 2009
Latest filing date: November 15, 2009

Secondary Application Required?: Yes
Sent to: All applicants
Contact: James J. Rosso
(716) 829-3466, jjrosso@buffalo.edu
Fee: Yes, $65
Fee waiver available: Yes
Earliest filing date: June 1, 2009
Latest filing date: December 15, 2009

MCAT® required?: Yes
Latest MCAT® considered: September 2009
Oldest MCAT® considered: April 2006

Early Decision Program: School does have EDP
Applicants notified: October 1, 2009
EDP available for: Both Residents and Non-residents

Regular Acceptance Notice
Earliest date: October 15, 2009
Latest date: Until class is full
Applicant's Response to Acceptance Offer – Maximum Time: Two weeks

Requests for Deferred Entrance Considered: Yes

Deposit to Hold Place in Class: Yes
Deposit (Resident): $100
Deposit (Non-resident): $100
Deposit due: With response to acceptance offer
Applied to tuition: Yes
Deposit refundable: Yes
Refundable by: May 15, 2010

Estimated number of new entrants: 135
EDP: 2, special program: 4

Start Month/Year: August 2010

Interview Format: Two, one-on-one interviews. Regional interviews are not available.

Other Programs

PREPARATORY PROGRAMS
Postbaccalaureate Program: No
Summer Program: No

COMBINED DEGREE PROGRAMS
Baccalaureate/M.D.: No
M.D./M.P.H.: Yes, James J. Rosso
(716) 829-3466, jjrosso@buffalo.edu
M.D./M.B.A.: Yes, James J. Rosso
(716) 829-3466, jjrosso@buffalo.edu
M.D./J.D.: No
M.D./Ph.D.: Yes, Arlene Albrecht
(716) 829-3398, ama7@buffalo.edu

Premedical Coursework

Course	Req.	Rec.	Lab.	Qtrs.
Inorganic Chemistry	•		•	2
Behavioral Sciences				
Biochemistry		•		
Biology	•		•	2
Biology/Zoology				
Calculus				
College English	•			2
College Mathematics				

Course	Req.	Rec.	Lab.	Qtrs.
Computer Science				
Genetics		•		
Humanities		•		
Organic Chemistry	•		•	2
Physics	•			2
Psychology				
Social Sciences		•		
Other				

Selection Factors: 2008 Accepted Applicants

Proportion of Accepted Applicants with Relevant Experience (Data Self-Reported to AMCAS®)		
Community Service/Volunteer		63%
Medically-Related Work		89%
Research		83%

Shaded bar represents school's accepted scores ranging from the 10th percentile to the 90th percentile ▨ ● School Median ● National Median

Overall GPA	2.0	2.1	2.2	2.3	2.4	2.5	2.6	2.7	2.8	2.9	3.0	3.1	3.2	3.3	3.4	3.5	3.6	(3.7)	3.8	3.9	4.0
Science GPA	2.0	2.1	2.2	2.3	2.4	2.5	2.6	2.7	2.8	2.9	3.0	3.1	3.2	3.3	3.4	3.5	(3.6)	3.7	3.8	3.9	4.0

MCAT® Total Numeric Score 9 10 11 12 13 14 15 16 17 18 19 20 21 22 23 24 25 26 27 28 29 30 (31) 32 33 34 35 36 37 38 39 40 41 42 43

Writing Sample			J	K	L	M	N	O	P	(Q)	R	S	T
Verbal Reasoning	3	4	5	6	7	8	9	(10)	11	12	13	14	15
Biological Sciences	3	4	5	6	7	8	9	10	(11)	12	13	14	15
Physical Sciences	3	4	5	6	7	8	9	10	(11)	12	13	14	15

Acceptance & Matriculation Data for 2008–2009 First Year Class

	Resident	Non-resident	International	Total
Applications	1760	1981	98	3839
Interviewed	423	219	0	642
Deferred	1	1	0	2
Matriculants				
Early Assurance Program	3	2	0	5
Early Decision Program	2	0	0	2
Baccalaureate/M.D.	n/a	n/a	n/a	n/a
M.D./Ph.D.	1	1	0	2
Matriculated	103	33	0	**136**

Applications accepted from International Applicants: No

Specialty Choice

2004, 2005, 2006 Graduates, Specialty Choice (As reported by program directors to GME Track™)	
Anesthesiology	5%
Emergency Medicine	7%
Family Practice	7%
Internal Medicine	17%
Obstetrics/Gynecology	6%
Orthopaedic Surgery	3%
Pediatrics	13%
Psychiatry	7%
Radiology	6%
Surgery	8%

Matriculant Demographics: 2008–2009 First Year Class

Men: 59   **Women:** 77

Matriculants' Self-Reported Race/Ethnicity

Mexican American	1	Korean	4
Cuban	0	Vietnamese	2
Puerto Rican	0	Other Asian	2
Other Hispanic	0	Total Asian	33
Total Hispanic	1	Native American	2
Chinese	14	Black	4
Asian Indian	9	Native Hawaiian	0
Pakistani	2	White	98
Filipino	2	Unduplicated Number	
Japanese	0	of Matriculants	136

Science and Math Majors: 74%
Matriculants with:
Baccalaureate degree: 99%
Graduate degree(s): 10%

Financial Information

Source: 2007–2008 LCME I-B survey and 2008–2009 AAMC TSF questionnaire

	Residents	Non-residents
Total Cost of Attendance	$45,460	$74,860
Tuition and Fees	$20,270	$34,970
Other (includes living expenses)	$23,585	$38,285
Health Insurance (can be waived)	$1,605	$1,605

Average 2008 Graduate Indebtedness: $128,738
% of Enrolled Students Receiving Aid: 87%

Criminal Background Check

This medical school requires a criminal background check prior to matriculation.

State University of New York
Downstate Medical Center College of Medicine
Brooklyn, New York

Admissions Office, State University of New York
Downstate Medical Center
450 Clarkson Avenue — Box 60
Brooklyn, New York 11203-2098
T 718 270 2446   **F** 718 270 4775

Admissions http://sls.downstate.edu/admissions/
medicine/index.html
Main www.downstate.edu/college_of_medicine
Financial http://sls.downstate.edu/financial_aid/costs/
cost_com.html
E-mail admissions@downstate.edu

Public Institution

*Dr. Ian L. Taylor, Dean and Senior
Vice President for Biomedical Education
and Research*

Dr. Marcia Gerber, Dean of Admissions

*Dr. Constance Hill, Associate Dean for
Minority Affairs*

Dr. Lorraine Terracina, VP for Students Affairs

*Dr. Shushawna DeOliveira, Director
of Admissions*

General Information

Current information about the college, curriculum, and admissions is available on the Web site at *www.downstate.edu.*

Mission Statement

To provide high quality education for the next generation of health professionals. Integral to our concept of professional education are both a commitment to confront the health problems of urban communities and a responsibility to advance the state of knowledge and practice in the health disciplines through basic and applied clinical research.

Curricular Highlights

Community Service Requirement: Optional.
Research/Thesis Requirement: Optional.

In preparing physicians to practice in the future health care system, the medical education process is under constant evaluation. The main goals of the curriculum are to improve the integration of basic and clinical science throughout the four years of medical school; to provide earlier exposure to patient care by introducing clinical experiences in the first and second years of medical school; to provide for small-group, self-directed and case-based learning; and to foster life-long learning skills through the introduction of new applications of information science, outcomes studies, and evidence-based medicine. An organ system approach is followed. The emphasis is on the development of clinical reasoning and problem-solving skills. During the first year, attention is focused on the basic components of human biology and behavior, as

well as on the essential aspects of the physician-patient relationship. The second year begins the study of human disease. The third and fourth years provide integrated clerkships and electives. See the Web site for more details. All courses are graded fail, conditional, pass, high pass and honors.

USMLE

Step 1: Required. Students must record a passing score for promotion.
Step 2: Clinical Skills (CS): Required. Students must only record a score.
Step 2: Clinical Knowledge (CK): Required. Students must only record a score.

Selection Factors

The Committee on Admissions considers the total qualifications of each applicant without regard to sex, sexual orientation, race, color, creed, religion, national origin, age, marital status, or disability. Decisions are based on multiple factors, including but not limited to, prior academic performance; completion of required courses for admission; the potential for academic success, including performance on standardized tests such as the MCAT; communication skills, character, and personal skills; health-related experiences; and motivation for medicine. The 2008 entering class attended 70 different colleges and universities. Matriculants' ages ranged from 20 to 40 years, with a mean age on matriculation of 23 years.

Financial Aid

The college is committed to help students meet their educational expenses. Aid is granted on the basis of need and, for some scholarships, on academic achievement. The major portion of assistance is derived from federal and state allocations: grants, scholarships, loans, and/or college work-study. Loans are the most common form of assistance. Financial aid application materials are sent to all accepted applicants, and students' financial aid needs are reviewed annually. Please refer to *http://sls.downstate.edu/financial_aid/costs/cost_com.html for current charges.*

Information about Diversity Programs

SUNY Downstate maintains a tradition of commitment to the enrollment of students

from groups underrepresented in medicine. The Office of Minority Affairs directs several programs targeted to furnish information and support to students from underrepresented and disadvantaged backgrounds. Entering students from groups underrepresented in medicine are matched with a faculty mentor. The Daniel Hale Williams Society also provides peer support for underrepresented students. Contact the Office of Minority Affairs at: oma@downstate.edu.

Campus Information

Setting
In NYC, 2.4 million people reside in Brooklyn. Downstate is located in central Brooklyn on an urban campus that includes a Basic Science Building, a Health Science Education Building, University Hospital, two residence halls, a student center, and a Biotech Center. The school is across the street from Kings County Hospital and three blocks from a subway station. More information is on the Web site.

Enrollment
For 2008, total enrollment was: 762

Special Features
The curriculum includes clinical exposure starting in the first year. Varied clinical settings throughout the curriculum prepare students superbly for their residency training (see Web site for more information). During the fourth year, 20–25 students participate in an international elective entitled, "Health Care in Developing Countries." A Clinical Neuroscience Pathway is available to provide enhanced exposure to neurosciences throughout the four years. Research opportunities are available throughout the four years and may lead to graduation honors. M.D./M.P.H. degrees may be earned concurrently within four years.

Housing
Two on-campus residence halls offer three different housing accommodations (see Web site for more information), while being conveniently located across the street from both academic buildings and recreational activities in the Student Center.

Application Process and Requirements 2010–2011

Primary Application Service: AMCAS
Earliest filing date: June 1, 2009
Latest filing date: December 15, 2009

Secondary Application Required?: Yes
Sent to: All applicants – download from Web site
URL: http://sls.downstate.edu/admissions/
medicine/programs/procedures/index.html
Fee: Yes, $80
Fee waiver available: Yes
Earliest filing date: June 1, 2009
Latest filing date: February 1, 2010

MCAT® required?: Yes
Latest MCAT® considered: September 2009
Oldest MCAT® considered: April 2007

Early Decision Program: School does have EDP
Applicants notified: October 1, 2009
EDP available for: Both Residents
and Non-residents

Regular Acceptance Notice
Earliest date: October 15, 2009
Latest date: Until class is full
Applicant's Response to Acceptance
Offer – Maximum Time: Two weeks

Requests for Deferred
Entrance Considered: Yes

Deposit to Hold Place in Class: Yes
Deposit (Resident): $100
Deposit (Non-resident): $100
Deposit due: Within two weeks of acceptance
Applied to tuition: Yes
Deposit refundable: Yes
Refundable by: May 14, 2010

Estimated number of new entrants: 185
EDP: 5, special program: n/a

Start Month/Year: August 2010

Interview Format: One-on-one, about
one hour in length. Regional interviews
are not available.

Other Programs

PREPARATORY PROGRAMS
Postbaccalaureate Program: No
Summer Program: n/a

COMBINED DEGREE PROGRAMS
Baccalaureate/M.D.: Yes, http://depthome. brook-
lyn.cuny.edu/bamd/bamdmain.html, Dr. Steven
Silbering, (718) 951-5471, silbering@brooklyn.cuny.edu
M.D./M.P.H.: Yes, www.downstate.edu/
publichealth/mdmph_about.html, (718) 270-1065,
PublicHealth@downstate.edu
M.D./M.B.A.: No
M.D./J.D.: No
M.D./Ph.D.: Yes, http://sls.downstate.edu/
admissions/medicine/mdpdh_program.html
Dr. Stanley Friedman, (718) 270-1335,
sfriedman@downstate.edu

Premedical Coursework

Course	Req.	Rec.	Lab.	Sems.	Course	Req.	Rec.	Lab.	Sems.
Inorganic Chemistry	•		•	8	Computer Science				
Behavioral Sciences					Genetics				
Biochemistry		•		4	Humanities				
Biology	•		•	8	Organic Chemistry	•		•	8
Biology/Zoology					Physics	•		•	8
Calculus					Psychology				
College English	•			6	Social Sciences				
College Mathematics					See website for recom.		•		

Selection Factors: 2008 Accepted Applicants

Proportion of Accepted Applicants with Relevant Experience (Data Self-Reported to AMCAS*)		Community Service/Volunteer	66%
		Medically-Related Work	87%
		Research	85%

Shaded bar represents school's accepted scores ranging from the 10th percentile to the 90th percentile — School Median ● National Median ●

Overall GPA 2.0 2.1 2.2 2.3 2.4 2.5 2.6 2.7 2.8 2.9 3.0 3.1 3.2 3.3 3.4 3.5 3.6 (3.7) 3.8 3.9 4.0
Science GPA 2.0 2.1 2.2 2.3 2.4 2.5 2.6 2.7 2.8 2.9 3.0 3.1 3.2 3.3 3.4 3.5 3.6 (3.7) 3.8 3.9 4.0

MCAT® Total Numeric Score 9 10 11 12 13 14 15 16 17 18 19 20 21 22 23 24 25 26 27 28 29 30 31 (32)(33) 34 35 36 37 38 39 40 41 42 43

Writing Sample			J	K	L	M	N	O	P	(Q)	R	S	T
Verbal Reasoning	3	4	5	6	7	8	9	(10)	11	12	13	14	15
Biological Sciences	3	4	5	6	7	8	9	10	(11)	12	13	14	15
Physical Sciences	3	4	5	6	7	8	9	10	(11)	12	13	14	15

Acceptance & Matriculation Data for 2008–2009 First Year Class

	Resident	Non-resident	International	Total
Applications	2171	3006	101	5278
Interviewed	695	379	0	1074
Deferred	2	1	0	3
Matriculants				
Early Assurance Program	n/a	n/a	n/a	n/a
Early Decision Program	2	1	0	3
Baccalaureate/M.D.	9	0	0	9
M.D./Ph.D.	2	1	0	3
Matriculated	147	36	0	**183**
Applications accepted from International Applicants: No				

Specialty Choice

2004, 2005, 2006 Graduates, Specialty Choice (As reported by program directors to GME Track™)	
Anesthesiology	8%
Emergency Medicine	6%
Family Practice	2%
Internal Medicine	26%
Obstetrics/Gynecology	4%
Orthopaedic Surgery	3%
Pediatrics	14%
Psychiatry	5%
Radiology	5%
Surgery	5%

Matriculant Demographics: 2008–2009 First Year Class

Men: 98   **Women:** 85

Matriculants' Self-Reported Race/Ethnicity

Mexican American	0	**Korean**	11
Cuban	0	**Vietnamese**	0
Puerto Rican	1	**Other Asian**	6
Other Hispanic	8	**Total Asian**	64
Total Hispanic	8	**Native American**	0
Chinese	24	**Black**	16
Asian Indian	11	**Native Hawaiian**	0
Pakistani	7	**White**	93
Filipino	4	**Unduplicated Number**	
Japanese	4	**of Matriculants**	183

Science and Math Majors: 58%
Matriculants with:
   Baccalaureate degree: 100%
   Graduate degree(s): 10%

Financial Information

Source: 2007–2008 LCME I-B survey
and 2008–2009 AAMC TSF questionnaire

	Residents	Non-residents
Total Cost of Attendance	$49,156	$66,091
Tuition and Fees	$20,705	$37,640
Other (includes living expenses)	$25,156	$25,156
Health Insurance (can be waived)	$3,295	$3,295

Average 2008 Graduate Indebtedness: $112,159
% of Enrolled Students Receiving Aid: 82%

Criminal Background Check

This medical school does not require a criminal
background check prior to matriculation.

State University of New York
Upstate Medical University College of Medicine
Syracuse, New York

Admissions Office
SUNY Upstate Medical University
766 Irving Ave.
Syracuse, New York 13210
T 315 464 4570   F 315 464 8867

Admissions www.upstate.edu/com/admissions.shtml
Main www.upstate.edu/com
Financial www.upstate.edu/prospective/tuition.php
E-mail admiss@upstate.edu

Public Institution
Dr. Steven J. Scheinman, Dean

Jennifer Welch, Director of Admissions

*Nakeia Chambers, Director
of Multicultural Affairs*

Mike Pede, Director of Financial Aid

Dr. Julie White, Dean, Student Affairs

General Information
The College of Medicine was established in 1834 as the Geneva Medical College. The college was transferred to the State University of New York (SUNY) system in 1950. In 1999, its name changed to SUNY Upstate Medical University to best reflect the college's academic mission in medical care, research, and education.

Mission Statement
The main mission of SUNY Upstate is the education of health professionals and to conduct biomedical research. Upstate's clinical faculty and health care professionals commit themselves to education and patient care, demonstrating excellence and compassion. In pursuing its mission, Upstate provides its faculty, staff, students, and volunteers an environment of mutual trust and respect, with opportunities to grow personally and professionally, and to make a positive difference in the lives of others.

Curricular Highlights
Community Service Requirement: Optional.
Research/Thesis Requirement: Optional.

The curriculum integrates the basic and clinical sciences and provides clinical exposure in the first semester. All courses are aligned by organ systems. The curriculum also addresses the humanistic aspects of medicine, including its ethical, legal, and social implications. During the third year, the students apply the principles of basic science to clinical problem-solving. Clerkships in subspecialty services are required. A research track is available, in which students spend the first two summers and elective time on a research project. Another interesting opportunity is the Rural Medical Education Program, which places students in rural communities for nine consecutive months of clinical

and didactic education during the 3rd and 4th year. A modified pass/fail grading system is used.

USMLE
Step 1: Required. Students must record a passing score for promotion.
Step 2: Clinical Skills (CS): Required. Students must only record a score.
Step 2: Clinical Knowledge (CK): Required. Students must only record a score.

Selection Factors
The Admissions Committee takes an applicant's total qualifications into consideration for the study and practice of medicine. Major factors in the selection of applicants include: review of college records, MCAT scores, letters of recommendation from premedical advisory committees, personal interview, communication skills, character, and motivation.

Financial Aid
Accepted applicants who are U.S. citizens or permanent residents are eligible to apply for financial aid. The Financial Aid Office generally sends out financial aid award letters beginning in March.

Information about Diversity Programs
Upstate is committed to making student enrollment reflective of the diverse New York State population. Disadvantaged students and students from groups underrepresented in medicine are actively sought. A summer Human Anatomy program is available for all students. For more information, please contact the Office of Admissions.

Campus Information
Setting
Located in Syracuse, New York's fourth largest city, SUNY Upstate is a compact, easy-to-navigate campus. We have a new human anatomy lab, an excellent library, and a teaching hospital that is connected to our main academic building. Syracuse is an affordable, medium-sized city with big-city sports, arts, and recreation. Just outside the city, you will find numerous parks, lakes, mountains, golf courses, ski slopes, hiking trails and beaches. University Hospital is a level-one trauma center and tertiary care hospital that services 17 different counties.

Enrollment
For 2008, total enrollment was: 646

Special Features
SUNY Upstate's teaching hospital, University Hospital, is the main clinical site in Syracuse. As the only Level I trauma and burn center in the region, University Hospital treats the most seriously ill and injured patients. University Hospital offers hundreds of specialty services and programs, including the Center for Children's Cancer and Blood Disorders, Clark Burn Center, CNY Gamma Knife Center, and the Joslin Diabetes Center. In 2009, we will open a Children's Hospital at University Hospital, the first children's hospital in the region. We also have a clinical campus in the city of Binghamton, which offers clinical training in a community-based setting.

Housing
Clark Tower, SUNY Upstate's residence hall, houses approximately 170 students from all four colleges in fully-furnished standard rooms, studio apartments, and two-bedroom suites. Clark Tower is located next door to the Campus Activities Building, one block from University Hospital and a short walk from the Library and the academic buildings.

Satellite Campuses/Facilities
At the beginning of the third year, one quarter of the class moves from SUNY Upstate's main campus in Syracuse to the Binghamton Campus. The Binghamton Campus is located 70 miles south of Syracuse. There, clinical training occurs in a community-based setting similar to the environment in which most physicians practice.

Application Process and Requirements 2010–2011

Primary Application Service: AMCAS
Earliest filing date: June 1, 2009
Latest filing date: October 15, 2009

Secondary Application Required?: Yes
Sent to: Information on how to access secondary application materials is sent to all verified AMCAS applicants.
URL: n/a
Fee: Yes, $100
Fee waiver available: Yes
Earliest filing date: Upon receipt of verified AMCAS application.
Latest filing date: December 1, 2009

MCAT® required?: Yes
Latest MCAT® considered: September 2009
Oldest MCAT® considered: 2006

Early Decision Program: School does have EDP
Applicants notified: October 1, 2009
EDP available for: Both Residents and Non-residents

Regular Acceptance Notice
Earliest date: October 15, 2009
Latest date: Until class is full
Applicant's Response to Acceptance Offer – Maximum Time: Two weeks

Requests for Deferred Entrance Considered: Yes

Deposit to Hold Place in Class: Yes
Deposit (Resident): $100
Deposit (Non-resident): $100
Deposit due: With response to acceptance offer
Applied to tuition: Yes
Deposit refundable: Yes
Refundable by: May 15, 2010

Estimated number of new entrants: 160
EDP: 2, special program: 15

Start Month/Year: August 2010

Interview Format: On campus with two individual interviewers. Regional interviews are not available.

Other Programs

PREPARATORY PROGRAMS
Postbaccalaureate Program: No
Summer Program: Yes, Jennifer Welch
(315) 464-4570, admiss@upstate.edu

COMBINED DEGREE PROGRAMS
Baccalaureate/M.D.: Yes
www.upstate.edu/com/admissions/options.php
M.D./M.P.H.: Yes, www.upstate.edu/cnymph/
M.D./M.B.A.: No
M.D./J.D.: No
M.D./Ph.D.: Yes, www.upstate.edu/mdphd/

Premedical Coursework

Course	Req.	Rec.	Lab.	Hrs.
Inorganic Chemistry	•		•	6-8
Behavioral Sciences				
Biochemistry		•		
Biology				
Biology/Zoology	•		•	6-8
Calculus		•		
College English	•			6
College Mathematics			•	

Course	Req.	Rec.	Lab.	Hrs.
Computer Science				
Genetics		•		
Humanities		•		
Organic Chemistry	•		•	6-8
Physics	•		•	6-8
Psychology				
Social Sciences				
Other				

Selection Factors: 2008 Accepted Applicants

Proportion of Accepted Applicants with Relevant Experience (Data Self-Reported to AMCAS)

Community Service/Volunteer	63%
Medically-Related Work	86%
Research	81%

Shaded bar represents school's accepted scores ranging from the 10th percentile to the 90th percentile. School Median ● National Median ●

Overall GPA 2.0 2.1 2.2 2.3 2.4 2.5 2.6 2.7 2.8 2.9 3.0 3.1 3.2 3.3 **3.4 3.5 3.6 (3.7) 3.8** 3.9 4.0
Science GPA 2.0 2.1 2.2 2.3 2.4 2.5 2.6 2.7 2.8 2.9 3.0 3.1 3.2 **3.3 3.4 3.5 3.6 (3.7) 3.8** 3.9 4.0

MCAT® Total Numeric Score 9 10 11 12 13 14 15 16 17 18 19 20 21 22 23 24 25 26 **27 28 29 30 31 (32) 33 34 35 36** 37 38 39 40 41 42 43

Writing Sample			J	K	L	**M N O P (Q) R**	S	T
Verbal Reasoning	3	4	5	6	7	**8 9 (10) 11 12** 13	14	15
Biological Sciences	3	4	5	6	7	8 **9 10 (11) 12 13**	14	15
Physical Sciences	3	4	5	6	7	8 **9 10 (11) 12 13**	14	15

Acceptance & Matriculation Data for 2008–2009 First Year Class

	Resident	Non-resident	International	Total
Applications	1874	2793	512	5179
Interviewed	595	225	103	923
Deferred	1	1	0	2
Matriculants				
Early Assurance Program	18	3	1	22
Early Decision Program	2	0	0	2
Baccalaureate/M.D.	3	1	0	4
M.D./Ph.D.	1	1	0	2
Matriculated	132	20	8	**160**

Applications accepted from International Applicants: Yes

Specialty Choice

2004, 2005, 2006 Graduates, Specialty Choice (As reported by program directors to GME Track™)

Anesthesiology	5%
Emergency Medicine	6%
Family Practice	6%
Internal Medicine	20%
Obstetrics/Gynecology	4%
Orthopaedic Surgery	4%
Pediatrics	13%
Psychiatry	5%
Radiology	7%
Surgery	7%

Matriculant Demographics: 2008–2009 First Year Class

Men: 83 **Women:** 77

Matriculants' Self-Reported Race/Ethnicity

Mexican American	1	Korean	2
Cuban	0	Vietnamese	1
Puerto Rican	1	Other Asian	2
Other Hispanic	1	Total Asian	24
Total Hispanic	3	Native American	1
Chinese	6	Black	20
Asian Indian	9	Native Hawaiian	0
Pakistani	3	White	106
Filipino	1	Unduplicated Number	
Japanese	1	of Matriculants	160

Science and Math Majors: 75%
Matriculants with:
Baccalaureate degree: 100%
Graduate degree(s): 13%

Financial Information

Source: 2007–2008 LCME I-B survey and 2008–2009 AAMC TSF questionnaire

	Residents	Non-residents
Total Cost of Attendance	$40,481	$55,181
Tuition and Fees	$19,956	$34,656
Other (includes living expenses)	$18,005	$18,005
Health Insurance (can be waived)	$2,520	$2,520

Average 2008 Graduate Indebtedness: $130,358
% of Enrolled Students Receiving Aid: 86%

Criminal Background Check

This medical school requires a criminal background check prior to matriculation.

Stony Brook University School of Medicine

Stony Brook, New York

Committee on Admissions
Level 4 Health Sciences Center
Stony Brook University School of Medicine
Stony Brook, New York 11794-8434
T 631 444 2113   **F** 631 444 6032

Admissions www.stonybrookmedicalcenter.org/
education/som_admissions.cfm
Main www.stonybrookmedicalcenter.org/
Financial www.hsc.stonybrook.edu/som/
student_affairs/index.cfm
E-mail somadmissions@stonybrook.edu

Public Institution

Dr. Richard N. Fine, Dean

Dr. Jack Fuhrer, Associate Dean for Admissions

Dr. Aldustus E. Jordan, Associate Dean for Student and Minority Affairs

Mary Jean Allen, Director of Financial Aid

Grace S. Agnetti, Assistant Dean for Admissions

General Information

Stony Brook University's School of Medicine accepted its first class in 1971. It is part of the Stony Brook University Medical Center, which includes the 540-bed University Hospital.

Mission Statement

The School of Medicine strives to improve the quality of health care by demonstrating national leadership in education, research, patient care, and community service. The School of Medicine prepares its students for careers in medical practice or research through its state-of-the-art curriculum and clinical and research opportunities.

Curricular Highlights

Community Service Requirement: Optional.
Research/Thesis Requirement: Optional.

The curriculum of the School of Medicine provides the opportunity for extensive training in the basic medical sciences and teaching in the clinical disciplines of medicine. The curriculum requires the acquisition and utilization of a variety of skills in basic and clinical sciences. The official grading system is honors/pass/fail. The first two years are devoted to basic sciences and the integrated Foundations of Medicine course. The Foundations course teaches medical ethics, patient assessment skills, preventive medicine, human behavior, and nutrition. The second year focuses on an organ system-based pathophysiology and therapeutics course. Third year students complete core clerkships in medicine, pediatrics, family medicine, obstetrics-gynecology, psychiatry, ambulatory medicine and surgery. One month of elective time is available. Fourth year students are offered selectives and electives. Core clerkships are completed at University Hospital or one of three teaching affiliates. Electives can be completed at other sites.

USMLE

Step 1: Required. Students must record a passing score for promotion.
Step 2: Clinical Skills (CS): Required. Students must record a passing total score to graduate.
Step 2: Clinical Knowledge (CK): Required. Students must record a passing total score to graduate.

Selection Factors

Grades, MCAT scores, letters of evaluation, and extracurricular and work experiences are carefully examined. Motivational and personal characteristics as indicated in the application and a personal interview are also a major part of the admissions assessment. There is no discrimination in the admissions process on the basis of sex, race, religion, national origin, age, marital status, or handicap. The school attempts to enroll a class representative of a variety of backgrounds and academic interests. Stony Brook hopes to attract a significant representation of persons from groups that have historically been underrepresented in medicine. Premedical coursework must be completed at an American college or university. While residents of New York constitute the majority of the applicants and entrants, out-of-state applicants are given due consideration. Required supporting documentation includes official transcripts of all college work and official letters of evaluation. Personal interviews will be arranged at the initiative of the school for candidates who appear to be serious contenders for admission. Stony Brook does not utilize a "cut-off" in grades or MCAT scores in making admission decisions. The school is committed to giving all applicants the individualized attention that they merit.

Financial Aid

Stony Brook participates in all financial aid programs available at the medical schools of the SUNY system. Financial aid and counseling are available through the Office of Student Affairs, as is assistance in securing housing and in meeting other personal needs. On-campus housing is available. Students are advised to have transportation available because there is no public transportation to outlying clinical facilities.

Information about Diversity Programs

Stony Brook is committed to admitting a diverse class each year. The school makes a concerted effort to enroll qualified students from groups underrepresented in medicine.

Campus Information

Setting

Stony Brook University and the School of Medicine are located 60 miles east of NYC on the north shore of Long Island. The campus is surrounded by a picturesque and historic community. The campus provides a wide spectrum of activities ranging from NCAA Division I sporting events to professional theatre and fine arts. Students can participate in a wide range of intramural athletic activities. The clinical campus includes Stony Brook University Hospital and three affiliates.

Enrollment

For 2008, total enrollment was: 474

Special Features

Stony Brook offers excellent research and clinical opportunities and has attracted a faculty of national and international renown. The University enjoys an outstanding research relationship with Cold Spring Harbor and Brookhaven National Laboratories. State-of-the-art Cancer and Heart Centers serve the needs of Long Islanders and a NIH-funded General Clinical Research Center offers cutting-edge clinical research.

Housing

There is limited on-campus housing and most medical students share apartments or houses in the surrounding communities. Housing costs range from $400–$900 per month with a median rent of $600.

Application Process and Requirements 2010–2011

Primary Application Service: AMCAS
Earliest filing date: June 1, 2009
Latest filing date: December 15, 2009

Secondary Application Required?: Yes
Sent to: All applicants.
URL: www.stonybrookmedicalcenter.org/education/som_admissions.cfm
Fee: Yes, $100
Fee waiver available: Yes
Earliest filing date: June 15, 2009
Latest filing date: December 30, 2009

MCAT® required?: Yes
Latest MCAT® considered: September 2009
Oldest MCAT® considered: 2005

Early Decision Program: School does have EDP
Applicants notified: October 1, 2009
EDP available for: Both Residents and Non-residents

Regular Acceptance Notice
Earliest date: October 15, 2009
Latest date: Until class is full
Applicant's Response to Acceptance
Offer – Maximum Time: 15 days, unless otherwise specified

Requests for Deferred
Entrance Considered: Yes

Deposit to Hold Place in Class: Yes
Deposit (Resident): $100
Deposit (Non-resident): $100
Deposit due: With response to acceptance offer
Applied to tuition: Yes
Deposit refundable: Yes
Refundable by: May 15, 2010

Estimated number of new entrants: 124
EDP: 2, special program: 8

Start Month/Year: August 2010

Interview Format: Two individual interviews with admission committee members. Regional interviews are not available.

Other Programs

PREPARATORY PROGRAMS
Postbaccalaureate Program: Yes
Summer Program: No

COMBINED DEGREE PROGRAMS
Baccalaureate/M.D.: Yes www.stonybrook.edu/honors, www.wise.sunysb.edu, www.stonybrook.edu/ugadmissions/programs/engsfmed.shtml
M.D./M.P.H.: Yes, www.stonybrookmedicalcenter.org/education/public_health/
M.D./M.B.A.: No
M.D./J.D.: No
M.D./Ph.D.: www.pharm.stonybrook.edu/mstp/index.html

Premedical Coursework

Course	Req.	Rec.	Lab.	Qtrs.
Inorganic Chemistry	•		•	2
Behavioral Sciences				
Biochemistry		•		1
Biology	•		•	2
Biology/Zoology				
Calculus				
College English	•			2
College Mathematics				

Course	Req.	Rec.	Lab.	Qtrs.
Computer Science				
Genetics				
Humanities				
Organic Chemistry	•		•	2
Physics	•		•	2
Psychology				
Social Sciences				
Other				

Selection Factors: 2008 Accepted Applicants

Proportion of Accepted Applicants with Relevant Experience (Data Self-Reported to AMCAS®)		
Community Service/Volunteer		63%
Medically-Related Work		89%
Research		88%

Shaded bar represents school's accepted scores ranging from the 10th percentile to the 90th percentile   School Median ●   National Median ●

Overall GPA	2.0	2.1	2.2	2.3	2.4	2.5	2.6	2.7	2.8	2.9	3.0	3.1	3.2	3.3	3.4	3.5	3.6	(3.7)	3.8	3.9	4.0
Science GPA	2.0	2.1	2.2	2.3	2.4	2.5	2.6	2.7	2.8	2.9	3.0	3.1	3.2	3.3	3.4	3.5	3.6	(3.7)	3.8	3.9	4.0

MCAT® Total Numeric Score 9 10 11 12 13 14 15 16 17 18 19 20 21 22 23 24 25 26 27 28 29 30 31 (32)(33) 34 35 36 37 38 39 40 41 42 43

Writing Sample			J	K	L	M	N	O	P	(Q)	R	S	T
Verbal Reasoning	3	4	5	6	7	8	9	(10)	11	12	13	14	15
Biological Sciences	3	4	5	6	7	8	9	10	(11)	12	13	14	15
Physical Sciences	3	4	5	6	7	8	9	10	(11)	12	13	14	15

Acceptance & Matriculation Data for 2008–2009 First Year Class

	Resident	Non-resident	International	Total
Applications	2010	1481	208	3699
Interviewed	497	115	0	612
Deferred	3	0	0	3
Matriculants				
Early Assurance Program	n/a	n/a	n/a	n/a
Early Decision Program	0	0	0	0
Baccalaureate/M.D.	2	0	0	2
M.D./Ph.D.	5	0	0	5
Matriculated	105	19	0	**124**

Applications accepted from International Applicants: No

Matriculant Demographics: 2008–2009 First Year Class

Men: 67   **Women:** 57

Matriculants' Self-Reported Race/Ethnicity

Mexican American	0	**Korean**	5
Cuban	6	**Vietnamese**	0
Puerto Rican	1	**Other Asian**	6
Other Hispanic	2	**Total Asian**	35
Total Hispanic	8	**Native American**	1
Chinese	10	**Black**	12
Asian Indian	11	**Native Hawaiian**	0
Pakistani	2	**White**	72
Filipino	2	**Unduplicated Number**	
Japanese	1	**of Matriculants**	124

Science and Math Majors: 66%
Matriculants with:
   Baccalaureate degree: 100%
   Graduate degree(s): 11%

Specialty Choice

2004, 2005, 2006 Graduates, Specialty Choice (As reported by program directors to GME Track™)	
Anesthesiology	8%
Emergency Medicine	8%
Family Practice	4%
Internal Medicine	24%
Obstetrics/Gynecology	5%
Orthopaedic Surgery	2%
Pediatrics	9%
Psychiatry	5%
Radiology	4%
Surgery	10%

Financial Information

Source: 2007–2008 LCME I-B survey and 2008–2009 AAMC TSF questionnaire

	Residents	Non-residents
Total Cost of Attendance	$44,818	$61,753
Tuition and Fees	$21,263	$38,198
Other (includes living expenses)	$20,765	$20,765
Health Insurance (can be waived)	$2,790	$2,790

Average 2008 Graduate Indebtedness: $139,175
% of Enrolled Students Receiving Aid: 84%

Criminal Background Check

This medical school requires a criminal background check prior to matriculation.

University of Rochester School of Medicine and Dentistry

Rochester, New York

Director of Admissions, University of Rochester
School of Medicine and Dentistry
601 Elmwood Avenue, Box 601A
Rochester, New York 14642
T 585 275 4539 F 585 756 5479

Admissions www.urmc.rochester.edu/education/
md/admissions
Main www.urmc.rochester.edu/
Financial www.urmc.rochester.edu/education/
financial-aid
E-mail mdadmish@urmc.rochester.edu

Private Institution

Dr. David S. Guzick, Dean

*Dr. John T. Hansen, Associate Dean
for Admissions*

*Adrienne Morgan, Senior Director, Center
for Advocacy, Community Health,
Education and Diversity*

Nancy Janson, Director, Financial Aid

Patricia Samuelson, Director of Admissions

General Information

The School of Medicine and Dentistry is an academic division of the University of Rochester, a privately endowed institution founded in 1850. The Medical Center includes the School of Medicine and Dentistry, School of Nursing, Eastman Dental Center, James P. Wilmot Cancer Center, Strong Memorial Hospital, and Golisano Children's Hospital at Strong.

Mission Statement

As the home of the biopsychosocial model, Rochester offers a student-centered educational program that prepares physicians for the 21st century. The curriculum fosters knowledge, skills, attitudes, and behaviors of the physician/scientist/humanist by combining cutting-edge, evidence-based medical science with the relationship-centered art that is medicine's distinctive trademark.

Curricular Highlights

Community Service Requirement: Required. Community Health Improvement Clerkship.
Research/Thesis Requirement: Optional. Graduate with "Distinction in Research" honors.

Rochester's Double Helix Curriculum captures the integrated strands of basic science and clinical medicine as they are woven throughout the four-year curriculum. The focus of the educational program is not merely the transfer of information, but the transformation of the learner in a culture providing that ingenious combination of support and challenge, which leads to education. Courses are interdisciplinary and clinical exposure begins during the first week of school with an introduction to clinical medicine and the start of the ambula-

tory care clerkship during the first spring semester. Inpatient clerkships focus on acute care experiences in adult medicine, women's and children's health, mind/brain/behavior, and urgent/emergent care. A formal tutoring system and assistance programs are available. A rich menu of opportunities is available to students, including a strong M.D./Ph.D. program (MSTP), a five-year Academic Research Track, Medical Humanities selectives, and community and international medicine experiences.

USMLE

Step 1: Required. Students must only record a score.
Step 2: Clinical Skills (CS): Required. Students must only record a score.
Step 2: Clinical Knowledge (CK): Required. Students must only record a score.

Selection Factors

Evaluation of applicants includes a careful examination of the entire academic record, letters of recommendation, and the candidate's personal statement. Demonstrated excellence in a demanding academic program, including a high level of achievement in the natural sciences, is a requirement for acceptance. Evidence of intrinsic intellectual drive and curiosity is highly valued since the program at Rochester emphasizes independent learning opportunities for individual students. Particular attention is given to achievements that demonstrate breadth and commitment, especially in areas of research, outreach, and clinical experience.

Financial Aid

The medical school offers scholarships and long-term loans to those students who demonstrate financial need. Entering students applying for institutional financial aid are required to provide a FAFSA, a more detailed financial statement including parent information, and the School of Medicine's financial aid application.

Information about Diversity Programs

The Center for Advocacy, Community Health, Education and Diversity represents a serious commitment on the part of the School of Medicine and Dentistry to meet the urgent need for diverse physicians in all aspects of the

medical profession. Rochester believes that a diverse class enriches the educational environment for all of its students. The office also coordinates numerous academic and cultural events for the education of all students.

Campus Information

Setting

The Medical Center is located adjacent to the University of Rochester which enrolls about 4,450 undergraduates and 3,890 graduate students. The Medical Center has new education and research facilities. Three affiliated hospitals, regional Veterans Affairs clinics, and community health centers are in close proximity to the Medical Center. The metropolitan area includes 1.1 million residents and is located in the scenic Finger Lakes region of upstate New York.

Enrollment

For 2008, total enrollment was: 395

Special Features

The University is consistently ranked among the top 30 institutions in federal funding for research and development, and it owns the Strong Memorial Hospital, which is a major referral center for upstate New York.

Housing

Campus housing is available and assigned by lottery; high quality, affordable housing is also located within a short distance of the Medical Center.

Satellite Campuses/Facilities

Students also rotate through three affiliated hospitals and community and private ambulatory clinics within a short distance of the Medical Center. Both inner city and rural clinic/hospital experiences are offered.

Application Process and Requirements 2010–2011

Primary Application Service: AMCAS
Earliest filing date: June 1, 2009
Latest filing date: October 15, 2009

Secondary Application Required?: Yes
Sent to: All applicants
URL: https://admissions.urmc.rochester.edu/StudentLogin.cfm
Fee: Yes, $75
Fee waiver available: Yes, (AMCAS FAP)
Earliest filing date: June 29, 2009
Latest filing date: November 15, 2009

MCAT® required?: Yes
Latest MCAT® considered: September 2009
Oldest MCAT® considered: August 2006

Early Decision Program: School does not have EDP
Applicants notified: n/a
EDP available for: n/a

Regular Acceptance Notice
Earliest date: October 15, 2009
Latest date: Until class is full
Applicant's Response to Acceptance Offer – Maximum Time: Two weeks

Requests for Deferred Entrance Considered: Yes

Deposit to Hold Place in Class: Yes
Deposit (Resident): $100
Deposit (Non-resident): $100
Deposit due: With response to acceptance offer
Applied to tuition: Yes
Deposit refundable: Yes
Refundable by: May 15, 2010

Estimated number of new entrants: 100
EDP: 0, special program: 12

Start Month/Year: August 2010

Interview Format: Two interviews.

Regional interviews are not available.

Other Programs

PREPARATORY PROGRAMS
Postbaccalaureate Program: No
Summer Program: No
One week pre-matriculation course:
John Hansen, (585) 275-4606,
John_Hansen@urmc.rochester.edu

COMBINED DEGREE PROGRAMS
Baccalaureate/M.D.: Yes, http://enrollment.rochester.edu/admissions/learning/programs.shtm
M.D./M.P.H.: Yes, www.urmc.rochester.edu/education/md/joint-degree.cfm
M.D./M.B.A.: Yes, www.urmc.rochester.edu/education/md/joint-degree.cfm
M.D./J.D.: No
M.D./Ph.D.: Yes, www.urmc.rochester.edu/education/md/joint-degree.cfm

Premedical Coursework

Course	Req.	Rec.	Lab.	Sems.
Inorganic Chemistry	•	•		2
Behavioral Sciences				
Biochemistry		•		
Biology				
Biology/Zoology	•		•	2
Calculus				
College English	•			2
College Mathematics				

Course	Req.	Rec.	Lab.	Sems.
Genetics		•		
Humanities	•			2
Organic Chemistry	•		•	2
Physics	•		•	2
Psychology				
Social Sciences	•			2
Anatomy/Physiology		•		
Biostatistics		•		

Selection Factors: 2008 Accepted Applicants

Proportion of Accepted Applicants with Relevant Experience (Data Self-Reported to AMCAS®)		
Community Service/Volunteer		73%
Medically-Related Work		84%
Research		88%

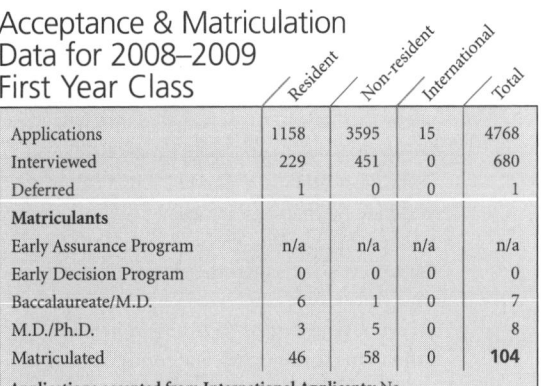

Shaded bar represents school's accepted scores ranging from the 10th percentile to the 90th percentile ■ School Median ● National Median ●

Overall GPA 2.0 2.1 2.2 2.3 2.4 2.5 2.6 2.7 2.8 2.9 3.0 3.1 3.2 3.3 **3.4** 3.5 3.6 3.7 (3.8) 3.9 4.0
Science GPA 2.0 2.1 2.2 2.3 2.4 2.5 2.6 2.7 2.8 2.9 3.0 3.1 3.2 **3.3** 3.4 3.5 3.6 (3.7) 3.8 3.9 4.0

MCAT® Total Numeric Score 9 10 11 12 13 14 15 16 17 18 19 20 21 22 23 24 25 26 27 28 29 30 31 (32) 33 (34) 35 36 37 38 39 40 41 42 43

Writing Sample			J	K	L	M	N	O	P	(Q)	R	S	T
Verbal Reasoning	3	4	5	6	7	8	9	(10)	(11)	12	13	14	15
Biological Sciences	3	4	5	6	7	8	9	10	(11)	(12)	13	14	15
Physical Sciences	3	4	5	6	7	8	9	10	(11)	12	13	14	15

Acceptance & Matriculation Data for 2008–2009 First Year Class

	Resident	Non-resident	International	Total
Applications	1158	3595	15	4768
Interviewed	229	451	0	680
Deferred	1	0	0	1
Matriculants				
Early Assurance Program	n/a	n/a	n/a	n/a
Early Decision Program	0	0	0	0
Baccalaureate/M.D.	6	1	0	7
M.D./Ph.D.	3	5	0	8
Matriculated	46	58	0	**104**

Applications accepted from International Applicants: No

Matriculant Demographics: 2008–2009 First Year Class

Men: 50 **Women:** 54

Matriculants' Self-Reported Race/Ethnicity

Mexican American	2	Korean	3	
Cuban	0	Vietnamese	2	
Puerto Rican	2	Other Asian	0	
Other Hispanic	6	Total Asian	17	
Total Hispanic	10	Native American	0	
Chinese	9	Black	12	
Asian Indian	1	Native Hawaiian	0	
Pakistani	1	White	69	
Filipino	0	Unduplicated Number		
Japanese	2	of Matriculants	104	

Science and Math Majors: 63%
Matriculants with:
   Baccalaureate degree: 100%
   Graduate degree(s): 7%

Specialty Choice

2004, 2005, 2006 Graduates, Specialty Choice (As reported by program directors to GME Track™)	
Anesthesiology	5%
Emergency Medicine	5%
Family Practice	3%
Internal Medicine	19%
Obstetrics/Gynecology	4%
Orthopaedic Surgery	3%
Pediatrics	14%
Psychiatry	5%
Radiology	5%
Surgery	7%

Financial Information

Source: 2007–2008 LCME I-B survey and 2008–2009 AAMC TSF questionnaire

	Residents	Non-residents
Total Cost of Attendance	$58,132	$58,132
Tuition and Fees	$40,204	$40,204
Other (includes living expenses)	$16,735	$16,735
Health Insurance (can be waived)	$1,193	$1,193

Average 2008 Graduate Indebtedness: $142,554
% of Enrolled Students Receiving Aid: 90%

Criminal Background Check

This medical school requires a criminal background check prior to matriculation.

The Brody School of Medicine at East Carolina University

Greenville, North Carolina

Associate Dean, Office of Admissions
The Brody School of Medicine
at East Carolina University
Greenville, North Carolina 27834
T 252 744 2202   **F** 252 744 1926

Admissions www.ecu.edu/bsomadmissions
Main www.ecu.edu/med
Financial www.ecu.edu/cs-dhs/bsomstudentaffairs/
Financial-Aid.cfm
E-mail somadmissions@ecu.edu

Public Institution

Dr. Paul R. G. Cunningham, Dean

Dr. James G. Peden Jr.,
Associate Dean for Admissions

Dr. Virginia D. Hardy, Senior Associate
Dean for Academic Affairs

Kelly Lancaster, Director of
Financial Aid and Student Services

Lynn S. Coward, Director of Admissions

General Information

In 1972, East Carolina University enrolled students in the First-Year Program in Medical Education. The Board of Governors and the State General Assembly authorized the expansion to a degree-granting School of Medicine in 1975, and the first class was enrolled in August 1977. The school's educational facilities are located in the nine-story Brody Medical Sciences Building on the 100-acre Health Sciences Center campus.

Mission Statement

Our mission is threefold: educating primary care physicians, making medical care more readily available to the people of eastern North Carolina, and providing opportunities for disadvantaged students.

Curricular Highlights

Community Service Requirement: Optional.
Research/Thesis Requirement: Optional.

The first year of the four-year curriculum is devoted to the study of the body through courses in anatomy, biochemistry, physiology, microbiology/immunology, and genetics. Courses in clinical skills, the psychosocial basis of medicine, and ethical and social issues in medicine and a primary care preceptorship are also presented. The second-year curriculum is directed toward clinical medicine, with courses including microbiology, pharmacology, pathology, psychiatry (including human sexuality and lifestyle abuse), ethical and social issues, clinical skills, and a primary care preceptorship. The third year is composed of six required clerkships in family medicine, internal medicine, obstetrics and gynecology, pedi-

atrics, psychiatry, and surgery and a two-week clinical elective. The fourth year is composed of 36 weeks of clinical and basic science electives, which must include blocks in primary care, medicine, and surgery. Student performance is evaluated by letter grade, and promotion to the next year's class is recommended to the Dean by the Promotions Committee of the respective year.

USMLE

Step 1: Required. Students must record a passing score for promotion.
Step 2: Clinical Skills (CS): Required. Students must record a passing total score to graduate.
Step 2: Clinical Knowledge (CK): Required. Students must record a passing total score to graduate.

Selection Factors

Factors considered in the selection process encompass the social, personal, and intellectual development of each applicant. All available application data are evaluated: MCAT scores; academic performance; comments contained in letters of reference/recommendation; and (for invited applicants) the results of two personal interviews, conducted only at the medical school campus, with two members of the Admissions Committee. The Brody School of Medicine at East Carolina University seeks competent students of diverse personalities and backgrounds, and all applicants are evaluated without discrimination based on race, religion, sex, color, national origin, age, or disability. Very strong preference is given to qualified residents of North Carolina. In conjunction with the undergraduate Office of Admissions, the Brody School of Medicine offers an Early Assurance Program for highly qualified high school seniors. Selected scholars enroll in the University and are assured of a spot in the medical school class after receiving their baccalaureate degree (provided certain academic standards are maintained). Qualified North Carolina residents from schools with similar medical curricula may be considered for transfer into the second- or third-year classes, but advanced standing positions are dependent on the very limited number of seats that become available through attrition. Interested students should send letters describ-

ing their circumstances to the Office of Admissions for further information.

Financial Aid

Many resources are available for loans and scholarships. Information on financial aid is given to every interviewee and accepted students who demonstrate a need for financial aid are given personal assistance in acquiring funds to meet the costs of their educational and living expenses. Awards are based on need as determined by confidential information supplied by the student. Merit awards, such as the Brody Medical Scholars Program, are also available.

Information about Diversity Programs

Persons from groups underrepresented in medicine who hold residence in North Carolina are encouraged to apply. There is diverse membership on the Admissions Committee, and the Academic Support and Enrichment Center offers a wide range of services to students desiring assistance or guidance.

Campus Information

Setting

The medical school is located in the 100-acre medical district and is adjacent to the primary clinical training site, Pitt County Memorial Hospital. Greenville is a short drive from several beaches, sounds, and other recreational areas.

Enrollment

For 2008, total enrollment was: 293

Special Features

The medical school houses an international robotic surgery training center and several clinical Centers of Excellence. A $180 million regional research center for cardiovascular disease, the East Carolina Heart Institute, will be completed in 2009. The newly-founded dental school is scheduled to begin operation in 2011.

Housing

There are many apartments, duplexes, and houses near the medical school.

Application Process and Requirements 2010–2011

Primary Application Service: AMCAS
Earliest filing date: June 1, 2009
Latest filing date: November 15, 2009

Secondary Application Required?: Yes
Sent to: All NC applicants
Contact: somadmissions@ecu.edu
Fee: Yes, $60
Fee waiver available: Yes
Earliest filing date: July 1, 2009
Latest filing date: November 15, 2009 or 2 weeks after receipt of AMCAS

MCAT® required?: Yes
Latest MCAT® considered: September 2009
Oldest MCAT® considered: April 2006

Early Decision Program: School does have EDP
Applicants notified: October 1, 2009
EDP available for: Residents only

Regular Acceptance Notice
Earliest date: October 15, 2009
Latest date: Varies
Applicant's Response to Acceptance Offer – Maximum Time: Three weeks

Requests for Deferred Entrance Considered: No

Deposit to Hold Place in Class: Yes
Deposit (Resident): $100
Deposit (Non-resident): $100
Deposit due: With response to acceptance offer
Applied to tuition: Yes
Deposit refundable: Yes
Refundable by: May 15, 2010

Estimated number of new entrants: 80
EDP: 8, special program: n/a

Start Month/Year: August 2010

Interview Format: Two semi-blind interviews by committee members. All interviews are conducted at the medical school.

Other Programs

PREPARATORY PROGRAMS
Postbaccalaureate Program: No
Summer Program: Yes www.ecu.edu/cs-dhs/ascc/SPFD.cfm

COMBINED DEGREE PROGRAMS
Baccalaureate/M.D.: No
M.D./M.P.H.: Yes, www.ecu.edu/mph
M.D./M.B.A.: Yes, www.ecu.edu/cs-dhs/med/MD_MBA.cfm
M.D./J.D.: No
M.D./Ph.D.: Yes, www.ecu.edu/cs-dhs/med/MD_PhD.cfm

Premedical Coursework

Course	Req.	Rec.	Lab.	Hrs.
Inorganic Chemistry	•		•	8
Behavioral Sciences				
Biochemistry				
Biology				
Biology/Zoology	•		•	8
Calculus				
College English	•			6
College Mathematics				

Course	Req.	Rec.	Lab.	Hrs.
Computer Science				
Genetics		•		
Humanities		•		
Organic Chemistry	•		•	8
Physics	•		•	8
Psychology				
Social Sciences		•		
Biostatistics				

Selection Factors: 2008 Accepted Applicants

Proportion of Accepted Applicants with Relevant Experience (Data Self-Reported to AMCAS®)		
Community Service/Volunteer		82%
Medically-Related Work		89%
Research		73%

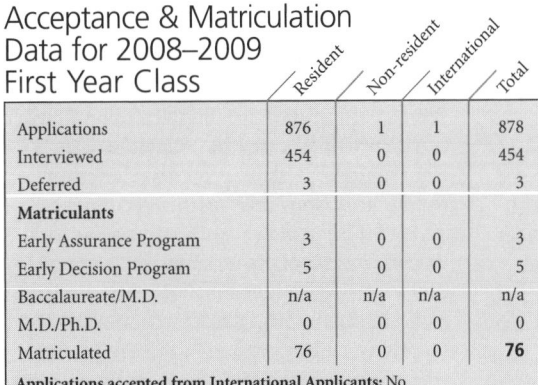

Shaded bar represents school's accepted scores ranging from the 10th percentile to the 90th percentile. School Median ● National Median ●

Overall GPA 2.0 2.1 2.2 2.3 2.4 2.5 2.6 2.7 2.8 2.9 3.0 3.1 3.2 3.3 3.4 3.5 3.6 (3.7) 3.8 3.9 4.0
Science GPA 2.0 2.1 2.2 2.3 2.4 2.5 2.6 2.7 2.8 2.9 3.0 3.1 3.2 3.3 3.4 3.5 (3.6) 3.7 3.8 3.9 4.0

MCAT® Total Numeric Score 9 10 11 12 13 14 15 16 17 18 19 20 21 22 23 24 25 26 27 28 (29) 30 31 (32) 33 34 35 36 37 38 39 40 41 42 43

Writing Sample			J	K	L	M	N	O	P	(Q)	R	S	T	
Verbal Reasoning	3	4	5	6	7	8	(9)	(10)	11	12	13	14	15	
Biological Sciences	3	4	5	6	7	8	9	(10)	(11)	12	13	14	15	
Physical Sciences	3	4	5	6	7	8	9	(10)	(11)	12	13	14	15	

Acceptance & Matriculation Data for 2008–2009 First Year Class

	Resident	Non-resident	International	Total
Applications	876	1	1	878
Interviewed	454	0	0	454
Deferred	3	0	0	3
Matriculants				
Early Assurance Program	3	0	0	3
Early Decision Program	5	0	0	5
Baccalaureate/M.D.	n/a	n/a	n/a	n/a
M.D./Ph.D.	0	0	0	0
Matriculated	76	0	0	**76**

Applications accepted from International Applicants: No

Matriculant Demographics: 2008–2009 First Year Class

Men: 38   **Women:** 38

Matriculants' Self-Reported Race/Ethnicity

Mexican American	0	**Korean**	1
Cuban	0	**Vietnamese**	1
Puerto Rican	0	**Other Asian**	2
Other Hispanic	1	**Total Asian**	10
Total Hispanic	1	**Native American**	2
Chinese	1	**Black**	11
Asian Indian	4	**Native Hawaiian**	0
Pakistani	2	**White**	49
Filipino	0	**Unduplicated Number**	
Japanese	0	**of Matriculants**	76

Science and Math Majors: 70%
Matriculants with:
Baccalaureate degree: 97%
Graduate degree(s): 18%

Specialty Choice

2004, 2005, 2006 Graduates, Specialty Choice (As reported by program directors to GME Track™)	
Anesthesiology	0%
Emergency Medicine	8%
Family Practice	18%
Internal Medicine	15%
Obstetrics/Gynecology	7%
Orthopaedic Surgery	2%
Pediatrics	14%
Psychiatry	1%
Radiology	2%
Surgery	4%

Financial Information

Source: 2007–2008 LCME I-B survey and 2008–2009 AAMC TSF questionnaire

	Residents	Non-residents
Total Cost of Attendance	$29,613	$54,603
Tuition and Fees	$9,034	$34,024
Other (includes living expenses)	$19,379	$19,379
Health Insurance (can be waived)	$1,200	$1,200

Average 2008 Graduate Indebtedness: $71,455
% of Enrolled Students Receiving Aid: 89%

Criminal Background Check

This medical school requires a criminal background check prior to matriculation.

Duke University School of Medicine
Durham, North Carolina

Committee on Admissions
Duke University School of Medicine
DUMC 3710
Durham, North Carolina 27710
T 919 684 2985   **F** 919 668 3714

Admissions http://dukemed.duke.edu/modules/
flash_articles/
Main http://medschool.duke.edu/
Financial http://medschool.duke.edu/modules/
som_finaid/index.php?id=1
E-mail medadm@mc.duke.edu

Private Institution

Dr. Nancy C. Andrews, Dean

Dr. Brenda E. Armstrong, Associate Dean and Director of Admissions

Dr. Delbert R. Wigfall, Associate Dean, Medical Education Director, Multicultural Resource Center

Stacey R. McCorison, Associate Dean of Medical Education, Director of Financial Aid and Registrar

Richard S. Wallace, Associate Director of Admissions

General Information
Duke University Health System is a world-class health care network dedicated to outstanding patient care, innovative medical education and biomedical research.

Mission Statement
DukeMed is a community of scholars devoted to understanding the causes, prevention and treatment of human disease. Our missions are to train scholars and leaders across a broad spectrum of careers in medicine. These missions are undertaken by students from diverse communities committed to the highest of academic goals: the generation, conservation, and dissemination of knowledge leading to the prevention and eradication of human disease throughout the world through innovative curricula, outstanding resources in education, clinical care, and basic and clinical research.

Curricular Highlights
Community Service Requirement: Optional.
Research/Thesis Requirement: Required. Required to complete the third year of medical school.

The curriculum stimulates rapid expansion of medical knowledge. First-year students study basic science principles alongside the first of two-years' introduction to clinical medicine. The second year is the clinical clerkship year. The third and fourth years are elective including half basic science/half clinical coursework with opportunities for mentored research. Students also elect from a number of dual-degree pro-

grams which begin during the third year. The fourth year is an advanced clinical clerkship year to prepare for postgraduate study. The MST Program provides MD/Ph.D degrees over a six-to-seven-year period. It is expected that candidates for this combined degree plan will have careers in academic medicine.

USMLE
Step 1: Required. Students must only record a score.
Step 2: Clinical Skills (CS): Required. Students must only record a score.
Step 2: Clinical Knowledge (CK): Required. Students must only record a score.

Selection Factors
Selection is based on evidence of outstanding academic and experiential preparation, including but not limited to outstanding curricular/extracurricular achievement, evidence of leadership, participation in volunteer/community service activities, excellent oral and written communications skills, supportive letters of recommendations from teachers/advisors, strong MCAT scores, exposure to and/or participation in scholarly research and the applicant's interview evaluation. Successful students have high GPAs/MCAT scores, demonstrated leadership on campus and in their respective communities. Duke Med does not discriminate on the basis of sex, race, religion, sexual orientation, creed, age, handicap, or national origin.

Financial Aid
The Office of Financial Aid requires the Need Access, the federal government's FAFSA obtained via Internet. Students applying for only Federal Stafford Loans only complete the FAFSA. Students are encouraged to submit the applications as soon as possible after acceptance. Prior year tax returns should be submitted. Accepted students receive award notices once all forms are received. Students with demonstrated need applying for institutional funds will receive approximately 50% Stafford and/or Duke loans and 50% institutional grants. 85% of currently enrolled medical students receive some type of financial aid. Admissions is need-blind. Seven Dean's Tuition Scholarships are awarded to academically excellent students from groups underrepresented in medicine. Students who

enter the Medical Scientist Training Program receive full tuition, fees, and a stipend.

Information about Diversity Programs
The Multicultural Resource Center is a resource-intensive repository providing opportunities for diverse learning experiences for all students and targeted pipeline programs for women, URM/disadvantaged, and students interested in careers in healthcare and biomedical research beginning as early as elementary school through undergraduate and graduate education. MRC integrates cross-cultural issues in medicine to the medical school curriculum and within the entirety of the medical school.

Campus Information
Setting
DukeMed is physically contiguous with the main campus of Duke University. Durham is one of three communities part of the Research Triangle Park, one of the nation's most prolific research centers and one rich in cultural, educational, and recreational opportunities.

Enrollment
For 2008, total enrollment was: 404

Special Features
DukeMed is consistently ranked among the top ten academic health centers in the country and has a national and international reputation for innovation and excellence.

Housing
Students choose from a number of affordable on- and off-campus housing units. Housing costs are extremely affordable.

Satellite Campuses/Facilities
Students are based throughout the Duke Health System at Duke University Hospital, the VA Hospital, Durham Regional Hospital, Lennox Baker Children's Hospital, Duke Children's Hospital, and more than 70 outpatient clinics located in Durham, Raleigh, Chapel Hill and surrounding communities.

Application Process and Requirements 2010–2011

Primary Application Service: AMCAS
Earliest filing date: June 1, 2009
Latest filing date: November 2, 2009

Secondary Application Required?: Yes
Sent to: All applicants
URL: http://dukemed.duke.edu
Fee: Yes, $80
Fee waiver available: Yes
Earliest filing date: Once AMCAS has verified application.
Latest filing date: November 16, 2009

MCAT® required?: Yes
Latest MCAT® considered: September 2009
Oldest MCAT® considered: August 2006

Early Decision Program: School does not have EDP
Applicants notified: n/a
EDP available for: n/a

**Regular Acceptance Notice
Earliest date:** March 1, 2010
Latest date: Until class is full
**Applicant's Response to Acceptance
Offer – Maximum Time:** Two weeks

**Requests for Deferred
Entrance Considered:** Yes

Deposit to Hold Place in Class: Yes
Deposit (Resident): $100
Deposit (Non-resident): $100
Deposit due: May 15, 2010
Applied to tuition: Yes
Deposit refundable: Yes
Refundable by: May 15, 2010

Estimated number of new entrants: 100
EDP: n/a, special program: n/a

Start Month/Year: August 2, 2010

Interview Format: One-on-one interviews on campus. Virtual interviews will be offered as an option in selected cases. Regional interviews are available.

Other Programs

PREPARATORY PROGRAMS
Postbaccalaureate Program: No
Summer Program: Yes, www.smdep.org Maureen Cullins, (919) 684-5882 mcullins@duke.edu

COMBINED DEGREE PROGRAMS
Baccalaureate/M.D.: No
M.D./M.P.H.: Yes, http://dukemed.duke.edu
M.D./M.B.A.: Yes, http://dukemed.duke.edu
M.D./J.D.: Yes, http://dukemed.duke.edu
M.D./Ph.D.: Yes, http://dukemed.duke.edu

Premedical Coursework

Course	Req.	Rec.	Lab.	Sems.
Inorganic Chemistry	•		•	2
Behavioral Sciences				
Biochemistry		•		1
Biology	•		•	1
Biology/Zoology	•			1
Calculus	•			1
College English				2
College Mathematics	•			1
Computer Science				

Course	Req.	Rec.	Lab.	Sems.
Genetics		•		1
Humanities				
Organic Chemistry	•		•	2
Physics	•		•	2
Psychology				
Social Sciences				
Statistics/Biostatistics		•		1
Spanish		•		1
Cell Biology		•		1

Selection Factors: 2008 Accepted Applicants

Proportion of Accepted Applicants with Relevant Experience (Data Self-Reported to AMCAS®)		
Community Service/Volunteer		76%
Medically-Related Work		83%
Research		94%

Shaded bar represents school's accepted scores ranging from the 10th percentile to the 90th percentile   **School Median** ●   **National Median** ●

Overall GPA	2.0	2.1	2.2	2.3	2.4	2.5	2.6	2.7	2.8	2.9	3.0	3.1	3.2	3.3	3.4	3.5	3.6	3.7	(3.8)	3.9	4.0
Science GPA	2.0	2.1	2.2	2.3	2.4	2.5	2.6	2.7	2.8	2.9	3.0	3.1	3.2	3.3	3.4	3.5	3.6	3.7	(3.8)	3.9	4.0

MCAT® Total Numeric Score 9 10 11 12 13 14 15 16 17 18 19 20 21 22 23 24 25 26 27 28 29 30 31 (32) 33 34 35 (36) 37 38 39 40 41 42 43

Writing Sample			J	K	L	M	N	O	P	(Q)	R	S	T
Verbal Reasoning	3	4	5	6	7	8	9	(10)	(11)	12	13	14	15
Biological Sciences	3	4	5	6	7	8	9	10	(11)	12	(13)	14	15
Physical Sciences	3	4	5	6	7	8	9	10	(11)	12	(13)	14	15

Acceptance & Matriculation Data for 2008–2009 First Year Class

	Resident	Non-resident	International	Total
Applications	381	4506	314	5201
Interviewed	91	648	31	770
Deferred	1	3	0	4
Matriculants				
Early Assurance Program	0	0	0	0
Early Decision Program	0	0	0	0
Baccalaureate/M.D.	n/a	n/a	n/a	n/a
M.D./Ph.D.	1	5	0	6
Matriculated	12	82	6	**100**

Applications accepted from International Applicants: Yes

Matriculant Demographics: 2008–2009 First Year Class

Men: 52   **Women:** 48

Matriculants' Self-Reported Race/Ethnicity

Mexican American	0	**Korean**	0
Cuban	3	**Vietnamese**	2
Puerto Rican	1	**Other Asian**	3
Other Hispanic	0	**Total Asian**	25
Total Hispanic	3	**Native American**	0
Chinese	12	**Black**	18
Asian Indian	8	**Native Hawaiian**	0
Pakistani	0	**White**	49
Filipino	2	**Unduplicated Number**	
Japanese	1	**of Matriculants**	100

Science and Math Majors: 65%
Matriculants with:

Baccalaureate degree: 100%
Graduate degree(s): 12%

Specialty Choice

2004, 2005, 2006 Graduates, Specialty Choice (As reported by program directors to GME Track™)

Anesthesiology	4%
Emergency Medicine	3%
Family Practice	2%
Internal Medicine	26%
Obstetrics/Gynecology	3%
Orthopaedic Surgery	5%
Pediatrics	7%
Psychiatry	2%
Radiology	10%
Surgery	8%

Financial Information
Source: 2007–2008 LCME I-B survey and 2008–2009 AAMC TSF questionnaire

	Residents	Non-residents
Total Cost of Attendance	$67,138	$67,138
Tuition and Fees	$43,985	$43,985
Other (includes living expenses)	$21,589	$21,589
Health Insurance (can be waived)	$1,564	$1,564

Average 2008 Graduate Indebtedness: $103,403
% of Enrolled Students Receiving Aid: 91%

Criminal Background Check

This medical school requires a criminal background check prior to matriculation.

University of North Carolina at Chapel Hill School of Medicine

Chapel Hill, North Carolina

Office of Admissions
CB #9500 1001 Bondurant Hall, First Floor
University of North Carolina at Chapel Hill
School of Medicine
Chapel Hill, North Carolina 27599-9500
T 919 962 8331   F 919 966 9930

Admissions www.med.unc.edu/admit
Main www.med.unc.edu
Financial www.med.unc.edu/md/financial-aid
E-mail Admis_UNC-SOM@listserv.med.unc.edu

Public Institution

Dr. William L. Roper, Dean,
Vice Chancellor for Medical Affairs

Dr. Robert A. Bashford,
Associate Dean for Admissions

Sheila M. Graham-McDonald,
Financial Aid Officer

Larry D. Keith, Assistant Dean for Admissions

General Information

The School of Medicine was established in 1879 and expanded to a four-year school in 1952. Other schools of health sciences are adjacent, allowing easy interaction and collaboration. The School of Medicine is continuing a major expansion and renovation of teaching and clinical facilities. Among other projects, three hospitals, Women's, Children's, and Neuroscience recently have been completed, and the North Carolina Cancer Hospital will be completed in 2009. Additional educational and clinical facilities are available throughout the State in Area Health Education Centers (AHEC) established in 1972 to provide clinical experiences and educational opportunities in community settings.

Mission Statement

The School of Medicine of the University of North Carolina at Chapel Hill exists to educate students and professionals of the health and biomedical sciences, to conduct scholarly investigation in biomedical, behavioral, and social sciences, and to render service to the people and institutions of the state, the region, the nation, and, as appropriate, throughout the world.

Curricular Highlights

Community Service Requirement: Optional.
Research/Thesis Requirement: Optional.

The curriculum offers an education that reflects our mission. The first year presents courses in basic biomedical science. Presentation is through a compilation of lectures, problem and case based small-group sessions, and electronic resource materials. Introduction to the profession of medicine begins in the first week of the first year through Introduction to Clinical Medicine (ICM). ICM provides a two-year continuum of weekly small-group seminars and experience

with simulated and real patients. A second weekly first-year seminar, Medicine and Society, focuses on health care issues. The second year presents the pathophysiology of disease in organ-based courses. Clinical skills development continues through the second year of ICM, and issues in social aspects of health care are presented through selectives offered by the Department of Social Medicine. The third and fourth year present a 2-year continuum of instruction in clinical medicine. Core clinical rotations, which are primarily completed in the third year, include internal medicine, surgery, family medicine, obstetrics and gynecology, pediatrics, and psychiatry. Some rotations are at AHEC sites. The advanced clinical curriculum of the 4th year builds more independence and increased responsibility into the base of the core. Students are assisted in choosing their interest in post graduate training through counseling and a broad choice of electives. Students conduct research with faculty mentorship support by school or grant funding, or through selection to the Distinguished Medical Scholars or Doris Duke programs (a year of funded study and research). Students pursue interests in rural and community medicine, public policy, or public health through Social Medicine selectives, fourth year Advance Practice Selectives, and Community Health Projects. The grading system is honors/pass/fail.

USMLE

Step 1: Required. Students must record a passing score for promotion.
Step 2: Clinical Skills (CS): Required. Students must only record a score.
Step 2: Clinical Knowledge (CK): Required. Students must record a passing total score to graduate.

Selection Factors

The Committee on Admissions evaluates the qualifications of all applicants to select those with the greatest potential for accomplishment in one of the many careers open to medical graduates. Preference is given to North Carolina residents. UNC does not discriminate on the basis of race, national origin, religion, sex, age, or handicap. In making its final selections from the group of qualified applicants, the committee considers evidence of each candidate's motivation,

maturity, leadership, integrity, and a variety of other personal qualifications and accomplishments in addition to the scholastic record. All information available about each applicant is considered without assigning priority to any single factor. No special admission tracks or quotas are applied among applicants. Undergraduate major is not an important consideration, but excellence in the chosen field is expected. Re-applications are compared to those previously submitted.

Financial Aid

Grants, school-based and Stafford loans are available to students with financial need. Awards are based on information obtained from the Free Application for Federal Student Aid (FAFSA) submitted by the student. A few scholarships are awarded for academic achievement and promise. Economically or environmentally disadvantaged state residents are eligible to apply to the Board of Governors Medical Scholarship-Loan Program. For more information call (919) 962-6118.

Information about Diversity Programs

The Medical Education Development Program acquaints disadvantaged students with the medical school curriculum and faculty. Academic counseling, including tutorial programs, the Learning and Assessment Laboratory, and other resources, are available. Summer review programs are also available.

Campus Information

Enrollment

For 2008, total enrollment was: 732

Application Process and Requirements 2010–2011

Primary Application Service: AMCAS
Earliest filing date: June 1, 2009
Latest filing date: November 15, 2009

Secondary Application Required?: Yes
Sent to: Screened applicants
URL: n/a
Fee: Yes, $68
Fee waiver available: Yes
Earliest filing date: August 1, 2009
Latest filing date: January 1, 2010

MCAT® required?: Yes
Latest MCAT® considered: September 2009
Oldest MCAT® considered: 2005

Early Decision Program: School does have EDP
Applicants notified: October 1, 2009
EDP available for: Both Residents and Non-residents

Regular Acceptance Notice
Earliest date: October 15, 2009
Latest date: Until class is full
Applicant's Response to Acceptance Offer – Maximum Time: Three weeks

Requests for Deferred Entrance Considered: Yes

Deposit to Hold Place in Class: Yes
Deposit (Resident): $100
Deposit (Non-resident): $100
Deposit due: With response to acceptance offer
Applied to tuition: Yes
Deposit refundable: Yes
Refundable by: May 15, 2010

Estimated number of new entrants: 160
EDP: 3, special program: 0

Start Month/Year: August 2010

Interview Format: One-on-one, open file. Regional interviews are not available.

Other Programs

PREPARATORY PROGRAMS
Postbaccalaureate Program: No
Summer Program: No

Combined Degree Programs
Baccalaureate/M.D.: No
M.D./M.P.H.: Yes, Available after completion of first two years.
M.D./M.B.A.: No
M.D./J.D.: No
M.D./Ph.D.: Yes, www.med.unc.edu/mdphd
Alison Regan, (919) 843-6507
aregan@med.unc.edu

Premedical Coursework

Course	Req.	Rec.	Lab.	Sems.	Course	Req.	Rec.	Lab.	Sems.
Inorganic Chemistry	•		•	8	Computer Science				
Behavioral Sciences					Genetics		•		
Biochemistry		•			Humanities		•		
Biology	•		•	7	Organic Chemistry	•		•	8
Biology/Zoology					Physics	•		•	8
Calculus					Psychology				
College English	•			6	Social Sciences		•		
College Mathematics					Other				

Selection Factors: 2008 Accepted Applicants

Proportion of Accepted Applicants with Relevant Experience (Data Self-Reported to AMCAS®)		
Community Service/Volunteer		74%
Medically-Related Work		90%
Research		83%

Shaded bar represents school's accepted scores ranging from the 10th percentile to the 90th percentile   School Median ●   National Median ●

Overall GPA	2.0	2.1	2.2	2.3	2.4	2.5	2.6	2.7	2.8	2.9	3.0	3.1	3.2	3.3	3.4	3.5	3.6	(3.7)	3.8	3.9	4.0
Science GPA	2.0	2.1	2.2	2.3	2.4	2.5	2.6	2.7	2.8	2.9	3.0	3.1	3.2	3.3	3.4	3.5	3.6	(3.7)	3.8	3.9	4.0

MCAT® Total Numeric Score 9 10 11 12 13 14 15 16 17 18 19 20 21 22 23 24 25 26 27 28 29 30 31 (32)(33) 34 35 36 37 38 39 40 41 42 43

Writing Sample				J	K	L	M	N	O	P	(Q)	R	S	T
Verbal Reasoning	3	4	5	6	7	8	9	(10)	(11)	12	13	14	15
Biological Sciences	3	4	5	6	7	8	9	10	(11)	12	13	14	15
Physical Sciences	3	4	5	6	7	8	9	10	(11)	12	13	14	15

Acceptance & Matriculation Data for 2008–2009 First Year Class

	Resident	Non-resident	International	Total
Applications	909	2949	164	4022
Interviewed	470	101	0	571
Deferred	4	1	0	5
Matriculants				
Early Assurance Program	n/a	n/a	n/a	n/a
Early Decision Program	3	0	0	3
Baccalaureate/M.D.	n/a	n/a	n/a	n/a
M.D./Ph.D.	13	35	0	48
Matriculated	135	25	0	**160**

Applications accepted from International Applicants: Canadian Only

Matriculant Demographics: 2008–2009 First Year Class

Men: 74   **Women:** 86

Matriculants' Self-Reported Race/Ethnicity

Mexican American	1	**Korean**	0
Cuban	0	**Vietnamese**	2
Puerto Rican	0	**Other Asian**	0
Other Hispanic	2	**Total Asian**	15
Total Hispanic	3	**Native American**	1
Chinese	7	**Black**	23
Asian Indian	5	**Native Hawaiian**	0
Pakistani	2	**White**	123
Filipino	0	**Unduplicated Number**	
Japanese	0	**of Matriculants**	160

Science and Math Majors: 59%
Matriculants with:
   Baccalaureate degree: 100%
   Graduate degree(s): 13%

Specialty Choice

2004, 2005, 2006 Graduates, Specialty Choice (As reported by program directors to GME Track™)	
Anesthesiology	6%
Emergency Medicine	6%
Family Practice	12%
Internal Medicine	18%
Obstetrics/Gynecology	5%
Orthopaedic Surgery	4%
Pediatrics	14%
Psychiatry	7%
Radiology	2%
Surgery	5%

Financial Information

Source: 2007–2008 LCME I-B survey and 2008–2009 AAMC TSF questionnaire

	Residents	Non-residents
Total Cost of Attendance	$39,564	$63,630
Tuition and Fees	$12,936	$37,002
Other (includes living expenses)	$24,828	$24,828
Health Insurance (can be waived)	$1,800	$1,800

Average 2008 Graduate Indebtedness: $100,090
% of Enrolled Students Receiving Aid: 85%

Criminal Background Check

This medical school requires a criminal background check prior to matriculation.

Wake Forest University School of Medicine

Winston-Salem, North Carolina

Office of Medical School Admissions
Wake Forest University School of Medicine
Medical Center Boulevard
Winston-Salem, North Carolina 27157-1090
T 336 716 4264   **F** 336 716 9593

Admissions www1.wfubmc.edu/MDProgram/
Admissions
Main www.wfubmc.edu/school
Financial www1.wfubmc.edu/FinancialAid
E-mail medadmit@wfubmc.edu

Private Institution

Dr. William B. Applegate, President and Dean

*Dr. Lewis H. Nelson III, Associate Dean
for Admissions*

*Dr. Brenda Latham-Sadler,
Assistant Dean, Director Diversity and
Development Initiatives*

Melissa Stevens, Financial Aid Director

Irene B. Tise, Coordinator, Student Admissions

General Information

The School of Medicine was established in 1902 at Wake Forest, North Carolina, and, of the existing 166 medical schools, it was one of 11 that required college preparation. Patient care, research, education, and community service remain the fourfold mission of the school as part of Wake Forest University. The name of the medical school was changed from The Bowman Gray School of Medicine to Wake Forest University School of Medicine, the Bowman Gray Campus, in 1997. The main teaching hospital of the medical school is the 880-bed North Carolina Baptist Hospital. Affiliated institutions include the 896-bed Forsyth Memorial Hospital, the Downtown Health Plaza of Baptist Hospital, and Northwest Area Health Education Center.

Mission Statement

The Medical Center is committed to serving society by providing a superior education; by rendering exemplary and efficient patient care; by fostering the discovery and application of new knowledge through research; and to improve the health and well-being of the nation.

Curricular Highlights

Community Service Requirement: Optional.
Research/Thesis Requirement: Optional.

WFUSM provides excellence in teaching in a collegial atmosphere. The curriculum is organized to meet the seven goals of the undergraduate medical education program: self-directed learning and life-long learning skills, core biomedical science knowledge, clinical skills, problem-solving/clinical-reasoning skills, interviewing and communication skills, informa-

tion management skills, and professional attitudes and behavior. Students study the basic and clinical sciences in an integrated fashion throughout the four-year curriculum utilizing small-group case centered learning, lectures, and labs which are closely integrated through the computer network. Early community-based clinical experience, as well as a focus on population health, are hallmarks of the curriculum. Professionalism issues are addressed longitudinally across the curriculum in formats designed to provide students with a clear understanding of the role and responsibilities of physicians within society. Information technology is integrated into the curriculum.

USMLE

Step 1: Required. Students must record a passing score for promotion.
Step 2: Clinical Skills (CS): Required. Students must record a passing total score to graduate.
Step 2: Clinical Knowledge (CK): Required. Students must record a passing total score to graduate.

Selection Factors

Candidates are selected on the basis of the quality of their academic records, MCAT scores, and general qualifications. There are no restrictions because of race, creed, sex, religion, age, physical disadvantages, marital status, or national origin. The Committee on Admissions (CoA) and/or the Associate Dean for Admissions evaluate each application. Secondary applications are selectively sent and all other applicants notified of their status. Applicants with completed secondaries are considered for interviews at the medical school. The School of Medicine may be able to accept an application for transfer from a student who is currently enrolled, and in good standing, in a medical school accredited by the Liaison Committee on Medical Education and who meets the prerequisite requirements. Early assurance of a place in medical school is offered to rising juniors who meet certain stringent requirements in an Early Assurance Program (EAP). More detailed information can be found on the Web site or by inquiry to the admissions office.

Financial Aid

Loans and scholarships are awarded to qualified applicants on the basis of financial need and academic standing. Applicants must complete required application forms prior to the April 1 deadline. Students receive a significant amount of their funding from federal student loan programs. Students should not work part-time because of the demands of medical study.

Information about Diversity Programs

The Office of Student Services/Diversity and Development Initiatives actively recruits students from groups underrepresented in medicine and has developed programs for academic enrichment, academic reinforcement, tutorial, and counseling services for enrolled students. Address inquiries to the Office of Diversity and Development Initiatives.

Campus Information

Setting

The school is located in a stable neighborhood near the heart of Winston-Salem, adjacent to hospital and medical facilities.

Enrollment

For 2008, total enrollment was: 465

Special Features

The Wake Forest University Health Sciences and the NC Baptist Hospital-associated medical center has more than 1,000 research studies and clinical trials underway, is home to NC's only Gamma Knife, and is establishing a 200-acre downtown research campus in biotechnology. One of the first tenants on the downtown campus is The Institute for Regenerative Medicine, where staff are working to grow 20 different organs and tissue types. The Anatomical Resource Clinical Training Center is a newly designed multidisciplinary learning center providing computational resources and both CT and MRI data acquired from actual cadavers dissected.

Housing

Available in the community surrounding the medical center. Listings are on Web site.

Application Process and Requirements 2010–2011

Primary Application Service: AMCAS
Earliest filing date: June 1, 2009
Latest filing date: November 1, 2009

Secondary Application Required?: Yes
Sent to: Screened applicants
E-mail: medadmit@wfubmc.edu
Fee: Yes, $55
Fee waiver available: Yes
Earliest filing date: July 15, 2009
Latest filing date: January 15, 2010

MCAT® required?: Yes
Latest MCAT® considered: September 2009
Oldest MCAT® considered: 2006

Early Decision Program: School does have EDP
Applicants notified: October 1, 2009
EDP available for: Both Residents and Non-residents

Regular Acceptance Notice
Earliest date: October 1, 2009
Latest date: Until class is full
Applicant's Response to Acceptance Offer – Maximum Time: Two weeks

Requests for Deferred Entrance Considered: Yes

Deposit to Hold Place in Class: Yes
Deposit (Resident): $100
Deposit (Non-resident): $100
Deposit due: With response to acceptance offer
Applied to tuition: Yes
Deposit refundable: Yes
Refundable by: May 1, 2010

Estimated number of new entrants: 120
EDP: 2, special program: 10

Start Month/Year: July 2010

Interview Format: Three individual 20-minute interviews with faculty. Regional interviews are not available.

Other Programs

PREPARATORY PROGRAMS

Postbaccalaureate Program: Yes, www1.wfubmc.edu/MDProgram/Student+Services/Diversity/Post+Graduate+Students/PostBacPreMed.htm
Summer Program: No
Additional Program:
MD/MS in Health Science Research
www1.wfubmc.edu/MDProgram/Admissions/Joint+Degree.htm

COMBINED DEGREE PROGRAMS

Baccalaureate/M.D.: No
M.D./M.P.H.: No
M.D./M.B.A.: Yes, www.mba.wfu.edu/default.aspx?id=141
M.D./J.D.: No
M.D./Ph.D.: Yes, www1.wfubmc.edu/MDProgram/Admissions/Joint+Degree.htm
Additional Program: Yes, www.wfu.edu/bioethics

Premedical Coursework

Course	Req.	Rec.	Lab.	Hrs.
Inorganic Chemistry	•			8
Behavioral Sciences				
Biochemistry				
Biology	•			8
Biology/Zoology				
Calculus				
College English				
College Mathematics				

Course	Req.	Rec.	Lab.	Hrs.
Computer Science				
Genetics				
Humanities				
Organic Chemistry	•			8
Physics	•			8
Psychology				
Social Sciences				
Other				

Selection Factors: 2008 Accepted Applicants

Proportion of Accepted Applicants with Relevant Experience (Data Self-Reported to AMCAS*)		
Community Service/Volunteer		76%
Medically-Related Work		88%
Research		84%

Shaded bar represents school's accepted scores ranging from the 10th percentile to the 90th percentile ▨   School Median ●   National Median ●

Overall GPA 2.0 2.1 2.2 2.3 2.4 2.5 2.6 2.7 2.8 2.9 3.0 3.1 3.2 3.3 **3.4 3.5 3.6 3.7** ⊙3.8 3.9 4.0
Science GPA 2.0 2.1 2.2 2.3 2.4 2.5 2.6 2.7 2.8 2.9 3.0 3.1 3.2 **3.3 3.4 3.5 3.6** ⊙3.7 3.8 3.9 4.0

MCAT® Total Numeric Score 9 10 11 12 13 14 15 16 17 18 19 20 21 22 23 24 25 26 27 28 29 30 3⬤32 33 34 35 36 37 38 39 40 41 42 43

Writing Sample			J	K	L	M	N	O	P	⊙Q	R	S	T
Verbal Reasoning	3	4	5	6	7	8	9	⊙10	11	12	13	14	15
Biological Sciences	3	4	5	6	7	8	9	10	⊙11	12	13	14	15
Physical Sciences	3	4	5	6	7	8	9	10	⊙11	12	13	14	15

Acceptance & Matriculation Data for 2008–2009 First Year Class

	Resident	Non-resident	International	Total
Applications	733	6380	389	7502
Interviewed	148	446	4	598
Deferred	2	5	0	7
Matriculants				
Early Assurance Program	1	5	0	6
Early Decision Program	5	0	0	5
Baccalaureate/M.D.	n/a	n/a	n/a	n/a
M.D./Ph.D.	0	1	1	2
Matriculated	46	71	3	**120**

Applications accepted from International Applicants: Only Canadian

Matriculant Demographics: 2008–2009 First Year Class

Men: 73   **Women:** 47

Matriculants' Self-Reported Race/Ethnicity

Mexican American	1	**Korean**	2
Cuban	0	**Vietnamese**	1
Puerto Rican	1	**Other Asian**	2
Other Hispanic	0	**Total Asian**	17
Total Hispanic	2	**Native American**	2
Chinese	3	**Black**	9
Asian Indian	9	**Native Hawaiian**	0
Pakistani	0	**White**	92
Filipino	1	**Unduplicated Number**	
Japanese	0	**of Matriculants**	120

Science and Math Majors: 66%
Matriculants with:
Baccalaureate degree: 100%
Graduate degree(s): 6%

Specialty Choice

2004, 2005, 2006 Graduates, Specialty Choice (As reported by program directors to GME Track™)	
Anesthesiology	10%
Emergency Medicine	7%
Family Practice	10%
Internal Medicine	16%
Obstetrics/Gynecology	5%
Orthopaedic Surgery	3%
Pediatrics	13%
Psychiatry	2%
Radiology	5%
Surgery	6%

Financial Information

Source: 2007–2008 LCME I-B survey and 2008–2009 AAMC TSF questionnaire

	Residents	Non-residents
Total Cost of Attendance	$58,164	$58,164
Tuition and Fees	$38,248	$38,248
Other (includes living expenses)	$17,276	$17,276
Health Insurance (can be waived)	$2,640	$2,640

Average 2008 Graduate Indebtedness: $149,793
% of Enrolled Students Receiving Aid: 93%

Criminal Background Check

This medical school requires a criminal background check prior to matriculation.

University of North Dakota
School of Medicine and Health Sciences
Grand Forks, North Dakota

Secretary, Committee on Admissions
University of North Dakota
School of Medicine and Health Sciences
501 North Columbia Road, Stop 9037
Grand Forks, North Dakota 58202-9037
T 701 777 4221   **F** 701 777 4942

Admissions http://smhs.med.und.nodak.edu/
UNDSMHS/admissions.html
Main www.med.und.nodak.edu
Financial www.med.und.edu/depts/saff/brochure.htm
E-mail jdheit@medicine.nodak.edu

Public Institution

Dr. H. David Wilson, Dean

*Judy L. DeMers, Associate Dean,
Student Affairs and Admissions*

Eugene DeLorme, Director, INMED Program

Sandra K. Elshaug, Financial Aid Administrator

General Information

The School of Medicine was established in 1905 as a basic science public medical school. In 1973, legislative action created an expanded curriculum and, in 1981, a full four-year medical education program was instituted in the state. The school is university-based and community-integrated.

Mission Statement

The mission of the University of North Dakota School of Medicine and Health Sciences is to educate and prepare physicians, medical scientists, and other health professionals for service to North Dakota and the nation, and to advance medical and biomedical knowledge through research.

Curricular Highlights

Community Service Requirement: Optional. A variety of activities is available.
Research/Thesis Requirement: Required during third year.

The School of Medicine's renewed curriculum was initiated during the 1998-99 academic year. Utilizing a "patient-centered learning" (PCL) approach, the number of lecture hours was reduced significantly, and greater emphasis was placed on small-group teaching and learning, active student participation, and early clinical experience. The curriculum is integrated across disciplines, consisting of four 10-week blocks of instruction during each of the first two years. Students either complete six 8-week clerkships in year 3 or they participate in the ROME (Rural Opportunities in Medical Education) Program, completing 7 months of clinical experience in a rural community. The school emphasizes the training of primary care physicians, but also offers a M.D.-Ph.D. program.

USMLE

Step 1: Required. Students must record a passing score for graduation, but not promotion.
Step 2: Clinical Skills (CS): Required. Students must only record a score.
Step 2: Clinical Knowledge (CK): Required. Students must only record a score.

Selection Factors

A student must maintain a GPA of 3.0 or better to be considered for admission. Selection is based upon the scholastic record, letters of recommendation, MCAT scores, and a personal interview. Interviews are conducted only at the medical school. In addition to high academic achievement, selection is based on a number of factors, including the demonstration of motivation and commitment to a medical career, empathy, compassion in interpersonal relationships, problem-solving, and the ability to work well in small groups. Qualified North Dakota residents are given preference in admission. The only exceptions include a limited number of Minnesota residents or admission through WICHE participation. Only persons who are U.S. citizens or legal permanent residents of the United States are eligible for consideration for admission. The school participates in the Professional Student Exchange Program administered by WICHE, under which legal residents of western states without a medical school may receive preference in admission. WICHE students who are certified and supported by their home state pay resident tuition. The school does not utilize AMCAS. Applications are ranked based on a combination of state of residency, grade-point average, and MCAT scores. The school is unable to accept transfer students from other medical schools except in very unique circumstances.

Financial Aid

The financial resources of applicants are not considered in the selection process. Immediately after acceptance into the School of Medicine, the applicant is sent all available financial aid information and is encouraged to apply. The awarding of financial aid is based on documented need. Loans and a limited number of scholarships and prizes are available. Some awards and scholarships are based on academics as well as need. Students are discouraged

from working. The financial aid office may be reached at (701) 777-2849.

Information about Diversity Programs

The INMED (Indians into Medicine) Program is a recruitment and retention program for American Indian students. It is a federally funded program that provides educational opportunities for fully qualified enrolled members of U.S. recognized tribes. State residency is not a consideration for admission through the INMED Program.

Campus Information

Setting

The medical school is located on the UND campus, a state-supported institution located in Grand Forks in the heart of the Red River Valley. The Grand Forks-East Grand Forks (MN) community has a total population of approximately 75,000. UND is classified by the Carnegie Foundation as a high research activity, doctoral/professional and engaged university, and offers a wide diversity of educational programs.

Enrollment

For 2008, total enrollment was: 242

Special Features

The Center for Rural Health is a recognized leader nationally. The school also has a Center of Excellence in Women's Health and a Center for Excellence in Neurosciences. A medical student exchange program exists with two medical schools in Norway.

Housing

On-campus housing is available in the form of residence halls and apartments for families and single students. A shuttle service runs between the housing area and the main campus. Rental housing also is plentiful in the community.

Satellite Campuses/Facilities

Students are assigned to one of four regional campuses statewide in Bismarck, Fargo, Grand Forks, and Minot for third- and fourth-year clinical experiences.

Application Process and Requirements 2010–2011

Primary Application Service: School specific
Earliest filing date: July 1, 2009
Latest filing date: November 1, 2009

Secondary Application Required?: No
Sent to: All qualified applicants
URL: www.med.und.nodak.edu/
Fee: Yes, $50
Fee waiver available: Yes
Earliest filing date: July 1, 2009
Latest filing date: November 1, 2009

MCAT® required?: Yes
Latest MCAT® considered: September 2009
Oldest MCAT® considered: August 2006

Early Decision Program: School does not have EDP
Applicants notified: n/a
EDP available for: n/a

Regular Acceptance Notice
Earliest date: January 15, 2010
Latest date: Until class is full
Applicant's Response to Acceptance Offer – Maximum Time: Four weeks

Requests for Deferred Entrance Considered: Yes

Deposit to Hold Place in Class: Yes
Deposit (Resident): $100
Deposit (Non-resident): $100
Deposit due: With response to acceptance offer
Applied to tuition: Yes
Deposit refundable: Yes
Refundable by: May 15, 2010

Estimated number of new entrants: 62
EDP: n/a, special program: n/a

Start Month/Year: August 2010

Interview Format: M.D. and Ph.D. faculty members and medical students conduct one-hour interviews.

Other Programs

PREPARATORY PROGRAMS
Postbaccalaureate Program: No
Summer Program: Yes, INMED Program
(701) 777-3039, edelorme@medicine.nodak.edu

COMBINED DEGREE PROGRAMS
Baccalaureate/M.D.: No
M.D./M.P.H.: Yes, Robert Beattie, M.D.
(701) 777-3264, beattie@medicine.nodak.edu
M.D./M.B.A.: No
M.D./J.D.: No
M.D./Ph.D.: Yes, www.med.und.nodak.edu, Edward Sauter, M.D., (701) 777-6226, esauter@medicine.nodak.edu

Premedical Coursework

Course	Req.	Rec.	Lab.	Hrs.
Inorganic Chemistry	•		•	8
Behavioral Sciences				
Biochemistry		•		
Biology				
Biology/Zoology	•		•	8
Calculus				
College English	•			6
College Mathematics	•			3

Course	Req.	Rec.	Lab.	Hrs.
Computer Science		•		
Genetics				
Humanities		•		
Organic Chemistry	•		•	8
Physics	•		•	8
Psychology	•			3
Social Sciences				
Other				

Selection Factors: 2008 Accepted Applicants

Proportion of Accepted Applicants with Relevant Experience (Data Self-Reported to AMCAS®)		
Community Service/Volunteer		90%
Medically-Related Work		87%
Research		84%

Shaded bar represents school's accepted scores ranging from the 10th percentile to the 90th percentile ■   School Median ● National Median ●

Overall GPA 2.0 2.1 2.2 2.3 2.4 2.5 2.6 2.7 2.8 2.9 3.0 3.1 3.2 3.3 3.4 3.5 3.6 3.7 (3.8) 3.9 4.0
Science GPA 2.0 2.1 2.2 2.3 2.4 2.5 2.6 2.7 2.8 2.9 3.0 3.1 3.2 3.3 3.4 3.5 3.6 (3.7) 3.8 3.9 4.0

MCAT® Total Numeric Score 9 10 11 12 13 14 15 16 17 18 19 20 21 22 23 24 25 26 27 (28) 29 30 31 (32) 33 34 35 36 37 38 39 40 41 42 43

Writing Sample			J	K	L	M	N	(O)	P	(Q)	R	S	T
Verbal Reasoning	3	4	5	6	7	8	(9)	(10)	11	12	13	14	15
Biological Sciences	3	4	5	6	7	8	9	(10)	(11)	12	13	14	15
Physical Sciences	3	4	5	6	7	8	(9)	10	(11)	12	13	14	15

Acceptance & Matriculation Data for 2008–2009 First Year Class

	Resident	Non-resident	International	Total
Applications	151	152	0	303
Interviewed	103	53	0	156
Deferred	4	1	0	5
Matriculants				
Early Assurance Program	0	0	0	0
Early Decision Program	0	0	0	0
Baccalaureate/M.D.	n/a	n/a	n/a	n/a
M.D./Ph.D.	0	0	0	0
Matriculated	46	16	0	**62**

Applications accepted from International Applicants: No

Specialty Choice

2004, 2005, 2006 Graduates, Specialty Choice (As reported by program directors to GME Track™)	
Anesthesiology	2%
Emergency Medicine	11%
Family Practice	16%
Internal Medicine	11%
Obstetrics/Gynecology	10%
Orthopaedic Surgery	4%
Pediatrics	11%
Psychiatry	2%
Radiology	6%
Surgery	7%

Matriculant Demographics: 2008–2009 First Year Class

Men: 26   **Women:** 36

Matriculants' Self-Reported Race/Ethnicity

Mexican American	1	**Korean**	0
Cuban	0	**Vietnamese**	0
Puerto Rican	0	**Other Asian**	0
Other Hispanic	0	**Total Asian**	4
Total Hispanic	1	**Native American**	8
Chinese	0	**Black**	0
Asian Indian	3	**Native Hawaiian**	0
Pakistani	0	**White**	49
Filipino	1	**Unduplicated Number**	
Japanese	0	**of Matriculants**	62

Science and Math Majors: 70%
Matriculants with:
      Baccalaureate degree: 100%
      Graduate degree(s): 13%

Financial Information

Source: 2007–2008 LCME I-B survey and 2008–2009 AAMC TSF questionnaire

	Residents	Non-residents
Total Cost of Attendance	$43,180	$62,340
Tuition and Fees	$24,077	$43,237
Other (includes living expenses)	$19,103	$19,103
Health Insurance (can be waived)	$0	$0

Average 2008 Graduate Indebtedness: $138,054
% of Enrolled Students Receiving Aid: 97%

Criminal Background Check

This medical school requires a criminal background check prior to matriculation.

Case Western Reserve University School of Medicine

Cleveland, Ohio

Office of Admissions
Case Western Reserve University School of Medicine
10900 Euclid Avenue
Cleveland, Ohio 44106-4920
T 216 368 3450   F 216 368 6011

Admissions http://casemed.case.edu/admissions
Main http://casemed.case.edu
Financial http://casemed.case.edu.edu/financial_aid
E-mail casemed-admissions@case.edu

Private Institution

Dr. Pamela B. Davis, Dean and Vice President for Medical Affairs

Dr. Lina Mehta, Associate Dean for Admissions

Joseph T. Williams, Director of Multicultural Programs

Wanda L. Rollins, Director of Financial Aid

Christian Essman, Director of Admissions

General Information

Since 1843, the Case Western Reserve University School of Medicine has been at the forefront of medical education and research. CWRU SOM is one of the nation's leaders in NIH funding. Current educational innovations include curricular reform within the University Program and partnership since 2002 with the Cleveland Clinic in the Cleveland Clinic Lerner College of Medicine (College Program), a distinct program to train physician-investigators.

Mission Statement

To advance the health of humankind through research, service and education.

Curricular Highlights

Community Service Requirement: Optional.
Research/Thesis Requirement: Required.

Case Western School of Medicine offers two types of M.D. programs, a Medical Scientist Training program (MSTP), and several dual-degree and master's programs. Applicants may choose one or more programs through AMCAS by applying to the CWRU School of Medicine, and must interview separately for each. The University Program (UP), a 4-year M.D. program designed to train physician-scholars, is based on four tenets: clinical mastery, research, leadership, and civic professionalism. The innovative curriculum integrates basic sciences, clinical medicine, and population health, focusing on the care of individual patients within social and environmental contexts. Students are introduced to basic sciences in a learner-centered environment which emphasizes small group and team-based learning. Learning is interactive with faculty and students as partners. Independent learning and

scholarship are emphasized. Material is organized in system-based blocks, with basic science and clinical integration throughout the four years. Early clinical experiences include rotating apprenticeships and a longitudinal outpatient preceptorship. A required, mentored research thesis is supported by the Office of Medical Student Research. Advising occurs in small groups by the Office of Student Affairs. The 5-year College Program (CP) admits 32 students, each of whom will graduate with an M.D. with Special Qualifications in Biomedical Research. A student-centered approach fosters critical thinking and self-directed learning. Basic sciences are taught in small groups using problem-based learning, interactive seminars, journal clubs, and labs; there are no formal lectures. Early clinical experiences include a longitudinal outpatient preceptorship throughout the first two years. A core research curriculum focuses on basic and clinical research and includes hands-on research during the first two summers. A master's level thesis is required. Students document their progress using a portfolio that details skills and expertise they achieve. A physician adviser ensures students' mastery of required competencies. A college level biochemistry course and research experience is required of all applicants to the College Program. Neither program utilizes grades or class rank.

USMLE

Step 1: Required. Students must record a passing score for promotion.
Step 2: Clinical Skills (CS): Required. Students must record a passing total score to graduate.
Step 2: Clinical Knowledge (CK): Required. Students must record a passing total score to graduate.

Selection Factors

The School of Medicine seeks a diverse student body. Students are selected without regard to age, nationality, race, religion, sex, sexual orientation, or state of residence. All candidates must have demonstrated exceptional academic strength and personal achievements. Written statements and letters of recommendation are also important. Transfer students are rarely accepted.

Financial Aid

Financial aid is based on demonstrated need. Merit scholarships may be awarded to some students with outstanding personal and academic achievement. College Program students do not pay tuition or continuation fees. Accepted students receive financial aid applications in January; awards are made by April.

Information about Diversity Programs

The Office of Multicultural Affairs offers academic and personal support for all underrepresented medical students. This office also recruits students for all programs, sponsors a rigorous, six-week, summer premed/predental program for college freshmen and sophomores and has an NIH-funded summer research program for undergraduate and medical students. The office supports the Case Western Student National Medical Association chapter and the Minority Graduate Student Organization.

Campus Information

Setting

The School of Medicine sits within the heart of the university's 150-acre campus in the city's University Circle area, a cultural and educational hub. Teaching affiliates are adjacent or nearby.

Enrollment

For 2008, total enrollment was: 711

Special Features

Center for Global Health and Diseases offers opportunities for students to study abroad. The Mt. Sinai Skills and Simulation Center offers a state-of-the-art clinical learning laboratory. Center for Reducing Health Disparities offers unique research and community outreach.

Housing

On campus housing is not available, but ample housing exists within walking distance. Rents average $400–$600 month.

Satellite Campuses/Facilities

Affiliate hospitals include University Hospitals Case Medical Center (including Rainbow Babies and Children's), Cleveland Clinic, MetroHealth, and the VA Hospital.

Application Process and Requirements 2010–2011

Primary Application Service: AMCAS
Earliest filing date: June 1, 2009
Latest filing date: November 1, 2009

Secondary Application Required?: Yes
Sent to: All applicants
URL: Sent when verified AMCAS application is received.
Fee: Yes, $85
Fee waiver available: Yes
Earliest filing date: July 1, 2009
Latest filing date: December 15, 2009

MCAT® required?: Yes
Latest MCAT® considered: September 2009
Oldest MCAT® considered: 2006

Early Decision Program: School does not have EDP
Applicants notified: n/a
EDP available for: n/a

Regular Acceptance Notice
Earliest date: October 15, 2009
Latest date: Until class is full
Applicant's Response to Acceptance Offer – Maximum Time: Four weeks

Requests for Deferred Entrance Considered: Yes

Deposit to Hold Place in Class: No
Deposit (Resident): n/a
Deposit (Non-resident): n/a
Deposit due: n/a
Applied to tuition: n/a
Deposit refundable: n/a
Refundable by: n/a

Estimated number of new entrants: 194
EDP: n/a, special program: 12

Start Month/Year: July 2010

Interview Format: UP: one faculty and one student. CP: two faculty and one student interview.

Other Program

PREPARATORY PROGRAMS
Postbaccalaureate Program: No
Summer Program: Yes, www.smdep.org
Joseph T. Williams, (216) 368-1914
joseph.williams@case.edu

COMBINED DEGREE PROGRAMS
Baccalaureate/M.D.: Yes, http://admission.case.edu/admissions/application/ppsp.asp, Christine Miller, (216) 368-5450, christine.miller@case.edu
M.D./M.P.H.: Yes, www.casemph.org
Kristina Knight, (216) 368-1967, info@casemph.org
MD/MBA: Yes, http://weatherhead.case.edu/mba/jointDegree/joint_mbaMd.cfm, Deborah Bibb, (216) 368-6702, deborah.bibb@case.edu
M.D./J.D.: Yes, http://law.case.edu/, Alyson Alber, 800-756-0036, alyson.alber@case.edu
M.D./Ph.D.: Yes, http://mstp.cwru.edu
Kathy Schultz, (216) 368-3404, mstp@case.edu
Additional Program: Yes, http://bme.case.edu/, Tiffany Thomas 216-368-4094, bmedept@case.edu

Premedical Coursework

Course	Req.	Rec.	Lab.	Sems.
Inorganic Chemistry	•		•	2
Behavioral Sciences				
Biochemistry		•		1
Biology	•		•	2
Biology/Zoology				
Calculus				
College English	•			1
College Mathematics				
Computer Science				

Course	Req.	Rec.	Lab.	Sems.
Genetics				
Humanities				
Organic Chemistry	•		•	2
Physics	•		•	2
Psychology				
Social Sciences				
Biochemistry for CP				1
Calculus for MSTP	•			2

Selection Factors: 2008 Accepted Applicants

Proportion of Accepted Applicants with Relevant Experience (Data Self-Reported to AMCAS®)		
Community Service/Volunteer		70%
Medically-Related Work		89%
Research		93%

Shaded bar represents school's accepted scores ranging from the 10th percentile to the 90th percentile   School Median ● National Median ●

Overall GPA	2.0	2.1	2.2	2.3	2.4	2.5	2.6	2.7	2.8	2.9	3.0	3.1	3.2	3.3	3.4	3.5	3.6	(3.7)	3.8 3.9 4.0
Science GPA	2.0	2.1	2.2	2.3	2.4	2.5	2.6	2.7	2.8	2.9	3.0	3.1	3.2	3.3	3.4	3.5	3.6	(3.7)	3.8 3.9 4.0

MCAT® Total Numeric Score 9 10 11 12 13 14 15 16 17 18 19 20 21 22 23 24 25 26 27 28 29 30 31 (32) 33 34 (35) 36 37 38 39 40 41 42 43

Writing Sample				J	K	L	M	N	O	P	(Q)	R	S	T
Verbal Reasoning	3	4	5	6	7	8	9	(10)	(11)	12	13	14	15
Biological Sciences	3	4	5	6	7	8	9	10	(11)	(12)	13	14	15
Physical Sciences	3	4	5	6	7	8	9	10	(11)	(12)	13	14	15

Acceptance & Matriculation Data for 2008–2009 First Year Class

	Resident	Non-resident	International	Total
Applications	731	4661	393	5785
Interviewed	149	1095	66	1310
Deferred	0	3	1	4
Matriculants				
Early Assurance Program	2	5	0	7
Early Decision Program	0	0	0	0
Baccalaureate/M.D.	n/a	n/a	n/a	0
M.D./Ph.D.	3	10	0	13
Matriculated	34	148	12	**194**

Applications accepted from International Applicants: Yes

Matriculant Demographics: 2008–2009 First Year Class

Men: 99   **Women:** 95

Matriculants' Self-Reported Race/Ethnicity

Mexican American	2	**Korean**	6
Cuban	1	**Vietnamese**	1
Puerto Rican	0	**Other Asian**	6
Other Hispanic	4	**Total Asian**	61
Total Hispanic	7	**Native American**	2
Chinese	27	**Black**	9
Asian Indian	21	**Native Hawaiian**	1
Pakistani	1	**White**	104
Filipino	2	**Unduplicated Number**	
Japanese	0	**of Matriculants**	194

Science and Math Majors: 73%
Matriculants with:
  Baccalaureate degree: 99%
  Graduate degree(s): 13%

Specialty Choice

2004, 2005, 2006 Graduates, Specialty Choice (As reported by program directors to GME Track™)

Anesthesiology	5%
Emergency Medicine	8%
Family Practice	4%
Internal Medicine	15%
Obstetrics/Gynecology	4%
Orthopaedic Surgery	5%
Pediatrics	11%
Psychiatry	6%
Radiology	7%
Surgery	4%

Financial Information

Source: 2007–2008 LCME I-B survey and 2008–2009 AAMC TSF questionnaire

	Residents	Non-residents
Total Cost of Attendance	$66,566	$66,566
Tuition and Fees	$43,966	$43,966
Other (includes living expenses)	$21,280	$21,280
Health Insurance (can be waived)	$1,320	$1,320

Average 2008 Graduate Indebtedness: $137,342
% of Enrolled Students Receiving Aid: 82%

Criminal Background Check

This medical school requires a criminal background check prior to matriculation.

University of Toledo College of Medicine

(Formerly Medical University of Ohio)

Toledo, Ohio

Admissions Office
3025 Arlington Avenue, Mail Stop 1043
Toledo, Ohio 43614
T 419 383 4229   **F** 419 383 3322

Admissions http://utoledo.edu/med/md
Main www.utoledo.edu/
Financial http://hsc.utoledo.edu/depts/stufnaid/sfamed.html
E-mail medadmissions@utnet.utoledo.edu

Public Institution

Dr. Jeffrey P. Gold, Dean

Dr. James F. Kleshinski, Associate Dean for Admissions

Dr. Samuel H. Hancock, Assistant to the President for Institutional Diversity

Carolyn Baumgartner, Director, Student Financial Aid

Dr. Robert S. Crissman, Assistant Dean for Admissions

Dr. Imran Ali, Associate Dean for Medical Education, Professionalism & Diversity

General Information

The Medical University of Ohio and the University of Toledo merged on July 1, 2006, thus creating the third largest university in Ohio, which is now known as The University of Toledo. Four health and research colleges are located on the Health Science Campus: the College of Medicine, the College of Health Science and Human Service, the College of Nursing, and the College of Graduate Studies.

Mission Statement

The mission of The University of Toledo College of Medicine is to improve the human condition. We do this by providing a world-class education for the next generation of physicians and scientists, by creating new knowledge that is translated into cutting-edge clinical practice, and by providing the highest level of professionalism and compassion as we deliver university quality health care.

Curricular Highlights

Community Service Requirement: Optional.
Research/Thesis Requirement: Optional.

The preclinical basic science content is integrated into the following interdisciplinary instructional units: Cellular and Molecular Biology, Human Structure and Development, Neurosciences/Behavioral Science, Immunity and Infection and Organ Systems. All students participate in a Clinical Decision Making course, which spans the first two years. This course provides medical students with the fundamental knowledge and skills necessary for clinical decision making. The third year of the curriculum is devoted to mandatory clerkships in internal medicine, surgery, pediatrics, obstetrics and gynecology, psychiatry and family medicine. The fourth year includes required clerkships in neurology, a basic science elective as well as 24 weeks of clinical electives. Most components of the curriculum are evaluated on an Honors, High Pass, Pass, Fail System.

USMLE

Step 1: Required. Students must record a passing score for promotion.
Step 2: Clinical Skills (CS): Required. Students must record a passing total score to graduate.
Step 2: Clinical Knowledge (CK): Required. Students must record a passing total score to graduate.

Selection Factors

Interviews are by invitation only. Re-applicants are not penalized. Preference is given to Ohio residents.

Financial Aid

Financial aid is awarded on the basis of demonstrated financial need according to federal methodology. Applicants for financial aid must file the FAFSA. Several full tuition Presidential Scholarships are available, as well as a number of both merit and need-based scholarships. Many students are employed during the academic year in the Federal Work-Study Program. Employment opportunities in research, community health, family practice, and acute care are also provided through the summer preceptorship programs.

Information about Diversity Programs

The University of Toledo is committed to increasing opportunities for individuals from traditionally underrepresented groups, as well as those from economically disadvantaged backgrounds. The Admissions Office works in cooperation with the Office of Faculty and Student Diversity, Recruitment and Retention, the Office for Institutional Diversity and the Office of Student Affairs and other campus departments in the recruitment, selection, and retention of qualified students.

Campus Information

Setting

The University of Toledo Health Science Campus is located on 475 acres in suburban south Toledo, approximately three miles south of the Main Campus. Toledo's many cultural attractions include the world famous Toledo Museum of Art, a symphony orchestra, opera company, zoological gardens, and an international institute serving the multicultural life of the city. Recreational activities include metroparks, boating, fishing, hiking, and cross-country skiing.

Enrollment

For 2008, total enrollment was: 642

Special Features

Four schools comprise the University of Toledo Health Science Campus: the College of Medicine, College of Nursing, College of Graduate Studies, and College of Health Science and Human Service. Researchers received more than $17 million in research grants and contracts in the 2008 fiscal year. Major areas of research include cellular and molecular neurobiology, molecular and cellular biology, and the molecular basis of diseases, covering such areas as cancer, diabetes, cardiovascular diseases, molecular and cellular immunology, and vaccine development.

Housing

On-campus housing is available on the main campus.

Satellite Campuses/Facilities

The clinical clerkships are completed at The University of Toledo Medical Center on the Health Science Campus, as well as at several other area teaching hospitals, including St. Vincent Mercy Medical Center, The Toledo Hospital, Mercy Children's Hospital, Toledo Children's Hospital, Flower Hospital, St. Charles Mercy Hospital and St. Luke's Hospital. All students complete a minimum of 8 weeks of clerkships in a rural Area Health Education Center. Opportunities are also available for students to do their required clerkships at Riverside Methodist Hospital in Columbus, Ohio, and at Henry Ford Health System in Detroit, Michigan. In the fourth year, students are able to complete up to several months of elective rotations at other approved institutions.

Application Process and Requirements 2010–2011

Primary Application Service: AMCAS
Earliest filing date: June 1, 2009
Latest filing date: November 1, 2009

Secondary Application Required?: Yes
Sent to: Screened applicants
URL: http://hsc.utoledo.edu/med/md/admissions/secondary.html
Fee: Yes, $80
Fee waiver available: Yes
Earliest filing date: June 15, 2009
Latest filing date: January 1, 2010

MCAT® required?: Yes
Latest MCAT® considered: September 2009
Oldest MCAT® considered: 2007

Early Decision Program: School does have EDP
Applicants notified: October 1, 2009
EDP available for: Residents only

Regular Acceptance Notice
Earliest date: October 15, 2009
Latest date: Until class is full
Applicant's Response to Acceptance
Offer – Maximum Time: Two weeks

Requests for Deferred
Entrance Considered: Yes

Deposit to Hold Place in Class: No
Deposit (Resident): n/a
Deposit (Non-resident): n/a
Deposit due: n/a
Applied to tuition: n/a
Deposit refundable: n/a
Refundable by: n/a

Estimated number of new entrants: 175
EDP: 5, special program: 25

Start Month/Year: August 2010

Interview Format: Two, one-on-one interviews with faculty. Regional interviews are not available.

Other Programs

PREPARATORY PROGRAMS
Postbaccalaureate Program: Yes, http://utoledo.edu/med/grad
Summer Program: Yes, www.hsc.utoledo.edu/med/md/admissions/srp.html
Additional Program: Yes, www.hsc.utoledo.edu/med/md/admissions.medstarz.html

COMBINED DEGREE PROGRAMS
Baccalaureate/M.D.: Yes, www.bioe.eng.utoledo.edu/undergraduate/programs/bsmd.html
M.D./M.P.H.: Yes, http://mph.bgsu.muo.utoledo.edu
MD/MBA: Yes, www.utoledo.edu/business
M.D./J.D.: No
M.D./Ph.D.: Yes, http://utoledo.edu/med/mdphd/index.html
Additonal Program: Yes, http://utoledo.edu/med/grad/pdfs/mdms2.pdf

Premedical Coursework

Course	Req.	Rec.	Lab.	Sems.	Course	Req.	Rec.	Lab.	Sems.
Inorganic Chemistry	•		•	2	Computer Science				
Behavioral Sciences					Genetics				
Biochemistry		•			Humanities		•		
Biology	•			2	Organic Chemistry	•		•	2
Biology/Zoology					Physics	•			2
Calculus					Psychology				
College English	•			2	Social Sciences		•		
College Mathematics	•			2	Other				

Selection Factors: 2008 Accepted Applicants

Proportion of Accepted Applicants with Relevant Experience (Data Self-Reported to AMCAS®)		
Community Service/Volunteer		68%
Medically-Related Work		81%
Research		80%

Shaded bar represents school's accepted scores ranging from the 10th percentile to the 90th percentile   School Median ●   National Median ●

Overall GPA	2.0	2.1	2.2	2.3	2.4	2.5	2.6	2.7	2.8	2.9	3.0	3.1	3.2	3.3	3.4	3.5	3.6	(3.7)	3.8	3.9	4.0
Science GPA	2.0	2.1	2.2	2.3	2.4	2.5	2.6	2.7	2.8	2.9	3.0	3.1	3.2	3.3	3.4	3.5	3.6	(3.7)	3.8	3.9	4.0

MCAT® Total Numeric Score 9 10 11 12 13 14 15 16 17 18 19 20 21 22 23 24 25 26 27 28 29 30 (31) 32 33 34 35 36 37 38 39 40 41 42 43

Writing Sample			J	K	L	M	N	O	(P)	(Q)	R	S	T
Verbal Reasoning	3	4	5	6	7	8	9	(10)	11	12	13	14	15
Biological Sciences	3	4	5	6	7	8	9	10	(11)	12	13	14	15
Physical Sciences	3	4	5	6	7	8	9	(10)	(11)	12	13	14	15

Acceptance & Matriculation Data for 2008–2009 First Year Class

	Resident	Non-resident	International	Total
Applications	1002	2407	22	3431
Interviewed	277	223	1	500
Deferred	30	4	0	34
Matriculants				
Early Assurance Program	17	2	0	19
Early Decision Program	2	0	0	2
Baccalaureate/M.D.	n/a	n/a	n/a	n/a
M.D./Ph.D.	2	0	0	2
Matriculated	113	62	1	**176**
Applications accepted from International Applicants: No				

Specialty Choice

2004, 2005, 2006 Graduates, Specialty Choice (As reported by program directors to GME Track™)	
Anesthesiology	5%
Emergency Medicine	8%
Family Practice	11%
Internal Medicine	18%
Obstetrics/Gynecology	5%
Orthopaedic Surgery	4%
Pediatrics	10%
Psychiatry	3%
Radiology	6%
Surgery	5%

Matriculant Demographics: 2008–2009 First Year Class

Men: 98   **Women:** 78

Matriculants' Self-Reported Race/Ethnicity

Mexican American	0	Korean	2
Cuban	2	Vietnamese	1
Puerto Rican	0	Other Asian	3
Other Hispanic	2	Total Asian	38
Total Hispanic	4	Native American	1
Chinese	7	Black	10
Asian Indian	20	Native Hawaiian	0
Pakistani	2	White	127
Filipino	3	Unduplicated Number	
Japanese	1	of Matriculants	176

Science and Math Majors: 72%
Matriculants with:
Baccalaureate degree: 100%
Graduate degree(s): 20%

Financial Information

Source: 2007–2008 LCME I-B survey and 2008–2009 AAMC TSF questionnaire

	Residents	Non-residents
Total Cost of Attendance	$41,328	$68,764
Tuition and Fees	$26,247	$53,683
Other (includes living expenses)	$13,075	$13,075
Health Insurance (can be waived)	$2,006	$2,006

Average 2008 Graduate Indebtedness: $145,238
% of Enrolled Students Receiving Aid: 91%

Criminal Background Check

This medical school requires a criminal background check prior to matriculation.

Northeastern Ohio Universities College of Medicine

Rootstown, Ohio

Office of Admissions and Student Services
Northeastern Ohio Universities College of Medicine
P.O. Box 95
Rootstown, Ohio 44272-0095
T 330 325 6270   F 330 325 8372

Admissions www.neoucom.edu/audience/applicants
Main www.neoucom.edu
Financial www.neoucom.edu/audience/students
E-mail admission@neoucom.edu

Public Institution

Dr. Lois Margaret Nora, President and Dean

Polly Moss, Assistant Dean, Student Affairs and Admissions

Michelle Cassetty Collins, Director, Admissions and Student Services

General Information

NEOUCOM is a state (public) medical school consisting of a basic medical sciences campus in Rootstown, a consortium of three major public universities and 20 community hospitals with more than 6,500 teaching beds in the greater Akron, Canton, and Youngstown areas. The clinical faculty numbers more than 1,800.

Mission Statement

The mission of the Northeastern Ohio Universities College of Medicine (NEOUCOM) is to graduate qualified physicians oriented to the practice of medicine at the community level, with an emphasis on primary care: family medicine, internal medicine, pediatrics, and obstetrics/gynecology.

Curricular Highlights

Community Service Requirement: Required.
Research/Thesis Requirement: Optional.

The integrated curriculum is offered in five steps during the four years. The four-year Doctoring course includes the biomedical, beavioral, social, population health, clinical sciences, and humanities to provide an understanding of the complex interplay of these disciplines in patient care. Step 1: Prologue addresses issues of professionalism, doctor-patient relationships, clinical skills, population health and college orientation requirements; Human Development and Structure emphasizes human anatomy; Molecules to Cells addresses biochemistry, molecular pathology, and genetics. Step 2: Physiological Basis of Medicine emphasizes physiological concepts in the practice of internal medicine; Brain, Mind and Behavior includes anatomy, physiology, and chemistry of the nervous system with basic clinical concepts and pathologies. Step 3: instruction is centered on systems and application in clinical settings. Step 4: core clerkships in family medicine, internal medicine, obstetrics/gynecology, pediatrics, psychiatry, and surgery, and a four-week exploratory experience. Step 5: electives and Clinical Epilogue and Capstone focusing on professionalism, humanities, social science disciplines, and provides vital skills needed as residents and interns.

USMLE

Step 1: Required. Students must record a passing score for promotion.
Step 2: Clinical Skills (CS): Required. Students must only record score.
Step 2: Clinical Knowledge (CK): Required. Students must record a passing total score to graduate.

Selection Factors

Applicants must demonstrate strong academic preparation as measured by GPAs and MCAT scores, and show appropriate personal characteristics and motivation for the practice of medicine. Interviews are by invitation only. Admission preference is given to Ohio residents. All applicants are considered; no formulas are used for the selection process. Only those who complete the supplementary applications are given full consideration. Early submission of application materials is strongly encouraged, particularly through the Early Decision Plan (EDP). NEOUCOM is an equal opportunity/affirmative action educator and employer, committed to preparing students for the practice of medicine in a multicultural environment by increasing the diversity of the student body, faculty, and staff and by enhancing policies, procedures, and practices that support a collaborative environment.

Financial Aid

Loan funds are available through federal sources to all students who qualify. Limited campus-based financial aid in the form of loans and grants are also available and is based on financial need as determined by the FAFSA. Parental information is required for all students seeking campus-based aid consideration. Limited scholarship opportunities are also available for disadvantaged and/or medical students from groups underrepresented in medicine. Application information is provided upon acceptance. Private counseling and debt management programs are offered to all students.

Information about Diversity Programs

NEOUCOM believes that diversity is a value that is central to its educational, research, service and health care missions. The Admissions Committee conducts a holistic review of all qualified applicants, striving to bring together a diverse student body constituted by academically gifted, highly motivated, resilient students who share a deep committment to the values and goals of our profession and the College.

Campus Information

Setting

Rootstown is 20 minutes from Akron and 50 minutes from Cleveland. The 105-acre NEOUCOM complex, centrally located among the consortium universities (The University of Akron, Kent State University and Youngstown State University) and clinical campuses, houses the College's administrative offices, and the divisions of basic medical sciences and community health sciences.

Enrollment

For 2008, total enrollment was: 456

Special Features

The state-of-the-art facilities on campus include the Wasson Center for Clinical Skills Training, Assessment, and Scholarship; newly renovated lecture halls; multidisciplinary labs; and the Regional Medical Informational Center, which houses more than 110,000 books and more than 725 journals. For relaxation, students can enjoy the workout room, student lounge, and basketball, tennis, and volleyball courts.

Housing

NEOUCOM maintains a listing of local housing options; no on-campus housing is available.

Satellite Campuses/Facilities

Rotations are completed among 20 associated hospitals, eight of which are major teaching facilities.

Application Process and Requirements 2010–2011

Primary Application Service: AMCAS
Earliest filing date: June 1, 2009
Latest filing date: November 1, 2009

Secondary Application Required?: Yes
Sent to: All Applicants
URL: www.neoucom.edu/audience/applicants
Admissions, (330) 325-6274
Fee: Yes, $75
Fee waiver available: Yes
Earliest filing date: July 1, 2009
Latest filing date: December 1, 2009

MCAT® required?: Yes
Latest MCAT® considered: December 2009
Oldest MCAT® considered: 2007

Early Decision Program: School does have EDP
Applicants notified: October 1, 2009
EDP available for: Both Residents
and Non-residents

Regular Acceptance Notice
Earliest date: November 1, 2009
Latest date: Until class is full
Applicant's Response to Acceptance
Offer – Maximum Time: Two weeks

Requests for Deferred
Entrance Considered: Yes

Deposit to Hold Place in Class: Yes
Deposit (Resident): $100
Deposit (Non-resident): $100
Deposit due: Two weeks after offer of acceptance
Applied to tuition: Yes
Deposit refundable: No
Refundable by: n/a

Estimated number of new entrants: 30
EDP: 5, special program: 80

Start Month/Year: August 2010

Interview Format: 30-minute interview by two faculty. Regional interviews are not available.

Other Programs

PREPARATORY PROGRAMS
Postbaccalaureate Program: No
Summer Program: No

COMBINED DEGREE PROGRAMS
Baccalaureate/M.D.: Yes www.neoucom.edu/audience/applicants
330-325-6270, admission@neoucom.edu
M.D./M.P.H.: Yes
MD/MBA: No
M.D./J.D.: No
M.D./Ph.D.: Yes
Additional Program: Yes,
www.neoucom.edu/PharmD
330-325-6270, pharmacy@neoucom.edu

Premedical Coursework

Course	Req.	Rec.	Lab.	Sems.	Course	Req.	Rec.	Lab.	Sems.
Inorganic Chemistry		•			Computer Science				
Behavioral Sciences		•			Genetics		•		
Biochemistry		•			Humanities		•		
Biology	•			1	Organic Chemistry	•			2
Biology/Zoology		•			Physics	•			2
Calculus		•			Psychology		•		
College English		•			Social Sciences		•		
College Mathematics		•			Other				

Selection Factors: 2008 Accepted Applicants

Proportion of Accepted Applicants with Relevant Experience (Data Self-Reported to AMCAS®)		
Community Service/Volunteer		44%
Medically-Related Work		41%
Research		39%

Shaded bar represents school's accepted scores ranging from the 10th percentile to the 90th percentile ●School Median ●National Median

Overall GPA 2.0 2.1 2.2 2.3 2.4 2.5 2.6 2.7 2.8 2.9 3.0 3.1 3.2 3.3 3.4 3.5 3.6 3.7 (3.8) 3.9 4.0
Science GPA 2.0 2.1 2.2 2.3 2.4 2.5 2.6 2.7 2.8 2.9 3.0 3.1 3.2 3.3 3.4 3.5 3.6 (3.7) 3.8 3.9 4.0

MCAT® Total Numeric Score 9 10 11 12 13 14 15 16 17 18 19 20 21 22 23 24 25 26 27 (28) 29 30 31 (32) 33 34 35 36 37 38 39 40 41 42 43

Writing Sample			J	K	L	M	N	(O)	P	(Q)	R	S	T
Verbal Reasoning	3	4	5	6	7	8	(9)	(10)	11	12	13	14	15
Biological Sciences	3	4	5	6	7	8	9	(10)	(11)	12	13	14	15
Physical Sciences	3	4	5	6	7	8	(9)	10	(11)	12	13	14	15

Acceptance & Matriculation Data for 2008–2009 First Year Class

	Resident	Non-resident	International	Total
Applications	819	1198	33	2050
Interviewed	128	6	0	134
Deferred	2	0	0	2
Matriculants				
Early Assurance Program	0	0	0	0
Early Decision Program	2	0	0	2
Baccalaureate/M.D.	76	4	0	80
M.D./Ph.D.	n/a	n/a	n/a	n/a
Matriculated	110	4	0	**114**

Applications accepted from International Applicants: No

Specialty Choice

2004, 2005, 2006 Graduates, Specialty Choice (As reported by program directors to GME Track™)	
Anesthesiology	6%
Emergency Medicine	7%
Family Practice	9%
Internal Medicine	20%
Obstetrics/Gynecology	6%
Orthopaedic Surgery	4%
Pediatrics	9%
Psychiatry	3%
Radiology	4%
Surgery	8%

Matriculant Demographics: 2008–2009 First Year Class

Men: 56   **Women:** 58

Matriculants' Self-Reported Race/Ethnicity

Mexican American	1	Korean	1
Cuban	0	Vietnamese	1
Puerto Rican	0	Other Asian	3
Other Hispanic	3	Total Asian	34
Total Hispanic	4	Native American	0
Chinese	4	Black	3
Asian Indian	22	Native Hawaiian	0
Pakistani	2	White	73
Filipino	2	Unduplicated Number	
Japanese	0	of Matriculants	114

Science and Math Majors: 66%
Matriculants with:
          Baccalaureate degree: 100%
          Graduate degree(s): 2%

Financial Information

Source: 2007–2008 LCME I-B survey
and 2008–2009 AAMC TSF questionnaire

	Residents	Non-residents
Total Cost of Attendance	$53,419	$81,820
Tuition and Fees	$29,847	$57,708
Other (includes living expenses)	$22,210	$22,210
Health Insurance (can be waived)	$1,362	$1,362

Average 2008 Graduate Indebtedness: $147,581
% of Enrolled Students Receiving Aid: 86%

Criminal Background Check

This medical school requires a criminal background check prior to matriculation.

The Ohio State University College of Medicine

Columbus, Ohio

Admissions Office, The Ohio State University
College of Medicine
I55D Meiling Hall, 370 West 9th Avenue
Columbus, Ohio 43210-1238
T 614 292 7137   F 614 247 7959

Admissions http://medicine.osu.edu/futurestudents/admissions
Main http://medicine.osu.edu
Financial www.medicine.osu.edu/futurestudents/financialaid/
E-mail medicine@osu.edu

Public Institution

Dr. Wiley Chip Souba, Dean

Dr. Don Batisky, Associate Dean, Admissions

Dr. Leon McDougle, Assistant Dean, Minority Affairs

Samuel Matheny, Director, Financial Services

Lorna Kenyon, Director, Admissions

General Information

Since 1914, The Ohio State University College of Medicine has blended traditional medical education, innovative learning opportunities, and a strong reputation in the preparation of students for primary care and specialized residencies, encouraging research interests and a strong emphasis on a biopsychosocial approach to patient care.

Mission Statement

To achieve distinction in education, scholarship and public service; to educate skilled professionals in the basic and clinical medical sciences, public health, and allied medical professions; to create, evaluate, and disseminate knowledge and technology; and, to provide innovative solutions for improving the health of our people.

Curricular Highlights

Community Service Requirement: Required. Clinical Assessment and Problem Solving component.
Research/Thesis Requirement: Optional.

Initial ten-week gross anatomy and embryology course, followed by choice of two preclinical pathways. Integrated Pathway features body systems-oriented content that fuses basic and clinical sciences using methods of student-centered active learning, small-group case-based discussion, and lectures. Independent Study Pathway students use highly structured objectives, resource guides, Web and computer-based materials to read, review, and learn on their own. Clinical experiences begin in the first year with the Clinical Assessment and Problem Solving course. Additionally, standardized patients help students build clinical proficiency in the state-of-the-art clinical skills

center. Third-year clerkships include family medicine, internal medicine, obstetrics and gynecology, pediatrics, psychiatry, neurology, and surgery. A clinical skills immersion experience ensures all students have an in-depth understanding of a core set of procedurally based clinical skills. Fourth-year selectives focus on caring for patients at various stages of illness and wellness: undifferentiated patient; patient with chronic care needs; and a sub-internship. In the fourth year, students also have 4 months of elective rotations and 3 months of vacation.

USMLE

Step 1: Required. Students must record a passing score for promotion.
Step 2: Clinical Skills (CS): Required. Students must record a passing total score to graduate.
Step 2: Clinical Knowledge (CK): Required. Students must record a passing total score to graduate.

Selection Factors

Completed applications are reviewed to ensure that excellent candidates who do not fit the general profile are not overlooked. Factors considered include clinical experiences, community service and leadership activities, research experience, recommendations, suitability for the study of medicine, and extracurricular activities.

Financial Aid

There is need-based financial aid assistance. Students participate in various scholarship and low-interest loan programs. Accepted candidates are mailed financial aid materials prior to entering to be considered with students already in school. Financial need is not a deterrent to acceptance. Every effort is made to assist each student in securing sufficient resources for continuing their education.

Information about Diversity Programs

Students whose previous educational and economic deprivation warrants special consideration are carefully evaluated and offered special help in the acquisition of additional resources. The Medpath Medical Careers Pathway is a postbaccalaureate program aimed at developing the academic knowledge base and skills of

students enhancing their preparation for medical school.

Campus Information

Setting
The Ohio State University has the nation's largest single college campus enrollment and the resources that go with it. Columbus offers diversity in the arts, cultural events, festivals, restaurants, sports, and nightlife.

Enrollment
For 2008, total enrollment was: 824

Special Features
The Ohio State University Medical Center is at the center of cutting-edge developments in the areas of clinical care, education, and research. Ohio State was the first U.S. medical center to perform a complete heart bypass using robotics. An Ohio State faculty member became the first physician in the U.S. to implant a digital pacemaker in a patient. In 2004, the National Cancer Institute awarded the University's cancer program a numerical score equivalent to its highest possible rating—outstanding. The Patient Centered Medicine course was recognized in 2004 by the Institute of Medicine of the National Academies as one of four exemplary curricula for teaching social and behavioral science components of medicine.

Housing
The Neil Building and the Gateway Center offer professional student housing. Victorian Village and Grandview Heights are also popular. Rent: $400–2000 monthly.

Satellite Campuses/Facilities
Clinical rotations occur within the Medical Center, at community hospitals within Columbus and Ohio, in rural settings in Ohio, and at locations outside of Ohio. About 35 percent of the fourth-year class gains exposure to international health care with the assistance of the College of Medicine Office of Global Health.

Application Process and Requirements 2010–2011

Primary Application Service: AMCAS
Earliest filing date: June 1, 2009
Latest filing date: November 1, 2009

Secondary Application Required?: Yes
Sent to: All applicants
Contact: Admissions Office
(614) 292-7137, medicine@osu.edu
Fee: Yes, $60
Fee waiver available: Yes
Earliest filing date: July 1, 2009
Latest filing date: Varies

MCAT® required?: Yes
Latest MCAT® considered: September 2009
Oldest MCAT® considered: 2007

Early Decision Program: School does have EDP
Applicants notified: October 1, 2009
EDP available for: Both Residents and Non-residents

Regular Acceptance Notice
Earliest date: October 16, 2009
Latest date: Varies
Applicant's Response to Acceptance
Offer – Maximum Time: Two weeks

Requests for Deferred
Entrance Considered: Yes

Deposit to Hold Place in Class: No
Deposit (Resident): n/a
Deposit (Non-resident): n/a
Deposit due: n/a
Applied to tuition: n/a
Deposit refundable: n/a
Refundable by: n/a

Estimated number of new entrants: 210
EDP: 10, special program: n/a

Start Month/Year: August 2010

Interview Format: Open-file conversation; one faculty interview and one student interview. Regional interviews are not available.

Other Programs

PREPARATORY PROGRAMS
Postbaccalaureate Program: Yes, http://medicine.osu.edu/odca/7277.cfm, Nikki Radcliffe, (614) 292-3161, nikki.radcliffe@osumc.edu
Summer Program: Yes, Nikki Radcliffe, (614) 292-3161, nikki.radcliffe@osumc.edu

COMBINED DEGREE PROGRAMS
Baccalaureate/M.D.: Yes, www.medicine.osu.edu/futurestudents/admissions/eap/index.cfm, Anne Krabacher, (614) 292-3951, krabacher.4@osu.edu
M.D./M.P.H.: Yes, http://cph.osu.edu/academic programs/dcd/, (614) 293-3907, sph@osu.edu
M.D./MBA: Yes, http://fisher.osu.edu/ftmba/index.php?page=MD-MBA, 292-8511, fishergrad@cob.osu.edu
M.D./J.D.: Yes, http://moritzlaw.osu.edu (614) 292-8810, lawadmit@osu.edu
M.D./Ph.D.: Yes, www.osumdphd.org, Ashley Bertran, (614) 292-7790

Premedical Coursework

Course	Req.	Rec.	Lab.	Sems.	Course	Req.	Rec.	Lab.	Sems.
Inorganic Chemistry	•		•	2	Computer Science				
Behavioral Sciences		•			Genetics		•		
Biochemistry		•			Humanities		•		
Biology	•			2	Organic Chemistry	•		•	2
Biology/Zoology					Physics	•		•	2
Calculus					Psychology		•		
College English		•			Social Sciences		•		
College Mathematics					Diversity/Ethics		•		

Selection Factors: 2008 Accepted Applicants

Proportion of Accepted Applicants with Relevant Experience (Data Self-Reported to AMCAS)		
Community Service/Volunteer		75%
Medically-Related Work		85%
Research		86%

Shaded bar represents school's accepted scores ranging from the 10th percentile to the 90th percentile. **School Median** ● **National Median** ●

Overall GPA	2.0	2.1	2.2	2.3	2.4	2.5	2.6	2.7	2.8	2.9	3.0	3.1	3.2	3.3	3.4	3.5	3.6	3.7	(3.8)	3.9	4.0
Science GPA	2.0	2.1	2.2	2.3	2.4	2.5	2.6	2.7	2.8	2.9	3.0	3.1	3.2	3.3	3.4	3.5	3.6	3.7	(3.8)	3.9	4.0

MCAT® Total Numeric Score 9 10 11 12 13 14 15 16 17 18 19 20 21 22 23 24 25 26 27 28 29 30 31 (32) 33 (34) 35 36 37 38 39 40 41 42 43

Writing Sample			J	K	L	M	N	O	P	(Q)	R	S	T
Verbal Reasoning	3	4	5	6	7	8	9	(10)	(11)	12	13	14	15
Biological Sciences	3	4	5	6	7	8	9	10	(11)	(12)	13	14	15
Physical Sciences	3	4	5	6	7	8	9	10	(11)	(12)	13	14	15

Acceptance & Matriculation Data for 2008–2009 First Year Class

	Resident	Non-resident	International	Total
Applications	1054	3352	40	4446
Interviewed	235	417	0	652
Deferred	7	8	0	15
Matriculants				
Early Assurance Program	0	0	0	0
Early Decision Program	0	0	0	0
Baccalaureate/M.D.	13	0	0	13
M.D./Ph.D.	1	3	0	4
Matriculated	106	105	0	**211**

Applications accepted from International Applicants: No

Matriculant Demographics: 2008–2009 First Year Class

Men: 120   **Women:** 91

Matriculants' Self-Reported Race/Ethnicity

Mexican American	6	Korean	5
Cuban	4	Vietnamese	3
Puerto Rican	1	Other Asian	3
Other Hispanic	1	Total Asian	55
Total Hispanic	12	Native American	2
Chinese	16	Black	10
Asian Indian	24	Native Hawaiian	0
Pakistani	4	White	141
Filipino	0	Unduplicated Number	
Japanese	1	of Matriculants	211

Science and Math Majors: 67%
Matriculants with:
    Baccalaureate degree: 100%
    Graduate degree(s): 4%

Specialty Choice

2004, 2005, 2006 Graduates, Specialty Choice (As reported by program directors to GME Track™)	
Anesthesiology	5%
Emergency Medicine	6%
Family Practice	9%
Internal Medicine	20%
Obstetrics/Gynecology	4%
Orthopaedic Surgery	4%
Pediatrics	7%
Psychiatry	3%
Radiology	3%
Surgery	8%

Financial Information

Source: 2007–2008 LCME I-B survey and 2008–2009 AAMC TSF questionnaire

	Residents	Non-residents
Total Cost of Attendance	$49,919	$65,057
Tuition and Fees	$28,563	$43,701
Other (includes living expenses)	$19,636	$19,636
Health Insurance (can be waived)	$1,720	$1,720

Average 2008 Graduate Indebtedness: $136,260
% of Enrolled Students Receiving Aid: 93%

Criminal Background Check

This medical school requires a criminal background check prior to matriculation.

University of Cincinnati College of Medicine

Cincinnati, Ohio

Office of Student Affairs/Admissions
University of Cincinnati College of Medicine
P.O. Box 670552
Cincinnati, Ohio 45267-0552
T 513 558 7314   **F** 513 558 1165

Admissions www.med.uc.edu/admissions/
Main www.med.uc.edu
Financial http://medonestop.uc.edu
E-mail comadmis@ucmail.uc.edu

Public Institution

Dr. David M. Stern, Dean

Dr. Laura Wexler Sr., Associate Dean for Student Affairs/Admissions

Dr. Charles W. Collins, Associate Dean for Diversity and Community Affairs

Dr. Daniel Burr, Assistant Dean for Student Financial Planning

Dr. R. Stephen Manuel, Assistant Dean for Admissions

General Information

The UCCOM provides both outstanding research facilities and superb clinical and teaching experiences. Graduates, ranked as highly competitive by national residency program directors, choose careers in a broad range of specialty areas. Extensive research opportunities are available. UCCOM is ranked in the top third among all public medical schools in NIH, research funding.

Mission Statement

The mission of the University of Cincinnati College of Medicine is to improve the health of the public by educating physicians and scientists and by producing new knowledge.

Curricular Highlights

Community Service Requirement: Optional.
Research/Thesis Requirement: Optional.

UCCOM provides a stimulating learning environment, creating the undifferentiated M.D. ready to excel in residency training and provide excellent patient care. Using an integrated curricular approach including lab, small-group discussion, and team-based learning and lectures, the first two years provide students with the scientific, clinical and humanistic principles of medicine. Year 1 focuses on the normal structure, function and development of the human body. Year 2 emphasizes the basis and mechanisms of human disease. During Year 3, students rotate through six core clerkships. Students also begin exploring career options by participating in three specialty clerkships of their choosing. In Year 4, students hone their clinical skills during their Acting Internship

and required Neuroscience selectives. Students can also choose from over 100 elective offerings.

USMLE

Step 1: Required. Students must record a passing score for promotion.
Step 2: Clinical Skills (CS): Required. Students must record a passing total score to graduate.
Step 2: Clinical Knowledge (CK): Required. Students must record a passing total score to graduate.

Selection Factors

After AMCAS, secondary applications and letters of recommendations are received, completed applicants are evaluated for interviews. The UCCOM Web site provides applicants with admissions progress information. The College utilizes the Multiple Mini Interview and the interview day consists of a description of the College and student services and includes: a presentation about the admissions process, curriculum, student services, financial aid, lunch, and tour. Acceptance offers are based on the overall and holistic evaluation of academic and personal qualities. Postbaccalaureate and graduate coursework will be considered. Personal characteristics include demonstrated motivation, maturity, coping skills, interpersonal skills, sensitivity and tolerance toward others and communication and critical-thinking skills. Students are admitted regardless of age, religion, sex, sexual orientation, race, color, national origin or disability.

Financial Aid

The College provides counseling to help students fund their medical education and make sound financial decisions. Accepted applicants receive a financial aid packet in February. Applicants with complete files are sent estimated award letters by May 15. To be considered for need-based aid, applicants must submit the Need Access application, which includes parental information. Further information at *www.medonestop.uc.edu.*

Information about Diversity Programs

UCCOM Office of Diversity & Community Affairs works to increase diversity of the medical student body, residency training programs and faculty through regional and national

recruitment efforts of underrepresented groups. The Office retention activities include mentoring, connections with community physicians, academic & psychological support and career development. Community partners support the office activities.

Campus Information

Setting

The clinical facilities of University Hospital, VA Medical Center, Cincinnati Children's Hospital Medical Center and Shriners Hospital for Children, along with the Cardiovascular Research Center and Vontz Center for Molecular Studies, are all within walking distance of the college. In 2008, the UCCOM opened the doors of the Care/Crawley Building. Easily accessible by free shuttle service to the main campus are other dining options, a convenience store and top-of-the-line recreation facilities.

Enrollment

For 2008, total enrollment was: 626

Special Features

The Medical Scholars Program (MSSP) provides students with extracurricular clinical and didactic experiences throughout their education in topical areas such as Neuroscience; Geriatrics; the Art of Family Medicine; Child and Adolescent Health; and Nutrition. Poverty, Justice and Health elective explores international health and includes lectures, discussions, and an opportunity to visit Honduras with a medical team. Cincinnati Children's Hospital Medical Center is one of the top pediatric hospitals in the country, providing research and outstanding clinical opportunities. The Center for Surgical Intervention (CSI) bridges new technology in biomedical and surgical care. Using robotics, medical simulation, telecommunications, and medical informatics, the CSI uses new technology in surgical procedures.

Housing

While graduate housing is available on campus, most medical school students reside off campus. Housing information is provided, and students are encouraged to look for housing early.

Application Process and Requirements 2010–2011

Primary Application Service: AMCAS
Earliest filing date: June 1, 2009
Latest filing date: November 15, 2009

Secondary Application Required?: Yes
Sent to: All applicants
URL: www.MedOneStop.uc.edu
Fee: Yes, $25
Fee waiver available: Yes
Earliest filing date: July 15, 2009
Latest filing date: December 15, 2009

MCAT® required?: Yes
Latest MCAT® considered: September 2009
Oldest MCAT® considered: April 2007

Early Decision Program: School does have EDP
Applicants notified: October 1, 2009
EDP available for: Both Residents and Non-residents

Regular Acceptance Notice
Earliest date: October 15, 2009
Latest date: Varies
Applicant's Response to Acceptance
Offer – Maximum Time: Two weeks

Requests for Deferred
Entrance Considered: Yes

Deposit to Hold Place in Class: No
Deposit (Resident): n/a
Deposit (Non-resident): n/a
Deposit due: n/a
Applied to tuition: n/a
Deposit refundable: n/a
Refundable by: n/a

Estimated number of new entrants: 160
EDP: 12, special program: n/a

Start Month/Year: August 2010

Interview Format: Multiple Mini Interview with a series of six-eight raters. Regional interviews are not available.

Other Programs

PREPARATORY PROGRAMS
Postbaccalaureate Program: Yes,
www.mcp.uc.edu, Karen Coleman, (513) 558-3104,
karen.coleman@uc.edu
Summer Program: Yes, www.med.uc.edu/admissions/summerenrich.cfm
Lathel Bryant, MA, (513) 558-0693, lathel.bryant@uc.edu
Summer Research Scholars (SRS):
www.med.uc.edu/admissions/summerenrich.cfm

COMBINED DEGREE PROGRAMS
Baccalaureate/M.D.: Yes,
www.med.uc.edu/HS2MD, Nikki Bibler,
(513) 558-5581, DualAdmissionsProgram@uc.edu
M.D./M.P.H.: Yes, www.med.uc.edu/publichealth/MPH_Degree.cfm, James Boex, Ph.D., MBA,
(513) 558-5613, james.boex@uc.edu
MD/MBA: Yes, www.business.uc.edu,
(513) 556-7024, graduate@uc.edu
M.D./Ph.D.: Yes, www.med.uc.edu/pstp, Patrick Tso,
Ph.D., (513) 558-2380, patrick.tso@uc.edu

Premedical Coursework

Course	Req.	Rec.	Lab.	Sems.	Course	Req.	Rec.	Lab.	Sems.
Inorganic Chemistry		•			Computer Science		•		
Behavioral Sciences		•			Genetics		•		
Biochemistry		•			Humanities		•		
Biology		•			Organic Chemistry		•		
Biology/Zoology		•			Physics		•		
Calculus		•			Psychology		•		
College English		•			Social Sciences		•		
College Mathematics		•			Other				

Selection Factors: 2008 Accepted Applicants

Proportion of Accepted Applicants with Relevant Experience (Data Self-Reported to AMCAS®)		Community Service/Volunteer	68%
		Medically-Related Work	77%
		Research	84%

Shaded bar represents school's accepted scores ranging from the 10th percentile to the 90th percentile.   School Median ●   National Median ●

Overall GPA 2.0 2.1 2.2 2.3 2.4 2.5 2.6 2.7 2.8 2.9 3.0 3.1 3.2 **3.3 3.4 3.5 3.6 (3.7) 3.8 3.9 4.0**

Science GPA 2.0 2.1 2.2 2.3 2.4 2.5 2.6 2.7 2.8 2.9 3.0 3.1 **3.2 3.3 3.4 3.5 3.6 (3.7) 3.8 3.9 4.0**

MCAT® Total Numeric Score 9 10 11 12 13 14 15 16 17 18 19 20 21 22 23 24 25 26 27 28 29 30 31 **32 33 (34) 35** 36 37 38 39 40 41 42 43

Writing Sample			J	K	L	M	N	O	P	(Q)	R	S	T
Verbal Reasoning	3	4	5	6	7	8	9	(10)	11	12	13	14	15
Biological Sciences	3	4	5	6	7	8	9	10	(11)	(12)	13	14	15
Physical Sciences	3	4	5	6	7	8	9	10	(11)	(12)	13	14	15

Acceptance & Matriculation Data for 2008–2009 First Year Class

	Resident	Non-resident	International	Total
Applications	1107	2766	25	3898
Interviewed	395	231	0	626
Deferred	1	3	0	4
Matriculants				
Early Assurance Program	18	3	0	21
Early Decision Program	8	0	0	8
Baccalaureate/M.D.	n/a	n/a	n/a	n/a
M.D./Ph.D.	3	2	0	5
Matriculated	98	61	0	**159**

Applications accepted from International Applicants: No

Specialty Choice

2004, 2005, 2006 Graduates, Specialty Choice (As reported by program directors to GME Track™)	
Anesthesiology	7%
Emergency Medicine	8%
Family Practice	8%
Internal Medicine	14%
Obstetrics/Gynecology	3%
Orthopaedic Surgery	4%
Pediatrics	13%
Psychiatry	6%
Radiology	5%
Surgery	9%

Matriculant Demographics: 2008–2009 First Year Class

Men: 107   **Women:** 52

Matriculants' Self-Reported Race/Ethnicity

Mexican American	3	Korean	5
Cuban	0	Vietnamese	3
Puerto Rican	1	Other Asian	4
Other Hispanic	1	Total Asian	35
Total Hispanic	5	Native American	1
Chinese	11	Black	11
Asian Indian	12	Native Hawaiian	0
Pakistani	1	White	106
Filipino	0	Unduplicated Number	
Japanese	0	of Matriculants	159

Science and Math Majors: 75%
Matriculants with:
 Baccalaureate degree: 100%
 Graduate degree(s): 16%

Financial Information

Source: 2007–2008 LCME I-B survey and 2008–2009 AAMC TSF questionnaire

	Residents	Non-residents
Total Cost of Attendance	$48,352	$63,552
Tuition and Fees	$27,987	$42,987
Other (includes living expenses)	$19,063	$19,263
Health Insurance (can be waived)	$1,302	$1,302

Average 2008 Graduate Indebtedness: $140,174
% of Enrolled Students Receiving Aid: 88%

Criminal Background Check

This medical school requires a criminal background check prior to matriculation.

Wright State University School of Medicine

Dayton, Ohio

Office of Student Affairs/Admissions
Wright State University
Boonshoft School of Medicine
P.O. Box 1751
Dayton, Ohio 45401-1751
T 937 775 2934　**F** 937 775 3322

Admissions www.med.wright.edu/admiss
Main www.med.wright.edu
Financial www.med.wright.edu/students/
financialaid.html
E-mail som_saa@wright.edu

Public Institution

Dr. Howard Part, Dean

Dr. Gary LeRoy, Associate Dean of Student Affairs/Admissions

Charlotta Taylor, Director of Recruitment

Dr. Gwen Sloas, Director of Financial Aid

Dr. Stephen Peterson, Assistant Dean of Student Affairs and Admissions

Dr. Kevin Watt, Assistant Dean of Diversity and Inclusion

General Information

The Boonshoft School of Medicine is a community-based medical school. Clinical facilities include seven major teaching hospitals with over 3,500 patient beds. A faculty of over 1,200 provides students with opportunities for individualized attention. The educational program emphasizes research, generalist training, community health care, community service, patient focused care, cultural competence, cultural diversity, health promotion, disease prevention, and the provision of care to underserved populations.

Mission Statement

The mission of the School is to educate culturally diverse students to become excellent physicians by focusing on generalist training that is integrated, supported, and strengthened by specialists and researchers. The faculty values patient-focused care, community service, research, and have passion for improving health in our communities. These goals and objectives are achieved through: opportunities to learn in clinical settings beginning in the first month; integration of basic and clinical science throughout four years; instruction in community-based, inpatient and outpatient settings; utilization of diverse learning strategies; interaction with faculty in an atmosphere that fosters teamwork, camaraderie, and collegiality; and diversity in the student body and patient population, reflecting many ethnic, racial, social, age, lifestyle, and gender differences.

Curricular Highlights

Community Service Requirement: Optional. Opportunities are Numerous
Research/Thesis Requirement: Optional.

Students are taught in an interdisciplinary fashion using diverse techniques. In the first year, basic principles, mechanisms of disease, social and ethical issues, and evidence-based medicine are taught. Throughout the first two years, students are instructed in medical history-taking, physical examination, and catastrophic illnesses. Each year includes a two-week clinical elective. In the second year, pathology, therapeutics and eight organ systems are taught. The year concludes with USMLE preparation and time for study. In the third year, students learn through six core clerkships. The fourth year includes two clerkships, six electives (some of which may be done away) and time for USMLE study.

USMLE

Step 1: Required. Students must record a passing score for promotion.
Step 2: Clinical Skills (CS): Required. Students must record a passing total score to graduate.
Step 2: Clinical Knowledge (CK): Required. Students must record a passing total score to graduate.

Selection Factors

The school seeks a student body of diverse social, ethnic, and educational backgrounds. Applicants are admitted solely on the basis of individual qualifications without regard to race, religion, gender, sexual orientation, disability, veteran status, national origin, age, or ancestry. Dedication to human concerns, compassion, intellectual capacity, and maturity are of greater importance than specific areas of preprofessional preparation. The School also values evidence of motivation, altruism, leadership, and communication skills. Also considered are one's academic record, MCAT performance, letters of recommendation, history of service, and the results of a personal interview (by invitation). Ohio residents are given preference, but non-residents are encouraged to apply.

Financial Aid

Scholarships and loans are available. The school offers financial counseling services and assists students in obtaining needed support. An emergency loan fund is available. Financial status has no effect on one's acceptance.

Information about Diversity Programs

The school and its faculty have a stated policy of providing educational opportunities to disadvantaged applicants and applicants from groups underrepresented in medicine. The admissions process gives careful consideration to all applicants. A pre-matriculation program, mentoring, big brother/big sister program, tutoring, USMLE preparation, and assistance in critical thinking and learning are available.

Campus Information

Setting

The first two years are spent primarily on the main campus in Fairborn, Ohio, a suburb of Dayton. The bucolic campus occupies 250 acres, with over half devoted to wooded acreage and preserve. Dayton is a mid-sized city within a metropolitan area of nearly one million residents.

Enrollment

For 2008, total enrollment was: 417

Special Features

The school's hallmarks include a focus on holistic physician training, dynamic partnerships with our community, community service, and collaborative research. Our curriculum niche puts us on the cutting edge of medical instruction, but retains the personal touch so important to our students' education.

Housing

Housing is readily available at reasonable costs adjacent to campus and throughout the Dayton area. The school assists students in finding housing and roommates.

Satellite Campuses/Facilities

The School partners with area hospitals, clinics, and other health care providers. Students spend time in federal hospitals, private hospitals, a children's hospital, neighborhood clinics, nursing homes, and private physician offices. Approximately 250 full time clinical faculty are located in affiliated health care institutions. Many of the School's outreach programs have received national recognition.

Application Process and Requirements 2010–2011

Primary Application Service: AMCAS
Earliest filing date: June 1, 2009
Latest filing date: October 15, 2009

Secondary Application Required?: Yes
Sent to: All applicants
URL: www.med.wright.edu/admiss/start.html
Fee: Yes, $45
Fee waiver available: Yes
Earliest filing date: June 15, 2009
Latest filing date: December 31, 2009

MCAT® required?: Yes
Latest MCAT® considered: September 2009
Oldest MCAT® considered: January 2006

Early Decision Program: School does have EDP
Applicants notified: October 1, 2009
EDP available for: Residents only

Regular Acceptance Notice
Earliest date: October 15, 2009
Latest date: Until class is full

Applicant's Response to Acceptance
Offer – Maximum Time: Two weeks for return of Committal Form

Requests for Deferred Entrance Considered: Yes

Deposit to Hold Place in Class: No
Deposit (Resident): n/a
Deposit (Non-resident): n/a
Deposit due: n/a
Applied to tuition: n/a
Deposit refundable: n/a
Refundable by: n/a

Estimated number of new entrants: 100
EDP: 5
Special Programs: 12

Start Month/Year: August 2010

Interview Format: Two one-on-one interviews, each lasting 30-40 minutes. Regional interviews are not available.

Other Programs

PREPARATORY PROGRAMS
Postbaccalaureate Program: No
Summer Program: No
Prematriculation Program:
(second and third weeks of July)
www.med.wright.edu

COMBINED DEGREE PROGRAMS
Baccalaureate/M.D.: No
M.D./M.P.H.: Yes, www.med.wright.edu/md-mph
MD/MBA: Yes, www.med.wright.edu/md-mba
M.D./J.D.: No
M.D./Ph.D.: Yes, www.med.wright.edu/md-phd

Premedical Coursework

Course	Req.	Rec.	Lab.	Sems.
Inorganic Chemistry	•	•		2
Behavioral Sciences				
Biochemistry		•		
Biology	•		•	2
Biology/Zoology				
Calculus		•		
College English	•			2
College Mathematics	•			2

Course	Req.	Rec.	Lab.	Sems.
Computer Science		•		
Genetics				
Humanities		•		
Organic Chemistry	•		•	2
Physics	•		•	2
Psychology		•		
Social Sciences		•		
Other				

Selection Factors: 2008 Accepted Applicants

Proportion of Accepted Applicants with Relevant Experience (Data Self-Reported to AMCAS®)		
Community Service/Volunteer		72%
Medically-Related Work		90%
Research		78%

Shaded bar represents school's accepted scores ranging from the 10th percentile to the 90th percentile. School Median ● National Median ●

Overall GPA 2.0 2.1 2.2 2.3 2.4 2.5 2.6 2.7 2.8 2.9 3.0 3.1 3.2 3.3 3.4 3.5 3.6 (3.7) 3.8 3.9 4.0
Science GPA 2.0 2.1 2.2 2.3 2.4 2.5 2.6 2.7 2.8 2.9 3.0 3.1 3.2 3.3 3.4 3.5 (3.6) 3.7 3.8 3.9 4.0

MCAT® Total Numeric Score 9 10 11 12 13 14 15 16 17 18 19 20 21 22 23 24 25 26 27 28 (29) 30 31 (32) 33 34 35 36 37 38 39 40 41 42 43

Writing Sample			J	K	L	M	N	O	(P)	(Q)	R S T
Verbal Reasoning	3	4	5	6	7	8	9	(10)	11	12	13 14 15
Biological Sciences	3	4	5	6	7	8	9	(10)	(11)	12	13 14 15
Physical Sciences	3	4	5	6	7	8	9	(10)	(11)	12	13 14 15

Acceptance & Matriculation Data for 2008–2009 First Year Class

	Resident	Non-resident	International	Total
Applications	981	2015	35	3031
Interviewed	374	69	0	443
Deferred	2	1	0	3
Matriculants				
Early Assurance Program	4	0	0	4
Early Decision Program	10	0	0	10
Baccalaureate/M.D.	n/a	n/a	n/a	n/a
M.D./Ph.D.	2	0	0	2
Matriculated	92	8	0	**100**

Applications accepted from International Applicants: No

Specialty Choice

2004, 2005, 2006 Graduates, Specialty Choice (As reported by program directors to GME Track™)

Anesthesiology	4%
Emergency Medicine	8%
Family Practice	16%
Internal Medicine	14%
Obstetrics/Gynecology	6%
Orthopaedic Surgery	4%
Pediatrics	15%
Psychiatry	4%
Radiology	1%
Surgery	6%

Matriculant Demographics: 2008–2009 First Year Class

Men: 53   **Women:** 47

Matriculants' Self-Reported Race/Ethnicity

Mexican American	2	Korean	4
Cuban	0	Vietnamese	1
Puerto Rican	0	Other Asian	1
Other Hispanic	0	Total Asian	19
Total Hispanic	2	Native American	1
Chinese	4	Black	8
Asian Indian	9	Native Hawaiian	0
Pakistani	1	White	74
Filipino	0	Unduplicated Number	
Japanese	0	of Matriculants	100

Science and Math Majors: 68%
Matriculants with:
Baccalaureate degree: 99%
Graduate degree(s): 15%

Financial Information

Source: 2007–2008 LCME I-B survey and 2008–2009 AAMC TSF questionnaire

	Residents	Non-residents
Total Cost of Attendance	$49,806	$60,276
Tuition and Fees	$27,311	$37,781
Other (includes living expenses)	$20,221	$20,221
Health Insurance (can be waived)	$2,274	$2,274

Average 2008 Graduate Indebtedness: $146,790
% of Enrolled Students Receiving Aid: 94%

Criminal Background Check

This medical school requires a criminal background check prior to matriculation.

University of Oklahoma College of Medicine

Oklahoma City, Oklahoma

Dotty Shaw Killam
University of Oklahoma College of Medicine
P.O. Box 26901
Oklahoma City, Oklahoma 73126
T 405 271 2331 F 405 271 8810

Admissions www.oumedicine.com/body.cfm?id=655
Main www.oumedicine.com/medschool
Financial http://w3.ouhsc.edu/sfs/
E-mail AdminMed@ouhsc.edu

Public Institution

Dr. Phebe Tucker, M.D., Associate Dean for Student Affairs

Dotty Shaw Killam, Director of Admissions

James Albertson, Director of Student Services

Pamela Jordan, Director of Financial Aid

Kate Stanton, Director for Student Affairs

Dr. Sherri S. Baker, M.D., Assistant Dean for Admissions

General Information

The University of Oklahoma College of Medicine offers students a quality education with added advantages. Access to modern patient care facilities and research are provided at a reasonable cost, with a proven record of choice residency placement. Students gain experience in a variety of clinical settings. The college is part of a modern health sciences complex that serves as the state's principal education and research facility for physicians, dentists, nurses, biomedical scientists, pharmacists, public health administrators, and allied health professionals.

Mission Statement

The University of Oklahoma provides our students the best educational experience through excellence in teaching, research and creative activity, and service to the state and society. New facilities and technology — plus an internationally prominent faculty — will undoubtedly make the University of Oklahoma Health Sciences Center and the College of Medicine one of the next century's regional leaders in education, research, and patient care. OU Medicine believes that caring for our patients with honesty and integrity is essential. We strive for teamwork, effective communication, respect and continual improvement in education and research.

Curricular Highlights

Community Service Requirement: Optional. The Community Health Alliance serves 11 clinics.
Research/Thesis Requirement: Optional.

The four-year curriculum consists of two years of study in basic sciences and two in clinical

sciences. Letter grades are awarded for all coursework on a course-hour basis rather than a credit-hour basis. The first two years are complemented by a Web-based on-line curriculum. All students are required to have a computer. There are 17 required courses in the basic science portion of the curriculum. They account for 1,636 hours of instruction or 33 percent of the total. First-year courses provide a strong basic science foundation, and second-year classes form a bridge leading directly into the clinical portion of the curriculum. A significant feature of the curriculum is early exposure to patients through the continuum courses: Principles of Clinical Medicine I and II. Courses in bioethical and legal issues in medicine are also offered, as well as Objective Structured Clinical Examinations (OSCEs). The clinical program provides training at two sites, each having university and community clinical experiences.

USMLE

Step 1: Required. Students must record a passing score for promotion.
Step 2: Clinical Skills (CS): Required. Students must only record a score.
Step 2: Clinical Knowledge (CK): Required. Students must only record a score.

Selection Factors

Acceptance into the College of Medicine is based on GPA, MCAT scores, letters of evaluation from faculty and premedical committees, and personal interviews conducted on campus by members of the Admissions Board. Emphasis is placed on self-awareness, self-discipline, empathy, personal competence, social competence, and an over-all evaluation of character. Non-residents can represent up to 15% of the student body. The University of Oklahoma College of Medicine does not discriminate on the basis of race, sex, creed, national origin, age, or handicap.

Financial Aid

The College of Medicine offers a number of financial assistance opportunities in addition to the federally sponsored programs. The most prominent scholarships are the Regents' Scholarship Fee Waiver, the Oklahoma Rural Medical Education Loan Scholarship Fund

(designed for residents wishing to practice in rural communities). The loan funds established by the Shepherd Foundation, Inc., and the Lew Wentz Foundation, along with over 20 other scholarships, also aid many students annually. Additional support for students from groups underrepresented in medicine is available through the State Regents for Higher Education, the Ungerman Trust, and the Belknap, Culpeper, Maurer, and Reid-Winnie scholarships. In a need or merit-based application process, the College of Medicine awards up to approximately $350,000.00 in scholarships to over 150 medical students.

Information about Diversity Programs

The University of Oklahoma has a strong commitment to identify, recruit, and educate qualified students from groups underrepresented in medicine. Applications are strongly encouraged from these groups, as well as from any candidate with a disadvantaged background.

Campus Information

Setting

The College of Medicine offers programs in Oklahoma City and Tulsa. The Health Sciences Center in Oklahoma City is part of a 200-acre complex of 28 public and private institutions known as the Oklahoma Health Center.

Enrollment

For 2008, total enrollment was: 657

Special Features

The OU College of Medicine and OU Medical Center operate the state's only American College of Surgeons Level-I Trauma Center. The Health Sciences Center also has an Oklahoma Diabetes Center and an Oklahoma Cancer Institute with new facilities being built.

Housing

The University of Oklahoma operates an on-campus apartment complex. Off-campus housing options are also available to students.

Satellite Campuses/Facilities

The College of Medicine's primary campus is in Oklahoma City, with a clinical campus in Tulsa.

Application Process and Requirements 2010–2011

Primary Application Service: AMCAS
Earliest filing date: June 1, 2009
Latest filing date: October 15, 2009

Secondary Application Required?: Yes
Sent to: All applicants
URL: https://app.applyyourself.com/?id=UOK-MED
Fee: Yes, $65
Fee waiver available: No
Earliest filing date: June 1, 2009
Latest filing date: November 1, 2009

MCAT® required?: Yes
Latest MCAT® considered: August 2009
Oldest MCAT® considered: 2006

Early Decision Program: School does not have EDP
Applicants notified: n/a
EDP available for: n/a

Regular Acceptance Notice
Earliest date: November 1, 2009
Latest date: Until class is full
Applicant's Response to Acceptance
Offer – Maximum Time: Two weeks

Requests for Deferred
Entrance Considered: No

Deposit to Hold Place in Class: Yes
Deposit (Resident): $100
Deposit (Non-resident): $100
Deposit due: Within two weeks with response to acceptance offer
Applied to tuition: Yes
Deposit refundable: Yes
Refundable by: May 15, 2010

Estimated number of new entrants: 162
EDP: n/a, special program: n/a

Start Month/Year: August 2010

Interview Format: Held October through February. Regional interviews are not available.

Other Programs

PREPARATORY PROGRAMS
Postbaccalaureate Program: No
Summer Program: No

COMBINED DEGREE PROGRAMS
Baccalaureate/M.D.: No
M.D./M.P.H.: Yes, www.oumedicine.com/body.cfm?id=702
MD/MBA: No
M.D./J.D.: No
M.D./Ph.D.: Yes, http://mdphd.ouhsc.edu/ Megan Meehan, (405) 271-2503, mdphd-program@ouhsc.edu

Premedical Coursework

Course	Req.	Rec.	Lab.	Sems.	Course	Req.	Rec.	Lab.	Sems.
Inorganic Chemistry	•			2	Computer Science				
Behavioral Sciences					Genetics	•			1
Biochemistry					Humanities	•			1
Biology					Organic Chemistry	•			2
Biology/Zoology	•		•	1	Physics	•			2
Calculus					Psychology		•		1
College English	•			3	Social Sciences		•		1
College Mathematics					Other				

Selection Factors: 2008 Accepted Applicants

Proportion of Accepted Applicants with Relevant Experience (Data Self-Reported to AMCAS®)		
Community Service/Volunteer		64%
Medically-Related Work		82%
Research		60%

Shaded bar represents school's accepted scores ranging from the 10th percentile to the 90th percentile   School Median ●   National Median ●

Overall GPA	2.0 2.1 2.2 2.3 2.4 2.5 2.6 2.7 2.8 2.9 3.0 3.1 3.2 3.3 3.4 **3.5 3.6 3.7** (3.8) 3.9 4.0
Science GPA	2.0 2.1 2.2 2.3 2.4 2.5 2.6 2.7 2.8 2.9 3.0 3.1 3.2 3.3 **3.4 3.5 3.6 3.7** (3.8) 3.9 4.0

MCAT® Total Numeric Score 9 10 11 12 13 14 15 16 17 18 19 20 21 22 23 24 25 26 **27 28 29** (30) 31 (32) 33 34 35 36 37 38 39 40 41 42 43

Writing Sample			J	K	L	**M N O** (P) (Q) **R** S T
Verbal Reasoning	3	4	5	6	7	**8 9** (10) **11 12** 13 14 15
Biological Sciences	3	4	5	6	7	**8 9** (10) (11) **12** 13 14 15
Physical Sciences	3	4	5	6	7	**8 9** (10) (11) **12** 13 14 15

Acceptance & Matriculation Data for 2008–2009 First Year Class

	Resident	Non-resident	International	Total
Applications	354	1126	7	1487
Interviewed	264	47	0	311
Deferred	0	0	0	0
Matriculants				
Early Assurance Program	0	0	0	0
Early Decision Program	0	0	0	0
Baccalaureate/M.D.	n/a	n/a	n/a	n/a
M.D./Ph.D.	0	2	0	2
Matriculated	149	17	0	**166**

Applications accepted from International Applicants: No

Specialty Choice

2004, 2005, 2006 Graduates, Specialty Choice (As reported by program directors to GME Track™)	
Anesthesiology	9%
Emergency Medicine	4%
Family Practice	14%
Internal Medicine	12%
Obstetrics/Gynecology	5%
Orthopaedic Surgery	3%
Pediatrics	10%
Psychiatry	6%
Radiology	6%
Surgery	7%

Matriculant Demographics: 2008–2009 First Year Class

Men: 102   **Women:** 64

Matriculants' Self-Reported Race/Ethnicity

Mexican American	2	Korean	3
Cuban	0	Vietnamese	6
Puerto Rican	1	Other Asian	3
Other Hispanic	3	Total Asian	21
Total Hispanic	5	Native American	9
Chinese	4	Black	1
Asian Indian	4	Native Hawaiian	0
Pakistani	0	White	138
Filipino	1	Unduplicated Number	
Japanese	0	of Matriculants	166

Science and Math Majors: 74%
Matriculants with:
    Baccalaureate degree: 99%
    Graduate degree(s): 4%

Financial Information

Source: 2007–2008 LCME I-B survey and 2008–2009 AAMC TSF questionnaire

	Residents	Non-residents
Total Cost of Attendance	$48,752	$72,870
Tuition and Fees	$20,312	$44,430
Other (includes living expenses)	$27,590	$27,590
Health Insurance (can be waived)	$850	$850

Average 2008 Graduate Indebtedness: $119,724
% of Enrolled Students Receiving Aid: 91%

Criminal Background Check

This medical school requires a criminal background check prior to matriculation.

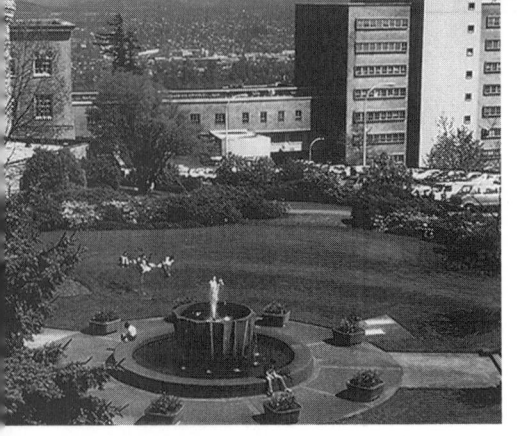

Oregon Health & Science University School of Medicine
Portland, Oregon

Oregon Health & Science University
Office of Education and Student Affairs, L102
3181 S.W. Sam Jackson Park Road
Portland, Oregon 97239-3098
T 503 494 2998   **F** 503 494 3400

Admissions www.ohsu.edu/ohsuedu/academic/
som/admissions.cfm
Main www.ohsu.edu/som
Financial www.ohsu.edu/finaid
E-mail n/a

Public Institution

Dr. Mark Richardson, Dean

*Dr. Cynthia Morris, Assistant Dean
for Admissions*

Debbie Melton, Director of Admissions

General Information
Oregon Health & Science University (OHSU) occupies a 101-acre site overlooking the city of Portland. Campus physical facilities include basic science, research, and laboratory buildings; two hospital units with a capacity of 509 beds; outpatient clinics. The 3rd and 4th year curriculum is regionalized throughout Oregon.

Mission Statement
The mission of the School of Medicine is to enhance human health through programs of excellence in education, research, health care, and public service to the larger community including underserved populations. In achieving these goals, the Oregon Health & Science University School of Medicine seeks to establish an educational environment that challenges students to strive for academic excellence and fosters development of compassion, humanism, professionalism, and cultural competence in the care of patients from their first days in the classroom to their final rotation in the hospitals and clinics. A priority throughout OHSU is to enable each student to fulfill his or her potential as a human being and as a health care professional while effectively meeting the health-related needs of the multiple communities he or she will serve.

Curricular Highlights
Community Service Requirement: Optional. Community service activities are encouraged.
Research/Thesis Requirement: Optional.

The preclincal integrated curriculum is devoted to the sciences basic to medicine, focusing on the normal structure and function of the body and continuing with the study of the pathophysiological basis of disease and its treatment. An early clinical experience is afforded through the Principles of Clinical Medicine, which teaches fundamental knowledge and skills in interviewing and physical diagnosis through a

continuity clinical preceptorship experience. Clinical clerkships are undertaken at OHSU Hospital and Clinics and affiliated hospitals in the Portland area. OHSU offers regional clinical experiences throughout Oregon.

USMLE
Step 1: Required. Students must only record a score.
Step 2: Clinical Skills (CS): Required. Students must only record a score.
Step 2: Clinical Knowledge (CK): Required. Students must only record a score.

Selection Factors
The Admissions Committee seeks students who have demonstrated academic excellence and readiness for the profession of medicine and who will contribute to the diversity necessary to enhance the medical education of all students. Applicants are selected on the basis of demonstrated motivation for medicine, humanistic attitudes, and a realistic understanding of the role of the physician in providing excellent health care to all communities in need of care. The ideal student will demonstrate evidence of strong communication skills; altruism, empathy, and personal integrity; self-appraisal and emotional maturity; and an ability to make a positive contribution to society and the profession. Attention is paid to achievements that demonstrate applicants' breadth of interests and experiences, commitment to others, leadership among their peers, and the ability to contribute diverse and innovative perspectives to problem-solving in medicine and health care. Evaluation of applicants includes the academic record as demonstration of scholarship; the MCAT; recommendations from undergraduate or graduate school faculty, employers, and those familiar with applicants' health care, volunteer, and community service experiences; and the personal interview. Preference is given to residents of Oregon, WICHE-certified residents of Montana and Wyoming, M.D./Ph.D. and M.D./M.P.H. candidates, and non-resident applicants with superior achievements in academics and other related experiences. The School of Medicine Admissions Committee fully recognizes the importance of diversity in its student body and in the physician workforce in providing for

effective delivery of health care. Accordingly, the OHSU School of Medicine strongly encourages applications from persons from all socioeconomic, racial, ethnic, religious, and educational backgrounds and persons from groups underrepresented in medicine. The committee adheres to a policy of equal opportunity and non-discrimination on the basis of sex, age, race, ethnic origin, religion, disability, or sexual orientation.

Financial Aid
Financial aid in the form of scholarships, grants, and loans is available based upon the demonstrated need of the student. For more information please review the Web site at *www.ohsu.edu/finaid.*

Information about Diversity Programs
Information may be obtained by contacting Leslie Garcia, MPA, Director, Center for Diversity & Multicultural Affairs, (503)494-5657 or email garcial@ohsu.edu. Web sites *www.ohsu.edu/academic/diversity/* and *www.ohsu.edu /ohsuedu/academic/som/diversity/index.cfm.*

Setting
University Hospital and the School of Medicine are located on a hilltop overlooking the city of Portland, Oregon. Students have easy access to the city center as well as the surrounding communities.

Campus Information
Enrollment
For 2008, total enrollment was: 528

Satellite Campuses/Facilities
Third and fourth year students may participate in required and elective clinical experiences in Eugene, Bend and Medford, Oregon.

Application Process and Requirements 2010–2011

Primary Application Service: AMCAS
Earliest filing date: June 1, 2009
Latest filing date: October 15, 2009

Secondary Application Required?: Yes
Sent to: All Applicants
URL: Sent via e-mail after verification of AMCAS application.
Fee: Yes, $100
Fee waiver available: Yes
Earliest filing date: July 1, 2009
Latest filing date: February 1, 2010

MCAT® required?: Yes
Latest MCAT® considered: September 2009
Oldest MCAT® considered: 2007

Early Decision Program: School does not have EDP
Applicants notified: n/a
EDP available for: n/a

Regular Acceptance Notice
Earliest date: October 15, 2009
Latest date: Until class is full
Applicant's Response to Acceptance Offer – Maximum Time: Two weeks

Requests for Deferred Entrance Considered: No

Deposit to Hold Place in Class: No
Deposit (Resident): n/a
Deposit (Non-resident): n/a
Deposit due: n/a
Applied to tuition: n/a
Deposit refundable: n/a
Refundable by: n/a

Estimated number of new entrants: 115
EDP: n/a, special program: n/a

Start Month/Year: August 2010

Interview Format: Two, one-on-one 30-45 minute interviews. Regional interviews are not available.

Other Programs

PREPARATORY PROGRAMS
Postbaccalaureate Program: No
Summer Program: No

COMBINED DEGREE PROGRAMS
Baccalaureate/M.D.: No
M.D./M.P.H.: Yes, www.ohsu.edu/public-health
MD/MBA: No
M.D./J.D.: No
M.D./Ph.D.: Yes, www.ohsu.edu/mdphd

Premedical Coursework

Course	Req.	Rec.	Lab.	Qtrs.	Course	Req.	Rec.	Lab.	Qtrs.
Inorganic Chemistry	•		•	1	Computer Science				
Behavioral Sciences					Genetics	•			1
Biochemistry	•		•	1	Humanities				
Biology	•		•	3	Organic Chemistry	•		•	1
Biology/Zoology					Physics	•		•	3
Calculus		•		1	Psychology				
College English	•			1	Statistics		•		1
College Mathematics	•			1	Humanities/Social Sciences	•			6

Selection Factors: 2008 Accepted Applicants

Proportion of Accepted Applicants with Relevant Experience (Data Self-Reported to AMCAS®)		
Community Service/Volunteer		69%
Medically-Related Work		94%
Research		81%

Shaded bar represents school's accepted scores ranging from the 10th percentile to the 90th percentile. School Median ● National Median ●

Overall GPA 2.0 2.1 2.2 2.3 2.4 2.5 2.6 2.7 2.8 2.9 3.0 3.1 3.2 3.3 **3.4 3.5 3.6 (3.7)** 3.8 3.9 4.0
Science GPA 2.0 2.1 2.2 2.3 2.4 2.5 2.6 2.7 2.8 2.9 3.0 3.1 **3.2 3.3 3.4 3.5 3.6 (3.7)** 3.8 3.9 4.0

MCAT® Total Numeric Score 9 10 11 12 13 14 15 16 17 18 19 20 21 22 23 24 25 26 **27 28 29 30 3(1 (32) 3** 34 35 36 37 38 39 40 41 42 43

Writing Sample			J	K	L	**M N O P (Q) R**	S	T
Verbal Reasoning	3	4	5	6	7	**8 9 (10) 11 12**	13	14	15
Biological Sciences	3	4	5	6	7	8 **9 10 (11) 12 13**	14	15
Physical Sciences	3	4	5	6	7	**8 9 10 (11) 12 13**	14	15

Acceptance & Matriculation Data for 2008–2009 First Year Class

	Resident	Non-resident	International	Total
Applications	390	3967	28	4385
Interviewed	203	333	0	536
Deferred	0	0	0	0
Matriculants				
Early Assurance Program	0	0	0	0
Early Decision Program	0	0	0	0
Baccalaureate/M.D.	0	0	0	0
M.D./Ph.D.	0	5	0	5
Matriculated	67	48	0	**115**

Applications accepted from International Applicants: No

Specialty Choice

2004, 2005, 2006 Graduates, Specialty Choice (As reported by program directors to GME Track™)	
Anesthesiology	4%
Emergency Medicine	9%
Family Practice	13%
Internal Medicine	22%
Obstetrics/Gynecology	6%
Orthopaedic Surgery	1%
Pediatrics	10%
Psychiatry	3%
Radiology	3%
Surgery	9%

Matriculant Demographics: 2008–2009 First Year Class

Men: 52   **Women:** 63

Matriculants' Self-Reported Race/Ethnicity

Mexican American	3	Korean	1
Cuban	0	Vietnamese	4
Puerto Rican	0	Other Asian	7
Other Hispanic	1	Total Asian	27
Total Hispanic	4	Native American	1
Chinese	4	Black	1
Asian Indian	5	Native Hawaiian	1
Pakistani	1	White	84
Filipino	2	Unduplicated Number	
Japanese	4	of Matriculants	115

Science and Math Majors: 63%
Matriculants with:
   Baccalaureate degree: 100%
   Graduate degree(s): 18%

Financial Information

Source: 2007–2008 LCME I-B survey and 2008–2009 AAMC TSF questionnaire

	Residents	Non-residents
Total Cost of Attendance	$56,247	$68,899
Tuition and Fees	$33,031	$45,683
Other (includes living expenses)	$19,474	$19,474
Health Insurance (can be waived)	$3,742	$3,742

Average 2008 Graduate Indebtedness: $170,137
% of Enrolled Students Receiving Aid: 95%

Criminal Background Check

This medical school requires a criminal background check prior to matriculation.

The Commonwealth Medical College

Scranton, Pennsylvania

The Commonwealth Medical College
P.O. Box 766
Scranton, Pennsylvania 18501
T 570 504 9068   F 570 504 2794

Admissions www.thecommonwealthmedical.
com/oth/Page.asp?PageID=OTH000007
Main www.thecommonwealthmedical.com
Financial www.thecommonwealthmedical.
com/oth/Page.asp?PageID=OTH000169
E-mail admissions@tcmedc.org

Private Institution

Dr. Robert M. D'Alessandri, President and Dean

Dr. David A. Axler, Associate Dean for Student Affairs

Ida Castro, Vice President for Diversity and Social Justice

Leo Danylak, Director of Financial Aid

Debra E. Stalk, Director of Admissions

General Information

The Commonwealth Medical College (TCMC) located in Scranton, Pennsylvania is the newest allopathic medical school in the United States. We are focused on developing diverse community physicians (both primary care and specialists) for the 21st century—those who are skilled in evidence-based medicine and the latest technology. We were conceived to respond to the regional decrease in physician availability, and to improve the health of community residents. TCMC has clinical campuses in Scranton, Wilkes-Barre and Williamsport covering sixteen counties. Each of these campuses is an integral part of the College's distributive model of medical education to provide students with experiences in diverse clinical settings. Students will be assigned a multi-generational family to follow from the beginning of the first year through the end of their medical school career. Aided by their physician mentor the student will experience the health care system through this family—many of whom will have chronic illnesses. Students also have the opportunity to work on a community public health issue as part of their Physician and Society Course. Students will also be encouraged to provide feedback about the curriculum and their entire educational experience giving them the opportunity to help shape the future of the College.

Mission Statement

The Commonwealth Medical College educates aspiring physicians and scientists to serve society using a community-based, patient-centered, interprofessional and evidence-based model of education that promotes discovery and utilizes innovative techniques.

Curricular Highlights

Community Service Requirement: Required.
Research/Thesis Requirement: Optional.

The curriculum was designed around the ACGME competencies and based on the characteristics we feel will make a physician successful in practice. The curriculum incorporates a variety of learning models but is less than 40% lecture based relying instead on small group, individual and case based learning. Clinical experiences are integrated into the first two years and the third and fourth year offer an longitudinal clerkship model instead of a block model. We feel this will increase learning and student satisfaction.

USMLE

Step 1: Required. Students must record a passing score for promotion.
Step 2: Clinical Skills (CS): Required. Students must record a passing total score to graduate.
Step 2: Clinical Knowledge (CK): Required. Students must record a passing total score to graduate.

Selection Factors

We are looking for students with a strong sense of social responsibility, who desire a sophisticated community-based practice caring for their patients, while improving the health of the community.

Financial Aid

Information about financial aid at TCMC may be found on the financial aid pages on the TCMC Web site. For additional information contact the TCMC Financial Aid office at our e-mail address: financialaid@tcmedc.org. The phone number for the Financial Aid Office is 570-504-7303. The administration has an aggressive fundraising strategy for scholarships for our students and scholarship opportunities will be posted on the College's Web site as they become available.

Information about Diversity Programs

The Center for Social Justice and Diversity represents the Commonwealth Medical College's commitment to meet the ever-increasing need for diverse quality physicians. A diverse environment enriches learning and the quality of the student's experience on campus and as

they reach out to serve the community. The Center works closely with Academic and Student affairs to develop programs that will support the student's experience on and off campus by imbedding cultural competencies in the curriculum, campus life and community-based service including the development of Clubs and special academic and cultural events for all students. TCMC will also develop a Global Health Center that will create hands on opportunities to visit with and work on health issues of global concern.

Setting

For the next two years the College will be located in temporary space while the new facilities are being constructed. These temporary facilties have had a $5 million investment to create a state of the art Clinical Skills and Simulation Center and Gross Anatomy Lab. All classrooms have audio and video capture capabilities to facilitate learning.

Campus Information

Enrollment

For 2008, total enrollment was: n/a

Special Features

Students will receive training in a wide variety of community practice settings—hospitals, private offices, and clinics.

Housing

Students will have access to many housing options on the Scranton campus for years 1 & 2 and on the clinical campuses for those years. Student Affairs has prepared housing guides for all campuses.

Satellite Campuses/Facilities

For years 3 & 4 students will select a clinical campus (Scranton, Wilkes-Barre or Williamsport). All campuses are student friendly and experienced with abundant and diverse clinical experiences.

Application Process and Requirements 2010–2011

Primary Application Service: AMCAS
Earliest filing date: June 1, 2009
Latest filing date: December 15, 2009

Secondary Application Required?: Yes
Sent to: Secondary application will be sent to all applicants upon receipt of verified AMCAS application.
Contact: Admissions Office, (570) 504-9068, admissions@tcmedc.org
Fee: Yes, $100
Fee waiver available: Yes
Earliest filing date: August 1, 2009
Latest filing date: January 15, 2010

MCAT® required?: Yes
Latest MCAT® considered: September 2009
Oldest MCAT® considered: 2007

Early Decision Program: School does not have EDP
Applicants notified: n/a
EDP available for: n/a

Regular Acceptance Notice
Earliest date: October 15, 2009
Latest date: Until class is full
Applicant's Response to Acceptance Offer – Maximum Time: Two weeks

Requests for Deferred Entrance Considered: Yes

Deposit to Hold Place in Class: Yes
Deposit (Resident): $100
Deposit (Non-resident): $100
Deposit due: With response to acceptance offer
Applied to tuition: Yes
Deposit refundable: Yes
Refundable by: May 15, 2010

Estimated number of new entrants: 60
EDP: n/a, special program: n/a

Start Month/Year: August 2010

Interview Format: Interviews are with a clinical faculty and a basic science faculty in a conversational format. Regional interviews are not available.

Other Programs

PREPARATORY PROGRAMS
Postbaccalaureate Program: No, www.thecommonwealthmedical.com/oth/Page.asp?PageID=OTH000030

COMBINED DEGREE PROGRAMS
Baccalaureate/M.D.: No
M.D./M.P.H.: No
MD/MBA: No
M.D./J.D.: No
M.D./Ph.D.: No

Premedical Coursework

Course	Req.	Rec.	Lab.	Sems.	Course	Req.	Rec.	Lab.	Sems.
Inorganic Chemistry	•		•	2	Computer Science				
Behavioral Sciences					Genetics		•		
Biochemistry		•			Humanities				
Biology	•		•	2	Organic Chemistry	•		•	2
Biology/Zoology					Physics	•		•	2
Calculus		•			Psychology				
College English	•			1	Social Sciences				
College Mathematics			•		Other1				

Selection Factors: 2008 Accepted Applicants

Proportion of Accepted Applicants with Relevant Experience (Data Self-Reported to AMCAS®)	Community Service/Volunteer Medically-Related Work Research	DATA NOT AVAILABLE

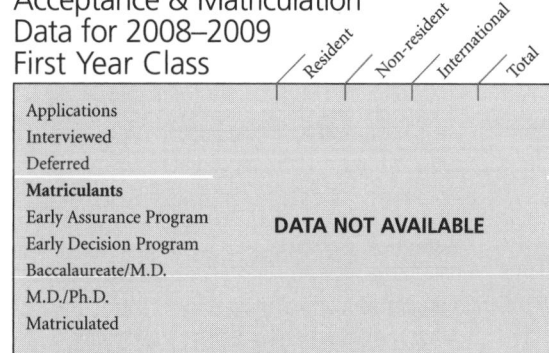

Shaded bar represents school's accepted scores ranging from the 10th percentile to the 90th percentile	School Median ● National Median ●
Overall GPA / Science GPA	DATA NOT AVAILABLE
MCAT® Total Numeric Score	DATA NOT AVAILABLE
Writing Sample / Verbal Reasoning / Biological Sciences / Physical Sciences	DATA NOT AVAILABLE

Acceptance & Matriculation Data for 2008–2009 First Year Class

	Resident	Non-resident	International	Total
Applications				
Interviewed				
Deferred				
Matriculants				
Early Assurance Program		DATA NOT AVAILABLE		
Early Decision Program				
Baccalaureate/M.D.				
M.D./Ph.D.				
Matriculated				

Applications accepted from International Applicants: Only Canadian

Specialty Choice

2004, 2005, 2006 Graduates, Specialty Choice (As reported by program directors to GME Track™)

Anesthesiology
Emergency Medicine
Family Practice

DATA NOT AVAILABLE

Psychiatry
Radiology
Surgery

Matriculant Demographics: 2008–2009 First Year Class

Men: n/a   **Women:** n/a

Matriculants' Self-Reported Race/Ethnicity

DATA NOT AVAILABLE

Science and Math Majors: n/a
Matriculants with:
    Baccalaureate degree: n/a
    Graduate degree(s): n/a

Financial Information

Source: 2007–2008 LCME I-B survey and 2008–2009 AAMC TSF questionnaire

	Residents	Non-residents
Total Cost of Attendance	$61,398	$66,398
Tuition and Fees	$38,550	$43,550
Other (includes living expenses)	$19,833	$19,833
Health Insurance (can be waived)	$3,015	$3,015

Average 2008 Graduate Indebtedness: 0
% of Enrolled Students Receiving Aid: n/a

Criminal Background Check

This medical school requires a criminal background check prior to matriculation.

Drexel University College of Medicine
Philadelphia, Pennsylvania

Admissions Office
Drexel University College of Medicine
2900 Queen Lane
Philadelphia, Pennsylvania 19129
T 215 991 8202   F 215 843 1766

Admissions www.drexelmed.edu/Admissions/
MDProgram/tabid/2289/Default.aspx
Main www.drexelmed.edu
Financial www.drexel.edu/provost/financialaid
E-mail medadmis@drexel.edu

Private Institution

Dr. Richard V. Homan, Dean

Dr. Samuel K. Parrish, Associate Dean for Admissions and Student Affairs

Dr. Anthony Rodriguez, Associate Dean of Student Affairs and Diversity

Elreo Campbell, Director of Financial Aid

General Information
Drexel University College of Medicine was formed when two historic Philadelphia medical schools joined their rich histories and resources. The Medical College of Pennsylvania (MCP) was founded in 1850 as the first medical school for women. Hahnemann University, a private nondenominational institution, was founded in 1848. Drexel offers a medical education rich in history and diversity, while providing the foundational curriculum and learning environment necessary for the scientific, technological, and ethical decisions required of physicians in the 21st century.

Mission Statement
Drexel is committed to providing our students with the finest possible medical education. Academic instruction in basic and clinical sciences, utilizing state-of-the-art technology, is enriched by an emphasis on compassionate patient care and community service.

Curricular Highlights
Community Service Requirement:
Required. 16 hours is required in year one.
Research/Thesis Requirement:
Optional. Though optional, many students conduct research.

Medical students are trained to consider each patient in a comprehensive, integrated manner, taking into account more factors than the presenting physiological condition. The school is dedicated to preparing "physician healers," who practice the art, science, and skill of medicine. Drexel offers a choice between two innovative curricula for the first two years of study. Interdisciplinary Foundations of Medicine (IFM) integrates basic science courses and presents them through symptom-based modules. Learning in IFM is faculty-driven; stu-

dents learn in lectures, labs, and small groups. Learning in the Program for Integrated Learning (PIL), a problem-based curriculum, is student-driven, supervised and facilitated by faculty. Students learn in small groups, labs, and resource sessions by focusing on case studies. Both options stress problem-solving, lifelong learning, and the coordinated training of basic science with clinical medicine. Both include the introduction of clinical skills training very early in the first year. The Pathway Program in the fourth year includes a balance of four week-long required and elective clinical experiences selected with the pathway advisors to be consistent with general medical training and the students ultimate career goals.

USMLE
Step 1: Required. Students must record a passing score for promotion.
Step 2: Clinical Skills (CS): Required. Students must record a passing total score to graduate.
Step 2: Clinical Knowledge (CK): Required. Students must record a passing total score to graduate.

Selection Factors
The academic factors taken into consideration for admission into the combined-degree program include SAT/ACT scores, high school GPA, and AP and honors courses. The average high school GPA for the 2008–2009 entering class was 3.9, with a mean score of 1470 on the SAT and a 33 Composite on the ACT. Medically related volunteer activities, leadership qualities, and community service are among the personal attributes sought in applicants. An interview at the college of medicine is also required. Once admitted into the program, students are expected to maintain an overall GPA of 3.5 in undergraduate studies; complete all prerequisite courses; and receive no grade less than a C in any course. Receive in a single examination a minimum MCAT score of "9" or better in the verbal section and "10s" or better in the physical or biological science section, or a total minimum score of 31 (with no individual subsection score less than an 8), and a letter score of "P" or higher in the MCAT written section. Apply through AMCAS in the second year. The MCAT is a factor in admittance and promotion to the medical school phase of the program.

Financial Aid
In addition to the Stafford Student Loan Program, the Primary Care Loan Program, other federally funded programs, and assistance in obtaining money from foundation sources, the Financial Affairs Office has at its disposal limited private grant and loan funds. A Work-Study Program for qualified students is available. Money allocated by the school is awarded on the basis of financial need. Fee waivers are only granted if approved by AMCAS.

Information about Diversity Programs
Applications are actively encouraged from groups underrepresented in medicine. Applications from women, those who come from Pennsylvania, and students interested in a career as a generalist physician are also encouraged.

Campus Information
Setting
Located in a largely residential section of Philadelphia, the college is only 15 minutes from Center City. Opened in 1992, this 15-acre site houses the education and research facility which is home for the first and second years of medical education. The campus features wireless internet access.

Enrollment
For 2008, total enrollment was: 1,070

Special Features
The medical school has a supportive environment that fosters a spirit of teamwork and personal interaction. Our state-of-the-art facility includes the CEAC Center with 10 exam rooms where students see standardized patients. Elective enrichment programs include Women's Health and Medical Humanities. Students in their clinical years use PDAs to record patient encounters and log procedures. The recently added 17,620 square-foot Student Activities Center greatly enhances the learning and living environment of the campus.

Housing
On-campus housing is not available. However, the college maintains an on-line list of rentals averaging $750 to $1,500 per month.

Satellite Campuses/Facilities
Students have the opportunity for clinical training in our extensive, integrated network of clinical campuses.

Application Process and Requirements 2010–2011

Primary Application Service: AMCAS
Earliest filing date: June 1, 2009
Latest filing date: December 15, 2009

Secondary Application Required?: Yes
Sent to: All applicants
URL: www.drexelmed.edu/Admissions/MDProgram/tabid/2289/Default.aspx
Fee: Yes, $75
Fee waiver available: Yes
Earliest filing date: Upon receipt of application
Latest filing date: January 1, 2010

MCAT® required?: Yes
Latest MCAT® considered: September 2009
Oldest MCAT® considered: 2007

Early Decision Program: School does have EDP
Applicants notified: October 1, 2009
EDP available for: Both Residents and Non-residents

Regular Acceptance Notice
Earliest date: October 15, 2009
Latest date: Until class is full
Applicant's Response to Acceptance Offer – Maximum Time: 21 days

Requests for Deferred Entrance Considered: Yes

Deposit to Hold Place in Class: Yes
Deposit (Resident): $100
Deposit (Non-resident): $100
Deposit due: 21 days from acceptance offer
Applied to tuition: Yes
Deposit refundable: Yes
Refundable by: May 15, 2010

Estimated number of new entrants: 255
EDP: n/a, special program: 80

Start Month/Year: August 2010

Interview Format: One faculty open-file, one student closed-file. Regional interviews are not available.

Other Programs

PREPARATORY PROGRAMS
Postbaccalaureate Program: Yes, www.drexelmed.edu/Home/AcademicPrograms/ProfessionalStudiesintheHealthSciences/Programs/InterdepartmentalMedicalScienceIMSProgram.aspx
Summer Program: No

Drexel links with a number of post-baccalaureate programs: www.drexelmed.edu/Home/Admissions/MDProgram/AcceleratedandEarlyAssuranceLinkagePrograms.aspx

COMBINED DEGREE PROGRAMS
Baccalaureate/M.D.: Yes, www.drexelmed.edu/Home/Admissions/MDProgram/AcceleratedandEarlyAssuranceLinkagePrograms.aspx
M.D./M.P.H.: Yes, http://publichealth.drexel.edu/
MD/MBA: Yes, www.lebow.drexel.edu/Prospects/MBA/MdMBA/index.php
M.D./J.D.: No
M.D./Ph.D.: Yes, www.drexelmed.edu/Home/AcademicPrograms/BiomedicalGraduateStudies/Programs/CombinedMDPhD.aspx
Additional Program: Yes, www.drexelmed.edu/Home/Admissions/MDProgram.aspx

Premedical Coursework

Course	Req.	Rec.	Lab.	Sems.
Inorganic Chemistry	•		•	2
Behavioral Sciences				
Biochemistry		•		
Biology	•		•	2
Biology/Zoology				
Calculus				
College English	•			2
College Mathematics				

Course	Req.	Rec.	Lab.	Sems.
Computer Science				
Genetics		•		
Humanities		•		
Organic Chemistry	•		•	2
Physics	•		•	2
Psychology				
Social Sciences				
Molecular Biology		•		

Selection Factors: 2008 Accepted Applicants

Proportion of Accepted Applicants with Relevant Experience (Data Self-Reported to AMCAS®)		
Community Service/Volunteer		65%
Medically-Related Work		84%
Research		81%

Shaded bar represents school's accepted scores ranging from the 10th percentile to the 90th percentile. School Median ● National Median ●

Overall GPA: 2.0 2.1 2.2 2.3 2.4 2.5 2.6 2.7 2.8 2.9 3.0 3.1 **3.2 3.3 3.4 3.5 (3.6) 3.7 3.8 3.9** 4.0

Science GPA: 2.0 2.1 2.2 2.3 2.4 2.5 2.6 2.7 2.8 2.9 3.0 **3.1 3.2 3.3 3.4 3.5 (3.6) 3.7 3.8 3.9** 4.0

MCAT® Total Numeric Score: 9 10 11 12 13 14 15 16 17 18 19 20 21 22 23 24 25 26 27 **28 29 30 (31) 32 33 34 35** 36 37 38 39 40 41 42 43

Writing Sample			J	K	L	**M N O P (Q) R S**				T
Verbal Reasoning	3	4	5	6	7	**8 9 (10) 11 12**	13	14			15
Biological Sciences	3	4	5	6	7	8	**9 10 (11) 12 13**	14			15
Physical Sciences	3	4	5	6	7	8	**9 (10) (11) 12 13**	14			15

Acceptance & Matriculation Data for 2008–2009 First Year Class

	Resident	Non-resident	International	Total
Applications	1136	10803	66	12005
Interviewed	344	987	0	1331
Deferred	0	3	0	3
Matriculants				
Early Assurance Program	3	4	0	7
Early Decision Program	3	1	0	4
Baccalaureate/M.D.	11	51	0	62
M.D./Ph.D.	1	3	0	4
Matriculated	78	178	0	**256**

Applications accepted from International Applicants: No

Specialty Choice

2004, 2005, 2006 Graduates, Specialty Choice (As reported by program directors to GME Track™)	
Anesthesiology	5%
Emergency Medicine	9%
Family Practice	10%
Internal Medicine	18%
Obstetrics/Gynecology	5%
Orthopaedic Surgery	5%
Pediatrics	10%
Psychiatry	5%
Radiology	6%
Surgery	8%

Matriculant Demographics: 2008–2009 First Year Class

Men: 130   **Women:** 126

Matriculants' Self-Reported Race/Ethnicity

Mexican American	4	Korean	7
Cuban	2	Vietnamese	1
Puerto Rican	0	Other Asian	2
Other Hispanic	10	Total Asian	105
Total Hispanic	16	Native American	3
Chinese	18	Black	21
Asian Indian	67	Native Hawaiian	1
Pakistani	5	White	129
Filipino	6	Unduplicated Number	
Japanese	1	of Matriculants	256

Science and Math Majors: 71%
Matriculants with:
  Baccalaureate degree: 99%
  Graduate degree(s): 19%

Financial Information
Source: 2007–2008 LCME I-B survey and 2008–2009 AAMC TSF questionnaire

	Residents	Non-residents
Total Cost of Attendance	$72,059	$72,059
Tuition and Fees	$43,800	$43,800
Other (includes living expenses)	$25,334	$25,334
Health Insurance (can be waived)	$2,925	$2,925

Average 2008 Graduate Indebtedness: $182,921
% of Enrolled Students Receiving Aid: 90%

Criminal Background Check

This medical school requires a criminal background check prior to matriculation.

Jefferson Medical College of Thomas Jefferson University

Philadelphia, Pennsylvania

Office of Admissions
Jefferson Medical College
of Thomas Jefferson University
1015 Walnut Street, Suite 110
Philadelphia, Pennsylvania 19107-5099
T 215 955 6983   **F** 215 955 5151

Admissions www.jefferson.edu/jmc/admissions
Main www.jefferson.edu/jmc
Financial www.jefferson.edu/financialaid
E-mail jmc.admissions@jefferson.edu

Private Institution

Dr. Mark L. Tykocinski, Dean

Dr. Clara Callahan, Dean of Students and Admissions

Dr. Edward Christian, Associate Dean for Diversity and Minority Affairs

Susan Batchelor McFadden, Director of Student Financial Aid

Dr. Elizabeth Brooks, Director of Admissions

General Information

As one of the oldest institutions of higher education in the nation, Thomas Jefferson University has, since its founding as the Jefferson Medical College in 1824, emphasized the attainment of clinical excellence in its educational programs. A recent significant expansion of the research programs has created a balanced institutional mission and has enhanced the clinical instruction at Thomas Jefferson University Hospital and its 17 affiliated hospitals.

Mission Statement

Jefferson's teaching mission centers on the education of outstanding individuals in the art and science of medicine. By helping these individuals to develop their medical knowledge, clinical and research skills, and professional values, attitudes, and behaviors, we strive to provide outstanding physicians for the United States and the world.

Curricular Highlights

Community Service Requirement: Required.
Research/Thesis Requirement: Optional.

The curriculum has been developed to enable students to acquire basic knowledge and skills in the biomedical sciences and to develop appropriate professional behaviors. The curriculum also allows students to pursue some of their special interests throughout their medical training. The tradition of providing a clinically balanced medical education, encouraged by the faculty, is that students support and cooperate with each other. In the first year, students focus on the function of human organism in its physical and psychosocial context. Clinical coursework focuses on the doctor-patient rela-

tionship, medical interviewing and history-taking, human development, behavioral science principles, and core clinical skills and reasoning. In addition to increasing emphasis on the study of clinical skills, the curriculum shifts in the second year to the study of pathophysioiogy and disease. The curriculum includes small-group sessions focusing on problem-solving, evidence-based medicine, and service-based learning. The clinical program consists of two 42-week phases. Phase I covers required clerkships. Advanced basic science, neurology/rehabilitation medicine, emergency medicine/advanced clinical skills, in- and outpatient subinternships, as well as 16 weeks of elective time, are included in Phase II.

USMLE

Step 1: Required. Students must record a passing score for promotion.
Step 2: Clinical Skills (CS): Required. Students must only record a score.
Step 2: Clinical Knowledge (CK): Required. Students must record a passing total score to graduate.

Selection Factors

Jefferson, in accordance with local, state, and federal law, is committed to providing equal educational and employment opportunities for all persons, without regard to race, color, national and ethnic origin, religion, sexual orientation, age, handicap, or veteran status. Jefferson complies with all relevant ordinances and state and federal statutes in the administration of its educational and employment policies and is an affirmative action employer. The selection of students is made after careful consideration of many factors, including the academic record, letters of recommendation, MCAT scores and interview results regarding the applicant's personal qualities, motivation, interpersonal skills, and achievement in nonacademic areas. Jefferson Medical College traditionally has given special consideration to the offspring of alumni and faculty, groups underrepresented in medicine, and applicants to Jefferson's special programs. International applicants must have a baccalaureate degree from an accredited U.S. or Canadian college or university.

Financial Aid

Financial aid awards are based on need determined by a confidential analysis of information provided by the student and the student's family to the designated needs analysis service. If need is established, the student is directed to obtain a federally subsidized Stafford loan. If need exists beyond this loan program, Jefferson will try to meet a portion of this need from loan and grant funds. Applications for financial aid are available after December from the Office of Student Financial Aid. Completed financial aid applications for the next academic year must be submitted before April 1 or within two weeks of the date of acceptance.

Information about Diversity Programs

Applications from qualified students from groups underrepresented in medicine are encouraged.

Campus Information

Setting

The medical school is proud to be situated near the most historic square mile in America. The campus is 13 square acres in the heart of Center City Philadelphia.

Enrollment

For 2008, total enrollment was: 999

Special Features

Thomas Jefferson University Hospital is one of the area's largest medical centers and includes both a Level I regional resource trauma center and a Spinal Cord Injury Center (SCI).

Housing

On-campus housing is available.

Application Process and Requirements 2010–2011

Primary Application Service: AMCAS
Earliest filing date: June 1, 2009
Latest filing date: November 16, 2009

Secondary Application Required?: Yes
Sent to: All applicants
URL: www.jefferson.edu/jmc/admissions/appforms.cfm
Fee: Yes, $80
Fee waiver available: Yes
Earliest filing date: June 1, 2009
Latest filing date: January 15, 2010

MCAT® required?: Yes
Latest MCAT® considered: September 2009
Oldest MCAT® considered: 2006

Early Decision Program: School does have EDP
Applicants notified: October 1, 2009
EDP available for: Both Residents and Non-residents

Regular Acceptance Notice
Earliest date: October 15, 2009
Latest date: Until class is full
Applicant's Response to Acceptance Offer – Maximum Time: Three weeks

Requests for Deferred Entrance Considered: Yes

Deposit to Hold Place in Class: Yes
Deposit (Resident): $100
Deposit (Non-resident): $100
Deposit due: at time of acceptance
Applied to tuition: Yes
Deposit refundable: Yes
Refundable by: May 15, 2010

Estimated number of new entrants: 255
EDP: 5, special program: 40

Start Month/Year: August 2010

Interview Format: One-on-one, open file (faculty) and closed file (student). Regional interview available on campus only.

Other Programs

PREPARATORY PROGRAMS
Postbaccalaureate Program: No
Summer Program: No

COMBINED DEGREE PROGRAMS
Baccalaureate/M.D.: Yes
www.science.psu.edu/premedmed/
M.D./M.P.H.: Yes, www.jefferson.edu/mph
M.D./M.B.A.: Yes, David Nash, M.D., M.B.A., (215) 955-6969, David.Nash@jefferson.edu
www.jefferson.edu/dhp/mdmbaprogram.cfm
M.D./J.D.: No
M.D./Ph.D.: Yes, www.jefferson.edu/jcgs/mdphd

Premedical Coursework

Course	Req.	Rec.	Lab.	Sems.
Inorganic Chemistry	•		•	2
Behavioral Sciences				
Biochemistry		•		1
Biology	•		•	2
Biology/Zoology				
Calculus				
College English		•		
College Mathematics				

Course	Req.	Rec.	Lab.	Sems.
Computer Science				
Genetics				
Humanities		•		
Organic Chemistry	•		•	2
Physics	•		•	2
Psychology				
Social Sciences		•		
Other				

Selection Factors: 2008 Accepted Applicants

Proportion of Accepted Applicants with Relevant Experience (Data Self-Reported to AMCAS®)		
Community Service/Volunteer		67%
Medically-Related Work		87%
Research		78%

Shaded bar represents school's accepted scores ranging from the 10th percentile to the 90th percentile ▪   School Median ●   National Median ●

Overall GPA 2.0 2.1 2.2 2.3 2.4 2.5 2.6 2.7 2.8 2.9 3.0 3.1 3.2 3.3 3.4 3.5 3.6 (3.7) 3.8 3.9 4.0

Science GPA 2.0 2.1 2.2 2.3 2.4 2.5 2.6 2.7 2.8 2.9 3.0 3.1 3.2 3.3 3.4 3.5 (3.6) 3.7 3.8 3.9 4.0

MCAT® Total Numeric Score 9 10 11 12 13 14 15 16 17 18 19 20 21 22 23 24 25 26 27 28 29 30 31 (32) 33 34 35 36 37 38 39 40 41 42 43

Writing Sample			J	K	L	M	N	O	P	(Q)	R	S	T
Verbal Reasoning	3	4	5	6	7	8	9	(10)	11	12	13	14	15
Biological Sciences	3	4	5	6	7	8	9	10	(11)	12	13	14	15
Physical Sciences	3	4	5	6	7	8	9	10	(11)	12	13	14	15

Acceptance & Matriculation Data for 2008–2009 First Year Class

	Resident	Non-resident	International	Total
Applications	1097	7714	512	9323
Interviewed	231	549	22	802
Deferred	3	1	1	5
Matriculants				
Early Assurance Program	6	6	0	12
Early Decision Program	3	4	0	7
Baccalaureate/M.D.	7	12	1	20
M.D./Ph.D.	2	3	0	5
Matriculated	98	143	14	**255**

Applications accepted from International Applicants: Yes

Matriculant Demographics: 2008–2009 First Year Class

Men: 132   **Women:** 123

Matriculants' Self-Reported Race/Ethnicity

Mexican American	3	Korean	9
Cuban	6	Vietnamese	7
Puerto Rican	2	Other Asian	2
Other Hispanic	6	Total Asian	57
Total Hispanic	16	Native American	0
Chinese	14	Black	3
Asian Indian	23	Native Hawaiian	0
Pakistani	0	White	172
Filipino	0	Unduplicated Number	
Japanese	3	of Matriculants	255

Science and Math Majors: 60%
Matriculants with:
Baccalaureate degree: 98%
Graduate degree(s): 6%

Specialty Choice

2004, 2005, 2006 Graduates, Specialty Choice (As reported by program directors to GME Track™)	
Anesthesiology	7%
Emergency Medicine	8%
Family Practice	10%
Internal Medicine	20%
Obstetrics/Gynecology	4%
Orthopaedic Surgery	4%
Pediatrics	8%
Psychiatry	4%
Radiology	4%
Surgery	8%

Financial Information

Source: 2007–2008 LCME I-B survey and 2008–2009 AAMC TSF questionnaire

	Residents	Non-residents
Total Cost of Attendance	$65,468	$65,468
Tuition and Fees	$43,033	$43,033
Other (includes living expenses)	$19,367	$19,367
Health Insurance (can be waived)	$3,068	$3,068

Average 2008 Graduate Indebtedness: $162,885
% of Enrolled Students Receiving Aid: 82%

Criminal Background Check

This medical school requires a criminal background check prior to matriculation.

Pennsylvania State University College of Medicine

Hershey, Pennsylvania

Pennsylvania State University College of Medicine
Office of Medical Student Affairs, H060
500 University Drive; P.O. Box 850
Hershey, Pennsylvania 17033
T 717 531 8755   F 717 531 6225

Admissions www.hmc.psu.edu/md/admissions
Main www.hmc.psu.edu/md
Financial www.hmc.psu.edu/md/financialaid
E-mail studentadmissions@hmc.psu.edu

Public Institution

Dr. Harold L. Paz, Dean, Senior Vice President for Health Affairs

Dr. Dwight Davis, Associate Dean for Admissions and Student Affairs

Dr. Alphonse E. Leure-duPree, Associate Dean for Academic Achievement

Dr. Joetta Bradica, Assistant Director for Financial Aid

Marc Lubbers, Assistant Director for Admissions

General Information

Penn State's Milton S. Hershey Medical Center opened its doors to the first class of medical students in 1967 and became the first medical school in the nation to establish a Department of Humanities, introducing humanistic disciplines into the required medical curriculum. The College of Medicine was also the first to start an independent Department of Family and Community Medicine. From its beginning, medical education and patient care have been guided by the institution's commitment to provide humane, compassionate, and expert care.

Mission Statement

Penn State College of Medicine is dedicated to the education of physicians and scientists in all of the disciplines of medicine and biomedical investigation for careers in practice, teaching, and research. Necessary to this educational mission are the provision of outstanding medical care and services and the enhancement of new knowledge through clinical and basic biomedical research.

Curricular Highlights

Community Service Requirement: Optional.
www.hmc.psu.edu/md/studentlife/studentorgs.html
Research/Thesis Requirement: Required.
Full details at: *www.hmc.psu.edu/msr*

A single integrated curriculum for years one and two combines elements of traditional medical teaching and case-based learning. The first-year curriculum and courses are interdisciplinary, combining case-based, student-centered learning with strategic lectures, laboratories, and small-group discussions. The second-year cur-

riculum is more heavily oriented to case-based learning in an organ/organ system approach to human health, pathophysiology, and disease. Year three includes a sequence of required core clinical clerkships in internal medicine, general surgery, pediatrics, obstetrics and gynecology, psychiatry, family and community medicine, and primary care supplemented by available selectives. In addition, there are week-long sessions in Advanced Clinical Diagnostics and Therapeutics, Communications and Professionalism, and Improving Healthcare. Year four consists of four elective rotations and four required advanced experiences. The College of Medicine offers a wide variety of both clinical and research electives. Students may select outpatient clinical rotations at teaching hospitals or in university-affiliated physicians' offices located in a variety of rural and metropolitan communities nationwide and abroad. All students participate in an individualized research program.

USMLE

Step 1: Required. Students must record a passing score for promotion.
Step 2: Clinical Skills (CS): Required. Students must record a passing total score to graduate.
Step 2: Clinical Knowledge (CK): Required. Students must record a passing total score to graduate.

Selection Factors

Applicants must show evidence of superior undergraduate achievement and outstanding personal characteristics. Each application is considered individually. A decision is reached after thorough evaluation of the applicant's academic record, letters of assessment, extracurricular activities, MCAT scores, and personal interviews. Since the practice of medicine requires a lifelong devotion to self-education, emphasis is placed on the excellence of the individual scholar no matter what the student's previous area of study.

Financial Aid

Financial aid is granted based upon need as determined by federal methodology. Parental income information is required for university scholarship and loan consideration, as well as some other financial assistance programs.

Additional financial aid information is available on the school's Web site.

Information about Diversity Programs

Students from groups underrepresented in medicine are encouraged to apply. Faculty members, with student support, are active in the recruitment of students from groups underrepresented in medicine.

Campus Information

Setting

The 550-acre campus is located in the rolling hills of southeastern Pennsylvania near the state capital, Harrisburg. The main facility houses the College of Medicine, the 500+ bed University Hospital and Children's Hospital, the Rehabilitation Center, the Biomedical Research Building, the Emergency Medical Center, and the Penn State Hershey Cancer Institute. The hospital serves as the only regional Level I Trauma Center for both adult and pediatric cases.

Enrollment

For 2008, total enrollment was: 592

Special Features

The College of Medicine has state-of-the art facilities, innovative programs, and an award-winning staff that combines medical expertise with compassionate patient care. Learn more at *www.hmc.psu.edu/md/admissions/eduexp.html*.

Housing

University Manor is a safe and affordable housing complex situated on campus with numerous ammenities. Learn more at *www.pennstatehersheyhousing.com*.

Satellite Campuses/Facilities

The College of Medicine has forged a large number of collaborations that provide extensive opportunities for its medical students. Students rotate at defined institutions that meet the College of Medicine's high standards of educational quality.

Application Process and Requirements 2010–2011

Primary Application Service: AMCAS
Earliest filing date: June 1, 2009
Latest filing date: November 15, 2009

Secondary Application Required?: Yes
Sent to: All applicants
Contact: Office of Medical Student Admissions, (717) 531-8755, studentadmissions@hmc.psu.edu
Fee: Yes, $70
Fee waiver available: Yes
Earliest filing date: Based on e-mail invitation
Latest filing date: January 15, 2010

MCAT® required?: Yes
Latest MCAT® considered: September 2009
Oldest MCAT® considered: 2007

Early Decision Program: School does have EDP
Applicants notified: October 1, 2009
EDP available for: Both Residents and Non-residents

Regular Acceptance Notice
Earliest date: October 16, 2009
Latest date: Until class is full
Applicant's Response to Acceptance Offer – Maximum Time: Two weeks

Requests for Deferred Entrance Considered: Yes

Deposit to Hold Place in Class: Yes
Deposit (Resident): $100
Deposit (Non-resident): $100
Deposit due: May 15, 2010
Applied to tuition: Yes
Deposit refundable: Yes
Refundable by: May 15, 2010

Estimated number of new entrants: 145
EDP: n/a, special program: n/a

Start Month/Year: August 2010

Interview Format: Interviews occur on campus by individual invitation. Regional interviews are not available.

Other Programs

PREPARATORY PROGRAMS
Postbaccalaureate Program: No
Summer Program: No
Early Assurance Program:
www.hmc.psu.edu/md/admissions/specialprog.html

Combined Degree Programs
Baccalaureate/M.D.: No
M.D./M.P.H.: No
MD/MBA: No
M.D./J.D.: No
M.D./Ph.D.: Yes, www.hmc.psu.edu/mdphd

Premedical Coursework

Course	Req.	Rec.	Lab.	Sems.	Course	Req.	Rec.	Lab.	Sems.
Inorganic Chemistry	•		•	2	Computer Science				
Behavioral Sciences	•			1	Genetics		•		1
Biochemistry		•			Humanities	•			1
Biology	•		•	2	Organic Chemistry	•		•	2
Biology/Zoology					Physics	•		•	2
Calculus		•			Psychology		•		
College English		•			Social Sciences		•		
College Mathematics	•			2	Other				

Selection Factors: 2008 Accepted Applicants

Proportion of Accepted Applicants with Relevant Experience (Data Self-Reported to AMCAS®)		
Community Service/Volunteer		73%
Medically-Related Work		86%
Research		87%

Shaded bar represents school's accepted scores ranging from the 10th percentile to the 90th percentile ▬   School Median ●   National Median ●

Overall GPA	2.0	2.1	2.2	2.3	2.4	2.5	2.6	2.7	2.8	2.9	3.0	3.1	3.2	3.3	3.4	3.5	3.6	3.7	(3.8)	3.9	4.0
Science GPA	2.0	2.1	2.2	2.3	2.4	2.5	2.6	2.7	2.8	2.9	3.0	3.1	3.2	3.3	3.4	3.5	3.6	(3.7)	3.8	3.9	4.0

MCAT® Total Numeric Score	9	10	11	12	13	14	15	16	17	18	19	20	21	22	23	24	25	26	27	28	29	30	3(32)33	34	35	36	37	38	39	40	41	42	43

Writing Sample			J	K	L	M	N	O	P	(Q)	R	S	T
Verbal Reasoning	3	4	5	6	7	8	9	(10)	11	12	13	14	15
Biological Sciences	3	4	5	6	7	8	9	10	(11)	12	13	14	15
Physical Sciences	3	4	5	6	7	8	9	10	(11)	12	13	14	15

Acceptance & Matriculation Data for 2008–2009 First Year Class

	Resident	Non-resident	International	Total
Applications	1043	5449	521	7013
Interviewed	270	562	19	851
Deferred	0	2	1	3
Matriculants				
Early Assurance Program	7	0	0	7
Early Decision Program	0	0	0	0
Baccalaureate/M.D.	n/a	n/a	n/a	n/a
M.D./Ph.D.	2	4	0	6
Matriculated	64	73	6	**143**

Applications accepted from International Applicants: Yes

Matriculant Demographics: 2008–2009 First Year Class

Men: 75   **Women:** 68

Matriculants' Self-Reported Race/Ethnicity

Mexican American	2	Korean	3
Cuban	1	Vietnamese	0
Puerto Rican	1	Other Asian	3
Other Hispanic	3	Total Asian	27
Total Hispanic	7	Native American	0
Chinese	9	Black	7
Asian Indian	10	Native Hawaiian	0
Pakistani	2	White	99
Filipino	1	Unduplicated Number	
Japanese	0	of Matriculants	143

Science and Math Majors: 80%
Matriculants with:
Baccalaureate degree: 99%
Graduate degree(s): 13%

Specialty Choice

2004, 2005, 2006 Graduates, Specialty Choice (As reported by program directors to GME Track™)	
Anesthesiology	8%
Emergency Medicine	9%
Family Practice	13%
Internal Medicine	16%
Obstetrics/Gynecology	6%
Orthopaedic Surgery	3%
Pediatrics	14%
Psychiatry	3%
Radiology	3%
Surgery	6%

Financial Information

Source: 2007–2008 LCME I-B survey and 2008–2009 AAMC TSF questionnaire

	Residents	Non-residents
Total Cost of Attendance	$50,254	$61,494
Tuition and Fees	$35,034	$46,274
Other (includes living expenses)	$14,060	$14,060
Health Insurance (can be waived)	$1,160	$1,160

Average 2008 Graduate Indebtedness: $160,064
% of Enrolled Students Receiving Aid: 91%

Criminal Background Check

This medical school requires a criminal background check prior to matriculation.

Temple University School of Medicine
Philadelphia, Pennsylvania

Office of Admissions
Temple University School of Medicine
3500 N. Broad Street, Suite 124
Philadelphia, Pennsylvania 19140
T 215 707 3656   F 215 707 6932

Admissions www.temple.edu/medicine/admissions
Main www.temple.edu/medicine
Financial www.temple.edu/sfs/med
E-mail medadmissions@temple.edu

Private Institution

Dr. John M. Daly, Dean

*Dr. Audrey B. Uknis,
Associate Dean for Admissions*

*Raul De La Cadena, Assistant Dean for
Recruitment, Admissions, and Retention*

General Information

A new 480,000 square foot 11-story medical school building will open in June 2009. This state of the art teaching and collaborative research space will transform the medical school campus and allow its continued growth as one of the nation's premier urban academic medical centers.

Mission Statement

A center of humanistic medicine, Temple University School of Medicine (TUSM) is known for its culture of service, diversity and collaboration. TUSM has three major interrelated missions: 1) provide excellent learner-centered education to a diverse body of medical and graduate students, instilling in them an ethic of human service and lifelong learning; 2) engage in research that advances medical science and clinical care; and 3) provide state-of-the-art health care.

Curricular Highlights

Community Service Requirement: Optional.
Research/Thesis Requirement: Optional.

In fall 2005, Temple introduced an Integrated Curriculum (IC), which provides integration among basic science disciplines and between basic science and clinical disciplines. The IC is competency-based, providing students with the opportunities to learn and practice the basic knowledge, clinical skills, and attitudes/behaviors essential to the medical profession. The curriculum incorporates state-of-the-art teaching technologies, including patient simulation. The IC is divided into a number of interdisciplinary blocks, each organized according to body or organ systems and taught by faculty from several basic science and clinical academic departments. The clerkships in years 3 and 4 will continue to provide exposure to a unique variety of clinical experiences, both inpatient and ambulatory. The IC facilitates the acquisi-

tion of an increasingly large body of biomedical information through the integration of basic science and medical information and places both in relevant clinical contexts.

USMLE

Step 1: Required. Students must record a passing score for promotion.
Step 2: Clinical Skills (CS): Required. Students must only record a score.
Step 2: Clinical Knowledge (CK): Required. Students must record a passing total score to graduate.

Selection Factors

An individualized holistic review of each completed application includes a variety of objective and subjective factors. The academic record, the college attended, MCAT scores, recommendations, extracurricular activities, work experience, medically related experience, and community service activities are all taken into account when selecting candidates for interview. While not required, many students have participated in research activities.
Approximately half of the matriculants are Pennsylvania residents, but non-residents with a particular interest in Temple and strong credentials are encouraged to apply. Students in the 2008 entering class attended 91 different colleges and Universities.

Financial Aid

Temple offers a variety of both merit and need-based scholarships. Students are encouraged to complete a FAFSA by March 1, including the parental section and submit tax returns to be considered for need-based University funds.

Information about Diversity Programs

The School of Medicine is committed to diversity in the faculty and student body. The Recruitment, Admissions, & Retention (RAR) program provides exceptional resources for professional academic guidance and counseling for applicants and students who are from disadvantaged backgrounds or groups underrepresented in medicine.

Campus Information

Setting

An urban institution, Temple serves a diverse population, drawing patients from the North Philadelphia community and from the greater Philadelphia region for specialized care. The School of Medicine shares a campus with Temple University Hospital and other health-related schools of the University. The campus is easily accessible by public transportation.

Enrollment

For 2008, total enrollment was: 703

Special Features

The Institute for Clinical Simulation and Patient Safety is a 10,000 sq foot learning laboratory which provides excellence in clinical skills training utilizing a combination of high-tech and traditional methods. The Clinical Simulation Center houses the programmable, anatomically detailed, and physiologically functional mannequins that are used to present a variety of clinical scenarios. The Clinical Skills Center houses the standardized patient program, which helps students learn to take histories, conduct physical examinations, make diagnoses, and communicate in a caring manner.

Housing

Students live about 20 minutes by car, in neighborhoods northwest of the campus or in downtown Philadelphia. The School of Medicine provides local housing information and hosts a blog for the incoming class.

Satellite Campuses/Facilities

Clinical experience and instruction are provided at Temple University Hospital, St. Christopher's Hospital for Children, Crozer-Chester Medical Center, Fox Chase Cancer Center, Abington Memorial Hospital, and other affiliated hospitals located throughout Pennsylvania. Clinical campuses have been established at the Western Pennsylvania Hospital in Pittsburgh, Geisinger Medical Center in Danville, and St. Luke's Hospital in Bethlehem. Students may elect to do all of the third and fourth-year rotations at one of the clinical campuses.

Application Process and Requirements 2010–2011

Primary Application Service: AMCAS
Earliest filing date: June 1, 2009
Latest filing date: December 15, 2009

Secondary Application Required?: Yes
Sent to: U.S. citizens, permanent residents or applicants who have refugee/asylee status.
URL: Sent when verified AMCAS application is received
Fee: Yes, $70
Fee waiver available: Yes
Earliest filing date: July 15, 2009
Latest filing date: January 15, 2010

MCAT® required?: Yes
Latest MCAT® considered: September 2009
Oldest MCAT® considered: January 2007

Early Decision Program: School does have EDP
Applicants notified: October 1, 2009
EDP available for: Both Residents and Non-residents

Regular Acceptance Notice
Earliest date: October 15, 2009
Latest date: Varies
Applicant's Response to Acceptance
Offer – Maximum Time: Two weeks

Requests for Deferred
Entrance Considered: Yes

Deposit to Hold Place in Class: Yes
Deposit (Resident): $100
Deposit (Non-resident): $100
Deposit due: Within two weeks of acceptance
Applied to tuition: Yes
Deposit refundable: Yes
Refundable by: May 15, 2010

Estimated number of new entrants: 200
EDP: 5, special program: 20

Start Month/Year: August 2010

Interview Format: Applicants have an interview with a faculty member and a student. Regional interviews are not available.

Other Programs

PREPARATORY PROGRAMS
Postbaccalaureate Program: Yes, www.temple.edu/medicine/postbac
Summer Program: Yes, www.temple.edu/medicine/rar
Early Assurance: Yes, www.temple.edu/medicine/admissions/special_admissions.htm

COMBINED DEGREE PROGRAMS
Baccalaureate/M.D.: Yes, www.temple.edu/medicine/admissions/special_admissions.htm
M.D./M.P.H.: Yes, www.temple.edu/medicine/education/dualdegree
MD/MBA: No
M.D./J.D.: No
M.D./Ph.D.: Yes, www.temple.edu/medicine/education/dualdegree/mdphd.htm

Premedical Coursework

Course	Req.	Rec.	Lab.	Hrs.
Inorganic Chemistry	•		•	8
Behavioral Sciences				
Biochemistry				
Biology	•	•	•	8
Biology/Zoology				
Calculus				
College English				
College Mathematics				

Course	Req.	Rec.	Lab.	Hrs.
Computer Science				
Genetics				
Humanities	•			6
Organic Chemistry	•		•	8
Physics	•		•	8
Psychology				
Social Sciences				
Other				

Selection Factors: 2008 Accepted Applicants

Proportion of Accepted Applicants with Relevant Experience (Data Self-Reported to AMCAS)		
Community Service/Volunteer		63%
Medically-Related Work		87%
Research		83%

Shaded bar represents school's accepted scores ranging from the 10th percentile to the 90th percentile   School Median ●   National Median ●

Overall GPA	2.0	2.1	2.2	2.3	2.4	2.5	2.6	2.7	2.8	2.9	3.0	3.1	3.2	3.3	3.4	3.5	3.6	(3.7)	3.8	3.9	4.0
Science GPA	2.0	2.1	2.2	2.3	2.4	2.5	2.6	2.7	2.8	2.9	3.0	3.1	3.2	3.3	3.4	3.5	3.6	(3.7)	3.8	3.9	4.0

MCAT® Total Numeric Score 9 10 11 12 13 14 15 16 17 18 19 20 21 22 23 24 25 26 27 28 29 30 (31) 32 33 34 35 36 37 38 39 40 41 42 43

Writing Sample			J	K	L	M	N	O	P	(Q)	R	S	T
Verbal Reasoning	3	4	5	6	7	8	9	(10)	11	12	13	14	15
Biological Sciences	3	4	5	6	7	8	9	10	(11)	12	13	14	15
Physical Sciences	3	4	5	6	7	8	9	10	(11)	12	13	14	15

Acceptance & Matriculation Data for 2008–2009 First Year Class

	Resident	Non-resident	International	Total
Applications	1117	8435	87	9639
Interviewed	269	678	0	947
Deferred	2	2	0	4
Matriculants				
Early Assurance Program	4	0	0	4
Early Decision Program	2	2	0	4
Baccalaureate/M.D.	2	1	0	3
M.D./Ph.D.	2	2	0	4
Matriculated	93	89	0	**182**

Applications accepted from International Applicants: No

Matriculant Demographics: 2008–2009 First Year Class

Men: 96   **Women:** 86

Matriculants' Self-Reported Race/Ethnicity

Mexican American	2	Korean	1
Cuban	4	Vietnamese	1
Puerto Rican	2	Other Asian	4
Other Hispanic	10	Total Asian	40
Total Hispanic	15	Native American	2
Chinese	16	Black	10
Asian Indian	16	Native Hawaiian	1
Pakistani	0	White	126
Filipino	3	Unduplicated Number	
Japanese	1	of Matriculants	182

Science and Math Majors: 67%
Matriculants with:
      Baccalaureate degree: 98%
      Graduate degree(s): 8%

Specialty Choice

2004, 2005, 2006 Graduates, Specialty Choice (As reported by program directors to GME Track™)	
Anesthesiology	5%
Emergency Medicine	9%
Family Practice	7%
Internal Medicine	27%
Obstetrics/Gynecology	3%
Orthopaedic Surgery	3%
Pediatrics	9%
Psychiatry	4%
Radiology	5%
Surgery	10%

Financial Information

Source: 2007–2008 LCME I-B survey and 2008–2009 AAMC TSF questionnaire

	Residents	Non-residents
Total Cost of Attendance	$63,629	$72,633
Tuition and Fees	$40,744	$49,778
Other (includes living expenses)	$20,397	$20,397
Health Insurance (can be waived)	$2,458	$2,458

Average 2008 Graduate Indebtedness: $173,712
% of Enrolled Students Receiving Aid: 91%

Criminal Background Check

This medical school requires a criminal background check prior to matriculation.

University of Pennsylvania School of Medicine

Philadelphia, Pennsylvania

Office of Admissions and Financial Aid
Suite 100, Edward J. Stemmler Hall
University of Pennsylvania School of Medicine
3450 Hamilton Walk
Philadelphia, Pennsylvania 19104-6056
T 215 898 8001   **F** 215 573 6645

Admissions www.med.upenn.edu/admiss
Main www.med.upenn.edu
Financial www.med.upenn.edu/financialaid/
E-mail admiss@mail.med.upenn.edu

Private Institution

Dr. Arthur H. Rubenstein, Dean

Dr. Gail Morrison, Vice Dean for Education

Gaye W. Sheffler, Director of Admissions and Financial Aid

Dr. Karen Hamilton, Assistant Dean for Diversity and Community Outreach in Undergraduate Medical Education

General Information

The School of Medicine, the first in the United States, was founded in 1765 and is a private, non-denominational school on the urban campus of the University of Pennsylvania. The one university concept enrolls medical students as members of the university as well as the School of Medicine community. Clinical education occurs in the Hospital of the University of Pennsylvania, Children's Hospital of Philadelphia, Veterans Administration Hospital of Philadelphia, Presbyterian Medical Center, and Pennsylvania Hospital.

Mission Statement

Our mission is to create the future of medicine through: Patient Care and Service Excellence, Educational Pre-eminence, New Knowledge and Innovation, and National and International Leadership.

Curricular Highlights

Community Service Requirement: Required. Three-year patient-centered experience.
Research/Thesis Requirement: Required. Three month scholarly pursuit and/or dual degree.

The four-year curriculum has three themes: Science of Medicine, Technology and Practice of Medicine, and Professionalism and Humanism. Module 1 (four months) provides the foundation of basic sciences and is divided into four blocks: Developmental and Molecular Biology; Cell Physiology and Metabolism: Human Body, Structure, and Function; and Host Defenses and Responses. Grades are pass/fail. Module 2 (40 weeks) integrates basic science across organ systems and ends in December of Year 2. Topics are organized by: Normal Development, Normal Processes, Abnormal Processes, Therapeutics and Disease

Management, Epidemiology/Evidenced-based Medicine, Prevention, and Nutrition. Grades are honors/pass/fail. Module 3, Technology and Practice of Medicine, runs concurrent with modules 1 and 2 and promotes competency in epidemiology and biostatistics, decision-making, health care economics, population-based medicine, managed care and quality assurance, and basic clinical medicine. Grades are pass/fail. Module 4, (clinical clerkships), runs from January of Year 2 through December of Year 3 and is composed of 48 weeks of required clinical clerkships divided into four three-month cross-disciplinary experiences. Basic science concepts are reinforced weekly in didactic sessions. Module 5 (16 months) begins in January of Year 3 and continues until graduation. It provides students flexibility in their elective/selective and scholarly pursuit experiences and exposure to upper level electives and mentors prior to residency selection. Grades are honors/high pass/pass/fail. Module 6, Professionalism and Humanism, runs concurrently throughout the curriculum and covers bioethics, multiculturalism, spirituality, research, ethics, and confidentiality. Grades are pass/fail. Detailed curriculum information can be found at *www.med.upenn. edu/admiss/curriculum.*

USMLE

Step 1: Required. Students must only record a score.
Step 2: Clinical Skills (CS): Required. Students must only record a score.
Step 2: Clinical Knowledge (CK): Required. Students must only record a score.

Selection Factors

Selection factors include academic excellence, out-of-classroom activities, and life experience, as well as community service, research, letters of recommendation, and leadership potential. Personal qualities of maturity, integrity, the ability to work with others, and humanistic interests are sought. The entering class of 2008 has representation from 61 undergraduate colleges. Applicants from all states are welcome, but some preference is given to PA residents. Penn does not discriminate on the basis of race, sex, sexual orientation, age, religion, national or ethnic origin, or physical handicap. There is no transfer admission program.

Financial Aid

Students come from all social, economic, and cultural backgrounds. Financial aid includes: need-based scholarship and loans restricted to U.S. citizens or permanent residents and 11-12 full-tuition merit scholarships awarded annually regardless of citizenship. Approximately 24 students annually are fully funded in the M.D./Ph.D. program.

Information about Diversity Programs

Penn values diversity in the student body, faculty, and health system. Its goal is to recruit, admit, and graduate students from groups underrepresented in medicine. The Office of Diversity and Community Outreach has programs and pipelines to assist in meeting the objectives of a diverse student body. There is a curriculum focus on cultural competency.

Campus Information

Setting

Penn's urban campus is located in Philadelphia, one of America's most historic and livable cities. The fact that all 12 of Penn's graduate schools are located within walking distance of one another supports and fosters Penn's interdisciplinary approach to education, scholarship, and research. The city is a vibrant cultural center of urban life.

Enrollment

For 2008, total enrollment was: 725

Special Features

Global health experiences throughout the world. Pediatrics at Children's Hospital of Philadelphia, a world-renowned pediatric center.

Housing

Housing is affordable. Campus resources help students find housing. University transit is available within boundaries.

Application Process and Requirements 2010–2011

Primary Application Service: AMCAS
Earliest filing date: June 1, 2009
Latest filing date: October 15, 2009, 12:00 a.m., EST

Secondary Application Required?: Yes
Sent to: All applicants
URL: n/a
Fee: Yes, $80
Fee waiver available: Yes
Earliest filing date: July 1, 2009
Latest filing date: November 15, 2009, 12 a.m. EST

MCAT® required?: Yes
Latest MCAT® considered: September 2009
Oldest MCAT® considered: September 2006

Early Decision Program: School does have EDP
Applicants notified: October 1, 2009
EDP available for: Both Residents and Non-residents

Regular Acceptance Notice
Earliest date: March 2010
Latest date: Until class is full
Applicant's Response to Acceptance
Offer – Latest Date: May 15, 2010, 5 p.m., EST

Requests for Deferred Entrance Considered: Yes

Deposit to Hold Place in Class: Yes
Deposit (Resident): $100
Deposit (Non-resident): $100
Deposit due: May 15, 2010 5 p.m. EST
Applied to tuition: Yes
Deposit refundable: Yes
Refundable by: May 15, 2010 5 p.m. EST

Estimated number of new entrants: 155
EDP: 5, special program: n/a

Start Month/Year: August 2010

Interview Format: Two individual interviews/faculty and student.
Regional interviews are not available.

Other Programs

PREPARATORY PROGRAMS
Postbaccalaureate Program: Yes, www.sas.upenn.edu/lps/postbac/
Summer Program: Yes, www.med.upenn.edu/bgs/suip
Clinical Epidemiology Program: www.cceb.upenn.edu/education/epidegree/msce.php
Master's in Translational Research: www.med.upenn.edu/mtr

COMBINED DEGREE PROGRAMS
Baccalaureate/M.D.: No
M.D./M.P.H.: Yes, www.publichealth.med.upenn.edu
MD/MBA: Yes, www.med.upenn.edu/educ_combdeg/mdmba.html
M.D./J.D.: Yes, www.med.upenn.edu/educ_combdeg/mdjd.html
M.D./Ph.D.: Yes, www.med.upenn.edu/mstp/
Additional Program: Yes, www.med.upenn.edu/mbe/

Premedical Coursework

Course	Req.	Rec.	Lab.	Hrs.	Course	Req.	Rec.	Lab.	Hrs.
Inorganic Chemistry		•			Computer Science		•		
Behavioral Sciences		•			Genetics		•		
Biochemistry		•			Humanities		•		
Biology		•	•		Organic Chemistry		•	•	
Biology/Zoology		•			Physics		•	•	
Calculus		•			Psychology		•		
College English		•			Social Sciences		•		
College Mathematics		•			Statistics		•		

Selection Factors: 2008 Accepted Applicants

Proportion of Accepted Applicants with Relevant Experience (Data Self-Reported to AMCAS®)		
Community Service/Volunteer		73%
Medically-Related Work		85%
Research		91%

Shaded bar represents school's accepted scores ranging from the 10th percentile to the 90th percentile. School Median ● National Median ●

Overall GPA	2.0	2.1	2.2	2.3	2.4	2.5	2.6	2.7	2.8	2.9	3.0	3.1	3.2	3.3	3.4	3.5	3.6	3.7	(3.8)	3.9	4.0
Science GPA	2.0	2.1	2.2	2.3	2.4	2.5	2.6	2.7	2.8	2.9	3.0	3.1	3.2	3.3	3.4	3.5	3.6	3.7	3.8	(3.9)	4.0

MCAT® Total Numeric Score 9 10 11 12 13 14 15 16 17 18 19 20 21 22 23 24 25 26 27 28 29 30 31 (32) 33 34 (35) 36 37 38 39 40 41 42 43

Writing Sample			J	K	L	M	N	O	P	(Q)	R	S	T
Verbal Reasoning	3	4	5	6	7	8	9	(10)	(11)	12	13	14	15
Biological Sciences	3	4	5	6	7	8	9	10	(11)	(12)	13	14	15
Physical Sciences	3	4	5	6	7	8	9	10	(11)	(12)	13	14	15

Acceptance & Matriculation Data for 2008–2009 First Year Class

	Resident	Non-resident	International	Total
Applications	675	5551	320	6546
Interviewed	147	707	12	866
Deferred	5	3	0	8
Matriculants				
Early Assurance Program	0	0	0	0
Early Decision Program	1	1	0	2
Baccalaureate/M.D.	n/a	n/a	n/a	n/a
M.D./Ph.D.	5	15	4	24
Matriculated	48	103	3	**154**

Applications accepted from International Applicants: Yes

Specialty Choice

2004, 2005, 2006 Graduates, Specialty Choice (As reported by program directors to GME Track™)

Anesthesiology	3%
Emergency Medicine	5%
Family Practice	2%
Internal Medicine	20%
Obstetrics/Gynecology	2%
Orthopaedic Surgery	4%
Pediatrics	11%
Psychiatry	5%
Radiology	8%
Surgery	5%

Matriculant Demographics: 2008–2009 First Year Class

Men: 81 **Women:** 73

Matriculants' Self-Reported Race/Ethnicity

Mexican American	3	Korean	0
Cuban	1	Vietnamese	1
Puerto Rican	1	Other Asian	3
Other Hispanic	13	Total Asian	31
Total Hispanic	17	Native American	2
Chinese	14	Black	13
Asian Indian	10	Native Hawaiian	0
Pakistani	1	White	106
Filipino	2	Unduplicated Number	
Japanese	2	of Matriculants	154

Science and Math Majors: 53%
Matriculants with:
Baccalaureate degree: 100%
Graduate degree(s): 7%

Financial Information

Source: 2007–2008 LCME I-B survey and 2008–2009 AAMC TSF questionnaire

	Residents	Non-residents
Total Cost of Attendance	$65,381	$65,381
Tuition and Fees	$44,251	$44,251
Other (includes living expenses)	$18,530	$18,530
Health Insurance (can be waived)	$2,600	$2,600

Average 2008 Graduate Indebtedness: $121,745
% of Enrolled Students Receiving Aid: 84%

Criminal Background Check

This medical school requires a criminal background check prior to matriculation.

University of Pittsburgh School of Medicine

Pittsburgh, Pennsylvania

Office of Admissions and Financial Aid
3550 Terrace Street, 518 Scaife Hall
University of Pittsburgh School of Medicine
Pittsburgh, Pennsylvania 15261
T 412 648 9891   F 412 648 8768

Admissions www.medschool.pitt.edu/future/future_02.asp
Main www.medschool.pitt.edu
Financial www.medschool.pitt.edu/future/future_04.asp
E-mail admissions@medschool.pitt.edu

Private Institution

Dr. Arthur S. Levine, Dean, Senior Vice Chancellor for Health Sciences

Dr. Beth Piraino, Associate Dean for Admissions and Financial Aid

Dr. Chenits Pettigrew, Jr. Assistant Dean for Student Affairs and Diversity Programs

Pamela Rikstad, Director of Financial Aid

Cynthia M. Bonetti, Executive Director of Admissions and Financial Aid

Connie Dobrich, Assistant Director of Admissions

General Information

Drawing patients from all over the nation and from more than 30 foreign countries, the University of Pittsburgh Medical Center (UPMC) is one of the largest non-profit academic health systems in the nation. UPMC sites and affiliates on the main campus in Oakland, or nearby, include Western Psychiatric Institute and Clinic, the University of Pittsburgh Cancer Institute, UPMC Presbyterian Hospital, UPMC Shadyside Hospital, Magee Women's Hospital, Eye and Ear Institute, the Benedum Geriatric Center, Children's Hospital of Pittsburgh, UPMC Mercy Hospital, and the University Drive VA Medical Center.

Mission Statement

The principal goal of the University of Pittsburgh School of Medicine remains the education of scholarly physicians. This goal is achieved by emphasizing the centrality of the patient, by providing a firm understanding of the sciences basic to medicine, and by fostering the application of principles of biomedical problem-solving to the care of patients. We feel that students must develop an understanding of ethical principles in medicine and the application of these principles to specific problems. Development, early in the student's career, of habits of self-education by methods that include problem-based and self-directed learning, communication skills, and computer-assisted education is critical to the learning process, which must occur throughout the professional life of a physician.

Curricular Highlights

Community Service Requirement: Optional. Participation in multiple activities possible.
Research/Thesis Requirement: Required. Performance of a longitudinal scholarly project.

Our multidisciplinary curriculum is organized by organ systems rather than by individual disciplines (e.g., physiology and biochemistry). It emphasizes problem-solving and learning in small groups. It also introduces students to clinical medicine in the first year. All students have required rotations in family medicine, internal medicine, obstetrics-gynecology, pediatrics, psychiatry/neurology, and surgery/anesthesia, surgical subspecialties and ambulatory care. Students may participate in electives during the third year before all core clerkships are completed and also have extensive elective time during the fourth year. All students complete a mentored scholarly project using the scientific method to examine a clinical, basic science or community-based problem. An Honors/Pass/Fail system is used for grading.

USMLE

Step 1: Required. Students must record a passing score for graduation, but not promotion.
Step 2: Clinical Skills (CS): Required. Students must record a passing total score to graduate.
Step 2: Clinical Knowledge (CK): Required. Students must record a passing total score to graduate.

Selection Factors

Applicants are chosen on the basis of intellect, integrity, maturity, and the ability to interact sensitively with people. Consideration is given to the past academic record and MCAT scores; evaluations of college preprofessional committees; letters of recommendation, preferably from faculty members with whom the student has interacted in scholarly pursuits; extracurricular activities; and personal interviews. Interviews are required and are conducted only at the medical school campus. All applicants are considered without regard to race, color, religion, ethnicity, national origin, age, sex, sexual orientation, marital, veteran, or handicap status.

Financial Aid

Most loans and scholarships are awarded on the basis of financial need as documented by information on the FAFSA. Parental income information is required to be considered for University need-based resources. Students are considered for academic scholarships during the admissions process. Additional financial aid information is available on the school's Web site.

Information about Diversity Programs

The School of Medicine is committed to maintaining a diverse student body; in the application process, students are asked how they might contribute to this diversity. The school hosts premedical summer enrichment programs, as well as a prematriculation program for all admitted students. Following admission, a broad range of support services are available to ensure retention. Specific information on the services provided to applicants from groups underrepresented in medicine can be obtained by contacting the Office of Student Affairs and Diversity Programs at (412) 648-8987.

Campus Information

Setting

Urban setting on the University of Pittsburgh campus; within a five-block radius of multiple UPMC hospitals and the Graduate School of Public Health.

Enrollment

For 2008, total enrollment was: 577

Special Features

The School of Medicine has continuous curricular revisions with considerable student involvement. The goal-oriented, integrated and centrally governed curriculum emphasizes general principles and encourages student self-learning based on actual clinical cases.

Housing

Housing is available on campus specifically for medical students. See: *www.ocl.pitt.edu/apartments/darragh.html.*

Satellite Campuses/Facilities

The School of Medicine is affiliated with UPMC, which operates 20 hospitals in western Pennsylvania. In addition, UPMC Palermo is a transplant hospital located in Sicily at which students may do a senior elective.

Application Process and Requirements 2010–2011

Primary Application Service: AMCAS
Earliest filing date: June 1, 2009
Latest filing date: November 1, 2009

Secondary Application Required?: Yes
Sent to: All applicants
URL: https://admissions.medschool.pitt.edu
Fee: Yes, $85
Fee waiver available: Yes
Earliest filing date: July 1, 2009
Latest filing date: December 1, 2009

MCAT® required?: Yes
Latest MCAT® considered: September 2009
Oldest MCAT® considered: 2006

Early Decision Program: School does not have EDP
Applicants notified: n/a
EDP available for: n/a

Regular Acceptance Notice
Earliest date: October 15, 2009
Latest date: Until class is full
Applicant's Response to Acceptance Offer – Maximum Time: Two weeks

Requests for Deferred Entrance Considered: Yes

Deposit to Hold Place in Class: Yes
Deposit (Resident): $100
Deposit (Non-resident): $100
Deposit due: May 17-21, 2010
Applied to tuition: Yes
Deposit refundable: No
Refundable by: n/a

Estimated number of new entrants: 148
EDP: n/a, special program: n/a

Start Month/Year: August 2010

Interview Format: A faculty and student interview are required. Regional interviews are not available.

Other Programs

PREPARATORY PROGRAMS
Postbaccalaureate Program: No
Summer Program: Yes, www.medschool.pitt.edu/future/future_03.asp

COMBINED DEGREE PROGRAMS
Baccalaureate/M.D.: No
M.D./M.P.H.: Yes, www.publichealth.pitt.edu/interior.php?pageID=203
MD/MBA: No
M.D./J.D.: No
M.D./Ph.D.: Yes, www.mdphd.pitt.edu
Additional Program: Yes, www.icre.pitt.edu/cstp-m/index.aspx; www.pstp.pitt.edu

Premedical Coursework

Course	Req.	Rec.	Lab.	Qtrs.	Course	Req.	Rec.	Lab.	Qtrs.
Inorganic Chemistry	•		•	2	Computer Science				
Behavioral Sciences					Genetics				
Biochemistry					Humanities				
Biology	•		•	2	Organic Chemistry	•		•	2
Biology/Zoology					Physics	•		•	2
Calculus					Psychology				
College English	•			2	Social Sciences				
College Mathematics					Other				

Selection Factors: 2008 Accepted Applicants

Proportion of Accepted Applicants with Relevant Experience (Data Self-Reported to AMCAS)	
Community Service/Volunteer	73%
Medically-Related Work	87%
Research	91%

Shaded bar represents school's accepted scores ranging from the 10th percentile to the 90th percentile.   School Median ●   National Median ●

Overall GPA 2.0 2.1 2.2 2.3 2.4 2.5 2.6 2.7 2.8 2.9 3.0 3.1 3.2 3.3 3.4 **3.5 3.6 3.7 (3.8)** 3.9 4.0
Science GPA 2.0 2.1 2.2 2.3 2.4 2.5 2.6 2.7 2.8 2.9 3.0 3.1 3.2 3.3 **3.4 3.5 3.6 3.7 (3.8)** 3.9 4.0

MCAT® Total Numeric Score 9 10 11 12 13 14 15 16 17 18 19 20 21 22 23 24 25 26 27 28 29 30 31 (32) 33 34 35 (36) 37 38 39 40 41 42 43

Writing Sample			J	K	L	M	N	O	P	(Q)	R	S	T	
Verbal Reasoning	3	4	5	6	7	8	9	(10)	(11)	12	13	14	15	
Biological Sciences	3	4	5	6	7	8	9	10	(11)	(12)	13	14	15	
Physical Sciences	3	4	5	6	7	8	9	10	(11)	(12)	13	14	15	

Acceptance & Matriculation Data for 2008–2009 First Year Class

	Resident	Non-resident	International	Total
Applications	846	4529	38	5413
Interviewed	199	815	0	1014
Deferred	0	2	0	2
Matriculants				
Early Assurance Program	4	0	0	4
Early Decision Program	0	0	0	0
Baccalaureate/M.D.	n/a	n/a	n/a	n/a
M.D./Ph.D.	1	8	0	9
Matriculated	46	101	0	**147**

Applications accepted from International Applicants: No

Specialty Choice

2004, 2005, 2006 Graduates, Specialty Choice (As reported by program directors to GME Track™)

Anesthesiology	6%
Emergency Medicine	11%
Family Practice	6%
Internal Medicine	16%
Obstetrics/Gynecology	6%
Orthopaedic Surgery	5%
Pediatrics	12%
Psychiatry	7%
Radiology	3%
Surgery	6%

Matriculant Demographics: 2008–2009 First Year Class

Men: 88   **Women:** 59

Matriculants' Self-Reported Race/Ethnicity

Mexican American	3	Korean	2
Cuban	1	Vietnamese	2
Puerto Rican	0	Other Asian	1
Other Hispanic	6	Total Asian	35
Total Hispanic	9	Native American	0
Chinese	16	Black	16
Asian Indian	12	Native Hawaiian	0
Pakistani	2	White	86
Filipino	1	Unduplicated Number	
Japanese	0	of Matriculants	147

Science and Math Majors: 63%
Matriculants with:
Baccalaureate degree: 100%
Graduate degree(s): 13%

Financial Information
Source: 2007–2008 LCME I-B survey and 2008–2009 AAMC TSF questionnaire

	Residents	Non-residents
Total Cost of Attendance	$57,268	$61,288
Tuition and Fees	$37,486	$41,506
Other (includes living expenses)	$17,782	$17,782
Health Insurance (can be waived)	$2,000	$2,000

Average 2008 Graduate Indebtedness: $138,601
% of Enrolled Students Receiving Aid: 88%

Criminal Background Check

This medical school requires a criminal background check prior to matriculation.

Ponce School of Medicine
Ponce, Puerto Rico

Admissions Office
Ponce School of Medicine
P.O. Box 7004
Ponce, Puerto Rico 00732
T 787 840 2575   **F** 787 842 0461

Admissions www.psm.edu/Student_Affairs/
Admissions/about_department.htm
Main www.psm.edu
Financial www.psm.edu/Student_Affairs/
Financial_Aid/fin_aid_about_department.htm
E-mail admissions@psm.edu

Private Institution

Dr. Raúl Armstrong, President and Dean

Dr. Wanda Vélez, Admissions Director

Pedro Barnés, Financial Aid Director

Arvin Báez, Assistant Dean for Student Affairs

General Information
The Ponce School of Medicine of the Ponce Medical School Foundation, Inc. (formerly the Catholic University of Puerto Rico School of Medicine) took over the school's operations on July 1, 1980, under the governance of a board of trustees. The school graduated its first class in June 1981. Clinical training is offered at the following facilities in Ponce: Damas Hospital, a private institution with 356 beds; La Playa Diagnostic Center, which serves as the main training area for community and family practice; Dr. Pila Hospital, with 160 beds; and St. Luke's Hospital, with 550 beds. Clinical training is also offered at the Concepcion Hospital, with 188 beds, located in San German, and at Yauco Regional Hospital, with 140 beds.

Mission Statement
Ponce School of Medicine has as its mission the provision of high quality education and graduate training, which shall strengthen students' character, moral fiber, and ethics, and prepare physicians and scientists for a fast-changing world in the area of healthcare delivery and research.

Curricular Highlights
Community Service Requirement: Optional.
Research/Thesis Requirement: Optional.

The medical program's basic objective is to provide the Commonwealth of Puerto Rico, especially the southern region of the island, with ethically motivated, professionally competent primary care physicians. The curriculum provides students with an early experience in family and community health needs. During the first two years, the basic medical sciences are thoroughly emphasized. Clinical experience takes precedence during the third and fourth years. The correlation between the basic and clinical sciences is achieved in a multidisciplinary program.

Throughout the four-year program great emphasis is placed on the student's contact with patients and their families as a complement to the student's academic-hospital experience. Every academic semester contains, in addition to the regular curriculum, a series of supplementary seminars dealing with the ethical and social components of medical practice, as well as with additional specific subjects that are incidental and relevant to the profession. A problem-based learning program has been introduced in clinical correlation sessions in the first year of medical studies and in the Pathophysiology course, where it is presented as a student-centered integrative exercise. Subject-oriented small-group discussions are included in basic sciences courses. The program seeks to develop well-balanced, mature general practitioners, equally well qualified in the professional and ethical aspects of medicine. Students' work is graded according to an Honor/Pass/Fail system.

USMLE
Step 1: Required. Students must record a passing score for promotion.
Step 2: Clinical Skills (CS): Required. Students must only record a score.
Step 2: Clinical Knowledge (CK): Required. Students must record a passing total score to graduate.

Selection Factors
Selection of applicants is made by the Admissions Committee on the basis of academic achievement, MCAT scores, evaluation letters, and personal interviews. The interviews are used to determine the motivation and character of the applicants. Only those who pass a preliminary screening, based on MCAT scores and college grades, are interviewed. Careful consideration is given to all applicants regardless of racial or ethnic background, religious affiliation, sex, or national origin. Residents of Puerto Rico are given preference, although a limited number of applicants who live in the United States are accepted. Candidates who do not have a functional knowledge of both English and Spanish are not encouraged to apply, since instruction is given in both languages. In the 2008 entering class, 77 percent of students were from Puerto Rico and 23 percent were from the continental United States.

Financial Aid
Students are admitted to Ponce School of Medicine without regard to financial circumstances. After acceptance, prospective students are informed of the necessary forms they must submit in order to complete the financial aid process.

Campus Information
Setting
The Ponce School of Medicine is located in the city of Ponce, adjacent to Damas Hospital where the majority of our clinical teaching activities take place. Ponce is the major city of the southwestern part of the island. It is seventy miles from San Juan, which is on the northern coast. The city and the surrounding area provide a population base sufficient for medical training.

Enrollment
For 2008, total enrollment was: 68

Housing
On-campus housing is not available. The university does maintain a list of affordable apartments within a 10-mile radius. Rents average $400-$1000 per month.

Application Process and Requirements 2010–2011

Primary Application Service: AMCAS
Earliest filing date: June 1, 2009
Latest filing date: December 15, 2009

Secondary Application Required?: No
Sent to: All applicants
URL: n/a
Fee: Yes, $100
Fee waiver available: No
Earliest filing date: September 1, 2009
Latest filing date: January 15, 2010

MCAT® required?: Yes
Latest MCAT® considered: March 2009
Oldest MCAT® considered: January 2007

Early Decision Program: School does have EDP
Applicants notified: October 1, 2009
EDP available for: Both Residents and Non-residents

Regular Acceptance Notice
Earliest date: November 15, 2009
Latest date: Until class is full
Applicant's Response to Acceptance
Offer – Maximum Time: Twenty days

Requests for Deferred
Entrance Considered: No

Deposit to Hold Place in Class: Yes
Deposit (Resident): $1,000
Deposit (Non-resident): $1,000
Deposit due: With response to acceptance offer
Applied to tuition: Yes
Deposit refundable: No
Refundable by: n/a

Estimated number of new entrants: 65
EDP: 3, special program: n/a

Start Month/Year: July 2010

Interview Format: Interviews are in groups or individually. Regional interviews are not available.

Other Programs

PREPARATORY PROGRAMS
Postbaccalaureate Program: No
Summer Program: No

COMBINED DEGREE PROGRAMS
Baccalaureate/M.D.: Yes
M.D./M.P.H.: No
MD/MBA: No
M.D./J.D.: No
M.D./Ph.D.: No

Premedical Coursework

Course	Req.	Rec.	Lab.	Hrs.
Inorganic Chemistry	•		•	8
Behavioral Sciences	•			12
Biochemistry		•		
Biology	•			8
Biology/Zoology			•	
Calculus				
College English	•			12
College Mathematics	•			6

Course	Req.	Rec.	Lab.	Hrs.
Computer Science				
Genetics				
Humanities				
Organic Chemistry	•		•	8
Physics	•		•	8
Psychology				
Social Sciences				
Spanish	•			6

Selection Factors: 2008 Accepted Applicants

Proportion of Accepted Applicants with Relevant Experience (Data Self-Reported to AMCAS®)		
Community Service/Volunteer	41%	
Medically-Related Work	46%	
Research	67%	

Shaded bar represents school's accepted scores ranging from the 10th percentile to the 90th percentile. **School Median** ○ **National Median** ○

Overall GPA 2.0 2.1 2.2 2.3 2.4 2.5 2.6 2.7 2.8 2.9 3.0 3.1 3.2 3.3 3.4 3.5 ③.⑥ 3.7 3.8 3.9 4.0
Science GPA 2.0 2.1 2.2 2.3 2.4 2.5 2.6 2.7 2.8 2.9 3.0 3.1 3.2 3.3 ③.④ 3.5 3.6 3.7 3.8 3.9 4.0

MCAT® Total Numeric Score 9 10 11 12 13 14 15 16 17 18 19 20 ㉑ 22 23 24 25 26 27 28 29 30 31 ㉜ 33 34 35 36 37 38 39 40 41 42 43

Writing Sample				J	K	L	Ⓜ	N	O	P	Ⓠ	R	S	T
Verbal Reasoning	3		4	5	6	⑦	8	9	⑩	11	12	13	14	15
Biological Sciences	3		4	5	6	7	⑧	9	10	⑪	12	13	14	15
Physical Sciences	3		4	5	6	⑦	8	9	10	⑪	12	13	14	15

Acceptance & Matriculation Data for 2008–2009 First Year Class

	Resident	Non-resident	International	Total
Applications	397	873	50	1320
Interviewed	145	35	0	180
Deferred	0	0	0	0
Matriculants				
Early Assurance Program	0	0	0	0
Early Decision Program	0	0	0	0
Baccalaureate/M.D.	2	0	0	2
M.D./Ph.D.	n/a	n/a	n/a	0
Matriculated	50	15	0	**65**

Applications accepted from International Applicants: Yes

Specialty Choice

2004, 2005, 2006 Graduates, Specialty Choice (As reported by program directors to GME Track™)	
Anesthesiology	3%
Emergency Medicine	6%
Family Practice	5%
Internal Medicine	22%
Obstetrics/Gynecology	8%
Orthopaedic Surgery	3%
Pediatrics	11%
Psychiatry	4%
Radiology	4%
Surgery	11%

Matriculant Demographics: 2008–2009 First Year Class

Men: 32   **Women:** 33

Matriculants' Self-Reported Race/Ethnicity

Mexican American	1	**Korean**	0
Cuban	3	**Vietnamese**	0
Puerto Rican	55	**Other Asian**	0
Other Hispanic	2	**Total Asian**	2
Total Hispanic	60	**Native American**	1
Chinese	1	**Black**	6
Asian Indian	1	**Native Hawaiian**	1
Pakistani	0	**White**	46
Filipino	0	**Unduplicated Number**	
Japanese	0	**of Matriculants**	65

Science and Math Majors: 74%
Matriculants with:
    Baccalaureate degree: 97%
    Graduate degree(s): 8%

Financial Information
Source: 2007–2008 LCME I-B survey and 2008–2009 AAMC TSF questionnaire

	Residents	Non-residents
Total Cost of Attendance	$36,601	$49,729
Tuition and Fees	$21,977	$31,475
Other (includes living expenses)	$13,324	$16,954
Health Insurance (can be waived)	$1,300	$1,300

Average 2008 Graduate Indebtedness: $132,411
% of Enrolled Students Receiving Aid: 89%

Criminal Background Check

This medical school requires a criminal background check prior to matriculation.

San Juan Bautista School of Medicine
Caguas, Puerto Rico

Admissions Office
P.O. Box 4968
Caguas, Puerto Rico 00726-4968
T 787 743 3038 x236   F 787 746 3093

Admissions www.sanjuanbautista.edu/
Admissions.aspx
Main www.sanjuanbautista.edu
Financial www.sanjuanbautista.edu/Admissions.aspx
E-mail admissions@sanjuanbautista.edu

Private Institution

Dr. Yocasta Brugal-Mena, President/Dean of Medicine

Dr. Myraida Rivera-Colon, Director of Admissions

Dr. Myraida Rivera-Colon, Minority Affairs Officer

Dr. Beatriz De Leon-Rivera, Financial Aid Officer

Dr. Salvador Santiago, Associate Dean for Student Affairs

Dr. Jaymi Sanchez-Cruz, Admissions Officer

General Information

The School of Medicine was founded in 1978 in San Juan, Puerto Rico, as a not-for-profit corporation, incorporated under the laws of the Commonwealth of Puerto Rico. It is located in Caguas, Puerto Rico, one of the most important urban centers. It is authorized by the Puerto Rico Council on Higher Education to offer studies leading to the M.D. degree. The MSCHE granted accreditation to the School in 2004. The LCME granted accreditation to the academic program in 2007. As of June 30, 2008, the School of Medicine has graduated a total of 915 medical doctors who have been successfully integrated in their communities as competent and caring health providers, both in Puerto Rico and abroad.

Mission Statement

The Mission of the School is to teach and train students to become primary care physicians that can provide holistic diagnosis and treatment to communities in need of health services in Puerto Rico. The School is committed to provide high quality medical education, service, and research, that will foster student's comprehensive development, so that they can become capable, competent, skilled, and honest professionals.

Curricular Highlights

Community Service Requirement: Required. 155 hrs required during the first three years
Research/Thesis Requirement: n/a

SJBSM had defined its curriculum within a student-centered approach, highlighting the values, attitudes, and social responsibility of the practice of medicine. It facilitates active learning and integration, offering early exposure to clinical scenarios and technological experiences in the learning process and using diverse assessment methodologies. The curriculum is structured in five emphases: medical knowledge, clinical skills, research and information literacy, professionalism and community awareness. These emphases are incorporated throughout the four years. The preclinical courses are offered during the first two years. The third year is devoted to core clinical clerkships, both inpatient and outpatient scenarios, including a research clerkship. The fourth year reinforces the practice of medicine with core and electives clinical clerkships, and a sub-specialties clerkship. Several curricular innovations strengthen the learning process: multidisciplinary exercises that promote vertical and horizontal integration, development of a research proposal throughout the four years, and different levels/types of community experiences, according to the School's mission.

USMLE

Step 1: Required. Must record a passing score for promotion.
Step 2: Clinical Skills (CS): Required. Students must record a passing total score to graduate.
Step 2: Clinical Knowledge (CK): Required. Students must record a passing total score to graduate.

Selection Factors

The Admissions office evaluates all applications, taking into consideration academic and personal qualifications. The analysis includes academic achievement, premedical studies required for admission to the program, and MCAT scores. The motivations to study medicine, leadership qualities, ability to relate to other people and deal with problems, and participation in community/scientific activities, are also taken into consideration by the Admissions Committee. Qualified applicants are required to appear for an interview.

Financial Aid

The Financial Aid Office counsels students regarding the availability of economic aid and the procedure to file applications. For further information, please refer to: *http://sanjuanbautista.edu/Admissions.aspx.*

Information about Diversity Programs

The School of Medicine is committed to diversity in the faculty and the student body. Its goal is to recruit, admit and graduate students that comply with the requirements. The office of Minority Affairs has programs to assist to help meeting the objectives of a diverse student body.

Campus Information

Setting

The School's facilities are located on the grounds of the San Juan Bautista Medical Center. The 52 acre campus is the location for the Hospital and the School, which houses administrative offices, the biomedical sciences faculty, and the Library/ Learning Resources Center, as well as the classrooms and laboratories for teaching and research. Clinical training at the SJBMC brings students into contact with a patient population drawn from many different socio-economic groups. The SJBMC is the principal clinical training facility for third and fourth year students.

Enrollment

For 2008, total enrollment was: 251

Special Features

Our School is a community-based institution, in which community service is a curricular axis. Courses and activities are patient-focused throughout the program.

Housing

The School provides information about available housing facilities in Caguas.

Satellite Campuses/Facilities

The School of Medicine has established several collaborations that provide opportunities for its students. Students rotate at hospitals and ambulatory health care systems that met the School's high standards of educational quality.

314   *Medical School Admission Requirements, 2010–2011*

Application Process and Requirements 2010–2011

Primary Application Service: AMCAS
Earliest filing date: June 1, 2009
Latest filing date: December 15, 2009

Secondary Application Required: Yes
URL: www.sanjuanbautista.edu/Admissions.aspx
Jaymi Sanchez-Cruz, (787) 743-3038 x236
admissions@sanjuanbautista.edu
Sent to: All applicants
Fee: Yes, $75
Fee Waiver Available: No
Earliest filing date: July 1, 2009
Latest filing date: April 15, 2010

MCAT® required?: Yes
Latest MCAT® considered: January 2009
Oldest MCAT® considered: January 2006

Early Decision Program: School does have EDP
Applicants notified: October 1, 2009
EDP available for: Both residents and non-residents

Regular Acceptance Notice
Earliest date: April 2010
Latest date: Until Class is Full

Applicant's Response to Acceptance
Offer – Maximum Time: Two weeks

Requests for deferred entrance considered: No

Deposit to Hold Place in Class: Yes,
Deposit (Resident): $300
Deposit (Non-resident): $300
Deposit due: Two weeks
Applied to tuition: Yes
Deposit refundable: No
Refundable by: n/a

Estimated number of new entrants: 60
EDP: 3, special program: n/a

Start month/year: August 2010

Interview format: Interviews occur individually or in groups on campus. Regional interviews are not available.

Other Programs

PREPARATORY PROGRAMS
Postbaccalaureate Program: No
Summer Program: No

COMBINED DEGREE PROGRAMS
Baccalaureate/M.D.: No
M.D./M.P.H.: No
MD/MBA: No
M.D./J.D.: No
M.D./Ph.D.: No

Premedical Coursework

Course	Req.	Rec.	Lab.	Sems.	Course	Req.	Rec.	Lab.	Sems.
Inorganic Chemistry	•			2	Computer Science				
Behavioral Sciences	•			4	Genetics				
Biochemistry		•			Humanities				
Biology	•			2	Organic Chemistry	•			2
Biology/Zoology					Physics	•			2
Calculus					Psychology				
College English	•			4	Social Sciences				
College Mathematics					Spanish	•			2
					Electives	•			6

Selection Factors: 2008 Accepted Applicants

Proportion of Accepted Applicants with Relevant Experience (Data Self-Reported to AMCAS®)			
Community Service/Volunteer			49%
Medically-Related Work			54%
Research			61%

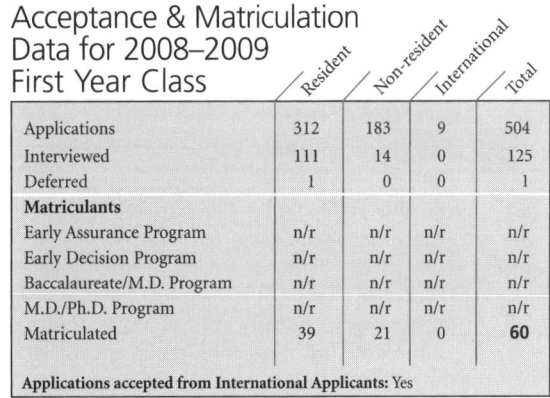

Shaded bar represents school's accepted scores ranging from the 10th percentile to the 90th percentile. School Median ● National Median ●

Overall GPA 2.0 2.1 2.2 2.3 2.4 2.5 2.6 2.7 2.8 2.9 3.0 3.1 3.2 ③.3 3.4 3.5 3.6 3.7 3.8 3.9 4.0
Science GPA 2.0 2.1 2.2 2.3 2.4 2.5 2.6 2.7 2.8 2.9 3.0 ③.1 3.2 3.3 3.4 3.5 3.6 3.7 3.8 3.9 4.0

MCAT® Total Numeric Score 9 10 11 12 13 14 15 16 17 18 19 ㉟ 21 22 23 24 25 26 27 28 29 30 31 ㉜ 33 34 35 36 37 38 39 40 41 42 43

	J	K	ⓛ	M	N	O	P	ⓠ	R	S	T
Writing Sample											

Verbal Reasoning	3	4	5	⑥	7	8	9	⑩	11	12	13	14	15
Biological Sciences	3	4	5	6	⑦	8	9	10	⑪	12	13	14	15
Physical Sciences	3	4	5	6	⑦	8	9	10	⑪	12	13	14	15

Acceptance & Matriculation Data for 2008–2009 First Year Class

	Resident	Non-resident	International	Total
Applications	312	183	9	504
Interviewed	111	14	0	125
Deferred	1	0	0	1
Matriculants				
Early Assurance Program	n/r	n/r	n/r	n/r
Early Decision Program	n/r	n/r	n/r	n/r
Baccalaureate/M.D. Program	n/r	n/r	n/r	n/r
M.D./Ph.D. Program	n/r	n/r	n/r	n/r
Matriculated	39	21	0	**60**

Applications accepted from International Applicants: Yes

Specialty Choice

2004, 2005, 2006 Graduates, Specialty Choice (As reported by program directors to GME Track™)

Anesthesiology
Emergency Medicine
Family Practice

DATA NOT AVAILABLE

Psychiatry
Radiology
Surgery

Matriculant Demographics: 2008–2009 First Year Class

Men: 27 **Women:** 33

Matriculants' Self-Reported Race/Ethnicity

Mexican American	1	Korean	1
Cuban	3	Vietnamese	0
Puerto Rican	41	Other Asian	2
Other Hispanic	6	Total Asian	5
Total Hispanic	49	Native American	0
Chinese	1	Black	8
Asian Indian	0	Native Hawaiian	2
Pakistani	1	White	46
Filipino	1	Unduplicated Number	
Japanese	0	of Matriculants	60

Science Majors: 80%
Matriculants with:
   Baccalaureate Degree: 98%
   Graduate Degree(s): 8%

Financial Information

Source: 2007–2008 LCME I-B survey and 2008–2009 AAMC TSF questionnaire

	Residents	Non-residents
Total Cost of Attendance	$41,767	$44,767
Tuition and Fees	$18,770	$21,770
Other (includes living expenses)	$21,525	$21,525
Health Insurance (can be waived)	$1,472	$1,472

Average 2008 Graduate Indebtedness: $84,323
% of Enrolled Students Receiving Aid: 97%

Criminal Background Check

This medical school requires a criminal background check prior to matriculation.

Universidad Central del Caribe
School of Medicine
Bayamón, Puerto Rico

Office of Admissions
Universidad Central del Caribe
School of Medicine,
P.O. Box 60-327
Bayamon, Puerto Rico 00960-6032
T 787 798 3001   F 787 269 7550

Admissions www.uccaribe.edu
Main www.uccaribe.edu
Financial www.uccaribe.edu
E-mail icordero@uccaribe.edu
edlopez@uccaribe.edu

Private Institution

Dr. Jose Ginel Rodriguez, Dean of Medicine

Irma L. Cordero, Admissions Officer

Ana M. Galan, Financial Aid Director

General Information
The Universidad Central del Caribe School of Medicine was founded in 1976 as a nonprofit private institution chartered under the laws of the Commonwealth of Puerto Rico. The new building for the basic sciences, library, animal house, and central administration was inaugurated in 1990 adjacent to Dr. Ramon Ruiz Arnau University Hospital, which serves as the principal teaching hospital. The school facilities are located in a 56-acre academic health center in the city of Bayamon.

Mission Statement
The mission of the School of Medicine is to develop competent physicians with an outstanding academic preparation within a humanistic and holistic framework. A guiding principle of our mission is to ensure that our graduates possess a strong sense of professionalism and commitment to social duties and service to Puerto Rico and Hispanic communities throughout the U.S. mainland.

Curricular Highlights
Community Service Requirement: Optional.
Research/Thesis Requirement: Optional.

The medical curriculum is organized in two years of preclinical and two years of clinical experiences. A longitudinal curriculum in bioethics and humanities in medicine characterizes the medical education program. Clinical correlations are included in the basic science courses. Exposure to real and standardized patients is provided beginning with the first year. Introduction to clinical medicine has as its foundation the biopsychosocial model. A problem-based course is structured around prevalent problems encountered in primary care. The third-year learning experience revolves around required clerkships in internal medicine, pediatrics, obstetrics-gynecology, general surgery, and family medicine. The latter takes place in the ambulatory setting. Also,

during the third year, students enroll in the surgical subspecialties and psychiatry clerkships. Eighteen weeks of electives are provided in the fourth year, plus three months in required courses in neurology, ambulatory medicine, selected topics, and bioethics and humanities in medicine. Individual student evaluation in all requisite basic science and clinical science courses is based on letter grade and Pass/Fail systems. Student evaluation in all elective courses is based on an Honors/Pass/Fail system.

USMLE
Step 1: Required. Students must record a passing score for promotion.
Step 2: Clinical Skills (CS): Required. Students must record a passing total score to graduate.
Step 2: Clinical Knowledge (CK): Required. Students must record a passing total score to graduate.

Selection Factors
The selection of candidates for admission is made exclusively by the Admissions Committee. The admission process does not discriminate against any individual on the basis of sex, age, race, religion, economic status, political ideology, or national origin. Applicants must demonstrate proficiency in both Spanish and English. Lectures may be in either language. Spanish is the predominant language of the institution. Major factors considered in the selection of candidates for admission include undergraduate academic record, overall GPA and science GPA, performance in all areas of the MCAT, results of a personal interview, and letters of recommendation. A personal interview is required prior to consideration for admission. All interviews are arranged by the Office of Admissions and are conducted at the medical school facilities in Bayamon. Rejected applicants are given the opportunity to reapply for admission.

Financial Aid
The Office of the Dean for Student Affairs provides financial aid counseling to all prospective students. Incoming students qualify for application to all pertinent federal and commonwealth scholarship and loan programs. Economic status of the applicant is not a consideration during the selection of candidates for admission.

Campus Information

Enrollment
For 2008, total enrollment was: 282

Housing
On-campus housing is not available. However, the Dean for Student Affairs maintains a list of affordable apartments in the vicinity.

Satellite Campuses/Facilities
Student rotations are divided between the University Hospital and a rich network of clinical settings in the metro area.

Application Process and Requirements 2010–2011

Primary Application Service: AMCAS
Earliest filing date: June 1, 2009
Latest filing date: December 15, 2009

Secondary Application Required?: No
Sent to: Several documents must be submitted.
Irma L. Cordero, (787) 798-3001 x 2403,
icordero@uccaribe.edu
Fee: Yes, $100
Fee waiver available: No
Earliest filing date: n/a
Latest filing date: n/a

MCAT® required?: Yes
Latest MCAT® considered: September 2009
Oldest MCAT® considered: January 2006

Early Decision Program: School does not have EDP
Applicants notified: n/a
EDP available for: n/a

Regular Acceptance Notice
Earliest date: January 2010
Latest date: Until class is full
Applicant's Response to Acceptance Offer – Maximum Time: Two weeks

Requests for Deferred Entrance Considered: No

Deposit to Hold Place in Class: Yes
Deposit (Resident): $100
Deposit (Non-resident): $100
Deposit due: 15 days after notification
Applied to tuition: No
Deposit refundable: No
Refundable by: n/a

Estimated number of new entrants: 60
EDP: n/a, special program: n/a

Start Month/Year: August 2010

Interview Format: Group interviews.

Other Programs

PREPARATORY PROGRAMS
Postbaccalaureate Program: Yes,
Edllian Lopez, (787) 798-3001 x2404,
edlopez@uccaribe.edu
Summer Program: No

COMBINED DEGREE PROGRAMS
Baccalaureate/M.D.: No
M.D./M.P.H.: No
MD/MBA: No
M.D./J.D.: No
M.D./Ph.D.: No

Premedical Coursework

Course	Req.	Rec.	Lab.	Hrs.
Inorganic Chemistry	•		•	8
Behavioral Sciences		•		
Biochemistry		•		
Biology		•		
Biology/Zoology	•		•	8
Calculus		•		
College English	•			12
College Mathematics	•			6

Course	Req.	Rec.	Lab.	Hrs.
Computer Science		•		
Genetics		•		
Humanities				
Organic Chemistry	•		•	8
Physics	•		•	8
Psychology		•		
Social Sciences		•		
Behavioral/Social Sciences	•			12
Spanish	•			6

Selection Factors: 2008 Accepted Applicants

Proportion of Accepted Applicants with Relevant Experience (Data Self-Reported to AMCAS®)		
Community Service/Volunteer		47%
Medically-Related Work		50%
Research		63%

Shaded bar represents school's accepted scores ranging from the 10th percentile to the 90th percentile. **School Median** ● **National Median** ●

Overall GPA	2.0	2.1	2.2	2.3	2.4	2.5	2.6	2.7	2.8	2.9	3.0	3.1	3.2	3.3	3.4	(3.5)	3.6	3.7	3.8	3.9	4.0
Science GPA	2.0	2.1	2.2	2.3	2.4	2.5	2.6	2.7	2.8	2.9	3.0	3.1	3.2	3.3	(3.4)	3.5	3.6	3.7	3.8	3.9	4.0

MCAT® Total Numeric Score 9 10 11 12 13 14 15 16 17 18 19 20 (21) 22 23 24 25 26 27 28 29 30 31 (32) 33 34 35 36 37 38 39 40 41 42 43

Writing Sample			J	K	L	(M)	N	O	P	(Q)	R	S	T
Verbal Reasoning	3	4	5	(6)	7	8	9	(10)	11	12	13	14	15
Biological Sciences	3	4	5	6	7	(8)	9	10	(11)	12	13	14	15
Physical Sciences	3	4	5	6	(7)	8	9	10	(11)	12	13	14	15

Acceptance & Matriculation Data for 2008–2009 First Year Class

	Resident	Non-resident	International	Total
Applications	380	618	23	1021
Interviewed	138	43	1	182
Deferred	0	0	0	0
Matriculants				
Early Assurance Program	0	0	0	0
Early Decision Program	0	0	0	0
Baccalaureate/M.D.	n/a	n/a	n/a	n/a
M.D./Ph.D.	n/a	n/a	n/a	n/a
Matriculated	49	15	1	**65**

Applications accepted from International Applicants: Yes

Specialty Choice

2004, 2005, 2006 Graduates, Specialty Choice (As reported by program directors to GME Track™)	
Anesthesiology	1%
Emergency Medicine	2%
Family Practice	4%
Internal Medicine	30%
Obstetrics/Gynecology	2%
Orthopaedic Surgery	0%
Pediatrics	8%
Psychiatry	14%
Radiology	3%
Surgery	4%

Matriculant Demographics: 2008–2009 First Year Class

Men: 37 **Women:** 28

Matriculants' Self-Reported Race/Ethnicity

Mexican American	0	Korean	0
Cuban	4	Vietnamese	0
Puerto Rican	49	Other Asian	1
Other Hispanic	4	Total Asian	3
Total Hispanic	56	Native American	0
Chinese	0	Black	4
Asian Indian	0	Native Hawaiian	0
Pakistani	2	White	40
Filipino	1	Unduplicated Number	
Japanese	0	of Matriculants	65

Science and Math Majors: 80%
Matriculants with:
Baccalaureate degree: 100%
Graduate degree(s): 9%

Financial Information

Source: 2007–2008 LCME I-B survey and 2008–2009 AAMC TSF questionnaire

	Residents	Non-residents
Total Cost of Attendance	$44,788	$51,788
Tuition and Fees	$25,120	$32,120
Other (includes living expenses)	$18,068	$18,068
Health Insurance (can be waived)	$1,600	$1,600

Average 2008 Graduate Indebtedness: $32,455
% of Enrolled Students Receiving Aid: 92%

Criminal Background Check

This medical school requires a criminal background check prior to matriculation.

University of Puerto Rico
School of Medicine

San Juan, Puerto Rico

Central Admissions Office
School of Medicine, Medical Sciences Campus
University of Puerto Rico, P.O. Box 365067
San Juan, Puerto Rico 00936-5067
T 787 758 2525 x5215   **F** 787 282 7117

Admissions www.md.rcm.upr.edu
Main www.md.rcm.upr.edu
Financial www.rcm.upr.edu/estudiantes/Asistencia
conomica/index.htm/
E-mail marrivera@rcm.upr.edu

Public Institution

Dr. Walter Frontera, Dean

*Dr. Gladys Gonzalez-Navarrete,
Assistant Dean for Student Affairs*

Margarita Rivera, Director, Admissions Office

Zoraida Cruz, Director, Financial Aid Office

General Information
The UPR-SOM was established in 1949. The affiliated hospitals of the P.R. Medical Center and the Hospital Consortium, which include the main health care facilities in other cities, serve the medical school for teaching purposes. On the Medical Sciences Campus, the School of Medicine works in close relation with the School of Dentistry, the College of Allied Health Professions, the Faculty of Biosocial Sciences and Graduate School of Public Health, the School of Nursing, and the School of Pharmacy in an interdisciplinary team approach. Its location, adjacent to the University District Hospital, permits integration of basic and clinical departments and an improved utilization of all Medical Sciences Campus resources.

Mission Statement
The mission of the UPR-SOM is to transmit, enrich, and increase knowledge in the medical sciences through teaching, research, and clinical service. The school is committed to achieve the ideals of personal and academic excellence through the interdisciplinary model for providing education and health services, especially at the primary level. The school will provide an academic and institutional environment conducive to the personal and professional development of both students and faculty.

Curricular Highlights
Community Service Requirement: Optional.
Research/Thesis Requirement: Optional.

The new curriculum is four academic years in length. The first two years include the fundamentals of biological, behavioral, and clinical sciences and are mostly handled by the basic sciences departments. Part of the sophomore year is dedicated to pathophysiology, physical diagnosis, and basic clerkship, which are offered by a multidisciplinary faculty. Small-group sessions utilizing the problem-based learning approach are introduced at the beginning of the medical studies. Human behavior, environmental factors, and public health concepts are integrated into the curriculum. The third and fourth years are dedicated to required clinical experiences and elective courses. Through the Hispanic Center of Excellence, the curriculum has been focused on community-oriented primary care exposure. Support services, counseling, tutorials, and other services are provided to students to assist in retention. Students are graded on a letter grade system during all four years.

USMLE
Step 1: Required. Students must record a passing score for promotion.
Step 2: Clinical Skills (CS): Optional.
Step 2: Clinical Knowledge (CK): Required. Students must record a passing total score to graduate.

Selection Factors
Since the UPR-SOM is a state-supported institution, preference will be given to qualified applicants who are legal residents of Puerto Rico. Foreign national applicants with an established residence in P.R. will be considered only if, at the time of application, they are either U.S. citizens or have been granted a permanent resident visa in the United States. In selecting students, the Admissions Committee considers the candidate's academic performance, MCAT scores, recommendations of instructors, attitudinal and other personality factors assessed in personal interviews, extracurricular activities, and any other pertinent information. Personal interviews are conducted only by invitation from the Admissions Committee for those students with high numerical ranks according to the admission formula. The admission formula gives equal weight to academic indices and MCAT scores, with somewhat less weight given to ratings derived from evaluations by premedical committees and interviewers. Rejected applicants are given the opportunity to reapply for admission. Applicants, without exception, must submit all application material and supporting documents by December 1 of the year preced-ing the school year for which they request admission. The UPR-SOM has the policy of giving equal opportunity for education and training in the practice of the health professions without regard to race, creed, sex, national origin, age, or handicap.

Financial Aid
Financial aid is available to students. Awards are made on the basis of confidential applications submitted by students. Financial need is the major criterion. Applicants who require scholarship assistance may make application in conjunction with the application for admission or before April 30. Financial need will not influence the selection process. Forms are available from the Financial Aid Office upon request. We do not offer financial assistance to foreign students.

Campus Information
Enrollment
For 2008, total enrollment was: 432

Application Process and Requirements 2010–2011

Primary Application Service: AMCAS
Earliest filing date: June 1, 2009
Latest filing date: December 1, 2009

Secondary Application Required?: Yes
Sent to: All applicants
URL: www.md.rcm.upr.edu
Fee: Yes, $20
Fee waiver available: No
Earliest filing date: June 1, 2009
Latest filing date: December 1, 2009

MCAT® required?: Yes
Latest MCAT® considered: September 2009
Oldest MCAT® considered: September 2007

Early Decision Program: School does not have EDP
Applicants notified: n/a
EDP available for: n/a

Regular Acceptance Notice
Earliest date: December 2009
Latest date: Varies
Applicant's Response to Acceptance Offer – Maximum Time: Two weeks

Requests for Deferred Entrance Considered: No

Deposit to Hold Place in Class: Yes
Deposit (Resident): $100
Deposit (Non-resident): $100
Deposit due: With response to acceptance offer
Applied to tuition: Yes
Deposit refundable: No
Refundable by: n/a

Estimated number of new entrants: 110
EDP: n/a, special program: n/a

Start Month/Year: August 2010

Interview Format: Regional interviews are not available.

Other Programs

PREPARATORY PROGRAMS
Postbaccalaureate Program: No
Summer Program: No

COMBINED DEGREE PROGRAMS
Baccalaureate/M.D.: No
M.D./M.P.H.: No
MD/MBA: No
M.D./J.D.: Yes, www.md.rcm.upr.edu
M.D./Ph.D.: Yes, www.md.rcm.upr.edu

Premedical Coursework

Course	Req.	Rec.	Lab.	Hrs.	Course	Req.	Rec.	Lab.	Hrs.
Inorganic Chemistry	•		•	8	Computer Science		•		
Behavioral Sciences	•			6	Genetics				
Biochemistry		•			Humanities		•		
Biology	•			8	Organic Chemistry	•		•	8
Biology/Zoology					Physics	•		•	8
Calculus					Psychology				
College English	•			12	Social Sciences	•			6
College Mathematics					Spanish	•			12

Selection Factors: 2008 Accepted Applicants

Proportion of Accepted Applicants with Relevant Experience (Data Self-Reported to AMCAS®)		Community Service/Volunteer	41%
		Medically-Related Work	46%
		Research	72%

Shaded bar represents school's accepted scores ranging from the 10th percentile to the 90th percentile.   School Median ●   National Median ●

Overall GPA	2.0	2.1	2.2	2.3	2.4	2.5	2.6	2.7	2.8	2.9	3.0	3.1	3.2	3.3	3.4	3.5	3.6	3.7	(3.8)	3.9	4.0
Science GPA	2.0	2.1	2.2	2.3	2.4	2.5	2.6	2.7	2.8	2.9	3.0	3.1	3.2	3.3	3.4	3.5	3.6	(3.7)	3.8	3.9	4.0

MCAT® Total Numeric Score 9 10 11 12 13 14 15 16 17 18 19 20 21 22 (23) 24 25 26 27 28 29 30 31 (32) 33 34 35 36 37 38 39 40 41 42 43

Writing Sample				J	K	L	(M)	N	O	P	(Q)	R	S	T
Verbal Reasoning	3	4	5	6	(7)	8	9	(10)	11	12	13	14	15
Biological Sciences	3	4	5	6	7	8	(9)	10	(11)	12	13	14	15
Physical Sciences	3	4	5	6	7	(8)	9	10	(11)	12	13	14	15

Acceptance & Matriculation Data for 2008–2009 First Year Class

	Resident	Non-resident	International	Total
Applications	324	602	16	942
Interviewed	142	0	0	142
Deferred	0	0	0	0
Matriculants				
Early Assurance Program	n/a	n/a	n/a	0
Early Decision Program	0	0	0	0
Baccalaureate/M.D.	n/a	n/a	n/a	0
M.D./Ph.D.	n/a	n/a	n/a	0
Matriculated	105	3	0	**108**

Applications accepted from International Applicants: No

Specialty Choice

2004, 2005, 2006 Graduates, Specialty Choice (As reported by program directors to GME Track™)	
Anesthesiology	1%
Emergency Medicine	4%
Family Practice	3%
Internal Medicine	23%
Obstetrics/Gynecology	4%
Orthopaedic Surgery	3%
Pediatrics	10%
Psychiatry	9%
Radiology	5%
Surgery	8%

Matriculant Demographics: 2008–2009 First Year Class

Men: 41   **Women:** 67

Matriculants' Self-Reported Race/Ethnicity

Mexican American	0	Korean	0
Cuban	1	Vietnamese	0
Puerto Rican	106	Other Asian	0
Other Hispanic	0	Total Asian	0
Total Hispanic	106	Native American	0
Chinese	0	Black	5
Asian Indian	0	Native Hawaiian	0
Pakistani	0	White	71
Filipino	0	Unduplicated Number	
Japanese	0	of Matriculants	108

Science and Math Majors: 69%
Matriculants with:
  Baccalaureate degree: 97%
  Graduate degree(s): 6%

Financial Information

Source: 2007–2008 LCME I-B survey and 2008–2009 AAMC TSF questionnaire

	Residents	Non-residents
Total Cost of Attendance	$31,382	$39,311
Tuition and Fees	$10,780	$18,709
Other (includes living expenses)	$20,602	$20,602
Health Insurance (can be waived)	$0	$0

Average 2008 Graduate Indebtedness: $52,770
% of Enrolled Students Receiving Aid: 72%

Criminal Background Check

This medical school does not require a criminal background check prior to matriculation.

The Warren Alpert Medical School of Brown University
Providence, Rhode Island

Office of Admissions
Alpert Medical School
97 Waterman Street, Box G-A213
Providence, Rhode Island 02912-9706
T 401 863 2149   F 401 863 2660

Admissions http://med.brown.edu/admissions
Main http://med.brown.edu
Financial http://med.brown.edu/financialaid/
E-mail MedSchool_Admissions@brown.edu

Private Institution

Dr. Edward J. Wing, Dean of Medicine and Biological Sciences

Barbara Fuller, Director of Admissions

Dr. Emma Simmons, Assistant Dean for Minority Medical Affairs

Linda A. Gillette, Director of Financial Aid

Dr. Philip Gruppuso, Associate Dean for Medical Education

John Deeley, Executive Dean for Administration

General Information
Since its accreditation in 1975, Alpert Medical School has become a national leader in medical education and biomedical research. The medical school and its eight affiliated hospitals receive $200 million annually in research funding. Brown is home to the state's only Master of Public Health degree program and to ten public health research centers. Entry into Alpert Medical School is possible through many admission routes, including a combined Baccalaureate/M.D. program, standard AMCAS admission, and an Early Identification Program for students from Tougaloo College (MS) and for Rhode Island residents enrolled at three Rhode Island Institutions of higher education.

Mission Statement
Our mission is to educate physicians in the scientific, ethical, and humanistic dimensions of medicine and to advance our ability to diagnose, treat, and prevent human illness.

Curricular Highlights
Community Service Requirement: Optional.
Research/Thesis Requirement: Optional.

The medical curriculum is demanding, yet flexible. The first year is devoted to core basic sciences in the form of two semester-length, integrated medical sciences courses and Doctoring, in which students encounter individual, community-based clinical skills teaching with group sessions on ethics, patient interviewing, and professional development topics. The second year consists of organ or system-based pathophysiology with integrated pharmacology, pathology, neurologic pathophysiology, epidemiology, and Doctoring. Students in the third and fourth-years are required to complete 50 weeks of clinical clerkships and 30 weeks of electives. Clinical clerkships include internal medicine, surgery, psychiatry, obstetrics and gynecology, pediatrics, family medicine, and community health. Elective requirements include an advanced clinical clerkship in medicine, surgery, or pediatrics, and an ambulatory longitudinal clerkship.

USMLE
Step 1: Required. Students must only record a score.
Step 2: Clinical Skills (CS): Required. Students must only record a score.
Step 2: Clinical Knowledge (CK): Required. Students must only record a score.

Selection Factors
Selection criteria are academic achievement, faculty evaluations, and evidence of maturity, leadership, integrity, and compassion. Applicants to the M.D./Ph.D. program are evaluated on the basis of their research accomplishment and potential. Eligible candidates generally must present a minimum cumulative grade point average of 3.00 (4.00 scale) in undergraduate courses. Applicants who have attended graduate school must achieve a cumulative grade point average of 3.00 (4.00 scale). Applicants must complete baccalaureate degree requirements before entry into medical school. Brown University adheres to a policy of equal opportunity in medical education and considers applicants without regard to sex, race, religion, age, disability, status as a veteran, national or ethnic origin, sexual orientation, or gender identity. An affirmative action program is maintained in all admission entry routes.

Financial Aid
Alpert Medical School assists students in meeting their educational expenses through a combination of low-interest loans and need-based institutional scholarships. Seventy-seven percent of students received financial aid awards in 2008-09. The average award was $44,847 and the average scholarship award was $20,259.

Information about Diversity Programs
Alpert Medical School invites applications from members of ethnic and racial groups underrepresented in medicine. The objective of the Office of Minority Medical Affairs (OMMA) is the recruitment, retention, and graduation of students from groups underrepresented in medicine. The OMMA provides academic and personal counseling, workshops, information on scholarship awards, and a program linking students from groups underrepresented in medicine with alumni/ae from such groups.

Campus Information
Setting
The medical school is located on the main campus of Brown University in an historic residential area of Providence. The revitalized downtown center, with its riverfront park, shopping mall, restaurants, train station, and arts and theater district, is within walking distance of the campus.

Enrollment
For 2008, total enrollment was: 409

Special Features
Alpert Medical School is affiliated with eight hospitals within a five-mile radius, including a Level I trauma center, a children's hospital, two community hospitals, separate adult and children's psychiatric hospitals, a Veterans Affairs Medical Center, and a women's hospital with the largest neonatal intensive care unit in the Northeast. Students gain global health experience through clinical electives or exchange programs in Germany, Kenya, Sweden, and Israel.

Housing
Affordable housing options are available in several neighborhoods within walking distance of campus. Students have an on-campus dorm option. The university leases and manages about 100 apartments and homes in the vicinity. Monthly rents range from $700 to $1,150 in Brown-owned housing.

Satellite Campuses/Facilities
Clinical training in all four years occurs in a variety of settings, from the affiliated hospitals to diverse community-based sites.

Application Process and Requirements 2010–2011

Primary Application Service: AMCAS
Earliest filing date: June 1, 2009
Latest filing date: November 1, 2009

Secondary Application Required?: Yes
Sent to: All verified AMCAS applicants
URL: http://bms.brown.edu/admissions/applications
Fee: Yes, $95
Fee waiver available: Yes
Earliest filing date: July 1, 2009
Latest filing date: December 15, 2009

MCAT® required?: No
Latest MCAT® considered: September 2009
Oldest MCAT® considered: 2005

Early Decision Program: School does not have EDP
Applicants notified: n/a
EDP available for: n/a

Regular Acceptance Notice
Earliest date: November 2009
Latest date: Until Class is Full
Applicant's Response to Acceptance Offer – Maximum Time: Three weeks

Requests for Deferred Entrance Considered: Yes

Deposit to Hold Place in Class: No
Deposit (Resident): n/a
Deposit (Non-resident): n/a
Deposit due: n/a
Applied to tuition: n/a
Deposit refundable: n/a
Refundable by: n/a

Estimated number of new entrants: 46
EDP: n/a, special program: 50

Start Month/Year: August 2010

Interview Format: Group session and two individual meetings. All interviews are at Alpert Medical School.

Other Programs

PREPARATORY PROGRAMS
Postbaccalaureate Program: No
Summer Program: No
Scholarly Concentrations Program: Yes, http://med.brown.edu/education/concentrations/index.php
Academic Enhancement Program: Yes, http://med.brown.edu/student_services/enhancement.html

COMBINED DEGREE PROGRAMS
Baccalaureate/M.D.: Yes, http://bms.brown.edu/plme/
M.D./M.P.H.: Yes, http://bms.brown.edu/pubhealth
MD/MBA: No
M.D./J.D.: No
M.D./Ph.D.: Yes, http://bms.brown.edu/mdphd/
Additional Program: Yes, www.brown.edu/Departments/Taubman_Center/minisite/grad/MD_MPP.html

Premedical Coursework

Course	Req.	Rec.	Lab.	Sems.
Inorganic Chemistry	•			2
Behavioral Sciences	•			1
Biochemistry		•		
Biology	•			1
Biology/Zoology				
Calculus	•			1
College English				
College Mathematics				

Course	Req.	Rec.	Lab.	Sems.
Computer Science				
Genetics				
Humanities				
Organic Chemistry	•		•	1
Physics	•		•	2
Psychology				
Social Sciences		•		1
Other				

Selection Factors: 2008 Accepted Applicants

Proportion of Accepted Applicants with Relevant Experience (Data Self-Reported to AMCAS®)		
Community Service/Volunteer	60%
Medically-Related Work	64%
Research	78%

Shaded bar represents school's accepted scores ranging from the 10th percentile to the 90th percentile. School Median ● National Median ●

Overall GPA: School median 3.8, National median 3.8
Science GPA: School median 3.8, National median 3.8

MCAT® Total Numeric Score: 32 (school), 35 (national)

Writing Sample: Q (school), R (national)
Verbal Reasoning: 10 (school), 11 (national)
Biological Sciences: 11 (school), 12 (national)
Physical Sciences: 11 (school), 12 (national)

Acceptance & Matriculation Data for 2008–2009 First Year Class

	Resident	Non-resident	International	Total
Applications	105	5258	539	5902
Interviewed	13	191	5	209
Deferred	0	0	0	0
Matriculants				
Early Assurance Program	2	2	0	4
Early Decision Program	n/a	n/a	n/a	n/a
Baccalaureate/M.D.	5	56	0	61
M.D./Ph.D.	1	1	0	2
Matriculated	10	84	0	**94**

Applications accepted from International Applicants: Yes

Matriculant Demographics: 2008–2009 First Year Class

Men: 41 **Women:** 53

Matriculants' Self-Reported Race/Ethnicity

Mexican American	7	Korean	3
Cuban	1	Vietnamese	0
Puerto Rican	0	Other Asian	3
Other Hispanic	2	Total Asian	35
Total Hispanic	9	Native American	3
Chinese	12	Black	10
Asian Indian	13	Native Hawaiian	1
Pakistani	2	White	38
Filipino	0	Unduplicated Number	
Japanese	3	of Matriculants	94

Science and Math Majors: 47%
Matriculants with:
Baccalaureate degree: 100%
Graduate degree(s): 3%

Specialty Choice

2004, 2005, 2006 Graduates, Specialty Choice (As reported by program directors to GME Track™)

Anesthesiology	2%
Emergency Medicine	6%
Family Practice	9%
Internal Medicine	20%
Obstetrics/Gynecology	3%
Orthopaedic Surgery	3%
Pediatrics	7%
Psychiatry	5%
Radiology	6%
Surgery	6%

Financial Information

Source: 2007–2008 LCME I-B survey and 2008–2009 AAMC TSF questionnaire

	Residents	Non-residents
Total Cost of Attendance	$60,150	$60,150
Tuition and Fees	$40,510	$40,510
Other (includes living expenses)	$17,128	$17,085
Health Insurance (can be waived)	$2,512	$2,512

Average 2008 Graduate Indebtedness: $124,982
% of Enrolled Students Receiving Aid: 77%

Criminal Background Check

This medical school does not require a criminal background check prior to matriculation.

Medical University of South Carolina
College of Medicine
Charleston, South Carolina

College of Medicine Dean's Office
Medical University of South Carolina
96 Jonathan Lucas Street, Suite 601
PO Box 250617, Charleston, South Carolina 29425
T 843 792 3283   F 843 792 0204

Admissions www.musc.edu/es/
Main www.musc.edu/com1
Financial www.musc.edu/financialmanagement/
E-mail taylorwl@musc.edu

Public Institution

Dr. Jerry Reves, Dean

Dr. Paul B. Underwood,
Associate Dean for Admissions

Willette Burnham, Executive Director of
Student Programs

Dr. Deborah Deas,
Associate Dean for Admissions

Wanda Taylor, Director of Admissions

General Information
The College of Medicine at MUSC was found-ed in Charleston in 1824 and is the South's oldest medical school. MUSC's Medical Center is comprised of four separate hospitals (the University Hospital, Ashley River Tower, the Institute of Psychiatry, and the Children's Hospital.) There are centers for specialized care (Heart Center, Transplantation Center, Hollings Cancer Center, Digestive Diseases Center, and Storm Eye Institute). The adjacent VA Hospital, with consortium/community hospitals in Greenville, Spartanburg, Columbia, and Florence, supply additional facilities for clinical teaching.

Mission Statement
The COM is committed to maintaining an educational environment for all students which prepares them for a career of excellence in the practice of medicine and service. It ensures optimal opportunities for all students, faculty, and administration, including all backgrounds and levels of diversity, to achieve full potential.

Curricular Highlights
Community Service Requirement: Required.
Research/Thesis Requirement: Optional.

The goal of the COM is to produce caring and competent physicians capable of choosing any postgraduate career. The curriculum in the first two years provides basic science concepts and problem-solving strategies, develops skills for taking histories and physical examinations, and introduces students to the role of the physician in society. Emphasis is placed on small-group instruction and independent, self-directed learning. The 3rd year consists of

clerkships in medicine, ob/gyn, pediatrics, family medicine, surgery, and psychiatry. Selectives in multiple disciplines are also pro-vided for students to gain exposure to major specialty areas. Emphasis is placed on the development of clinical, interpersonal, and professional competence. In the 4th year, stu-dents are required to take additional training in surgery and internal medicine and up to seven elective rotations in a wide variety of subspecialties.

USMLE
Step 1: Required. Students must record a passing score for promotion.
Step 2: Clinical Skills (CS): Required. Students must only record a score.
Step 2: Clinical Knowledge (CK): Required. Students must record a passing total score to graduate.

Selection Factors
Selection is based on a total evaluation of a student. Screening for interviews is based on the cumulative GPA and best total MCAT score. SC residency is a primary admission consideration. Non-residents must have close SC ties and superior records to be interviewed. Noncognitive traits, accomplishments, and cri-teria for added value are evaluated during interviews. Interpersonal skills, motivation, judgment, and compassion are important as well as the quality of recommendations, leader-ship, and volunteer/clinical/work experiences. Applicants with unique qualities or experiences important for diversity may be considered for added value. Early Decision is encouraged for SC applicants with a GPA of 3.5 or above and MCAT scores of 27 or higher. Foreign students must have a permanent resident visa to be con-sidered.

Financial Aid
Financial need is not a factor in the initial selection process. Loan programs and scholar-ships are available for entering students. A financial aid counselor advises new and current students on loan opportunities and debt man-agement. Merit scholarships are awarded by the Scholarship Board and are based on out-standing academic and personal achievement.

Information about Diversity Programs
Students from groups underrepresented in medicine are encouraged to apply; an active recruitment program is in place. PREP is an individually tailored undergraduate course of study prescribed for a few underprepared, but promising SC students who seek admission through AMCAS. The curriculum at the College of Charleston spans two semesters and is full time. No separate application is required. Students considered are those who apply through AMCAS and are denied admission. Students are selected annually; stipends are provided. A Summer Institute, devoted to underrepresented or rural students, focuses on MCAT/test-taking skills. The COM and the Center for Academic Excellence provide coun-seling and support services for Summer Institute students.

Campus Information

Setting
MUSC's 67-acre campus is located in historic Charleston, SC. Charleston combines the best that life has to offer: historic homes, art, music, museums, libraries, restaurants, beaches, and some of the country's finest golf courses. Within a short walk from the city's main street are all the hospitals, research centers, clinical, and basic science buildings that make up the MUSC complex.

Enrollment
For 2008, total enrollment was: 642

Special Features
MUSC has distinguished programs in neuro-science, substance abuse, cardiovascular medi-cine, drug sciences, perinatal medicine, oph-thalmology, hearing loss, genetics, rheumatol-ogy and cancer care. The newly opened MUSC Simulation Center gives students a wide range of learning experiences.

Housing
On-campus housing is not available. The MUSC Office of Student Programs maintains an online listing of affordable apartments near the MUSC campus. Rents average $600-$800 per month.

Application Process and Requirements 2010–2011

Primary Application Service: AMCAS
Earliest filing date: June 1, 2009
Latest filing date: December 1, 2009

Secondary Application Required?: Yes
Sent to: All applicants
URL: www.musc.edu/em/admissions/apply.html
Fee: Yes, $75
Fee waiver available: No
Earliest filing date: July 13, 2009
Latest filing date: January 15, 2010

MCAT® required?: Yes
Latest MCAT® considered: September 2009
Oldest MCAT® considered: August 2007

Early Decision Program: School does have EDP
Applicants notified: October 1, 2009
EDP available for: Residents only

Regular Acceptance Notice
Earliest date: November 1, 2009
Latest date: Until class is full
Applicant's Response to Acceptance
Offer – Maximum Time: Four weeks

Requests for Deferred
Entrance Considered: Yes

Deposit to Hold Place in Class: Yes
Deposit (Resident): $400
Deposit (Non-resident): $400
Deposit due: Within four weeks of response to acceptance offer
Applied to tuition: No
Deposit refundable: Yes
Refundable by: May 15, 2010

Estimated number of new entrants: 155
EDP: 28, special program: 4

Start Month/Year: August 2010

Interview Format: Three one-on-one interviews are required. Regional physicians assist with interviews.

Other Programs

PREPARATORY PROGRAMS
Postbaccalaureate Program: No
Summer Program: No
PREP - Postbaccalaureate Reapplication Education Program: Wanda Taylor, (843) 792-2055, taylorwl@musc.edu
MUSC Summer Institute: Wanda Taylor, (843) 792-2055, taylorwl@musc.edu

COMBINED DEGREE PROGRAMS
Baccalaureate/M.D.: No
M.D./M.P.H.: Yes, Dr. Lynn Manfred, (843) 792-1184, manfred@musc.edu
MD/MBA: Yes, Dr. Lynn Manfred, (843) 792-1184, manfred@musc.edu
M.D./J.D.: No
M.D./Ph.D.: Yes, www.musc.edu/grad/mstp/ Dr. Perry Halushka, (843) 792-3012, halushpv@musc.edu
Additional Program: Yes, Dr. Lynn Manfred, (843) 792-1184, manfred@musc.edu

Premedical Coursework

Course	Req.	Rec.	Lab.	Sems.
Inorganic Chemistry		•	•	2
Behavioral Sciences				
Biochemistry		•		2
Biology		•	•	2
Biology/Zoology				
Calculus				
College English		•		2
College Mathematics				
Computer Science				
Genetics				

Course	Req.	Rec.	Lab.	Sems.
Humanities				
Organic Chemistry		•	•	2
Physics		•		2
Psychology				
Social Sciences				
Other				
Cell Biology		•		2
Physiology		•		2
Anatomy		•		2

Selection Factors: 2008 Accepted Applicants

Proportion of Accepted Applicants with Relevant Experience (Data Self-Reported to AMCAS®)		
Community Service/Volunteer		65%
Medically-Related Work		78%
Research		76%

Shaded bar represents school's accepted scores ranging from the 10th percentile to the 90th percentile. School Median ● National Median ●

Overall GPA 2.0 2.1 2.2 2.3 2.4 2.5 2.6 2.7 2.8 2.9 3.0 3.1 3.2 3.3 3.4 3.5 3.6 (3.7) 3.8 3.9 4.0
Science GPA 2.0 2.1 2.2 2.3 2.4 2.5 2.6 2.7 2.8 2.9 3.0 3.1 3.2 3.3 3.4 3.5 (3.6) 3.7 3.8 3.9 4.0

MCAT® Total Numeric Score 9 10 11 12 13 14 15 16 17 18 19 20 21 22 23 24 25 26 27 28 (29) 30 31 32 33 34 35 36 37 38 39 40 41 42 43

			J	K	L	M	N	O	P	Q	R	S	T
Writing Sample			J	K	L	M	N	(O)	P	(Q)	R	S	T
Verbal Reasoning	3	4	5	6	7	8	9	(10)	11	12	13	14	15
Biological Sciences	3	4	5	6	7	8	9	(10)	(11)	12	13	14	15
Physical Sciences	3	4	5	6	7	8	9	(10)	(11)	12	13	14	15

Acceptance & Matriculation Data for 2008–2009 First Year Class

	Resident	Non-resident	International	Total
Applications	464	1741	40	2245
Interviewed	347	45	0	381
Deferred	1	0	0	1
Matriculants				
Early Assurance Program	0	0	0	0
Early Decision Program	42	0	0	42
Baccalaureate/M.D.	n/a	n/a	n/a	n/a
M.D./Ph.D.	2	3	0	5
Matriculated	150	14	1	**165**
Applications accepted from International Applicants: No				

Specialty Choice

2004, 2005, 2006 Graduates, Specialty Choice (As reported by program directors to GME Track™)

Anesthesiology	6%
Emergency Medicine	4%
Family Practice	11%
Internal Medicine	17%
Obstetrics/Gynecology	10%
Orthopaedic Surgery	5%
Pediatrics	13%
Psychiatry	4%
Radiology	4%
Surgery	7%

Matriculant Demographics: 2008–2009 First Year Class

Men: 96 **Women:** 69

Matriculants' Self-Reported Race/Ethnicity

Mexican American	1	Korean	1
Cuban	0	Vietnamese	0
Puerto Rican	0	Other Asian	1
Other Hispanic	0	Total Asian	13
Total Hispanic	1	Native American	2
Chinese	1	Black	21
Asian Indian	7	Native Hawaiian	0
Pakistani	1	White	128
Filipino	1	Unduplicated Number	
Japanese	1	of Matriculants	165

Science and Math Majors: 72%
Matriculants with:
  Baccalaureate degree: 100%
  Graduate degree(s): 12%

Financial Information

Source: 2007–2008 LCME I-B survey and 2008–2009 AAMC TSF questionnaire

	Residents	Non-residents
Total Cost of Attendance	$49,310	$96,092
Tuition and Fees	$26,976	$73,758
Other (includes living expenses)	$21,344	$21,344
Health Insurance (can be waived)	$990	$990

Average 2008 Graduate Indebtedness: $144,428
% of Enrolled Students Receiving Aid: 90%

Criminal Background Check

This medical school requires a criminal background check prior to matriculation.

University of South Carolina School of Medicine
Columbia, South Carolina

Associate Dean for Medical Education
and Academic Affairs
University of South Carolina School of Medicine
Columbia, South Carolina 29208
T 803 733 3325   F 803 733 3328

Admissions http://medicaleducationoffice.med.sc.edu/
AdmissionsHomePage.htm
Main www.med.sc.edu
Financial www.sc.edu/financialaid
E-mail jeanette.ford@uscmed.sc.edu

Public Institution

Dr. Donald J. DiPette, Dean

Dr. Jeanette H. Ford, Registrar, Administrator, Office of Admissions

Dr. Carol L. McMahon, Assistant Dean for Minority Affairs

Jerel Arceneaux, Assistant Director of Student Services and Financial Aid

Dr. Richard A. Hoppmann, Associate Dean for Medical Education and Academic Affairs

Dr. Donald J. Kenney, Director, Student Services

General Information
The USC SOM was established in 1977 and is located in the state's capital city. The school offers a wide range of educational and professional opportunities to its students, featuring a small class size, a nationally recognized Senior Mentor Program, and a state-of-the-art ultrasound curriculum. The school works closely with its three major affiliated hospitals to provide students valuable clinical experience.

Mission Statement
The mission of the USC SOM is to improve the health of the people of the state of SC through the development and implementation of programs for medical education, research, and the delivery of health care. Programs will be developed in collaboration with affiliated institutions, and allocation of resources will be based upon the physician manpower and health care needs of SC, the effectiveness and efficiency of specific programs, and the accreditation requirements of all appropriate organizations. Medical education and graduate education at all levels are conducted in a highly personal atmosphere that emphasizes a balance among scientific disciplines, humanistic concerns, and societal needs.

Curricular Highlights
Community Service Requirement: Optional.
Research/Thesis Requirement: Optional.

The SOM offers a program of study designed to provide education and training in the art and science of medicine and to prepare stu-

dents for a wide variety of medical career choices. Each of the first two years consists of two academic semesters of both basic science and clinically relevant coursework in which students are exposed to patients in various inpatient, outpatient, community, and rural settings. The correlation between basic and clinical science information in the first two years is emphasized by means of an interdisciplinary, four-semester Introduction to Clinical Medicine course continuum. The third year consists of required clinical clerkships in medicine, surgery, pediatrics, obstetrics-gynecology, family medicine, and psychiatry. The fourth year is devoted to advanced clinical work, including 20 weeks each of required and elective rotations, during which students have the opportunity to strengthen their clinical skills and pursue individual academic interests and career goals in preparation for the lifelong study of medicine. An integrated ultrasound curriculum (iUSC) has been introduced in both the basic science and clinical years.

USMLE
Step 1: Required. Students must record a passing score for promotion.
Step 2: Clinical Skills (CS): Required. Students must record a passing total score to graduate.
Step 2: Clinical Knowledge (CK): Required. Students must record a passing total score to graduate.

Selection Factors
The selection process involves the comparative evaluation and review of all available application data, including MCAT scores, undergraduate academic performance, letters of evaluation, and the results of personal interviews with Admissions Committee members. The opportunity for admission is greatest for legal residents of South Carolina. Applications are only accepted from permanent residents or U.S. citizens. The ultimate selection of a student is based upon a total and comparative appraisal of the applicant's suitability for the successful practice of medicine. The AMCAS application is used for preliminary screening. After this initial review, the Admissions Committee may extend an invitation for personal interviews. Each applicant is evaluated on the basis of individual qualifications without regard to age, race,

creed, national origin, sex, or disability.

Financial Aid
The SOM participates in all federally funded loan and scholarship programs. A SOM-sponsored low-interest loan program is available to students with proven need. Every effort is made to provide information and assistance to help students meet their financial obligations. Students seeking part-time employment during medical school should have the prior approval of the director of student services.

Information about Diversity Programs
The SOM actively encourages applications from members of groups underrepresented in the medical profession. There is diverse membership on the Admissions Committee. For additional information, contact the assistant dean for minority affairs at (803) 733-3319.

Campus Information
Setting
The beautiful USC SOM campus, with its spacious lawns and trees, and convenient parking, is located four miles east of the USC Columbia campus and adjacent to the Dorn V.A. Medical Center.

Enrollment
For 2008, total enrollment was: 319

Special Features
Students enjoy 24-hour secure access to USC SOM laboratories and library facilities. They participate in the extensive intramural athletic and recreational sports programs. The fitness center is located on-campus. USC SOM students also have access to all facilities and programs available to USC students.

Housing
The majority of USC SOM students choose housing in the area adjacent to the campus. Housing information can be obtained from the Student Services Office.

Satellite Campuses/Facilities
Students have the option of completing core clinical training in the third and fourth years at the Greenville Hospital System; 24 positions are available.

Application Process and Requirements 2010–2011

Primary Application Service: AMCAS
Earliest filing date: June 1, 2009
Latest filing date: December 1, 2009

Secondary Application Required?: Yes
Sent to: All applicants
URL: n/a
Fee: Yes, $75
Fee waiver available: Yes
Earliest filing date: June 1, 2009
Latest filing date: January 15, 2010

MCAT® required?: Yes
Latest MCAT® considered: September 2009
Oldest MCAT® considered: 2004

Early Decision Program: School does have EDP
Applicants notified: October 1, 2009
EDP available for: Residents only

Regular Acceptance Notice
Earliest date: October 15, 2009
Latest date: Until class is full
**Applicant's Response to Acceptance
Offer – Maximum Time:** Two weeks

**Requests for Deferred
Entrance Considered:** Yes

Deposit to Hold Place in Class: Yes
Deposit (Resident): $100
Deposit (Non-resident): $100
Deposit due: With response within two weeks
Applied to tuition: Yes
Deposit refundable: Yes
Refundable by: May 15, 2010 with written request

Estimated number of new entrants: 85
EDP: 5, special program: n/a

Start Month/Year: August 2010

Interview Format: Two 30-minute interviews. Regional interviews are available in Greenville, South Carolina.

Other Programs

PREPARATORY PROGRAMS
Postbaccalaureate Program: Yes
Summer Program: No

COMBINED DEGREE PROGRAMS
Baccalaureate/M.D.: No
M.D./M.P.H.: Yes, www.sc.edu/bulletin/SOM/admissions.html
MD/MBA: No
M.D./J.D.: No
M.D./Ph.D.: Yes, www.sc.edu/bulletin/SOM/admissions.html

Premedical Coursework

Course	Req.	Rec.	Lab.	Hrs.
Inorganic Chemistry	•		•	8
Behavioral Sciences				
Biochemistry		•		
Biology				
Biology/Zoology	•		•	8
Calculus				
College English				6
College Mathematics				

Course	Req.	Rec.	Lab.	Hrs.
Computer Science				
Genetics				
Humanities				
Organic Chemistry	•		•	8
Physics		•		
Psychology				
Social Sciences				
Other				

Selection Factors: 2008 Accepted Applicants

Proportion of Accepted Applicants with Relevant Experience (Data Self-Reported to AMCAS®)		
Community Service/Volunteer		71%
Medically-Related Work		83%
Research		69%

Shaded bar represents school's accepted scores ranging from the 10th percentile to the 90th percentile. School Median ● National Median ●

Overall GPA 2.0 2.1 2.2 2.3 2.4 2.5 2.6 2.7 2.8 2.9 3.0 3.1 **3.2 3.3 3.4 3.5 3.6 (3.7) 3.8 3.9 4.0**

Science GPA 2.0 2.1 2.2 2.3 2.4 2.5 2.6 2.7 2.8 2.9 **3.0 3.1 3.2 3.3 3.4 3.5 3.6 (3.7) 3.8 3.9 4.0**

MCAT® Total Numeric Score 9 10 11 12 13 14 15 16 17 18 19 20 21 22 23 24 25 26 27 28 (29) 30 31 (32) 33 34 35 36 37 38 39 40 41 42 43

	J	K	L	M	N	O	(P)	(Q)	R	S	T
Writing Sample											

Verbal Reasoning	3	4	5	6	7	8	9	(10)	11	12	13	14	15
Biological Sciences	3	4	5	6	7	8	9	(10)	(11)	12	13	14	15
Physical Sciences	3	4	5	6	7	8	(9)	10	(11)	12	13	14	15

Acceptance & Matriculation Data for 2008–2009 First Year Class

	Resident	Non-resident	International	Total
Applications	381	1549	30	1960
Interviewed	237	99	0	336
Deferred	2	1	0	3
Matriculants				
Early Assurance Program	n/a	n/a	n/a	n/a
Early Decision Program	2	0	0	2
Baccalaureate/M.D.	n/a	n/a	n/a	n/a
M.D./Ph.D.	0	0	0	0
Matriculated	67	16	0	**83**

Applications accepted from International Applicants: No

Specialty Choice

2004, 2005, 2006 Graduates, Specialty Choice (As reported by program directors to GME Track™)	
Anesthesiology	4%
Emergency Medicine	11%
Family Practice	12%
Internal Medicine	24%
Obstetrics/Gynecology	4%
Orthopaedic Surgery	1%
Pediatrics	15%
Psychiatry	7%
Radiology	1%
Surgery	7%

Matriculant Demographics: 2008–2009 First Year Class

Men: 43 **Women:** 40

Matriculants' Self-Reported Race/Ethnicity

Mexican American	0	Korean	0
Cuban	0	Vietnamese	3
Puerto Rican	0	Other Asian	0
Other Hispanic	1	Total Asian	12
Total Hispanic	1	Native American	1
Chinese	2	Black	6
Asian Indian	6	Native Hawaiian	1
Pakistani	0	White	66
Filipino	0	Unduplicated Number	
Japanese	1	of Matriculants	83

Science and Math Majors: 73%
Matriculants with:
Baccalaureate degree: 100%
Graduate degree(s): 11%

Financial Information

Source: 2007–2008 LCME I-B survey and 2008–2009 AAMC TSF questionnaire

	Residents	Non-residents
Total Cost of Attendance	$49,807	$85,489
Tuition and Fees	$25,576	$61,258
Other (includes living expenses)	$23,241	$23,241
Health Insurance (can be waived)	$990	$990

Average 2008 Graduate Indebtedness: $119,848
% of Enrolled Students Receiving Aid: 93%

Criminal Background Check

This medical school requires a criminal background check prior to matriculation.

Sanford School of Medicine of the University of South Dakota

Vermillion, South Dakota

Medical School Admissions
Sanford School of Medicine
University of South Dakota
414 East Clark Street
Vermillion, South Dakota 57069
T 605 677 6886   F 605 677 5109

Admissions www.usd.edu/med/md/prospective
students/admissions.cfm
Main www.usd.edu/med/md
Financial www.usd.edu/med/md/prospective
students/tuition.cfm
E-mail usdsmsa@usd.edu

Public Institution

Dr. Rodney R. Parry, Dean

Dr. Paul C. Bunger, Dean, Medical Student Affairs

Dr. Gerald J. Yutrzenka, Director, Diversity Affairs

Carol Hemmingson, Program Assistant, Financial Aid

Jill Christopherson, Program Assistant – Admissions

General Information

The School of Medicine was established in 1907 as a two-year school for the basic sciences and in 1974 became a four-year, M.D. degree program with the first class of graduates in 1977. The first two years are located in Vermillion, with years three and four available on campuses in Sioux Falls, Yankton or Rapid City. In 2005, the name was changed to Sanford School of Medicine of the University of South Dakota.

Mission Statement

The mission of the Sanford School of Medicine of the University of South Dakota is to provide the opportunity for South Dakota residents to receive a quality, broad-based medical education with an emphasis on family medicine. The curriculum is to be established to encourage graduates to serve people living in medically underserved areas of South Dakota and to require excellence in the basic sciences and in all clinical disciplines. The School of Medicine is to provide to its students and to the people of South Dakota excellence in education, research, and service. (Complete mission statement on Web site.)

Curricular Highlights

Community Service Requirement: Required. A community based, cultural diversity program.
Research/Thesis Requirement: Optional.

The first two years use traditional courses, problem/case-based teaching, and clinical experiences. To cap year two, students spend four weeks with a physician in a primary care setting in a South Dakota community. At the Sioux Falls and Rapid City sites, the third year is hospital-based, with clerkships in family medicine, internal medicine, pediatrics, ob/gyn, psychiatry, neurology, and surgery. Students also take clinical colloquium, ambulatory program and radiology. At the Yankton site, the third year is an ambulatory-based program, with students rotating through all six of the clerkships throughout the year. Year four requirements are rural family medicine, emergency medicine, surgical subspecialties and a sub-internship. Students also have 22 weeks of electives; many take 4–8 weeks outside the state. Grading is A-B-C-D-F. Students must pass USMLE Step 1 for promotion, and Step 2-CK and a school OSCE to graduate. They must also take Step 2-CS.

USMLE

Step 1: Required. Students must record a passing score for promotion.
Step 2: Clinical Skills (CS): Required. Students must only record a score.
Step 2: Clinical Knowledge (CK): Required. Students must record a passing total score to graduate.

Selection Factors

Applicants are chosen on the basis of intellect, character, and motivation. The Admissions Committee considers: academic achievement as indicated by scholastic records; recall, reading comprehension, and ability to perform within time constraints as reflected by MCAT scores; intellectual curiosity, work ethic, and fitness for a career in medicine as viewed by the applicant's former instructors; assessments of personal factors of the applicant as determined by interviews conducted by the committee. Applicants invited to interview must meet in person with at least two committee members. Interviews are conducted at the office or clinic of the interviewer or at the Vermillion campus. The school does not discriminate on the basis of race, color, creed, national origin, ancestry, citizenship, gender, sexual orientation, religion, age, or disability. Priority for supplemental applications and interviews is given to legal residents of South Dakota, non-residents with strong ties to South Dakota, and Native Americans affiliated with federally recognized tribes in the region. The School of Medicine does not sponsor an Early Decision Program. An Alumni Student Scholars Program (ASSP) offers a limited number of provisional acceptances to South Dakota high school seniors who meet strict criteria. The School of Medicine will consider applications for transfer only into Year 2 or Year 3 and only from students who are currently in good standing at an LCME-accredited medical school. Transfer opportunities are limited, with priority given to South Dakota residents.

Financial Aid

Financial aid is administered through the office of Medical Student Affairs. Loans are available to matriculated students on the basis of demonstrated financial need.

Information about Diversity Programs

The Sanford School of Medicine is committed to training a diverse group of students to meet the needs of the diverse population of the state. Interested applicants may contact the Director of Diversity Affairs for information about programs for premedical and medical students.

Campus Information

Setting
The first two years are based in Vermillion. The clinical years are based in Sioux Falls (1/2 of the class), Yankton (1/4 of the class), and Rapid City (1/4 of the class).

Enrollment
For 2008, total enrollment was: 205

Special Features
Students have significant one-on-one teaching from clinical faculty, numerous experiences in clinical and surgical procedures, many options for cultural immersion experiences, participation in the Scholarship Pathways program, and research opportunities.

Housing
See USD Web site at *www.usd.edu*.

Satellite Campuses/Facilities
Besides the four major campuses, students have options to rotate through many hospitals/clinics throughout the state.

Application Process and Requirements 2010–2011

Primary Application Service: AMCAS
Earliest filing date: June 1, 2009
Latest filing date: November 15, 2009

Secondary Application Required?: Yes
Sent to: SD residents and selected non-residents with ties to SD
Name: Jill Christopherson
Phone: (605) 677-6886
E-mail: Jill.Christopherson@usd.edu
Fee: Yes, $35
Fee waiver available: No
Earliest filing date: July 15, 2009
Latest filing date: Two weeks after invitation to submit Secondary Application

MCAT® required?: Yes
Latest MCAT® considered: September 2009
Oldest MCAT® considered: January 2007

Early Decision Program: School does not have EDP
Applicants notified: n/a
EDP available for: n/a

Regular Acceptance Notice
Earliest date: November 18, 2009
Latest date: Until class is full
Applicant's Response to Acceptance
Offer – Maximum Time: Two weeks after offer

Requests for Deferred
Entrance Considered: Yes

Deposit to Hold Place in Class: Yes
Deposit (Resident): $100
Deposit (Non-resident): $100
Deposit due: With response to acceptance offer
Applied to tuition: Yes
Deposit refundable: Yes
Refundable by: June 1, 2010

Estimated number of new entrants: 45
EDP: n/a, special program: 9

Start Month/Year: August 2, 2010

Interview Format: Open file, two individual face-to-face interviews. Regional interviews are not available.

Other Programs

PREPARATORY PROGRAMS
Postbaccalaureate Program: No
Summer Program: No

COMBINED DEGREE PROGRAMS
Baccalaureate/M.D.: No
M.D./M.P.H.: No
MD/MBA: No
M.D./J.D.: No
M.D./Ph.D.: Yes, www.usd.edu/mdphd
Jill Christopherson (605) 677-6886
Jill.Christopherson@usd.edu

Premedical Coursework

Course	Req.	Rec.	Lab.	Qtrs.	Course	Req.	Rec.	Lab.	Qtrs.
Inorganic Chemistry	•		•	2	Computer Science				
Behavioral Sciences		•			Genetics		•		
Biochemistry		•			Humanities		•		
Biology		•			Organic Chemistry	•		•	2
Biology/Zoology	•		•	2	Physics	•		•	2
Calculus		•			Psychology				
College English		•			Social Sciences				
College Mathematics	•			2	Other				

Selection Factors: 2008 Accepted Applicants

Proportion of Accepted Applicants with Relevant Experience (Data Self-Reported to AMCAS®)	
Community Service/Volunteer	63%
Medically-Related Work	67%
Research	70%

Shaded bar represents school's accepted scores ranging from the 10th percentile to the 90th percentile.   School Median ●   National Median ●

Overall GPA 2.0 2.1 2.2 2.3 2.4 2.5 2.6 2.7 2.8 2.9 3.0 3.1 3.2 3.3 **3.4 3.5 3.6 3.7 (3.8) 3.9 4.0**

Science GPA 2.0 2.1 2.2 2.3 2.4 2.5 2.6 2.7 2.8 2.9 3.0 3.1 3.2 3.3 **3.4 3.5 3.6 3.7 (3.8) 3.9 4.0**

MCAT® Total Numeric Score 9 10 11 12 13 14 15 16 17 18 19 20 21 22 23 24 25 **26 27 28 29 (30) 31 (32) 33 34** 35 36 37 38 39 40 41 42 43

Writing Sample			J	K	L	**M**	**N**	**(O)**	**P**	**(Q)**	**R**	S	T	
Verbal Reasoning	3	4	5	6	7	**8**	**9**	**(10)**	**(11)**	**12**	13	14	15	
Biological Sciences	3	4	5	6	7	8	**9**	**(10)**	**(11)**	**12**	13	14	15	
Physical Sciences	3	4	5	6	7	**8**	**9**	**(10)**	**(11)**	**12**	13	14	15	

Acceptance & Matriculation Data for 2008–2009 First Year Class

	Resident	Non-resident	International	Total
Applications	144	471	26	641
Interviewed	133	37	0	170
Deferred	2	0	0	2
Matriculants				
Early Assurance Program	2	0	0	2
Early Decision Program	0	0	0	0
Baccalaureate/M.D.	n/a	n/a	n/a	n/a
M.D./Ph.D.	1	3	0	4
Matriculated	44	10	0	**54**

Applications accepted from International Applicants: Can be Accepted from among South Dakota Residents only

Matriculant Demographics: 2008–2009 First Year Class

Men: 30   **Women:** 24

Matriculants' Self-Reported Race/Ethnicity

Mexican American	0	**Korean**	0
Cuban	0	**Vietnamese**	1
Puerto Rican	0	**Other Asian**	1
Other Hispanic	0	**Total Asian**	2
Total Hispanic	0	**Native American**	0
Chinese	0	**Black**	0
Asian Indian	0	**Native Hawaiian**	0
Pakistani	0	**White**	51
Filipino	0	**Unduplicated Number**	
Japanese	0	**of Matriculants**	54

Science and Math Majors: 69%
Matriculants with:
  Baccalaureate degree: 96%
  Graduate degree(s): 11%

Specialty Choice

2004, 2005, 2006 Graduates, Specialty Choice (As reported by program directors to GME Track™)	
Anesthesiology	10%
Emergency Medicine	10%
Family Practice	9%
Internal Medicine	11%
Obstetrics/Gynecology	10%
Orthopaedic Surgery	5%
Pediatrics	5%
Psychiatry	5%
Radiology	3%
Surgery	12%

Financial Information

Source: 2007–2008 LCME I-B survey and 2008–2009 AAMC TSF questionnaire

	Residents	Non-residents
Total Cost of Attendance	$40,221	$61,543
Tuition and Fees	$19,765	$41,087
Other (includes living expenses)	$18,248	$18,248
Health Insurance (can be waived)	$2,208	$2,208

Average 2008 Graduate Indebtedness: $126,766
% of Enrolled Students Receiving Aid: 98%

Criminal Background Check

This medical school requires a criminal background check prior to matriculation.

East Tennessee State University
James H. Quillen College of Medicine

Johnson City, Tennessee

Assistant Dean for Admissions and Records
East Tennessee State University
James H. Quillen College of Medicine
P.O. Box 70580, Johnson City, Tennessee 37614-1708
T 423 439 2033   **F** 423 439 2110

Admissions www.etsu.edu/com/sa/admissions/
default.aspx
Main www.etsu.edu/com
Financial www.etsu.edu/com/sa/finaid/
default.aspx
E-mail sacom@etsu.edu

Public Institution

Dr. Philip C. Bagnell, Dean of Medicine

*Edwin D. Taylor, Assistant Dean
for Admissions and Records*

Linda Embree, Director, Financial Services

*Dr. Thomas Kwasigroch, Associate Dean
for Student Affairs*

General Information

Since its beginning in 1978, ETSU's Quillen College of Medicine has established itself as a national leader in primary care and rural medicine. ETSU students enjoy an exceptional success rate in the national residency match, and over 60 percent of graduates choose a career in primary care. ETSU's Community Partnerships Program is nationally recognized, and the Rural Primary Care Track has exceeded all expectations. Student input and participation are encouraged in all facets of their medical education. A collegial atmosphere is encouraged at all levels. The campus is unified on the grounds of the VA Medical Center pictured above. The school is located in Tennessee's fourth largest metropolitan area (population 1.2 million) and on the campus of the state's fourth largest university (enrollment 14,000). It is supported by modern and convenient medical centers and clinics throughout the Tri-Cities area, as well as by hospitals and clinics located in small, rural communities such as Rogersville and Mountain City. The school enrolls one class of 60 new students in August of each year.

Mission Statement

The primary mission of Quillen College of Medicine is to educate future physicians, especially those with an interest in primary care, to practice in underserved rural communities. In addition, the college is committed to excellence in biomedical research and is dedicated to the improvement of health care in Northeast Tennessee and the surrounding Appalachian Region.

Curricular Highlights

Community Service Requirement: Optional.
Research/Thesis Requirement: Optional.

Quillen College of Medicine enjoys a dynamic and ever-changing curriculum. The curriculum includes a mix of traditional, systems-based, and case-based learning, as well as a wide range of educational experiences, patient populations, and hospitals. The highly diversified faculty considers students as colleagues. Patient contact comes early in the curriculum and continues throughout. Flexibility is allowed for students to decelerate a portion of the curriculum for elective courses, including research and advanced clinical studies. Student input is a key component in curricular change, along with the rapidly changing body of knowledge and the needs of the profession. The goals of the curriculum are to prepare students to be well-grounded in the science and art of medicine, capable practitioners of their profession, and self-directed, lifelong learners.

USMLE

Step 1: Required. Students must record a passing score for promotion.
Step 2: Clinical Skills (CS): Required. Students must record a passing total score to graduate.
Step 2: Clinical Knowledge (CK): Required. Students must record a passing total score to graduate.

Selection Factors

To be admitted, an applicant must be a U.S. or Canadian citizen or possess a U.S. permanent resident visa. Admission is based upon a competitive selection process involving those applicants who meet the minimum requirements for admission. The Admissions Committee selects students who give the promise of being not merely satisfactory medical students, but also capable, responsible physicians of high ethical standards. The Admissions Committee screens applicants on the basis of academic achievement, MCAT scores, letters of recommendation, pertinent extracurricular research and work experiences, and evidence of non-scholastic accomplishments. After a general screening, the Admissions Committee may request supplementary information and a personal interview with the applicant. Interviews are held only on the campus and are at the applicant's expense. Admission preferences are for residents of the state of Tennessee who are U.S. citizens, veterans of U.S. military service, and recipients of baccalaureate degrees prior to enrollment. Marginally qualified non-residents should not apply.

Financial Aid

The need for student financial assistance is not a consideration in the selection process. Scholarships, grants, and loans are available for students who demonstrate need as defined by a federal needs analysis and who meet the specific criteria set forth by the various agencies. Additional information may be obtained by writing directly to the medical school Director for Financial Services.

Information about Diversity Programs

The College of Medicine actively seeks applicants of both sexes and members of groups underrepresented in medicine. African-American matriculants may be eligible for financial awards from the state of Tennessee. Support services are available to matriculants to assist in the timely completion of the medical curriculum. ETSU does not discriminate on the basis of race, sex, creed, national origin, age, or disability. The university is an equal opportunity/affirmative action employer.

Campus Information

Enrollment
For 2008, total enrollment was: 245

Application Process and Requirements 2010–2011

Primary Application Service: AMCAS
Earliest filing date: June 1, 2009
Latest filing date: November 15, 2009

Secondary Application Required?: Yes
Sent to: Selected applicants
URL: n/a
Fee: Yes, $50
Fee waiver available: Yes
Earliest filing date: June 1, 2009
Latest filing date: Twenty-one days from request

MCAT® required?: Yes
Latest MCAT® considered: September 2009
Oldest MCAT® considered: January 2007

Early Decision Program: School does have EDP
Applicants notified: October 1, 2009
EDP available for: Both Residents and Non-residents

Regular Acceptance Notice
Earliest date: October 16, 2009
Latest date: Until class is full
Applicant's Response to Acceptance Offer – Maximum Time: Two weeks

Requests for Deferred Entrance Considered: Yes

Deposit to Hold Place in Class: Yes
Deposit (Resident): $100
Deposit (Non-resident): $100
Deposit due: With response to acceptance offer
Applied to tuition: Yes
Deposit refundable: Yes
Refundable by: May 15, 2010

Estimated number of new entrants: 64
EDP: 3, special program: n/a

Start Month/Year: August 2010

Interview Format: Two, one-hour interviews with an admissions committee member. Regional interviews are not available.

Other Programs

PREPARATORY PROGRAMS
Postbaccalaureate Program: No
Summer Program: No

COMBINED DEGREE PROGRAMS
Baccalaureate/M.D.: No
M.D./M.P.H.: No
M.D./M.B.A.: No
M.D./J.D.: No
M.D./Ph.D.: No

Premedical Coursework

Course	Req.	Rec.	Lab.	Hrs.	Course	Req.	Rec.	Lab.	Hrs.
Inorganic Chemistry	•		•	8	Computer Science				
Behavioral Sciences					Genetics				
Biochemistry					Humanities				
Biology	•		•	8	Organic Chemistry	•		•	8
Biology/Zoology					Physics	•		•	8
Calculus					Psychology				
College English					Comm. Skills Courses				9
College Mathematics					Electives				49

Selection Factors: 2008 Accepted Applicants

Proportion of Accepted Applicants with Relevant Experience (Data Self-Reported to AMCAS®)		Community Service/Volunteer	70%
		Medically-Related Work	83%
		Research	66%

Shaded bar represents school's accepted scores ranging from the 10th percentile to the 90th percentile | School Median ● | National Median ●

Overall GPA	2.0	2.1	2.2	2.3	2.4	2.5	2.6	2.7	2.8	2.9	3.0	3.1	3.2	3.3	3.4	3.5	3.6	(3.7)	3.8	3.9	4.0
Science GPA	2.0	2.1	2.2	2.3	2.4	2.5	2.6	2.7	2.8	2.9	3.0	3.1	3.2	3.3	3.4	3.5	3.6	(3.7)	3.8	3.9	4.0

MCAT® Total Numeric Score 9 10 11 12 13 14 15 16 17 18 19 20 21 22 23 24 25 26 27 28 29 (30) 31 (32) 33 34 35 36 37 38 39 40 41 42 43

			J	K	L	M	N	O	(P)	(Q)	R	S	T
Writing Sample			J	K	L	M	N	O	(P)	(Q)	R	S	T
Verbal Reasoning	3	4	5	6	7	8	9	(10)	11	12	13	14	15
Biological Sciences	3	4	5	6	7	8	9	(10)	(11)	12	13	14	15
Physical Sciences	3	4	5	6	7	8	9	(10)	(11)	12	13	14	15

Acceptance & Matriculation Data for 2008–2009 First Year Class

	Resident	Non-resident	International	Total
Applications	562	1018	61	1641
Interviewed	180	79	0	259
Deferred	1	0	0	1
Matriculants				
Early Assurance Program	0	0	0	0
Early Decision Program	1	0	0	1
Baccalaureate/M.D.	n/a	n/a	n/a	n/a
M.D./Ph.D.	n/a	n/a	n/a	n/a
Matriculated	50	10	0	**60**

Applications accepted from International Applicants: Canadian only

Specialty Choice

2004, 2005, 2006 Graduates, Specialty Choice (As reported by program directors to GME Track™)	
Anesthesiology	1%
Emergency Medicine	5%
Family Practice	16%
Internal Medicine	10%
Obstetrics/Gynecology	9%
Orthopaedic Surgery	1%
Pediatrics	14%
Psychiatry	4%
Radiology	3%
Surgery	13%

Matriculant Demographics: 2008–2009 First Year Class

Men: 36   **Women:** 24

Matriculants' Self-Reported Race/Ethnicity

Mexican American	1	**Korean**	0
Cuban	0	**Vietnamese**	0
Puerto Rican	0	**Other Asian**	1
Other Hispanic	0	**Total Asian**	7
Total Hispanic	1	**Native American**	0
Chinese	0	**Black**	1
Asian Indian	5	**Native Hawaiian**	0
Pakistani	2	**White**	51
Filipino	0	**Unduplicated Number**	
Japanese	0	**of Matriculants**	60

Science and Math Majors: 63%
Matriculants with:
Baccalaureate degree: 100%
Graduate degree(s): 15%

Financial Information

Source: 2007–2008 LCME I-B survey and 2008–2009 AAMC TSF questionnaire

	Residents	Non-residents
Total Cost of Attendance	$41,190	$63,188
Tuition and Fees	$22,081	$44,079
Other (includes living expenses)	$18,003	$18,003
Health Insurance (can be waived)	$1,106	$1,106

Average 2008 Graduate Indebtedness: $115,594
% of Enrolled Students Receiving Aid: 92%

Criminal Background Check

This medical school requires a criminal background check prior to matriculation.

Meharry Medical College
School of Medicine
Nashville, Tennessee

Director, Admissions and Recruitment
Meharry Medical College
1005 Dr. D. B. Todd Boulevard
Nashville, Tennessee 37208
T 615 327 6223   F 615 327 6228

Admissions www.mmc.edu/admissions/index.html
Main www.mmc.edu
Financial www.mmc.edu/students/student
financialaid.html
E-mail admissions@mmc.edu

Private Institution

*Dr. Valerie Montgomery Rice, Dean
and Senior Vice President for Health Affairs*

*Allen D. Mosley, Director,
Admissions and Recruitment*

Barbara Tharpe, Director, Student Financial Aid

Dr. Pamela C.Williams, Executive Vice Dean

Deborah Davis, Senior Admissions Manager

General Information
In 1876, Meharry Medical College was founded and established as the Meharry Medical Department of Central Tennessee College by the Freedmen's Aid Society of the Methodist Episcopal Church. Meharry's inception was part of the society's continuing effort to educate freed slaves and to provide health care services for the poor and underserved. Today, the School of Medicine continues to provide excellent educational opportunities to promising students from groups underrepresented in medicine. Clinical teaching facilities include the Metropolitan Nashville General Hospital; Blanchfield Army Hospital; Veterans Affairs Tennessee Valley Health Care System, Nashville Campus and the Alvin C. York Murfreesboro Campus; Vanderbilt's Monroe Carrell Children's Hospital; and a number of affiliated hospitals and clinics. The provision of primary care, particularly in medically underserved areas, is a special emphasis, as is health disparities research.

Mission Statement
Meharry Medical College exists to improve the health and health care of minority and underserved communities by offering excellent education and training programs in the health sciences placing special emphasis on providing opportunities to people of color and individuals from disadvantaged backgrounds, regardless of race or ethnicity; delivering high quality health services; and conducting research that fosters the elimination of health disparities.

Curricular Highlights
Community Service Requirement: Optional.
Research/Thesis Requirement: Optional.
Encouraged in areas of health disparities.

The school has an integrated curriculum for the freshman year in which instruction is organized into modules that include basic, clinical, and social sciences. The modules include Principles and Practice Of Medicine, Molecular Cell Biology, Genetics, Gross Anatomy, and Embryology; also included are Integrated Neuroscience, Immunology, Principles of Infectious Disease, and Foundations in Human Disease and Treatment. The sophomore year is organized around a series of organ systems. The clinical years consist of the following blocks: family medicine, psychiatry, obstetrics and gynecology, pediatrics, internal medicine, surgery, an ambulatory rotation served in an urban or rural underserved area, internal medicine subinternship, capstone, and radiology, as well as guided electives.

USMLE
Step 1: Required. Students must record a passing score for promotion.
Step 2: Clinical Skills (CS): Required. Students must record a passing total score to graduate.
Step 2: Clinical Knowledge (CK): Required. Students must record a passing total score to graduate.

Selection Factors
Applicants are selected on a competitive basis with regard to cognitive and non-cognitive skills that denote probable success in medical school. Performance in the basic science prerequisite subjects and MCAT scores form the basis for screening for the interview process in which the non-cognitive aspects of the applicant are assessed. While special empathy is held for minority and disadvantaged applicants of all origins, Meharry Medical College seeks to attract a wide demographic, cultural, and educational population to reflect the caliber of social interchange in which the eventual practice of medicine will occur. Meharry Medical College does not discriminate on the basis of race, sex, creed, national origin, age, or handicap.

Financial Aid
Financial aid awards are based on analyses of student needs and academic achievement. The limited financial aid program includes scholarships, grants, and loans. Because of fluctuations in federal and private support for

financial aid programs, the types and amounts of awards are revised and adjusted on a continuing basis. Therefore, it is necessary that applicants plan their financial program as carefully as their academic program.

Information about Diversity Programs
For over 130 years, Meharry has produced a large percentage of the minority health professionals in the United States and abroad.

Campus Information
Setting
Its campus in North Nashville places Meharry at the epicenter of Middle Tennessee's most vulnerable citizens. As such, Meharry students, faculty, staff, and residents provide services where they are most needed. Located off Nashville's historic Jefferson Street, nestled between two neighboring historically black universities and near Nashville's thriving downtown, Meharry provides students with a full-range of auxiliary services to make their experience intellectually stimulating and socially comfortable and enjoyable.

Enrollment
For 2008, total enrollment was: 409

Special Features
Through several Centers of Excellence, the college and its faculty are working to unlock the mysteries behind health disparities in a variety of areas, most notably in women's health, cancer, and HIV/AIDS.

Housing
On campus there is the Meharry Towers, a 10-story residential complex which contains 156 apartments and Dorothy Brown Hall, which houses 70 students. The college also maintains a list of available off-campus accommodations in the Nashville area.

Application Process and Requirements 2010–2011

Primary Application Service: AMCAS
Earliest filing date: June 1, 2009
Latest filing date: December 15, 2010

Secondary Application Required?: Yes
Sent to: Screened applicants
Contact: Deborah Davis,
(615) 327-6223, ddavis@mmc.edu
Fee: Yes, $65
Fee waiver available: Yes
Earliest filing date: August 1, 2009
Latest filing date: February 15, 2010

MCAT® required?: Yes
Latest MCAT® considered: January 2010
Oldest MCAT® considered: April 2007

Early Decision Program: School does have EDP
Applicants notified: October 1, 2009
EDP available for: Both Residents
and Non-residents

Regular Acceptance Notice
Earliest date: November 1, 2009
Latest date: Until class is full
Applicant's Response to Acceptance
Offer – Maximum Time: Three weeks

Requests for Deferred
Entrance Considered: Yes

Deposit to Hold Place in Class: Yes
Deposit (Resident): $300
Deposit (Non-resident): $300
Deposit due: With response to acceptance offer
Applied to tuition: Yes
Deposit refundable: Yes
Refundable by: $200 refundable prior
to April 15, 2010

Estimated number of new entrants: 78
EDP: 2, special program: 20

Start Month/Year: July 2010

Interview Format: Two 30-minute interviews.
Regional interviews are available.

Other Programs

PREPARATORY PROGRAMS
Postbaccalaureate Program: Yes,
By invitation only (20 places)
Summer Program: Yes, Pre-Baccalaureate
program, Sharon Turner-Friley, (615) 327-5966,
sfriley@mmc.edu

COMBINED DEGREE PROGRAMS
Baccalaureate/M.D.: Yes,
Allen Mosley, (615) 327-6223, amosley@mmc.edu
M.D./M.P.H.: No
M.D./M.B.A.: No
M.D./J.D.: No
M.D./Ph.D.: Yes, Dr. Fatima Lima, (615) 327-6533,
admissions@mmc.edu

Premedical Coursework

Course	Req.	Rec.	Lab.	Hrs.
Inorganic Chemistry	•		•	8
Behavioral Sciences				
Biochemistry		•		4
Biology				
Biology/Zoology	•		•	8
Calculus				
College English	•			6
College Mathematics	•			3

Course	Req.	Rec.	Lab.	Hrs.
Computer Science				
Genetics				
Humanities				
Organic Chemistry	•		•	8
Physics	•		•	8
Psychology				
Social Sciences				
Other				

Selection Factors: 2008 Accepted Applicants

Proportion of Accepted Applicants with Relevant Experience (Data Self-Reported to AMCAS')		
Community Service/Volunteer	66%
Medically-Related Work	72%
Research	74%

Shaded bar represents school's accepted scores ranging from the 10th percentile to the 90th percentile. School Median ● National Median ●

Overall GPA 2.0 2.1 2.2 2.3 2.4 2.5 2.6 2.7 2.8 2.9 3.0 3.1 3.2 3.3 3.4 (3.5) 3.6 3.7 3.8 3.9 4.0

Science GPA 2.0 2.1 2.2 2.3 2.4 2.5 2.6 2.7 2.8 2.9 3.0 3.1 3.2 (3.3) 3.4 3.5 3.6 3.7 3.8 3.9 4.0

MCAT® Total Numeric Score 9 10 11 12 13 14 15 16 17 18 19 20 21 22 23 24 (25) 26 27 28 29 30 31 (32) 33 34 35 36 37 38 39 40 41 42 43

Writing Sample		J	K	L	M	N	(O)	P	(Q)	R	S	T
Verbal Reasoning	3	4	5	6	7	(8)	9	(10)	11	12	13	14	15
Biological Sciences	3	4	5	6	7	8	(9)	10	(11)	12	13	14	15
Physical Sciences	3	4	5	6	7	(8)	9	10	(11)	12	13	14	15

Acceptance & Matriculation Data for 2008–2009 First Year Class

	Resident	Non-resident	International	Total
Applications	259	3997	273	4529
Interviewed	54	341	10	405
Deferred	0	1	0	1
Matriculants				
Early Assurance Program	0	0	0	0
Early Decision Program	0	0	0	0
Baccalaureate/M.D.	0	2	0	2
M.D./Ph.D.	0	0	0	0
Matriculated	10	88	2	**100**

Applications accepted from International Applicants: Canadian Only

Matriculant Demographics: 2008–2009 First Year Class

Men: 49 **Women:** 51

Matriculants' Self-Reported Race/Ethnicity

Mexican American	2	Korean	0
Cuban	1	Vietnamese	3
Puerto Rican	2	Other Asian	0
Other Hispanic	1	Total Asian	8
Total Hispanic	5	Native American	1
Chinese	0	Black	82
Asian Indian	3	Native Hawaiian	0
Pakistani	1	White	6
Filipino	1	Unduplicated Number	
Japanese	0	of Matriculants	100

Science and Math Majors: 69%
Matriculants with:
    Baccalaureate degree: 98%
    Graduate degree(s): 19%

Specialty Choice

2004, 2005, 2006 Graduates, Specialty Choice (As reported by program directors to GME Track™)	
Anesthesiology	4%
Emergency Medicine	2%
Family Practice	11%
Internal Medicine	17%
Obstetrics/Gynecology	10%
Orthopaedic Surgery	2%
Pediatrics	11%
Psychiatry	9%
Radiology	3%
Surgery	6%

Financial Information

Source: 2007–2008 LCME I-B survey
and 2008–2009 AAMC TSF questionnaire

	Residents	Non-residents
Total Cost of Attendance	$66,193	$66,193
Tuition and Fees	$32,508	$32,508
Other (includes living expenses)	$31,087	$31,087
Health Insurance (can be waived)	$2,598	$2,598

Average 2008 Graduate Indebtedness: $131,721
% of Enrolled Students Receiving Aid: 94%

Criminal Background Check

This medical school does not require a criminal
background check prior to matriculation.

University of Tennessee Health Science Center College of Medicine
Memphis, Tennessee

University of Tennessee,
Health Science Center College of Medicine
910 Madison Avenue, Suite 500
Memphis, Tennessee 38163
T 901 448 5559   F 901 448 1740

Admissions www.utmem.edu/Medicine/Admissions
Main www.utmem.edu/Medicine
Financial www.utmem.edu/finaid
E-mail nstrother@utmem.edu

Public Institution

Dr. Steve J. Schwab, Executive Dean

E. Nelson Strother Jr., Assistant Dean for Admissions and Student Affairs

Dr. Gerald J. Presbury, Representative to Minority Affairs Section

John H. Lewis, IV, Director of Financial Aid

General Information
The UTHSC College of Medicine traces its origin to 1851 as the Medical Department of the University of Nashville. Today, the college utilizes over 20 facilities statewide for its training programs, including the Boston-Baskin Cancer Group, Campbell Orthopaedic Clinic, LeBonheur Children's Medical Center, Methodist University Hospital, Regional Medical Center, Semmes-Murphy Clinic, St. Jude Children's Research Hospital, UT Medical Group, VA Medical Center, Baptist Hospital-Memphis, St. Francis Hospital, UT Knoxville Medical Center, Erlanger Medical Center-Chattanooga, Baptist Hospital-Nashville, and Family Practice Center-Jackson.

Mission Statement
The Faculty of the College of Medicine is committed to educating physicians whose primary responsibilities will be evaluating, treating and preventing disease. The educational program is designed to prepare students to become knowledgeable, skillful, and compassionate physicians. Students are imbued with both the ideal that the study of medicine is a lifelong process and the sense of a physician's deep commitment to high moral and ethical standards regarding patients, colleagues, and society.

Curricular Highlights
Community Service Requirement: Required. Community service project.
Research/Thesis Requirement: Optional.

Year 1 of the curriculum begins in August with Gross Anatomy; Prevention, Community and Culture (PCC); Doctoring: Recognizing Signs and Symptoms (DRS); Molecular Basis of Disease; and Physiology, and runs through March. In April and May of year 1, some concepts from the Pathophysiology, Microbiology, Pathology, and Pharmacology courses are pre-

sented. Year 2 begins in August with Pharmacology, Microbiology, Pathology, Pathophysiology, Neurosciences, PCC and DRS. Students are introduced to clinical medicine in their first semester through PCC and DRS. These courses expose students to the practice of medicine by placing them in a community physician's office and emphasizing professionalism. The third-year clerkships focus on patient problem-solving with an increasing level of responsibility. The fourth year is composed of six 4-week clerkships and four 4-week electives.

USMLE
Step 1: Required. Students must record a passing score for promotion.
Step 2: Clinical Skills (CS): Required. Students must record a passing total score to graduate.
Step 2: Clinical Knowledge (CK): Required. Students must record a passing total score to graduate.

Selection Factors
The criteria the Committee on Admissions uses in the selection process are the academic record, MCAT scores, preprofessional evaluations, and personal interviews. Personal interviews by members of the committee provide candidates with an opportunity to review their curricular and extracurricular activities. More important, the interviewers gain insight into the character of the applicants, as well as how they have formulated their plans for the study and practice of medicine. Applicants must be citizens or permanent residents of the U.S. at the time of application. Applications are considered from Tennessee and its contiguous states (Mississippi, Arkansas, Missouri, Kentucky, Virginia, North Carolina, Georgia, and Alabama). Children of UT alumni may also be considered, regardless of their state of residence. Since priority is given to qualified Tennesseans, non-residents must possess superior qualifications to be considered by the committee. Only 10 percent of the entering class may be non-residents. Upon initial review of the AMCAS application, a supplemental application will be sent to applicants considered competitive for further review. Advanced standing applications will be considered for year 3 only. Applicants for transfer must be residents of Tennessee, be attending LCME-accredited schools, have successfully completed the basic science curriculum, and have passed

USMLE Step 1. Applicants must also provide evidence of circumstances necessitating a transfer. Deadline for transfer applications is April 1.

Financial Aid
Aid consists of loans, scholarships, and work-study. Merit-based scholarships are available to highly qualified students.

Information about Diversity Programs
The College of Medicine actively encourages applications from members of groups underrepresented in medicine. The Committee on Admissions evaluates both academic and non-academic factors in the selection process, with consideration given to the unique backgrounds and challenges of these applicants. Among American medical schools, the college is a national leader in the admission, matriculation, and graduation of students from groups underrepresented in medicine.

Campus Information
Setting
UTHSC is situated in one of the largest medical centers in the nation and close to vibrant downtown Memphis, home of NBA basketball, AAA baseball, the Symphony, Broadway plays, Beale Street blues and barbecue.

Enrollment
For 2008, total enrollment was: 598

Special Features
Please go to *www.utmem.edu/Medicine*.

Housing
UTHSC has one dormitory. An abundance of affordable off-campus housing is available. See *www.UTMemOffCampus.com*.

Satellite Campuses/Facilities
Rotations are available at all three UT College of Medicine campuses: Memphis, Knoxville and Chattanooga.

Application Process and Requirements 2010–2011

Primary Application Service: AMCAS
Earliest filing date: June 1, 2009
Latest filing date: November 15, 2009

Secondary Application Required?: Yes
Sent to: Screened applicants
Contact: Nelson Strother
(901) 448-5561, nstrother@utmem.edu
Fee: Yes, $50
Fee waiver available: Yes
Earliest filing date: July 2009
Latest filing date: February 2010

MCAT® required?: Yes
Latest MCAT® considered: September 2009
Oldest MCAT® considered: April 2004

Early Decision Program: School does not have EDP
Applicants notified: n/a
EDP available for: n/a

Regular Acceptance Notice
Earliest date: October 15, 2009
Latest date: Varies
Applicant's Response to Acceptance Offer – Maximum Time: Two weeks

Requests for Deferred Entrance Considered: Yes

Deposit to Hold Place in Class: No
Deposit (Resident): n/a
Deposit (Non-resident): n/a
Deposit due: n/a
Applied to tuition: n/a
Deposit refundable: n/a
Refundable by: n/a

Estimated number of new entrants: 150
EDP: 0, special program: n/a

Start Month/Year: August 2010

Interview Format: Two individual interviews with admissions committee members. May have 1 in Memphis and 1 regional.

Other Programs

PREPARATORY PROGRAMS
Postbaccalaureate Program: No
Summer Program: Yes
www.utmem.edu/HCP

COMBINED DEGREE PROGRAMS
Baccalaureate/M.D. : No
M.D./M.P.H.: No
M.D./M.B.A.: No
M.D./J.D.: No
M.D./Ph.D.: Yes, Dr. Don Thomason,
(901) 448-7224, thomason@physio1.utmem.edu

Premedical Coursework

Course	Req.	Rec.	Lab.	Sems.
Inorganic Chemistry	•		•	8
Behavioral Sciences				
Biochemistry		•		
Biology	•		•	8
Biology/Zoology				
Calculus				
College English	•			6
College Mathematics				

Course	Req.	Rec.	Lab.	Sems.
Computer Science				
Genetics		•		
Humanities				
Organic Chemistry	•		•	8
Physics	•		•	8
Psychology				
Social Sciences				

Selection Factors: 2008 Accepted Applicants

Proportion of Accepted Applicants with Relevant Experience (Data Self-Reported to AMCAS®)		
Community Service/Volunteer		78%
Medically-Related Work		84%
Research		70%

Shaded bar represents school's accepted scores ranging from the 10th percentile to the 90th percentile. School Median ○ National Median ◉

Overall GPA 2.0 2.1 2.2 2.3 2.4 2.5 2.6 2.7 2.8 2.9 3.0 3.1 3.2 **3.3** 3.4 3.5 3.6 (3.7) 3.8 3.9 4.0
Science GPA 2.0 2.1 2.2 2.3 2.4 2.5 2.6 2.7 2.8 2.9 3.0 3.1 **3.2** 3.3 3.4 3.5 3.6 (3.7) 3.8 3.9 4.0

MCAT® Total Numeric Score 9 10 11 12 13 14 15 16 17 18 19 20 21 22 23 24 25 26 27 28 29 (30) 31 (32) 33 34 35 36 37 38 39 40 41 42 43

Writing Sample			J	K	L	M	N	O	(P)	(Q)	R	S	T
Verbal Reasoning	3	4	5	6	7	8	9	(10)	11	12	13	14	15
Biological Sciences	3	4	5	6	7	8	9	(10)	(11)	12	13	14	15
Physical Sciences	3	4	5	6	7	8	9	(10)	(11)	12	13	14	15

Acceptance & Matriculation Data for 2008–2009 First Year Class

	Resident	Non-resident	International	Total
Applications	654	772	6	1432
Interviewed	438	49	0	487
Deferred	6	1	0	7
Matriculants				
Early Assurance Program	n/a	n/a	n/a	n/a
Early Decision Program	0	0	0	0
Baccalaureate/M.D.	n/a	n/a	n/a	n/a
M.D./Ph.D.	0	0	0	0
Matriculated	144	6	0	**150**

Applications accepted from International Applicants: No

Specialty Choice

2004, 2005, 2006 Graduates, Specialty Choice (As reported by program directors to GME Track™)	
Anesthesiology	8%
Emergency Medicine	4%
Family Practice	7%
Internal Medicine	14%
Obstetrics/Gynecology	7%
Orthopaedic Surgery	5%
Pediatrics	10%
Psychiatry	4%
Radiology	9%
Surgery	8%

Matriculant Demographics: 2008–2009 First Year Class

Men: 86   **Women:** 64

Matriculants' Self-Reported Race/Ethnicity

Mexican American	1	**Korean**	2
Cuban	0	**Vietnamese**	0
Puerto Rican	2	**Other Asian**	1
Other Hispanic	0	**Total Asian**	25
Total Hispanic	3	**Native American**	0
Chinese	2	**Black**	11
Asian Indian	18	**Native Hawaiian**	0
Pakistani	2	**White**	114
Filipino	0	**Unduplicated Number**	
Japanese	0	**of Matriculants**	150

Science and Math Majors: 67%
Matriculants with:
Baccalaureate degree: 99%
Graduate degree(s): 9%

Financial Information

Source: 2007–2008 LCME I-B survey and 2008–2009 AAMC TSF questionnaire

	Residents	Non-residents
Total Cost of Attendance	$47,174	$65,624
Tuition and Fees	$20,405	$38,855
Other (includes living expenses)	$25,705	$25,705
Health Insurance (can be waived)	$1,064	$1,064

Average 2008 Graduate Indebtedness: $129,311
% of Enrolled Students Receiving Aid: 88%

Criminal Background Check

This medical school requires a criminal background check prior to matriculation.

Vanderbilt University School of Medicine

Nashville, Tennessee

Office of Admissions
215 Light Hall
Vanderbilt University School of Medicine
Nashville, Tennessee 37232-0685
T 615 322 2145   **F** 615 343 8397

Admissions www.mc.vanderbilt.edu/medschool/
admissions
Main www.mc.vanderbilt.edu/medschool
Financial www.mc.vanderbilt.edu/medschool/
finaid/finaid1.php
E-mail pat.sagen@vanderbilt.edu

Private Institution

Dr. Jeff Balser, Dean and Associate Vice Chancellor for Health Affairs

Dr. John A. Zic, Associate Dean for Admissions

Dr. George C. Hill, Associate Dean for Diversity in Medical Education

Vicky L. Cagle, Director of Student Financial Services

Dr. Patricia Sagen, Director of Admissions

General Information

Vanderbilt University School of Medicine is a private medical school located on the campus of Vanderbilt University. The Vanderbilt University Medical Center and affiliated hospitals provide a total of over 5,000 beds for diversified, comprehensive clinical experience. These hospitals share common goals of education, research, patient care, and community service.

Mission Statement

VUSM seeks to matriculate a diverse group of academically exceptional students whose attributes and accomplishments suggest that they will be future leaders and/or scholars in medicine to begin the process of lifelong learning in the science and practice of medicine.

Curricular Highlights

Community Service Requirement: Optional.
Research/Thesis Requirement: Optional.

Medical education at Vanderbilt is oriented toward promoting the intellectual development of students and equipping them with the disciplined approach, knowledge, and skills required of both a physician and scientist. The curriculum provides the student with a fundamental knowledge of basic medical principles, but flexibility is stressed. Changes in curriculum content and teaching methods continually evolve from Vanderbilt's focus upon new ways to assist students in their preparation for a lifetime of learning. The curriculum offers a productive blend of required and elective courses throughout all four years of the program. The Emphasis Program, whose primary goal is to develop leadership potential, is scheduled for the first two years of the curriculum, including

eight weeks during the intervening summer. Areas of focus include: laboratory-based research, patient-oriented research, healthcare research, community health initiatives, international medicine, biomedical informatics, medical education, law and medicine, and medical humanities.

USMLE

Step 1: Required. Student must record a score.
Step 2: Clinical Skills (CS): Required. Student must record a score.
Step 2: Clinical Knowledge (CK): Required. Student must record a score.

Selection Factors

Applicants are invited without regard to race, sex, religion, national origin, sexual orientation, or state of residence. Applicants must possess sufficient intellectual ability, emotional stability, and sensory and motor functions to meet the academic requirements of the school of medicine without fundamental alteration in the nature of this program. Applications are reviewed in two stages. The initial review is made from material provided through AMCAS. Competitive strength of credentials reflecting preparation for medical studies, motivation, personal qualities, and educational background are evaluated by the Admissions Committee and determine the recipients of secondary applications and invitations to interview. There is a holistic review of academic performance and non-academic factors (patient care experience, research experience, extracurricular involvement, leadership roles, sports activities, relationship to the medical school, and applicants from underserved populations). Interviews are held at Vanderbilt. AP credit, CLEP credit, and PASS/FAIL credit are not accepted for any required courses. In lieu of required courses with AP credit, higher level coursework should be taken. Vanderbilt undergraduates with at least a 3.5 GPA are eligible to apply for the binding Early Acceptance Program during the spring of the sophomore year. Those accepted are encouraged to broaden their curricular experiences. Acceptance for transfer is limited to third year with places made available by attrition only. Those students who have completed the second year in good standing at an LCME-accredited U.S. or

Canadian medical school are eligible to apply. The deadline for applying is March 1.

Financial Aid

Every effort is made to see that each student who applies has sufficient funds to meet the total estimated cost of attendance by utilizing a variety of loans and scholarships. Thirty-three percent of the class receives full tuition scholarships on merit or through the MST program.

Information about Diversity Programs

Matriculation of a diverse student body is a central goal of VUSM. Diversity is defined in the broadest sense (gender, race, ethnicity, sexual preference, socio-economic background, geographic origin).

Campus Information

Setting

The medical school is part of a 323-acre campus that also serves as a national arboretum.

Enrollment

For 2008, total enrollment was: 442

Special Features

The Monroe Carell, Jr. Children's Hospital at Vanderbilt is a state-of-the-art pediatric facility. VUSM has an NIH-sponsored Comprehensive Cancer Center. The Vanderbilt Transplant Center is one of the leaders in the field. The new Center for Experiential Learning and Assessment describes state-of-the-art simulation technologies and standardized patient learning environments to master clinical skills. The new anatomy lab features plasma screen computers to enhance learning.

Housing

There is limited on-campus housing. The university does maintain a list of affordable apartments within a 10-mile radius. Rents average $500–$900 per month.

Satellite Campuses/Facilities

Student rotations are divided between Vanderbilt Hospital and the Nashville VA Hospital. Clinical opportunities also exist at Meharry Medical School as part of a formal collaboration.

Application Process and Requirements 2010–2011

Primary Application Service: AMCAS
Earliest filing date: June 1, 2009
Latest filing date: November 15, 2009

Secondary Application Required?: Yes
Sent to: Screened applicants invited to interview
URL: www.mc.vanderbilt.edu/medschool/admissions
Fee: Yes, $50
Fee waiver available: Yes
Earliest filing date: August 1, 2009
Latest filing date: December 31, 2009

MCAT® required?: Yes
Latest MCAT® considered: September 2009
Oldest MCAT® considered: 2006

Early Decision Program: School does have EDP
Applicants notified: October 1, 2009
EDP available for: Both Residents
and Non-residents

Regular Acceptance Notice
Earliest date: October 16, 2009
Latest date: Until class is full
Applicant's Response to Acceptance
Offer – Maximum Time: Two weeks

Requests for Deferred
Entrance Considered: Yes

Deposit to Hold Place in Class: No
Deposit (Resident): n/a
Deposit (Non-resident): n/a
Deposit due: n/a
Applied to tuition: n/a
Deposit refundable: n/a
Refundable by: n/a

Estimated number of new entrants: 110
EDP: 2, special program: 10

Start Month/Year: August 2010

Interview Format: Individual interview
with faculty member. Regional interviews
are not available.

Other Programs

PREPARATORY PROGRAMS
Postbaccalaureate Program: No
Summer Program: Yes, https://medschool.mc.
vanderbilt.edu/summer_academy/

COMBINED DEGREE PROGRAMS
Baccalaureate/M.D.: No
M.D./M.P.H.: Yes, Wayne A. Ray, M.D.,
(615) 322-2017, wayne.ray@vanderbilt.edu
M.D./M.B.A.: Yes, Nancy L. Hyer,
(615) 322-2530, nancy.l.hyer.2@vanderbilt.edu
M.D./J.D.: Yes, Nancy J. King,
(615) 343-9836, nancy.king@vanderbilt.edu
M.D./Ph.D.: Yes, Michelle S. Grundy, Ph.D.,
(615) 343-2573, michelle.grundy@vanderbilt.edu
Additional Program: Yes, MD/MDiv.,
Rev. Angela D. Davis, (615) 343-3963,
angela.d.davis@vanderbilt.edu

Premedical Coursework

Course	Req.	Rec.	Lab.	Qtrs.
Inorganic Chemistry	•		•	8
Behavioral Sciences				
Biochemistry		•		
Biology				
Biology/Zoology	•		•	8
Calculus				
College English	•			6
College Mathematics				

Course	Req.	Rec.	Lab.	Qtrs.
Computer Science				
Genetics				
Humanities				
Organic Chemistry	•		•	8
Physics	•		•	8
Psychology				
Social Sciences				
Other				

Selection Factors: 2008 Accepted Applicants

Proportion of Accepted Applicants with Relevant Experience (Data Self-Reported to AMCAS*)	
Community Service/Volunteer	77%
Medically-Related Work	89%
Research	95%

Shaded bar represents school's accepted scores ranging from the 10th percentile to the 90th percentile   School Median ●   National Median ●

Overall GPA 2.0 2.1 2.2 2.3 2.4 2.5 2.6 2.7 2.8 2.9 3.0 3.1 3.2 3.3 3.4 3.5 3.6 3.7 (3.8) 3.9 4.0

Science GPA 2.0 2.1 2.2 2.3 2.4 2.5 2.6 2.7 2.8 2.9 3.0 3.1 3.2 3.3 3.4 3.5 3.6 3.7 (3.9) 4.0

MCAT® Total Numeric Score 9 10 11 12 13 14 15 16 17 18 19 20 21 22 23 24 25 26 27 28 29 30 31 (32) 33 34 (35) 36 37 38 39 40 41 42 43

Writing Sample		J	K	L	M	N	O	P	(Q)	R	S	T
Verbal Reasoning	3	4	5	6	7	8	9	(10)	(11)	12	13	14	15
Biological Sciences	3	4	5	6	7	8	9	10	(11)	(12)	13	14	15
Physical Sciences	3	4	5	6	7	8	9	10	(11)	(12)	13	14	15

Acceptance & Matriculation Data for 2008–2009 First Year Class

	Resident	Non-resident	International	Total
Applications	345	4390	297	5032
Interviewed	50	815	42	907
Deferred	0	3	0	3
Matriculants				
Early Assurance Program	3	6	0	9
Early Decision Program	0	0	0	0
Baccalaureate/M.D.	n/a	n/a	n/a	n/a
M.D./Ph.D.	0	9	1	10
Matriculated	14	84	7	**105**

Applications accepted from International Applicants: Yes

Specialty Choice

2004, 2005, 2006 Graduates, Specialty Choice (As reported by program directors to GME Track™)	
Anesthesiology	3%
Emergency Medicine	6%
Family Practice	0%
Internal Medicine	20%
Obstetrics/Gynecology	3%
Orthopaedic Surgery	5%
Pediatrics	11%
Psychiatry	6%
Radiology	7%
Surgery	9%

Matriculant Demographics: 2008–2009 First Year Class

Men: 54   **Women:** 51

Matriculants' Self-Reported Race/Ethnicity

Mexican American	3	Korean	1
Cuban	1	Vietnamese	0
Puerto Rican	1	Other Asian	3
Other Hispanic	2	Total Asian	16
Total Hispanic	6	Native American	1
Chinese	3	Black	12
Asian Indian	10	Native Hawaiian	1
Pakistani	0	White	70
Filipino	0	Unduplicated Number	
Japanese	0	of Matriculants	105

Science and Math Majors: 64%
Matriculants with:
     Baccalaureate degree: 100%
     Graduate degree(s): 6%

Financial Information

Source: 2007–2008 LCME I-B survey
and 2008–2009 AAMC TSF questionnaire

	Residents	Non-residents
Total Cost of Attendance	$58,920	$58,920
Tuition and Fees	$39,291	$39,291
Other (includes living expenses)	$17,671	$17,671
Health Insurance (can be waived)	$1,958	$1,958

Average 2008 Graduate Indebtedness: $119,637
% of Enrolled Students Receiving Aid: 86%

Criminal Background Check

This medical school requires a criminal background
check prior to matriculation.

Baylor College of Medicine
Houston, Texas

Office of Admissions
Baylor College of Medicine
One Baylor Plaza, MS BCM 110
Houston, Texas 77030
T 713 798 4842   **F** 713 798 5563

Admissions www.bcm.edu/admissions
Main www.bcm.edu
Financial www.bcm.edu/osa/osa-financial.html
E-mail admissions@bcm.edu

Private Institution

Dr. William T. Butler, Interim President

Dr. Florence Eddins-Folensbee, Associate Dean, Admissions

Dr. Stephen B. Greenberg, Senior Vice President and Dean of Education

Graciela B. Villarreal, Associate Dean

General Information

Baylor College of Medicine (BCM) is a private, nonsectarian institution governed by an independent Board of Trustees composed of community leaders. BCM is the academic center around which the 1000-acre Texas Medical Center was developed. The Baylor faculty currently is composed of 1,832 full-time members and 1,414 voluntary members. Facilities include teaching and research buildings and seven affiliated teaching hospitals (including private, county, and Veterans Affairs hospitals).

Mission Statement

The mission of BCM is to promote health for all people through education, research, and public service. The college pursues this mission by sustaining excellence in educating medical and graduate students, primary care and specialty physicians, biomedical scientists and allied health professionals; by advancing basic and clinical biomedical research; by fostering public awareness of health and the prevention of disease; and by promoting patient care of the highest standard.

Curricular Highlights

Community Service Requirement: Required.
Research/Thesis Requirement: Required.

The educational program is structured to prepare graduates to pursue careers as primary care physicians, specialists, research scientists, academic physicians, or physicians involved in public health policy. The integration of basic and clinical sciences includes direct patient-care experiences early in the first year and a focus on core basic science topics prior to graduation. This integration also includes special courses featuring integrated problem-solving and clinical skills training that encourages application of content learned in lectures and labs. The BCM curriculum is unique in that the basic sciences are taught in slightly less than one and a half years, giving students more time to take advantage of a wealth of clinical experiences. During the clinical curriculum, students have flexibility in organizing their schedules to complete 56 weeks of required clinical clerkships, four weeks of selectives, and 20 weeks of elective experiences. All students will be expected to develop and execute with faculty mentorship a scholarly project of their choice during their medical education. Interested students are given the opportunity to do research or to apply for a combined M.D./Ph.D. program. Students with an interest in ethics, research, international health, or geriatrics may participate in tracks designed for the specific topic. There are several joint degree programs: a 5-year M.D./M.B.A. program with a health care focus with the Jones School of Management at Rice University; a six-year M.D./J.D. program with the University of Houston Law Center and a 5-year M.D./M.P.H. with the University of Texas School of Public Health.

USMLE

Step 1: Required. Students must only record a score.
Step 2: Clinical Skills (CS): Required. Students must only record a score.
Step 2: Clinical Knowledge (CK): Required. Students must only record a score.

Selection Factors

All applicants offered places in the class are interviewed at BCM. All available information is utilized in the selection process. Attention is paid to course selections and the academic challenge imposed by the student's curriculum. Intellectual ability and academic achievement alone are not sufficient to support the development of the ideal physician. To work effectively in a profession dependent upon interpersonal relationships, physicians should possess those traits of personality and character which permit them to communicate effectively with warmth and compassion. Written requests for deferred matriculation from accepted students will be reviewed on an individual basis. BCM does not discriminate on the basis of race, sex, marital status, creed, national origin, age, or disability.

Financial Aid

Financial need is not a factor in the selection of students. Aid funds are provided by private donors, the Board of Trustees, and various state and federal loan, scholarship, and work-study programs. Financial aid information and application materials are sent to all accepted applicants, and a financial aid officer is available for consultation with students and parents.

Information about Diversity Programs

BCM encourages applications from members of groups underrepresented in medicine. Students from these groups comprise a substantial portion of the student body; they also serve as Admissions Committee members. For additional information, contact Dr. Graciela Villarreal, Associate Dean for Admissions, at 713-798-4842, or Dr. James L. Phillips, Senior Associate Dean.

Campus Information

Setting

BCM is located at the center of the Texas Medical Center, next door to Hermann Park, the zoo, and a public golf course. To the west are Rice University and the Village Shopping Center. The Museum District is to the north and offers more than 16 art organizations.

Enrollment

For 2008, total enrollment was: 664

Housing

There are many homes, apartments, townhouses, and condominiums for lease or purchase near the Texas Medical Center. Many of these living options are close to a light rail system that provides access to TMC at little or no cost to BCM students.

Application Process and Requirements 2010–2011

Primary Application Service: AMCAS
Earliest filing date: June 1, 2009
Latest filing date: November 1, 2009

Secondary Application Required?: Yes
Sent to: All applicants
URL: www.bcm.edu/admissions/?PMID=1776
Fee: Yes, $80
Fee waiver available: Yes
Earliest filing date: July 1, 2009
Latest filing date: December 1, 2009

MCAT® required?: Yes
Latest MCAT® considered: September 2009
Oldest MCAT® considered: 2005

Early Decision Program: School does have EDP
Applicants notified: October 1, 2009
EDP available for: Both Residents and Non-residents

Regular Acceptance Notice
Earliest date: October 15, 2009
Latest date: Until class is full
Applicant's Response to Acceptance Offer – Maximum Time: n/a

Requests for Deferred Entrance Considered: Yes

Deposit to Hold Place in Class: Yes
Deposit (Resident): $300
Deposit (Non-resident): $300
Deposit due: May 15, 2010
Applied to tuition: Yes
Deposit refundable: Yes
Refundable by: April 15, 2010

Estimated number of new entrants: 184
EDP: 5, special program: 40

Start Month/Year: July 2010

Interview Format: Two 30-minute one-on-one interviews. Regional interviews are not available.

Other Programs

PREPARATORY PROGRAMS
Postbaccalaureate Program: No
Summer Program: No
Additional Programs: Yes, www.bcm.edu/smart www.debakeydepartmentofsurgery.org/home/content.cfm?menu_id=17

Combined Degree Programs
Baccalaureate/M.D.: Yes, www.bcm.edu/medschool/baccmd.htm
M.D./M.P.H.: Yes, www.bcm.edu/education/dual_programs.cfm#md_mph, admissions@bcm.tmc.edu
M.D./M.B.A.: Yes, admissions@bcm.tmc.edu, www.bcm.edu/education/dual_programs.cfm#MD_MBA
M.D./J.D.: Yes, admissions@bcm.tmc.edu
M.D./Ph.D.: Yes, www.bcm.edu/mstp

Premedical Coursework

Course	Req.	Rec.	Lab.	Sems.	Course	Req.	Rec.	Lab.	Sems.
Inorganic Chemistry	•		•	2	Computer Science				
Behavioral Sciences					Genetics				
Biochemistry					Humanities				
Biology	•		•	2	Organic Chemistry	•		•	2
Biology/Zoology					Physics				
Calculus					Psychology				
College English	•			2	Social Sciences				
College Mathematics					Other				

Selection Factors: 2008 Accepted Applicants

Proportion of Accepted Applicants with Relevant Experience (Data Self-Reported to AMCAS)	Community Service/Volunteer	73%
	Medically-Related Work	82%
	Research	88%

Shaded bar represents school's accepted scores ranging from the 10th percentile to the 90th percentile   School Median ●   National Median ●

Overall GPA	2.0	2.1	2.2	2.3	2.4	2.5	2.6	2.7	2.8	2.9	3.0	3.1	3.2	3.3	3.4	3.5	3.6	3.7	3.8	3.9	4.0
Science GPA	2.0	2.1	2.2	2.3	2.4	2.5	2.6	2.7	2.8	2.9	3.0	3.1	3.2	3.3	3.4	3.5	3.6	3.7	3.8	3.9	4.0

MCAT® Total Numeric Score 9 10 11 12 13 14 15 16 17 18 19 20 21 22 23 24 25 26 27 28 29 30 31 **32** 33 34 35 **36** 37 38 39 40 41 42 43

Writing Sample			J	K	L	M	N	O	P	**Q**	R	S	T
Verbal Reasoning	3	4	5	6	7	8	9	**10**	**11**	12	13	14	15
Biological Sciences	3	4	5	6	7	8	9	10	**11**	**12**	13	14	15
Physical Sciences	3	4	5	6	7	8	9	**10**	**11**	12	**13**	14	15

Acceptance & Matriculation Data for 2008–2009 First Year Class

	Resident	Non-resident	International	Total
Applications	1446	3218	215	4879
Interviewed	394	357	0	751
Deferred	6	3	0	9
Matriculants				
Early Assurance Program	n/a	n/a	n/a	n/a
Early Decision Program	4	0	0	4
Baccalaureate/M.D.	38	4	1	43
M.D./Ph.D.	9	2	1	12
Matriculated	140	36	0	**176**

Applications accepted from International Applicants: Yes

Specialty Choice

2004, 2005, 2006 Graduates, Specialty Choice (As reported by program directors to GME Track™)	
Anesthesiology	8%
Emergency Medicine	2%
Family Practice	3%
Internal Medicine	19%
Obstetrics/Gynecology	4%
Orthopaedic Surgery	4%
Pediatrics	15%
Psychiatry	4%
Radiology	6%
Surgery	6%

Matriculant Demographics: 2008–2009 First Year Class

Men: 90   **Women:** 86

Matriculants' Self-Reported Race/Ethnicity

Mexican American	15	Korean	1
Cuban	3	Vietnamese	2
Puerto Rican	1	Other Asian	6
Other Hispanic	5	Total Asian	74
Total Hispanic	23	Native American	6
Chinese	24	Black	9
Asian Indian	36	Native Hawaiian	1
Pakistani	3	White	86
Filipino	2	Unduplicated Number	
Japanese	2	of Matriculants	176

Science and Math Majors: 73%
Matriculants with:
Baccalaureate degree: 99%
Graduate degree(s): 5%

Financial Information

Source: 2007–2008 LCME I-B survey and 2008–2009 AAMC TSF questionnaire

	Residents	Non-residents
Total Cost of Attendance	$39,443	$52,543
Tuition and Fees	$12,803	$25,903
Other (includes living expenses)	$24,165	$24,165
Health Insurance (can be waived)	$2,475	$2,475

Average 2008 Graduate Indebtedness: $73,803
% of Enrolled Students Receiving Aid: 79%

Criminal Background Check

This medical school requires a criminal background check prior to matriculation.

Texas A&M University System Health Science Center College of Medicine

College Station, Texas

Office of Student Affairs and Admissions
The Texas A&M Health Science Center
College of Medicine, 159 Joe Reynolds Medical Bldg.
College Station, Texas 77843-1114
T 979 845 7743   F 979 845 5533

Admissions http://medicine.tamhsc.edu/
admissions/index.htm
Main http://medicine.tamhsc.edu/
Financial http://tamhsc.edu/academics/finaid
E-mail admissions@medicine.tamhsc.edu

Public Institution

Dr. Christopher C. Colenda, Dean

*Filomeno G. Maldonado,
Associate Dean for Admissions*

*Wanda J. Watson, Director of Recruitment
and Special Programs*

*Harold Whitis, Executive Director of
Student Financial Aid*

*Dr. Kathleen F. Fallon, Associate Dean
for Student Affairs and Admissions*

Leila E. Diaz, Director of Admissions

General Information

Established in 1973, the College of Medicine is part of The Texas A&M Health Science Center, a public health sciences university. The College is affiliated with Scott & White Hospital and Clinic and the Olin E. Teague Veterans Center of the Central Texas Health Care System in Temple Texas. Combined, these clinical facilities provide 1,976 teaching beds and treat approximately 2,389,000 outpatients and another 45,500 inpatients each year.

Mission Statement

The College of Medicine is dedicated to the education of humane and highly skilled physicians and to the development of knowledge in the biomedical and clinical sciences. In order to improve the quality and efficacy of medical care through its programs of medical education and research, the College of Medicine maintains a personalized educational experience for medical students. The College's overarching goals are building signature research and clinical programs and reaffirming its land grant heritage of community outreach and service.

Curricular Highlights

Community Service Requirement: Optional.
Research/Thesis Requirement: Optional.

The goal of the curriculum is to produce undifferentiated physicians of the highest caliber. Years 1 and 2 taught at both the College Station and Temple campuses include an organ systems curriculum, which integrates the traditional basic sciences along with instruction in

behavioral science, working with patients, physical diagnosis, humanities in medicine, community medicine, leadership in medicine, evidence-based medicine, and epidemiology. Correlation of the basic sciences with clinical medicine is achieved from the start, with clinical instruction in both years 1 and 2. Years 3 and 4 consist of traditional clerkships and a mixed rotation of ambulatory care experiences.

USMLE

Step 1: Required. Students must record a passing score for graduation, but not promotion.
Step 2: Clinical Skills (CS): Required. Students must record a passing total score to graduate.
Step 2: Clinical Knowledge (CK): Required. Students must record a passing total score to graduate.

Selection Factors

Academic ability, grades in college courses, and performance on the MCAT are important selection criteria. Equally important are interpersonal and communication skills, maturity, motivation, and compassion. Careful consideration is given to other factors such as dedication to service, disadvantaged circumstances, socioeconomic background, race/ethnicity, faculty support, primary care interest, and/or service in a rural/underserved area. Knowledge of and experiences in the medical profession are important. Admission is open to qualified individuals regardless of race, color, religion, gender, age, national origin, or disability. Applicants are invited for personal interviews based upon their competeness in the review process.

Financial Aid

Scholarship and loan funds are available to students with financial need from local, state, and national sources. Financial needs of the applicant are not a consideration in the admission process.

Information about Diversity Programs

The college believes that diversity enhances its ability to provide care and to serve communities across a broad range of racial and ethnic groups. As part of its commitment to this effort, the college administers several programs for students who are disadvantaged or from groups underrepresented in medicine. The

Joint Admissions Medical Program is open to economically disadvantaged students, and the Partnership for Primary Care Program is open to students from rural/underserved communities in Texas. Also, the adjustment and retention of minority students is facilitated through the college's chapter of the Student National Medical Association (SNMA).

Campus Information

Setting
The college is located on the west campus of Texas A&M University in College Station, Texas. College Station and Bryan, its neighboring city to the north, are home to 124,493 people. College Station-Bryan is located in East-Central Texas between the Brazos and Navasota Rivers and 100 miles northwest of Houston.

Enrollment
For 2008, total enrollment was: 413

Special Features
The College of Medicine's primary clinical partner, Scott & White Hospital and Clinic, is one of the largest integrated multi-specialty health care systems in the U.S. and ranked for the fourth straight year among the 100 Top Hospitals in the country and the 15 Top Teaching Hospitals in the country.

Housing
Although on-campus housing is not available, the Coordinator of Student Services provides access to apartment listings and roommate search options. Rents for unfurnished apartments range from $290 to $1,200 per month.

Satellite Campuses/Facilities
Traditional clerkships and ambulatory care experiences are conducted predominantly at Scott & White and the Teague Veterans Center. The college is also affiliated with four other hospitals and clinics in College Station, Round Rock, Corpus Christi, Houston, Fort Worth, Waco, Austin, and Fort Hood, Texas.

Application Process and Requirements 2010–2011

Primary Application Service: TMDSAS
Earliest filing date: May 1, 2009
Latest filing date: October 1, 2009

Secondary Application Required?: Yes
Sent to: All applicants
URL: http://medicine.tamhsc.edu/admissions/index.htm
Fee: Yes, $50
Fee waiver available: Yes
Earliest filing date: May 1, 2009
Latest filing date: October 1, 2009

MCAT® required?: Yes
Latest MCAT® considered: September 2009
Oldest MCAT® considered: August 2005

Early Decision Program: School does not have EDP
Applicants notified: n/a
EDP available for: n/a

Regular Acceptance Notice
Earliest date: November 15, 2009 for Texas residents; October 15, 2009 for non-residents
Latest date: Until class is full
Applicant's Response to Acceptance Offer – Maximum Time: Two weeks

Requests for Deferred Entrance Considered: Yes

Deposit to Hold Place in Class: No
Deposit (Resident): n/a
Deposit (Non-resident): n/a
Deposit due: n/a
Applied to tuition: n/a
Deposit refundable: n/a
Refundable by: n/a

Estimated number of new entrants: 170
EDP: n/a, special program: n/a

Start Month/Year: July 2010

Interview Format: Two individual 30-minute interviews. Regional interviews are not available.

Other Programs

PREPARATORY PROGRAMS
Postbaccalaureate Program: No
Summer Program: Yes, www.utsystem.edu/jamp/
Partnership for Primary Care: Yes, http://medicine.tamhsc.edu/admissions/ppc/index.html
Summer Research Program: Yes, http://medicine.tamhsc.edu/research/student/index.html

COMBINED DEGREE PROGRAMS
Baccalaureate/M.D.: No
M.D./M.P.H.: No
M.D./M.B.A.: Yes, http://medicine.tamhsc.edu/admissions/dualdegree.htm
Dr. Gary McCord, (979) 845-7743 or (254) 724-0242, McCord@medicine.tamhsc.edu
M.D./J.D.: No
M.D./Ph.D.: Yes, http://medicine.tamhsc.edu/admissions/dualdegree.htm
Dr. Julian Leibowitz, (979) 845-7288, leibowit@medicine.tamhsc.edu

Premedical Coursework

Course	Req.	Rec.	Lab.	Hrs.
Inorganic Chemistry	•		•	8
Behavioral Sciences				
Biochemistry		•		3
Biology	•		•	14
Biology/Zoology				
Calculus	•			3
College English	•			6
College Mathematics				

Course	Req.	Rec.	Lab.	Hrs.
Computer Science				
Genetics				
Humanities				
Organic Chemistry	•		•	8
Physics	•		•	8
Psychology				
Social Sciences				
Math-based Statistics	•			3

Selection Factors: 2008 Accepted Applicants

Proportion of Accepted Applicants with Relevant Experience (Data Self-Reported to AMCAS*)		
Community Service/Volunteer		92%
Medically-Related Work		95%
Research		63%

Shaded bar represents school's accepted scores ranging from the 10th percentile to the 90th percentile. **School Median** ● **National Median** ●

Overall GPA	2.0	2.1	2.2	2.3	2.4	2.5	2.6	2.7	2.8	2.9	3.0	3.1	3.2	3.3	3.4	3.5	3.6	3.7	(3.8)	3.9	4.0
Science GPA	2.0	2.1	2.2	2.3	2.4	2.5	2.6	2.7	2.8	2.9	3.0	3.1	3.2	3.3	3.4	3.5	3.6	3.7	(3.8)	3.9	4.0

MCAT® Total Numeric Score 9 10 11 12 13 14 15 16 17 18 19 20 21 22 23 24 25 26 27 28 29 30 (31) 32 33 34 35 36 37 38 39 40 41 42 43

Writing Sample			J	K	L	M	N	O	(P)	(Q)	R	S	T
Verbal Reasoning	3	4	5	6	7	8	9	(10)	11	12	13	14	15
Biological Sciences	3	4	5	6	7	8	9	10	(11)	12	13	14	15
Physical Sciences	3	4	5	6	7	8	9	(10)	(11)	12	13	14	15

Acceptance & Matriculation Data for 2008–2009 First Year Class

	Resident	Non-resident	International	Total
Applications	2605	420	63	3088
Interviewed	708	41	2	751
Deferred	1	0	0	1
Matriculants				
Early Assurance Program	16	0	0	16
Early Decision Program	0	0	0	0
Baccalaureate/M.D.	n/a	n/a	n/a	n/a
M.D./Ph.D.	1	3	0	4
Matriculated	125	10	4	**139**

Applications accepted from International Applicants: Yes

Specialty Choice

2004, 2005, 2006 Graduates, Specialty Choice (As reported by program directors to GME Track™)	
Anesthesiology	8%
Emergency Medicine	5%
Family Practice	13%
Internal Medicine	14%
Obstetrics/Gynecology	10%
Orthopaedic Surgery	3%
Pediatrics	12%
Psychiatry	5%
Radiology	5%
Surgery	10%

Matriculant Demographics: 2008–2009 First Year Class

Men: 81   **Women:** 58

Matriculants' Self-Reported Race/Ethnicity

Mexican American	12	**Korean**	2
Cuban	0	**Vietnamese**	4
Puerto Rican	1	**Other Asian**	5
Other Hispanic	3	**Total Asian**	45
Total Hispanic	16	**Native American**	0
Chinese	10	**Black**	8
Asian Indian	20	**Native Hawaiian**	0
Pakistani	3	**White**	80
Filipino	0	**Unduplicated Number**	
Japanese	2	**of Matriculants**	139

Science and Math Majors: 44%
Matriculants with:
    Baccalaureate degree: 63%
    Graduate degree(s): 10%

Financial Information

Source: 2007–2008 LCME I-B survey and 2008–2009 AAMC TSF questionnaire

	Residents	Non-residents
Total Cost of Attendance	$34,936	$48,036
Tuition and Fees	$11,231	$24,331
Other (includes living expenses)	$23,705	$23,705
Health Insurance (can be waived)	$0	$0

Average 2008 Graduate Indebtedness: $103,826
% of Enrolled Students Receiving Aid: 90%

Criminal Background Check

This medical school requires a criminal background check prior to matriculation.

Texas Tech University Health Sciences Center School of Medicine

Lubbock, Texas

Texas Tech University Health Sciences Center
School of Medicine
Office of Admissions, Room 2B116
3601 4th Street
Lubbock, Texas 79430
T 806 743 2297   **F** 806 743 2725

Admissions www.ttuhsc.edu/som/admissions
Main www.ttuhsc.edu
Financial www.ttuhsc.edu/FinancialAid/
E-mail somadm@ttuhsc.edu

Public Institution

Dr. Steven L. Berk, Dean

Dr. Bernell K. Dalley, Associate Dean, Admissions and Minority Affairs

Dr. German Nunez, Vice President for Diversity and Multicultural Affairs

E. Marcus Wilson, Director, Financial Aid

Linda Prado, Director, Office of Admissions

Dr. Kimberly Peck, Interim Assistant Dean, Admissions

General Information

The TTUHSC School of Medicine was established in 1969. All medical students spend the first two years at the Lubbock campus; third and fourth year students receive their clinical training in Lubbock, Amarillo, or Midland/Odessa (Permian Basin). Affiliations with teaching hospitals provide over 2,900 beds for clinical teaching. The medical school has 553 full-time and 48 part-time faculty members and more than 902 volunteer clinical faculty members. Agreements have been developed with four area universities to provide early acceptance of qualified students into TTUHSC School of Medicine. Applicants must be academically talented. Following satisfactory interview, the Admissions Committee recommends acceptance of the applicant. Applicants who continue to maintain the required GPA are guaranteed admission to Texas Tech School of Medicine in the fall following graduation. The MCAT is waived for these applicants.

Mission Statement

TTUHSC School of Medicine provides the highest standard of excellence in higher education, while pursuing continuous quality improvement. The school is committed to health care delivery for its 135,000 square mile service area. At the same time and as part of improvement of health care, its efforts include support of meaningful academic research for the betterment of future health care.

Curricular Highlights

Community Service Requirement: Optional.
Research/Thesis Requirement: Optional.

The new four-year curriculum provides a broad innovative integration of basic and clinical care, with emphasis on developing the student's analytical problem-solving skills. The first two years blend core concepts of basic sciences with early clinical experience. Introduction to patience care skills begins in the first month. The second year now follows an overall systems approach, again aligned with supervised patient care experiences. Teaching formats include small group discussions, PBL, and team learning. Summer preceptorships are also available. The third and fourth years include clerkships in family medicine, internal medicine, neurology, obstetric-gynecology, pediatrics, psychiatry, and surgery. The fourth year combines required and elective rotations. Research opportunities include summer preceptorships, a Research Honors Program, and an integrated M.D.–Ph.D. program. Joint degree programs in the M.B.A./M.D. and J.D./M.D. are also offered. Students are graded using a categorical grading system: Honors, High Pass, Pass, Marginal Pass and Fail.

USMLE

Step 1: Required. Students must record a passing score for promotion.
Step 2: Clinical Skills (CS): Required. Students must only record a score.
Step 2: Clinical Knowledge (CK): Required. Students must only record a score.

Selection Factors

Applications are invited from qualified Texas residents and service area counties of New Mexico and Oklahoma. Only U.S. citizens or applicants with permanent resident visas are considered. Application forms and procedural information may be obtained from the Texas Medical and Dental Schools Application Service (*www.utsystem.edu/tmdsas*). A secondary application to TTUHSC School of Medicine is also required. The Admissions Committee carefully reviews all applications. Evidence of high intellectual ability and a record of strong academic achievement are essential for success in the study of medicine. Qualities such as compassion, motivation, the ability to communicate with people, maturity, and personal integrity are also important. There is no discrimination on the basis of race, sex, creed,

national origin, age, or disability. It is the goal of the institution to recruit a diverse medical class exhibiting the qualities promising academic success and to meet the needs of an increasingly diverse population. Personal interviews are offered to those candidates deemed competitive for admission. Interviews are conducted on the Lubbock campus.

Financial Aid

After an applicant has been accepted, financial aid assistance can be obtained from the Office of Student Financial Aid. Employment, other than during the summer, is discouraged.

Information about Diversity Programs

In an effort to recruit a highly qualified and diverse student body, which reflects the demographics of the West Texas region, race/ethnicity as well as a socioeconomically disadvantaged background, is among the many factors considered in the admission process.

Campus Information

Setting

The medical school is situated at the north edge of the city of Lubbock. It is adjacent to Texas Tech University, which makes it one of the few medical schools in the country to be on or adjacent to a major undergraduate campus and law school. The Lubbock campus is across the street from a number of apartment complexes and is within easy driving distance of shopping, recreational and cultural areas.

Enrollment

For 2008, total enrollment was: 568

Satellite Campuses/Facilities

All students spend the first two years of medical school on the Lubbock campus. The in-depth clinical training for medical students is divided among three campuses: to Lubbock, Amarillo, or Midland/Odessa (Permian Basin).

Application Process and Requirements 2010–2011

Primary Application Service: TMDSAS
Earliest filing date: May 1, 2009
Latest filing date: October 1, 2009

Secondary Application Required?: Yes
Sent to: Required of all applicants
URL: www.ttuhsc.edu/som/admissions
Fee: Yes, $50
Fee waiver available: No
Earliest filing date: May 1, 2009
Latest filing date: October 1, 2009

MCAT® required?: Yes
Latest MCAT® considered: September 2009
Oldest MCAT® considered: 2005

Early Decision Program: School does have EDP
Applicants notified: October 1, 2009
EDP available for: Residents only

Regular Acceptance Notice
Earliest date: November 15, 2009
Latest date: Until class is full
Applicant's Response to Acceptance
Offer – Maximum Time: Two weeks

Requests for Deferred
Entrance Considered: Yes

Deposit to Hold Place in Class: Yes
Deposit (Resident): $100
Deposit (Non-resident): $100
Deposit due: May 15, 2010
Applied to tuition: No
Deposit refundable: Yes
Refundable by: May 15, 2010

Estimated number of new entrants: 140
EDP: 3, special program: n/a

Start Month/Year: August 2010

Interview Format: Two individual thirty-minute interviews. Regional interviews are not available.

Other Programs

PREPARATORY PROGRAMS
Postbaccalaureate Program: No
Summer Program: Yes
www.ttuhsc.edu/som/admissions
**Joint Admission to Medicine Program
(JAMP):** www.utsystem.edu/jamp

COMBINED DEGREE PROGRAMS
Baccalaureate/M.D.: No
M.D./M.P.H.: No
M.D./M.B.A.: Yes,
www.ttuhsc.edu/som/admissions
M.D./J.D.: Yes, www.ttuhsc.edu/som/admissions,
www.law.ttu.edu/prospective
M.D./Ph.D.: Yes,
www.ttuhsc.edu/som/admissions

Premedical Coursework

Course	Req.	Rec.	Lab.	Qtrs.
Inorganic Chemistry	•		•	8
Behavioral Sciences				
Biochemistry				
Biology				
Biology/Zoology	•		•	14
Calculus	•			3
College English	•			6
College Mathematics				

Course	Req.	Rec.	Lab.	Qtrs.
Computer Science				
Genetics				
Humanities				
Organic Chemistry	•		•	8
Physics	•		•	8
Psychology				
Social Sciences				
Statistics	•			3

Selection Factors: 2008 Accepted Applicants

Proportion of Accepted Applicants with Relevant Experience (Data Self-Reported to AMCAS®)		
Community Service/Volunteer		90%
Medically-Related Work		97%
Research		64%

Shaded bar represents school's accepted scores ranging from the 10th percentile to the 90th percentile   School Median ●   National Median ●

Overall GPA	2.0	2.1	2.2	2.3	2.4	2.5	2.6	2.7	2.8	2.9	3.0	3.1	3.2	3.3	3.4	3.5	3.6	3.7	(3.8)	3.9	4.0
Science GPA	2.0	2.1	2.2	2.3	2.4	2.5	2.6	2.7	2.8	2.9	3.0	3.1	3.2	3.3	3.4	3.5	3.6	(3.7)	3.8	3.9	4.0

MCAT® Total Numeric Score 9 10 11 12 13 14 15 16 17 18 19 20 21 22 23 24 25 26 27 28 29 (30) 31 (32) 33 34 35 36 37 38 39 40 41 42 43

Writing Sample			J	K	L	M	N	O	(P)	(Q)	R	S	T
Verbal Reasoning	3	4	5	6	7	8	9	(10)	11	12	13	14	15
Biological Sciences	3	4	5	6	7	8	9	10	(11)	12	13	14	15
Physical Sciences	3	4	5	6	7	8	9	(10)	(11)	12	13	14	15

Acceptance & Matriculation Data for 2008–2009 First Year Class

	Resident	Non-resident	International	Total
Applications	2559	359	48	2966
Interviewed	727	34	0	761
Deferred	8	0	0	8
Matriculants				
Early Assurance Program	3	0	0	3
Early Decision Program	0	0	0	0
Baccalaureate/M.D.	n/a	n/a	n/a	n/a
M.D./Ph.D.	2	0	0	2
Matriculated	133	5	2	**140**

Applications accepted from International Applicants: No

Matriculant Demographics: 2008–2009 First Year Class

Men: 84   **Women:** 56

Matriculants' Self-Reported Race/Ethnicity

Mexican American	6	**Korean**	3
Cuban	1	**Vietnamese**	3
Puerto Rican	0	**Other Asian**	17
Other Hispanic	3	**Total Asian**	39
Total Hispanic	10	**Native American**	2
Chinese	3	**Black**	2
Asian Indian	12	**Native Hawaiian**	0
Pakistani	1	**White**	90
Filipino	1	**Unduplicated Number**	
Japanese	0	**of Matriculants**	140

Science and Math Majors: 36%
Matriculants with:
   Baccalaureate degree: 100%
   Graduate degree(s): 1%

Specialty Choice

2004, 2005, 2006 Graduates, Specialty Choice (As reported by program directors to GME Track™)	
Anesthesiology	8%
Emergency Medicine	5%
Family Practice	12%
Internal Medicine	14%
Obstetrics/Gynecology	8%
Orthopaedic Surgery	5%
Pediatrics	12%
Psychiatry	4%
Radiology	5%
Surgery	8%

Financial Information

Source: 2007–2008 LCME I-B survey and 2008–2009 AAMC TSF questionnaire

	Residents	Non-residents
Total Cost of Attendance	$34,772	$47,872
Tuition and Fees	$12,736	$25,836
Other (includes living expenses)	$21,136	$21,136
Health Insurance (not applicable)	$900	$900

Average 2008 Graduate Indebtedness: $137,374
% of Enrolled Students Receiving Aid: 91%

Criminal Background Check

This medical school requires a criminal background check prior to matriculation.

Paul L. Foster School of Medicine at Texas Tech University Health Sciences Center at El Paso

El Paso, Texas

Paul L. Foster School of Medicine at Texas Tech
University Health Sciences Center at El Paso
5001 El Paso Drive
El Paso, Texas 79905
T 915 783 1250   **F** 915 783 1265

Admissions www.ttuhsc.edu/fostersom/admissions/
Main www.ttuhsc.edu/fostersom/
Financial www.ttuhsc.edu/financialaid/
E-mail fostersom.admissions@ttuhsc.edu

Public Institution

Dr. Jose Manuel de la Rosa, Dean

Dr. Manuel Schydlower, Associate Dean for Admissions

Dr. German R. Nunez, Vice President for Diversity and Multicultural Affairs

E. Marcus Wilson, Director, Financial Aid

John Snelling, Director of Admissions

Lorraine James, M.B.A., Assistant Director of Admissions

General Information

In 1999, then Texas Tech System Chancellor John T. Montford shared with the Board of Regents a vision for a full four-year medical school in El Paso by expanding the existing third and fourth-year clinical program. The addition of the first two years of the medical school would allow students from El Paso and nearby regions to complete their education near home and help retain doctors in the area. On December 9, 2003, the ground breaking for El Paso Medical Science Building I took place and two years later, on January 31, 2006, a ribbon cutting followed. This $38 million, 93,000 sq.-ft. facility houses research on diabetes, cancer, environmental health and infectious diseases, as well as a repository dedicated to data on Hispanic health and a genomic facility to link hereditary diseases in families. The medical classroom building was completed in November 2007. This $48 million 125,000 sq.-ft. building has four floors and a partial penthouse. Included in the building are classrooms, library, small group rooms, a clinical skills area for students, faculty and administrative areas, basic science labs, gross anatomy lab, a student services area, and food services. The School of Medicine's graduates will have seen diseases that only a small fraction of medical students ever come across in their medical school clinical learning experiences. El Paso students may encounter diseases and other ailments that have virtually been wiped out in the United States, but flourish in many emerging nations. The variety and diversity of patients that our students see allow our future doctors to learn so much more than classic "text book" cases.

Mission Statement

The school's mission is to provide exceptional opportunities for students, trainees, and physicians; to advance knowledge through innovative scholarship and research in medicine with a focus on international health and health care disparities; and to provide exemplary patient care and service to the entire El Paso community and beyond.

Curricular Highlights

Community Service Requirement: Required. As part of Society, Community and the Individual.
Research/Thesis Requirement: Optional.

Among the goals of the Paul L. Foster School of Medicine is the provision of a medical education that is consistent with modern scientific principles, supportive of strong ethical principles, sensitive to the needs of the community, and committed to excellence. The school offers an integrated curriculum that is permeated with clinical presentations assigned to organ-system based courses. Clinical presentations are the ways in which a patient presents to a physician. Students learn anatomy, biochemistry, physiology and other basic science concepts and content needed to understand specific clinical presentations at the time that the presentation is being addressed. This approach enhances knowledge comprehension and has been shown to improve retention of the basic sciences and to promote the acquisition of diagnostic reasoning skills that are more like those of the expert practicing physician. During the clinical science years students participate in a unique and rich variety of clinical patient-care learning experiences that include not only traditional medicine, but also international, bi-national, bicultural, and border health medicine.

USMLE

Step 1: Required. Students must record a passing score for promotion.
Step 2: Clinical Skills (CS): Required. Students must record a passing total score to graduate.
Step 2: Clinical Knowledge (CK): Required. Students must record a passing total score to graduate.

Selection Factors

Candidates who are considered to be competitive for admission, based on criteria established by the school, will be invited to interview. These criteria include scores from the MCAT; academic performance as reflected by the science and overall GPA; rigor of the undergraduate curriculum, extracurricular activities (medical and non-medical) and employment and their impact on performance and maturation; recommendations from premedical advisors or faculty; socioeconomic and disadvantaged background; personal statement and its reflection of communication skills, personal qualities, leadership, maturity, determination, and motivation for a career in medicine; and regional origin. The interview evaluates the applicant's interest and knowledge of the health care field and motivation for a medical career; personal characteristics; and problem solving skills.

Financial Aid

Once accepted, financial aid assistance can be obtained from the Office of Student Financial Aid. Employment is discouraged, except in summer.

Information about Diversity Programs

In an effort to recruit a qualified and diverse student body that reflects the demographics of the West Texas region, ethnicity, as well as socioeconomically disadvantaged background is among the many factors considered in the admissions process.

Campus Information

Setting

The school is located in South Central El Paso just a few hundred yards north of the international border with Mexico.

Enrollment

For 2008, total enrollment was: 108

Housing

No on campus housing. Ample affordable housing available within 20 minute radius.

Application Process and Requirements 2010–2011

Primary Application Service: TMDSAS
Earliest filing date: May 1, 2009
Latest filing date: October 1, 2009

Secondary Application:
URL: n/a
Sent to: n/a
Fee: n/a
Fee Waiver Available: n/a
Earliest filing date: n/a
Latest filing date: n/a

MCAT® required?: Yes
Latest MCAT® considered: September 2009
Oldest MCAT® considered: 2005

Early Decision Program: School does not have EDP
Applicants notified: n/a
EDP available for: n/a

Regular Acceptance Notice
Earliest date: November 15, 2009
Latest date: Until class is full
Applicant's Response to Acceptance Offer – Maximum Time: Two weeks

Requests for deferred entrance considered: Yes

Deposit to Hold Place in Class: Yes,
Deposit (Resident): Yes, $100
Deposit (Non-resident): Yes, $100
Deposit due: May 15, 2010
Applied to tuition: No
Deposit refundable: Yes
Refundable by: May 15, 2010

Estimated number of new entrants: 60
EDP: n/a, special program: n/a

Start month/year: July 2010

Interview format: Two individual 30-minute interviews. Regional interviews are not available.

Other Programs

PREPARATORY PROGRAMS
Postbaccalaureate Program: No
Summer Program: No

COMBINED DEGREE PROGRAMS
Baccalaureate/M.D.: No
M.D./M.P.H.: No
M.D./M.B.A.: No
M.D./J.D.: No
M.D./Ph.D.: No

Premedical Coursework

Course	Req.	Rec.	Lab.	Hrs.	Course	Req.	Rec.	Lab.	Hrs.
Inorganic Chemistry	•		•	8	Computer Science				
Behavioral Sciences		•			Genetics				
Biochemistry		•			Humanities		•		
Biology	•		•	14	Organic Chemistry	•		•	8
Biology/Zoology					Physics	•		•	8
Calculus	•			3	Psychology				
College English	•			6	Social Sciences		•		
College Mathematics									

Selection Factors: 2008 Accepted Applicants

Proportion of Accepted Applicants with Relevant Experience (Data Self-Reported to AMCAS)	**DATA NOT AVAILABLE**

Shaded bar represents school's accepted scores ranging from the 10th percentile to the 90th percentile ▬   School Median ●   National Median ●

Overall GPA	DATA NOT AVAILABLE
Science GPA	

MCAT® Total Numeric Score 9 10 11 12 13 14 15 16 17 18 19 20 21 22 23 24 25 26 27 28 29 30 31 32 33 34 35 36 37 38 39 40 41 42 43

Writing Sample

Verbal Reasoning

Biological Sciences   **DATA NOT AVAILABLE**

Physical Sciences

Acceptance & Matriculation Data for 2008–2009 First Year Class

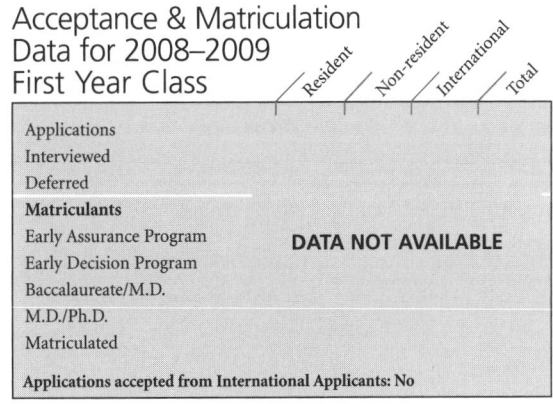

	Resident	Non-resident	International	Total
Applications				
Interviewed				
Deferred				
Matriculants				
Early Assurance Program		DATA NOT AVAILABLE		
Early Decision Program				
Baccalaureate/M.D.				
M.D./Ph.D.				
Matriculated				

Applications accepted from International Applicants: No

Specialty Choice

2004, 2005, 2006 Graduates, Specialty Choice (As reported by program directors to GME Track™)

Anesthesiology
Emergency Medicine
Family Practice

DATA NOT AVAILABLE

Psychiatry
Radiology
Surgery

Matriculant Demographics: 2008–2009 First Year Class

Men: n/a   **Women:** n/a

Matriculants' Self-Reported Race/Ethnicity

Mexican American   Korean
Cuban   Vietnamese
Puerto Rican   Other Asian
Other
Total
Chine   **DATA NOT AVAILABLE**
Asian
Pakis
Filipino   **Unduplicated Number**
Japanese   **of Matriculants**

Science Majors: n/a
Matriculants with:
        Baccalaureate Degree: n/a
        Graduate Degree(s): n/a

Financial Information
Source: 2007–2008 LCME I-B survey
and 2008–2009 AAMC TSF questionnaire

	Residents	Non-residents
Total Cost of Attendance	$33,736	$46,836
Tuition and Fees	$12,736	$25,836
Other (includes living expenses)	$21,000	$21,000
Health Insurance (not applicable)	$0	$0

Average 2008 Graduate Indebtedness: n/a
% of Enrolled Students Receiving Aid: n/a

Criminal Background Check

This medical school requires a criminal background check prior to matriculation.

University of Texas
Medical Branch at Galveston
Galveston, Texas

Office of Student Affairs & Admissions
University of Texas Medical Branch
301 University Boulevard
Galveston, Texas 77555-0807
T 409 772 1442 **F** 409 747 5148

Admissions www.utmb.edu/somstudentaffairs
Main www.som.utmb.edu
Financial www.utmb.edu/enrollmentservices
E-mail tsilva@utmb.edu

Public Institution

Dr. Garland Anderson, IV, Dean and Provost

Dr. Lauree Thomas, Associate Dean for Student Affairs and Admissions

Melvin Williams, Director, Equal Opportunity and Diversity

Vickie Brewer, Director, Enrollment Services and University Financial Aid

Dr. Jeffrey Rabek, Assistant Dean for Student Affairs and Admissions

General Information
The University of Texas Medical Branch (UTMB), established in 1891, is a state-owned academic health center with seven hospitals, 797 teaching beds, and 147 specialty and subspecialty clinics directed by UTMB's administration. It is comprised of four schools (Medicine, Graduate School of Biomedical Sciences, Nursing, and Allied Health Sciences) and three institutes (Marine Biomedical, Medical Humanities, and Human Infections and Immunity).

Mission Statement
The mission of UTMB is to provide scholarly teaching, innovative scientific investigation, and state-of-the-art patient care in a learning environment to better the health of society. UTMB's education programs enable the state's talented individuals to become outstanding practitioners, teachers, and investigators in the health care sciences. Its comprehensive primary, specialty, and subspecialty clinics support the educational mission of the SOM, which is committed to the health care of all Texans through the delivery of state-of-the-art preventive, diagnostic, and treatment services.

Curricular Highlights
Community Service Requirement: Optional.
Research/Thesis Requirement: Optional.

The Integrated Medical Curriculum (IMC) is a four-year program that emphasizes continuous integration of the basic medical sciences with clinical medicine, early clinical skills and clinical experiences, and professionalism. In this student-centered curriculum, which utilizes small-group problem-based learning, computer-assisted instruction, lectures, and labs, the basic medical sciences are learned in clinical contexts. Its organ system-based approach and clinical science contexts promote basic science integration across disciplines. The third and fourth years of the IMC are centered on ambulatory and inpatient experiences in emergency medicine, family medicine, internal medicine, neurology, obstetrics and gynecology, pediatrics, psychiatry, and surgery. A unique feature of the third-year curriculum is an elective month, which allows students to expand their experience in a primary care field or explore potential career interests in a medical specialty. The fourth year also includes an acting internship, community-based ambulatory medicine, and a scholarly project in which a basic science or medical humanities topic is explored in depth. UTMB employs a grading system of Honors, High Pass, Pass, and Fail for required core courses and Pass/Fail for elective courses.

USMLE
Step 1: Required. Students must record a passing score for promotion.
Step 2: Clinical Skills (CS): Required. Students must record a passing total score to graduate.
Step 2: Clinical Knowledge (CK): Required. Students must record a passing total score to graduate.

Selection Factors
UTMB includes race and ethnicity to the broad range of criteria considered for student admission and for scholarship awards. All information available is utilized in the selection process such as intellect, achievement, character, interpersonal skills, and motivation. In evaluating candidates, consideration is given to the total academic record, the results of aptitude and achievement tests, college preprofessional committee evaluations, and the personal interview.

Financial Aid
Long-term, low-interest and short-term loans are available to students with financial need. In addition, a number of scholarships are available which are based on need, disadvantaged status and academic merit.

Information about Diversity Programs
UTMB is committed to increasing the number of disadvantaged students in medicine. Each applicant is reviewed holistically and individually by experienced members of the Admissions Committee with particular emphasis on the applicant's potential. Both cognitive and non-cognitive factors are considered. Following admission, a broad range of support services are available to assist students in completing the medical curriculum. UTMB does not discriminate on the basis of race, sex, creed, national origin, age, or handicap.

Campus Information

Setting
UTMB is located on an island in the Gulf of Mexico, 50 miles south of Houston. It is a 99-acre campus with 77 major modern buildings, including the state-of-the-art Truman Blocker, Jr. Medical Research Building, Trauma Center, and Shriners Burns Hospital. Clinical training takes place in seven teaching hospitals; UTMB owns and operates all of the facilities, and they are physically located on the campus.

Enrollment
For 2008, total enrollment was: 890

Special Features
UTMB is one of two medical schools that received NIH funding for a Biosafety Level 4 Laboratory, which is currently under construction. The Galveston National Laboratory will house the new Institute for Human Infections and Immunity.

Housing
Student housing is available on campus and in the surrounding Galveston community.

Satellite Campuses/Facilities
A limited number of clerkship positions are available for third year students to spend their entire year in Austin, Texas. However, all third and fourth year students can choose to do a portion of their clerkships at this additional training site.

Application Process and Requirements 2009–2010

Primary Application Service: TMDSAS
Earliest filing date: May 1, 2009
Latest filing date: October 1, 2009

Secondary Application Required?: No
Sent to: n/a
URL: n/a
Fee: No
Fee waiver available: No
Earliest filing date: n/a
Latest filing date: n/a

MCAT® required?: Yes
Latest MCAT® considered: September 2009
Oldest MCAT® considered: April 2005

Early Decision Program: School does not have EDP
Applicants notified: n/a
EDP available for: n/a

Regular Acceptance Notice
Earliest date: November 15, 2009
Latest date: Until class is full
Applicant's Response to Acceptance Offer – Maximum Time: varies

Requests for Deferred Entrance Considered: Yes

Deposit to Hold Place in Class: No
Deposit (Resident): n/a
Deposit (Non-resident): n/a
Deposit due: n/a
Applied to tuition: n/a
Deposit refundable: n/a
Refundable by: n/a

Estimated number of new entrants: 230
EDP: n/a, special program: 20

Start Month/Year: August 2010

Interview Format: Two interviews, presentation, and tour. Regional interviews are not available.

Other Programs

PREPARATORY PROGRAMS
Postbaccalaureate Program: No
Summer Program: Yes, www.utmb.edu/somstudentaffairs/specialprograms
Lisa Cain, Ph.D., (409) 772-5397, ldcain@utmb.edu
Early Medical School Acceptance Program (EMSAP): www.utmb.edu/somstudentaffairs/specialprograms
Prematriculation Reinforcement & Enrichment Program:
www.utmb.edu/somstudentaffairs/specialprograms

COMBINED DEGREE PROGRAMS
Baccalaureate/M.D.: No
M.D./M.P.H.: Yes, Nelson Avery, M.D., (409) 747-0971, navery@utmb.edu
M.D./M.B.A.: No
M.D./J.D.: No
M.D./Ph.D.: Yes, www.utmb.edu/mdphd
Ana McAfee, (409) 772-5446, abmcafee@utmb.edu
Additional Program: Yes, www.mdphd.utexas.edu
Robin Dusek, (512) 471-0934, mdphd@austin.utexas.edu

Premedical Coursework

Course	Req.	Rec.	Lab.	Sems.	Course	Req.	Rec.	Lab.	Sems.
Inorganic Chemistry	•	•		2	Computer Science				
Behavioral Sciences					Genetics		•		
Biochemistry		•		4	Humanities				
Biology	•		•	4	Organic Chemistry	•		•	2
Biology/Zoology					Physics	•		•	2
Calculus	•			1	Psychology				
College English	•			2	Social Sciences				
College Mathematics					Other				

Selection Factors: 2008 Accepted Applicants

Proportion of Accepted Applicants with Relevant Experience (Data Self-Reported to AMCAS®)		
Community Service/Volunteer		73%
Medically-Related Work		87%
Research		77%

Shaded bar represents school's accepted scores ranging from the 10th percentile to the 90th percentile   School Median ●   National Median ●

Overall GPA	2.0	2.1	2.2	2.3	2.4	2.5	2.6	2.7	2.8	2.9	3.0	3.1	3.2	3.3	3.4	3.5	**3.6**	**3.7**	3.8	(3.9)	4.0
Science GPA	2.0	2.1	2.2	2.3	2.4	2.5	2.6	2.7	2.8	2.9	3.0	3.1	3.2	3.3	3.4	**3.5**	**3.6**	**3.7**	3.8	(3.9)	4.0

MCAT® Total Numeric Score 9 10 11 12 13 14 15 16 17 18 19 20 21 22 23 24 25 **26 27 28 29 30** (31) 32 33 34 35 36 37 38 39 40 41 42 43

Writing Sample			J	K	L	**M**	**N**	**O**	(P)	(Q)	R	S	T
Verbal Reasoning	3	4	5	6	7	**8**	**9**	(10)	11	12	13	14	15
Biological Sciences	3	4	5	6	7	**8**	**9**	10	(11)	12	13	14	15
Physical Sciences	3	4	5	6	7	**8**	**9**	10	(11)	12	13	14	15

Acceptance & Matriculation Data for 2008–2009 First Year Class

	Resident	Non-resident	International	Total
Applications	2915	584	81	3580
Interviewed	916	70	4	990
Deferred	5	0	0	5
Matriculants				
Early Assurance Program	0	0	0	0
Early Decision Program	0	0	0	0
Baccalaureate/M.D.	n/a	n/a	n/a	n/a
M.D./Ph.D.	6	0	0	6
Matriculated	210	18	3	**231**

Applications accepted from International Applicants: Yes

Matriculant Demographics: 2008–2009 First Year Class

Men: 133   **Women:** 98

Matriculants' Self-Reported Race/Ethnicity

Mexican American	30	Korean	2
Cuban	0	Vietnamese	5
Puerto Rican	3	Other Asian	9
Other Hispanic	7	Total Asian	37
Total Hispanic	39	Native American	1
Chinese	10	Black	24
Asian Indian	9	Native Hawaiian	0
Pakistani	1	White	142
Filipino	1	Unduplicated Number	
Japanese	0	of Matriculants	231

Science and Math Majors: 45%
Matriculants with:
    Baccalaureate degree: 63%
    Graduate degree(s): 3%

Specialty Choice

2004, 2005, 2006 Graduates, Specialty Choice (As reported by program directors to GME Track™)	
Anesthesiology	9%
Emergency Medicine	7%
Family Practice	10%
Internal Medicine	15%
Obstetrics/Gynecology	3%
Orthopaedic Surgery	4%
Pediatrics	11%
Psychiatry	6%
Radiology	6%
Surgery	7%

Financial Information

Source: 2007–2008 LCME I-B survey and 2008–2009 AAMC TSF questionnaire

	Residents	Non-residents
Total Cost of Attendance	$38,155	$51,255
Tuition and Fees	$13,353	$26,452
Other (includes living expenses)	$24,056	$24,056
Health Insurance (can be waived)	$746	$746

Average 2008 Graduate Indebtedness: $122,556
% of Enrolled Students Receiving Aid: 82%

Criminal Background Check

This medical school requires a criminal background check prior to matriculation.

University of Texas Medical School at Houston

Houston, Texas

Office of Admissions—Room G.420
University of Texas Medical School at Houston
6431 Fannin, MSB G.420
Houston, Texas 77030
T 713 500 5116   **F** 713 500 0604

Admissions http://med.uth.tmc.edu/administration/admissions/
Main http://med.uth.tmc.edu
Financial http://sfs.uth.tmc.edu
E-mail msadmissions@uth.tmc.edu

Public Institution

Dr. Giuseppe N. Colasurdo, Dean

Dr. Margaret McNeese, Associate Dean for Admissions and Student Affairs

Wanda K. Williams, Director, Student Financial Services

Dr. Judianne Kellaway, Assistant Dean for Admissions

Yvette Sanders, Coordinator for Admissions

General Information

UT-Houston Medical School is located in the Texas Medical Center in Houston. Memorial Hermann Hosp., a 650-bed general medical and surgical hospital, and Level I trauma center, is the school's primary teaching hospital. Other major teaching hospitals include the U. of Texas M.D. Anderson Cancer Ctr., the LBJ Hosp., the Harris County Psychiatric Center, Texas Heart Inst., St. Luke's Episcopal Hosp., Methodist Hosp. and others.

Mission Statement

The mission of the University of Texas Medical School at Houston is to provide the highest quality of education and training of future physicians for the state of Texas and to conduct the highest caliber of research in the biomedical and health sciences.

Curricular Highlights

Community Service Requirement: Optional.
Community Service: Unlimited opportunities
Research Thesis: Unlimited opportunities
Research/Thesis Requirement: Optional.

The first two academic years are divided into four semesters, with three months of vacation between the first and second years. The initial four semesters are devoted to preparing the student for clerkship experiences in the clinical years. During the first two years the student becomes familiar with the basic and applied biomedical sciences. The student progresses from a study of the morphology of the human body and the fundamentals of molecular and cellular biology to that of the normal and abnormal structure and function of the various organ systems. Taking a history and con-

ducting a physical examination are emphasized. After completion of this sequence, the student progresses through a series of clinical clerkships in the major disciplines for the next 12 months. In the fourth year, there are four required months and five to seven months of electives. Medical jurisprudence and technical skills are taught. In consultation with faculty, each student devises an educational sequence that relates specifically to ultimate career goals and postgraduate educational plans.

USMLE

Step 1: Required. Students must only record a score.
Step 2: Clinical Skills (CS): Required. Students must only record a score.
Step 2: Clinical Knowledge (CK): Required. Students must only record a score.

Selection Factors

Applicants are selected with an emphasis on motivation and potential for service, especially in the state of Texas. Emphasis is given to students who have a broad education as well as academic achievement. A command of the English language with the ability to write and speak well is essential. The applicant's academic record is evaluated with special attention to the subjects taken and the demonstration of a broad-based comprehensive educational experience regardless of undergraduate institution. Significant attention is given to humanitarian endeavors, achievement in a nonacademic field of activity, and the applicant's specific interest in The University of Texas Medical School at Houston. Admission decisions are made in light of the school's mission, with preference given to Texas residents and those who will practice in underserved areas in the state and in needed specialties. Veteran status is also considered. The University of Texas Medical School at Houston does not discriminate on the basis of race, sex, creed, national origin, age, or handicap. For more information, go to *med.uth.tmc.edu.*

Financial Aid

Scholarship and loan funds from federal, state, and local sources are available to students with financial need as determined by the FAFSA.

Information about Diversity Programs

Numerous student organizations create an inclusive and supportive environment at UTH. All are aligned under the broad "Alliance for Diversity and Culture." The primary goal of the Office of Cultural and Institutional Diversity is to enhance success and promote retention of all students through early identification of stress factors and personal challenges, information which is then provided with the student's consent to academic advisors. Workshops and individual consultations are offered to enhance specific skills and time management, and diagnostic testing is available to help identify learning difficulties.

Campus Information

Setting

The Medical School Building (MSB), located in the Texas Medical Center, was built in 1976 and, at 875,365 gross sq. ft., comprises the school's largest facility. A state-of-the-art Surgical and Clinical Skills Center is one of this building's latest additions. Adjoining the MSB, a six-story building dedicated to research was completed in 2007.

Enrollment

For 2008, total enrollment was: 909

Special Features

Our location in the Texas Medical Center and membership in the UT Health Science Ctr. (comprising dentistry, nursing, public health, graduate school, and health informatics) provide many opportunities for students to engage in research, dual-degree programs, and specialty exploration with first-rate physicians and scientists.

Housing

Apartment-living managed by the UTHSC is available to students at two facilities. Various floor plans are available. Many other residential options are located near the Texas Medical Center, convenient shuttle or light rail available.

Satellite Campuses/Facilities

Student rotations are completed at several hospitals and clinics in the Texas Medical Center and nearby.

Application Process and Requirements 2009–2010

Primary Application Service: TMDSAS
Earliest filing date: May 1, 2009
Latest filing date: October 1, 2009

Secondary Application Required?: No
Sent to: n/a
URL: n/a
Fee: No
Fee waiver available: Yes
Earliest filing date: n/a
Latest filing date: n/a

MCAT® required?: Yes
Latest MCAT® considered: September 2009
Oldest MCAT® considered: August 2004

Early Decision Program: School does not have EDP
Applicants notified: October 15, 2009
November 15, 2009
EDP available for: Both Residents and Non-residents

Regular Acceptance Notice
Earliest date: October 15, 2009
Latest date: Until class is full
Applicant's Response to Acceptance Offer – Maximum Time: Two weeks

Requests for Deferred Entrance Considered: No

Deposit to Hold Place in Class: No
Deposit (Resident): n/a
Deposit (Non-resident): n/a
Deposit due: n/a
Applied to tuition: n/a
Deposit refundable: n/a
Refundable by: n/a

Estimated number of new entrants: 230
EDP: n/a, special program: n/a

Start Month/Year: August 2010

Interview Format: Personal interview with two faculty members. Regional interviews are not available.

Other Programs

PREPARATORY PROGRAMS
Postbaccalaureate Program: No
Summer Program: Yes, http://med.uth.tmc.edu/administration/admissions/
Pre-Entry Program: http://med.uth.tmc.edu/administration/edu_programs/ep/summer_programs.htm, Wai-San Johansson, (713) 500-7869, wai-san.johansson@uth.tmc.edu

COMBINED DEGREE PROGRAMS
Baccalaureate/M.D.: No
M.D./M.P.H.: Yes, http://med.uth.tmc.edu/administration/admissions/MDMPH.html
M.D./M.B.A.: No
M.D./J.D.: No
M.D./Ph.D.: Yes, www.uth.tmc.edu/gsbs/programs/mdphd/

Premedical Coursework

Course	Req.	Rec.	Lab.	Hrs.
Inorganic Chemistry	•		•	8
Behavioral Sciences				
Biochemistry				
Biology	•		•	14
Biology/Zoology				
Calculus				
College English	•			6
College Mathematics				

Course	Req.	Rec.	Lab.	Hrs.
Computer Science				
Genetics				
Humanities		•		
Organic Chemistry	•		•	8
Physics	•		•	8
Psychology				
Social Sciences				
Other				

Selection Factors: 2008 Accepted Applicants

Proportion of Accepted Applicants with Relevant Experience (Data Self-Reported to AMCAS)		
Community Service/Volunteer		72%
Medically-Related Work		83%
Research		76%

Shaded bar represents school's accepted scores ranging from the 10th percentile to the 90th percentile   School Median ●   National Median ●

Overall GPA	2.0	2.1	2.2	2.3	2.4	2.5	2.6	2.7	2.8	2.9	3.0	3.1	3.2	3.3	3.4	3.5	3.6	(3.7)	3.8	3.9	4.0
Science GPA	2.0	2.1	2.2	2.3	2.4	2.5	2.6	2.7	2.8	2.9	3.0	3.1	3.2	3.3	3.4	3.5	3.6	(3.7)	3.8	3.9	4.0

MCAT® Total Numeric Score 9 10 11 12 13 14 15 16 17 18 19 20 21 22 23 24 25 26 27 28 29 30 31 (32) 33 34 35 36 37 38 39 40 41 42 43

Writing Sample				J	K	L	M	N	O	(P)	(Q)	R	S	T
Verbal Reasoning	3		4	5	6	7	8	9	(10)	11	12	13	14	15
Biological Sciences	3		4	5	6	7	8	9	10	(11)	12	13	14	15
Physical Sciences	3		4	5	6	7	8	9	10	(11)	12	13	14	15

Acceptance & Matriculation Data for 2008–2009 First Year Class

	Resident	Non-resident	International	Total
Applications	3006	593	0	3599
Interviewed	1040	100	0	1140
Deferred	0	0	0	0
Matriculants				
Early Assurance Program	0	0	0	0
Early Decision Program	0	0	0	0
Baccalaureate/M.D.	n/a	n/a	n/a	00
M.D./Ph.D.	1	2	0	3
Matriculated	121	18	0	**230**

Applications accepted from International Applicants: Yes

Matriculant Demographics: 2008–2009 First Year Class

Men: 137   **Women:** 93

Matriculants' Self-Reported Race/Ethnicity

Mexican American	24	**Korean**	1
Cuban	1	**Vietnamese**	4
Puerto Rican	3	**Other Asian**	8
Other Hispanic	17	**Total Asian**	29
Total Hispanic	45	**Native American**	2
Chinese	10	**Black**	10
Asian Indian	6	**Native Hawaiian**	1
Pakistani	0	**White**	170
Filipino	2	**Unduplicated Number**	
Japanese	0	**of Matriculants**	230

Science and Math Majors: 49%
Matriculants with:
    Baccalaureate degree: 100%
    Graduate degree(s): 4%

Specialty Choice

2004, 2005, 2006 Graduates, Specialty Choice (As reported by program directors to GME Track™)	
Anesthesiology	9%
Emergency Medicine	6%
Family Practice	10%
Internal Medicine	14%
Obstetrics/Gynecology	6%
Orthopaedic Surgery	5%
Pediatrics	10%
Psychiatry	7%
Radiology	3%
Surgery	8%

Financial Information

Source: 2007–2008 LCME I-B survey and 2008–2009 AAMC TSF questionnaire

	Residents	Non-residents
Total Cost of Attendance	$35,696	$48,796
Tuition and Fees	$11,009	$24,109
Other (includes living expenses)	$23,568	$23,568
Health Insurance (can be waived)	$1,119	$1,119

Average 2008 Graduate Indebtedness: $116,197
% of Enrolled Students Receiving Aid: 82%

Criminal Background Check

This medical school requires a criminal background check prior to matriculation.

University of Texas School of Medicine at San Antonio

San Antonio, Texas

Medical School Admissions, Office of the Dean
Univ. of Texas School of Medicine at San Antonio
7703 Floyd Curl Drive
San Antonio, Texas 78229-3900
T 210 567 6080   F 210 567 6962

Admissions http://som.uthscsa.edu/admissions/index.asp
Main http://som.uthscsa.edu
Financial http:// studentservices.uthscsa.edu/financialaid.aspx
E-mail medadmissions@uthscsa.edu

Public Institution

Dr. Glen A. Halff, Acting Dean

Dr. David J. Jones, Associate Dean for Admissions

Belinda Chapa, Director of Admissions and Special Programs

General Information

The University of Texas School of Medicine at San Antonio graduated its first class in 1970. The main campus is located at the South Texas Medical Center in NW San Antonio. Clinical instruction is carried out at the University Hospital, University Health Center, Audie Murphy Veterans Hospital, Santa Rosa Children's Hospital, and affiliated hospitals including Wilford Hall USAF Hospital and Brooke Army Hospital.

Mission Statement

The mission of the School of Medicine is to serve the needs of the citizens of Texas by providing medical education and training to medical students and physicians at all career levels and fostering an environment of life-long learning that is flexible and emphasizes professionalism, with special commitment to the preparation of physicians in both the art and science of medical practice; conducting biomedical and other health-related research, with particular attention to translational research; delivering exemplary health care; and providing a responsive resource in health-related affairs for the nation and the state, with particular emphasis on South Texas.

Curricular Highlights

Community Service Requirement: Optional.
Research/Thesis Requirement: Optional.

A four-year curriculum is offered. The first year is devoted to an organ systems-based presentation of anatomy, histology, biochemistry, physiology, and microbiology. The second year is anchored by the pathology course, and it incorporates pharmacology, medicine, pediatrics, obstetrics and gynecology, and surgery coordinated by organ systems. Behavioral sciences and an introduction to psychiatry are also included. Throughout the first two years,

one-half day per week is devoted to clinical integration activities. The third academic year is spent entirely in the clinical setting in eight consecutive assignments of six weeks each in family practice, medicine, the medical specialties, surgery, the surgical specialties, obstetrics and gynecology, psychiatry, and pediatrics. The senior year includes a didactic period of two months, with the rest of the academic year consisting of elective courses. A letter grading system is used.

USMLE

Step 1: Required. Must record a passing score for graduation, but not promotion.
Step 2: Clinical Skills (CS): Required. Students must only record a score.
Step 2: Clinical Knowledge (CK): Required. Students must only record a score.

Selection Factors

Ranking of applicants considers GPA, MCAT section scores, evaluation by premedical advisors, and judgment by the Committee on Admissions of the candidate's nonacademic achievements and personal qualifications, such as responsibility, integrity, maturity, and motivation. In addition, bilingual language ability, hometown or county of residence that has been designated a medically underserved area, socioeconomic history, positions of leadership held, communication skills, and clinical/volunteer experiences are considered. No person shall be excluded from participation in, denied the benefits of, or subject to discrimination under any program or activity sponsored or conducted by the University of Texas System on the basis of age, race, national origin, religion, or sex. Two hundred thirty five acceptances were offered to obtain a class of 200 first-year students. All procedural information including electronic submission of applications is available through the Texas Medical and Dental Schools Application Service. Questions related to completeness of an application or other information should be directed to the Admissions Office at the medical school (medadmissions@uthscsa.edu). Additional information is available at (210) 567-6080.

Financial Aid

Financial assistance for students in need is available in the form of loans and scholarships. Accepted applicants can obtain complete information regarding financial assistance from the Financial Aid Administrator in the Office of Student Services *http://studentservices.uthscsa.edu/financialinfo/financialaid2.html*.

Information about Diversity Programs

Diversity of the student body is a compelling interest of the University of Texas School of Medicine at San Antonio. With this in mind, race and ethnicity is among the factors considered for acceptance of students.

Campus Information

Setting

The University of Texas School of Medicine at San Antonio is located in the South Texas Medical Center in northwest San Antonio.

Enrollment

For 2008, total enrollment was: 884

Special Features

The HEB Clinical Skills Center offers students 20 state-of-the-art examination rooms to develop patient examination skills.

Housing

On campus housing is not available. Homes, apartments, and condominiums are available within walking distance of the school of medicine and teaching hospitals.

Satellite Campuses/Facilities

The Regional Academic Health Center located in the Rio Grande Valley in Harlingen, Texas, is a second clinical education campus. At the end of their second year, up to 24 students move to Harlingen to complete their third and fourth years of medical school. Third-year clerkships are completed at Valley Baptist Hospital and Su Clinica Familiar. Fourth-year students participate in the same didactic and externship opportunities available at the San Antonio campus.

Application Process and Requirements 2010–2011

Primary Application Service: TMDSAS
Earliest filing date: May 1, 2009
Latest filing date: October 1, 2009

Secondary Application Required?: No
Sent to: n/a
URL: n/a
Fee: n/a
Fee waiver available: n/a
Earliest filing date: n/a
Latest filing date: n/a

MCAT® required?: Yes
Latest MCAT® considered: September 2009
Oldest MCAT® considered: 2006

Early Decision Program: School does not have EDP
Applicants notified: n/a
EDP available for: n/a

Regular Acceptance Notice
Earliest date: October 15, 2009 (non-residents)
November 15, 2009 (residents)
Latest date: Until class is full
Applicant's Response to Acceptance
Offer – Maximum Time: Two weeks

Requests for Deferred
Entrance Considered: Yes

Deposit to Hold Place in Class: No
Deposit (Resident): n/a
Deposit (Non-resident): n/a
Deposit due: n/a
Applied to tuition: n/a
Deposit refundable: n/a
Refundable by: n/a

Estimated number of new entrants: 220
EDP: 0, special program: 5

Start Month/Year: July 28, 2010

Interview Format: Two 30-minute interviews; interviewers have only personal essays. Regional interviews are not available.

Other Programs

PREPARATORY PROGRAMS
Postbaccalaureate Program: No
Summer Program: No

COMBINED DEGREE PROGRAMS
Baccalaureate/M.D.: Yes, http://som.uthscsa.edu/
Admissions/earlyMatriculationProgram.asp
Belinda Chapa, (210) 567-6080,
chapab@uthscsa.edu
M.D./M.P.H.: Yes, http://som.uthscsa.edu/
AcademicAffairs/mdmph.asp, Dr. Claudia Miller,
(210) 567-7457, millercs@uthscsa.edu
M.D./M.B.A.: No
M.D./J.D.: No
M.D./Ph.D.: Yes, http://som.uthscsa.edu/
Admissions/MDPhD.asp
Dr. Martin Adamo, (210) 567-3742,
adamo@uthscsa.edu

Premedical Coursework

Course	Req.	Rec.	Lab.	Hrs.	Course	Req.	Rec.	Lab.	Hrs.
Inorganic Chemistry	•		•	8	Computer Science				
Behavioral Sciences					Genetics				
Biochemistry	•			3	Humanities				
Biology	•		•	11	Organic Chemistry	•		•	8
Biology/Zoology					Physics	•		•	8
Calculus	•			3	Psychology				
College English	•			6	Social Sciences				
College Mathematics					Other				

Selection Factors: 2008 Accepted Applicants

Proportion of Accepted Applicants with Relevant Experience (Data Self-Reported to AMCAS®)		
Community Service/Volunteer		76%
Medically-Related Work		88%
Research		79%

Shaded bar represents school's accepted scores ranging from the 10th percentile to the 90th percentile. School Median ● National Median ●

Overall GPA 2.0 2.1 2.2 2.3 2.4 2.5 2.6 2.7 2.8 2.9 3.0 3.1 3.2 3.3 3.4 3.5 3.6 (3.7) 3.8 3.9 4.0
Science GPA 2.0 2.1 2.2 2.3 2.4 2.5 2.6 2.7 2.8 2.9 3.0 3.1 3.2 3.3 3.4 3.5 3.6 (3.7) 3.8 3.9 4.0

MCAT® Total Numeric Score 9 10 11 12 13 14 15 16 17 18 19 20 21 22 23 24 25 26 27 28 29 30 (31) 32 33 34 35 36 37 38 39 40 41 42 43

Writing Sample			J	K	L	M	N	O	(P)	(Q)	R	S	T
Verbal Reasoning	3	4	5	6	7	8	9	(10)	11	12	13	14	15
Biological Sciences	3	4	5	6	7	8	9	(10)	(11)	12	13	14	15
Physical Sciences	3	4	5	6	7	8	9	(10)	(11)	12	13	14	15

Acceptance & Matriculation Data for 2008–2009 First Year Class

	Resident	Non-resident	International	Total
Applications	2887	585	57	3529
Interviewed	918	100	0	1018
Deferred	4	0	0	4
Matriculants				
Early Assurance Program	0	0	0	0
Early Decision Program	0	0	0	0
Baccalaureate/M.D.	9	0	0	9
M.D./Ph.D.	5	0	0	5
Matriculated	197	24	0	**221**

Applications accepted from International Applicants: Only Canadian

Matriculant Demographics: 2008–2009 First Year Class

Men: 111 **Women:** 110

Matriculants' Self-Reported Race/Ethnicity

Mexican American	28	Korean	3
Cuban	1	Vietnamese	1
Puerto Rican	0	Other Asian	16
Other Hispanic	11	Total Asian	39
Total Hispanic	38	Native American	0
Chinese	12	Black	11
Asian Indian	7	Native Hawaiian	0
Pakistani	3	White	152
Filipino	1	Unduplicated Number	
Japanese	0	of Matriculants	221

Science and Math Majors: 41%
Matriculants with:
Baccalaureate degree: 68%
Graduate degree(s): 5%

Specialty Choice

2004, 2005, 2006 Graduates, Specialty Choice (As reported by program directors to GME Track™)	
Anesthesiology	11%
Emergency Medicine	4%
Family Practice	10%
Internal Medicine	17%
Obstetrics/Gynecology	7%
Orthopedic Surgery	4%
Pediatrics	11%
Psychiatry	4%
Radiology	4%
Surgery	9%

Financial Information
Source: 2007–2008 LCME I-B survey and 2008–2009 AAMC TSF questionnaire

	Residents	Non-residents
Total Cost of Attendance	$37,566	$52,753
Tuition and Fees	$13,450	$28,637
Other (includes living expenses)	$23,387	$23,387
Health Insurance (can be waived)	$729	$729

Average 2008 Graduate Indebtedness: $125,521
% of Enrolled Students Receiving Aid: 87%

Criminal Background Check

This medical school requires a criminal background check prior to matriculation.

University of Texas Southwestern Medical Center at Dallas Southwestern Medical School

Dallas, Texas

University of Texas
Southwestern Medical Center at Dallas
5323 Harry Hines Boulevard
Dallas, Texas 75390-9162
T 214 648 5617   **F** 214 648 3289

Admissions www.utsouthwestern.edu/admissions
Main www.utsouthwestern.edu
Financial www.utsouthwestern.edu
E-mail admissions@utsouthwestern.edu

Public Institution

Dr. Alfred G. Gilman, Dean

Anne P. McLane, Associate Director of Admissions

Dr. Byron Cryer, Associate Dean for Minority Student Affairs

Charles L. Kettlewell, Director of Student Financial Aid

Dr. James Wagner, Associate Dean for Student Affairs

Dr. Angela Mihalic, Associate Dean for Student Affairs

General Information

Founded in 1943, UT Southwestern is a multifaceted academic health science center nationally recognized for its excellence in educating physicians, biomedical scientists, and other health care professionals.

Mission Statement

UT Southwestern is dedicated to educating physicians who are thoroughly grounded in the scientific basis of modern medicine, who are inspired to maintain lifelong medical scholarship, and who care for patients in a responsible and compassionate manner. UT Southwestern's mission emphasizes the importance of training primary care physicians, educating doctors who will practice in underserved areas of Texas, and preparing physician-scientists who seek careers in academic medicine and research.

Curricular Highlights

Community Service Requirement: Optional.
Research/Thesis Requirement: Optional.

UT Southwestern offers a four-year curriculum based on departmental as well as interdisciplinary teaching. The purpose of the first two years is to provide a strong background in the basic sciences and an introduction to clinical medicine. The first-year curriculum is designed to begin the study of the normal human body and its processes at the molecular and cellular levels. The second year is an organ system-based curriculum that integrates pharmacology, microbiology, pathology, and clinical medicine. Contact with patients begins early in the second

year with history-taking and physical examination, as well as visits to outpatient clinics. The third and fourth years provide intense clinical experiences involving the student in direct inpatient and outpatient care in a variety of clinical settings. Specific information about the UT Southwestern medical curriculum is available at *http://medschool.swmed.edu/*.

USMLE

Step 1: Required. Students must record a passing score for graduation, but not promotion.
Step 2: Clinical Skills (CS): Required. Students must record a passing total score to graduate.
Step 2: Clinical Knowledge (CK): Required. Students must record a passing total score to graduate.

Selection Factors

The following factors are considered in evaluating each applicant's acceptability: MCAT scores; undergraduate GPA; rigor of the undergraduate curriculum; letters of recommendation; research experience; extracurricular activities; socioeconomic background; time spent in outside employment; personal integrity and compassion for others; race/ethnicity; the ability to communicate in English; other personal qualities and individual factors such as leadership, social/family support, self-appraisal, maturity/coping skills, and determination; and motivation for a career in medicine. In addition, applicants are evaluated with regard to the mission of Southwestern Medical School. State law requires that at least 90 percent of the class be residents of Texas. Therefore, the minimum credentials for non-residents are more stringent than are those for Texas residents. Early application is strongly advised. A personal on-campus interview is required; interviews are held on Saturdays between early September and early January.

Financial Aid

UT Southwestern works directly with students to obtain funding for their medical education. Most of the financial aid available is obtained through federal and state loan programs. However, a limited number of scholarships from private sources are available. Non-residents are eligible to pay resident tuition on receipt of a competitive academic scholarship. Students

rarely discontinue school for financial reasons.

Information about Diversity Programs

The Admissions Committee at Southwestern Medical School recognizes the need for increased numbers of physicians from groups underrepresented in medicine and encourages applications from Texas residents who are members of these groups. UT Southwestern uses race/ethnicity as one of the criteria for evaluating applicants in an effort to provide a diverse educational environment.

Campus Information

Setting

Located just north of downtown Dallas, the 150-acre campus includes an extensive medical library, 45,000-square-foot student recreation center, tennis and outdoor basketball courts, jogging paths, and a 6-acre wooded bird sanctuary. Four hospitals are adjacent to the campus: Parkland Hospital, Children's Medical Center Dallas, University Hospital, University Hospital-Zale Lipshy, and UT Southwestern University Hospital.

Enrollment

For 2008, total enrollment was: 923

Special Features

UT Southwestern Medical School offers an M.D. with Research Distinction program to recognize students who distinguish themselves in the conduct of meaningful clinical or basic research activities.

Housing

Ample and affordable housing opportunities are available within 5 to 10 miles of the campus. Additionally, UT Southwestern's Medical Park Apartments is a gated community with one- and two-bedroom units with individually monitored security, clubhouse, study center, exercise room, and pool.

Satellite Campuses/Facilities

Clinical training takes place at university sites and affiliated hospitals and clinics throughout the North Texas area, including Parkland Memorial Hospital, Children's Medical Center Dallas, the Dallas VA Medical Center, University Hospital, and University Hospital-Zale Lipshy.

Application Process and Requirements 2010–2011

Primary Application Service: TMDSAS
Earliest filing date: May 1, 2009
Latest filing date: October 1, 2009

Secondary Application Required?: Yes
Sent to: All applicants
URL: www.utsouthwestern.edu/admissions
Fee: No
Fee waiver available: n/a
Earliest filing date: May 1, 2009
Latest filing date: October 1, 2009

MCAT® required?: Yes
Latest MCAT® considered: September 2009
Oldest MCAT® considered: September 2005

Early Decision Program: School does not have EDP
Applicants notified: n/a
EDP available for: n/a

Regular Acceptance Notice
Earliest date: November 15, 2009
Latest date: Varies
Applicant's Response to Acceptance
Offer – Maximum Time: Three weeks

Requests for Deferred
Entrance Considered: Yes

Deposit to Hold Place in Class: No
Deposit (Resident): n/a
Deposit (Non-resident): n/a
Deposit due: n/a
Applied to tuition: n/a
Deposit refundable: n/a
Refundable by: n/a

Estimated number of new entrants: 230
EDP: n/a, special program: n/a

Start Month/Year: August 2010

Interview Format: Two 25-minute faculty interviews. Regional interviews are not available.

Other Programs

PREPARATORY PROGRAMS
Postbaccalaureate Program: No
Summer Program: No

COMBINED DEGREE PROGRAMS
Baccalaureate/M.D.: No
M.D./M.P.H.: Yes, www.sph.uth.tmc.edu
M.D./M.B.A.: Yes, www.utsouthwestern.edu/md-mba
M.D./J.D.: No
M.D./Ph.D.: Yes, www.utsouthwestern.edu/md-phd
Dr. Andrew Zinn, (800) 633-6787
MSTP@UTSouthwestern.edu
Additional Program: Yes, www.utsouthwestern.edu/md-ms
Dr. Michael McPhaul, (214) 648-3465
michael.mcphaul@utsouthwestern.edu

Premedical Coursework

Course	Req.	Rec.	Lab.	Sems.	Course	Req.	Rec.	Lab.	Sems.
Inorganic Chemistry	•		•	2	Computer Science				
Behavioral Sciences					Genetics				
Biochemistry		•		1	Humanities				
Biology	•		•	4	Organic Chemistry	•		•	2
Biology/Zoology					Physics	•		•	2
Calculus	•			1	Psychology				
College English	•			2	Social Sciences				
College Mathematics					Other				

Selection Factors: 2008 Accepted Applicants

Proportion of Accepted Applicants with Relevant Experience (Data Self-Reported to AMCAS®)

Community Service/Volunteer	73%
Medically-Related Work	85%
Research	79%

Shaded bar represents school's accepted scores ranging from the 10th percentile to the 90th percentile. School Median ● National Median ●

Overall GPA: 2.0 2.1 2.2 2.3 2.4 2.5 2.6 2.7 2.8 2.9 3.0 3.1 3.2 3.3 3.4 3.5 3.6 3.7 3.8 (3.9) 4.0
Science GPA: 2.0 2.1 2.2 2.3 2.4 2.5 2.6 2.7 2.8 2.9 3.0 3.1 3.2 3.3 3.4 3.5 3.6 3.7 3.8 (3.9) 4.0

MCAT® Total Numeric Score: 9 10 11 12 13 14 15 16 17 18 19 20 21 22 23 24 25 26 27 28 29 30 31 (32) 33 (34) 35 36 37 38 39 40 41 42 43

Writing Sample			J	K	L	M	N	O	P	(Q)	R	S	T
Verbal Reasoning	3	4	5	6	7	8	9	(10)	(11)	12	13	14	15
Biological Sciences	3	4	5	6	7	8	9	10	(11)	(12)	13	14	15
Physical Sciences	3	4	5	6	7	8	9	10	(11)	(12)	13	14	15

Acceptance & Matriculation Data for 2008–2009 First Year Class

	Resident	Non-resident	International	Total
Applications	2743	607	94	3444
Interviewed	739	80	14	833
Deferred	6	4	1	11
Matriculants				
Early Assurance Program	0	0	0	0
Early Decision Program	0	0	0	0
Baccalaureate/M.D.	n/a	n/a	n/a	n/a
M.D./Ph.D.	3	3	0	6
Matriculated	192	22	6	**220**

Applications accepted from International Applicants: Yes

Matriculant Demographics: 2008–2009 First Year Class

Men: 109   **Women:** 111

Matriculants' Self-Reported Race/Ethnicity

Mexican American	19	Korean	5
Cuban	0	Vietnamese	13
Puerto Rican	1	Other Asian	15
Other Hispanic	4	Total Asian	85
Total Hispanic	24	Native American	0
Chinese	28	Black	8
Asian Indian	24	Native Hawaiian	0
Pakistani	3	White	115
Filipino	2	Unduplicated Number	
Japanese	0	of Matriculants	220

Science and Math Majors: 60%
Matriculants with:
   Baccalaureate degree: 98%
   Graduate degree(s): 5%

Specialty Choice

2004, 2005, 2006 Graduates, Specialty Choice (As reported by program directors to GME Track™)

Anesthesiology	5%
Emergency Medicine	4%
Family Practice	8%
Internal Medicine	21%
Obstetrics/Gynecology	7%
Orthopaedic Surgery	3%
Pediatrics	12%
Psychiatry	3%
Radiology	7%
Surgery	9%

Financial Information

Source: 2007–2008 LCME I-B survey and 2008–2009 AAMC TSF questionnaire

	Residents	Non-residents
Total Cost of Attendance	$35,477	$48,577
Tuition and Fees	$13,515	$26,615
Other (includes living expenses)	$21,962	$21,962
Health Insurance (not applicable)	$0	$0

Average 2008 Graduate Indebtedness: $88,679
% of Enrolled Students Receiving Aid: 85%

Criminal Background Check

This medical school requires a criminal background check prior to matriculation.

University of Utah
School of Medicine

Salt Lake City, Utah

Office of Admissions
University of Utah School of Medicine
30 North 1900 East Room 1C029
Salt Lake City, Utah 84132-2101
T 801 581 7498   **F** 801 581 2931

Admissions http://medicine.utah.edu/admissions/
Main http://medicine.utah.edu/
Financial http://medicine.utah.edu/financialaid/
E-mail deans.admissions@hsc.utah.edu

Public Institution

Dr. David J. Bjorkman, Dean

Dr. Wayne M. Samuelson, Associate Dean for Admissions

Dr. Edward Junkins, Assistant Dean for Diversity & Community Outreach

Dr. A. Lorris Betz, Senior Vice President for Health Sciences, Executive Dean

General Information

A minimum of 75% of positions are offered to Utah residents. The school contracts with the State of Idaho to accept eight Idaho residents each year. Nonresident applicants must have significant ties to Utah or be specifically recognized as a member of a population group underrepresented in the physician workforce. (Africans and African Americans, American Indians, Alaska Natives, Chamorros, Polynesians including Native Hawaiians, Tongans, Samoans, Filipinos, Tahitians, Maoris, Fijians, Niueans, Palauans; Chicanos/as and Latinos/as including Puerto Ricans, Mexican Americans, Central Americans and South Americans), or apply to the M.D./Ph.D. program. M.D./Ph.D. applicants must be U.S. citizens or U.S. permanent residents. Application may be made for three consecutive years. Applicants who have been dismissed from, or on probation or under suspension at, another medical school will not be considered. Transfers are not available unless the transferring student meets all of the following criteria: must be the spouse of a medical school faculty member or of a person accepted into one of the School of Medicine's postgraduate training programs; must be enrolled and in good standing in the third year at a fully LCME accredited U.S. or Canadian medical school; must have taken Step 1 of the USMLE. The school does not discriminate with respect to applicants' age, color, gender, sexual orientation, race, national origin, religion, status as a person with a disability, or status as a veteran or a disabled veteran. The University of Utah provides reasonable accommodation to known disabilities of applicants.

Mission Statement

The School of Medicine has three major missions: education, research, and clinical service. The three missions are closely interrelated. Each supports and, in turn, benefits from the others. All are considered to be of equal importance.

Curricular Highlights

Community Service Requirement: Optional.
Research/Thesis Requirement: Optional.

The four years of formal medical education constitute but a brief introduction to a broad, deep, and rapidly changing discipline. The mastery of medical knowledge and technical skills requires lifelong self-education. The curriculum is designed to provide students with the knowledge, skills and attitudes necessary to practice medicine.

USMLE

Step 1: Required. Students must record a passing score for promotion.
Step 2: Clinical Skills (CS): Required. Students must record a passing total score to graduate.
Step 2: Clinical Knowledge (CK): Required. Students must record a passing total score to graduate.

Selection Factors

The school's goal is to select the most capable students who will excel in the art and science of medicine. A diverse student body promotes an atmosphere of creativity, experimentation, and discussion that is conducive to learning. Exposure to a variety of perspectives and experiences prepares students to care for patients in every segment of society. The Admissions Committee considers how the applicant balances outside activities and responsibilities with schoolwork to be an indicator of ability to deal with the rigors of life as a physician. The committee is interested in applicants' motivation for attending medical school and their understanding of the medical profession. Commitment to service, ethics, compassion, leadership ability, and communication skills are important characteristics of physicians. Applicants with a science, nonscience, or overall GPA below 3.0 will not be considered. The minimum score for each section of the MCAT is 7. If the test is taken more than once within

three years of application, the best score for each section will be considered. Note: Premedical Course - Biology: 2 courses. 1 course must be in cellular biology or biochemistry.

Financial Aid

In addition to federal loans, a limited number of institutional loans and scholarships are available. All awards are based on need. Financial aid supplements the contribution of the student and/or family, who are expected to provide the maximum assistance possible.

Information about Diversity Programs

The Office of Diversity and Community Outreach assists in recruiting and graduating a diverse student body. The office presents a series of pre-college and premedical educational outreach programs throughout the state.

Campus Information

Setting

The medical school is situated on the east bench of the Salt Lake Valley with the Wasatch Mountains as a backdrop. Public transportation connects the school with downtown Salt Lake City and surrounding areas.

Enrollment

For 2008, total enrollment was: 412

Special Features

University Hospital is home to many centers and clinics that provide research and specialized care to patients from all over the world.

Housing

Housing is available on and off campus.

Satellite Campuses/Facilities

Rotations are performed at University and Intermountain Healthcare hospitals including Children's Medical Center. Primary care rotations may be in community settings.

Application Process and Requirements 2010–2011

Primary Application Service: AMCAS
Earliest filing date: June 1, 2009
Latest filing date: November 1, 2009

Secondary Application Required?: Yes
Sent to: Screened applicants
E-mail: deans.admissions@hsc.utah.edu
Fee: Yes, $100
Fee waiver available: Yes
Earliest filing date: August 2009
Latest filing date: January 2010

MCAT® required?: Yes
Latest MCAT® considered: September 2009
Oldest MCAT® considered: 2007

Early Decision Program: School does not have EDP
Applicants notified: n/a
EDP available for: n/a

Regular Acceptance Notice
Earliest date: October 15, 2009
Latest date: Until class is full
Applicant's Response to Acceptance Offer – Maximum Time: Two weeks

Requests for Deferred Entrance Considered: Yes

Deposit to Hold Place in Class: Yes
Deposit (Resident): $100
Deposit (Non-resident): $100
Deposit due: With response to acceptance offer
Applied to tuition: Yes
Deposit refundable: Yes
Refundable by: May 15, 2010

Estimated number of new entrants: 102
EDP: 0, special program: n/a

Start Month/Year: August 2010

Interview Format: Each applicant will have two interviews. Regional interviews are not available.

Other Programs

PREPARATORY PROGRAMS
Postbaccalaureate Program: No
Summer Program: No

COMBINED DEGREE PROGRAMS
Baccalaureate/M.D.: No
M.D./M.P.H.: Yes, http://medicine.utah.edu/dfpm
M.D./M.B.A.: No
M.D./J.D.: No
M.D./Ph.D.: Yes, http://medicine.utah.edu/mdphd

Premedical Coursework

Course	Req.	Rec.	Lab.	Sems.
Inorganic Chemistry	•		•	2
Behavioral Sciences		•		1
Biochemistry	•			1
Biology	•			1
Biology/Zoology		•		1
Calculus		•		1
College English	•			2
College Mathematics		•		1
Computer Science				

Course	Req.	Rec.	Lab.	Sems.
Genetics		•		1
Humanities	•			1
Organic Chemistry	•		•	2
Physics	•		•	2
Psychology		•		1
Social Sciences	•			1
Diversity	•			1
Anatomy		•		1
Cellular Biology	•			1

Selection Factors: 2008 Accepted Applicants

Proportion of Accepted Applicants with Relevant Experience (Data Self-Reported to AMCAS®)		Community Service/Volunteer	89%
		Medically-Related Work	94%
		Research	98%

Shaded bar represents school's accepted scores ranging from the 10th percentile to the 90th percentile. School Median ● National Median ●

Overall GPA	2.0	2.1	2.2	2.3	2.4	2.5	2.6	2.7	2.8	2.9	3.0	3.1	3.2	3.3	3.4	3.5	3.6	(3.7)	3.8	3.9	4.0
Science GPA	2.0	2.1	2.2	2.3	2.4	2.5	2.6	2.7	2.8	2.9	3.0	3.1	3.2	3.3	3.4	3.5	(3.6)	3.7	3.8	3.9	4.0

MCAT® Total Numeric Score 9 10 11 12 13 14 15 16 17 18 19 20 21 22 23 24 25 26 27 28 (29) 30 31 (32) 33 34 35 36 37 38 39 40 41 42 43

Writing Sample			J	K	L	M	N	O	(P)	Q	R	S	T
Verbal Reasoning	3	4	5	6	7	8	(9)	(10)	11	12	13	14	15
Biological Sciences	3	4	5	6	7	8	9	(10)	(11)	12	13	14	15
Physical Sciences	3	4	5	6	7	8	9	(10)	(11)	12	13	14	15

Acceptance & Matriculation Data for 2008–2009 First Year Class

	Resident	Non-resident	International	Total
Applications	458	865	13	1336
Interviewed	337	209	2	548
Deferred	0	0	0	0
Matriculants				
Early Assurance Program	0	0	0	0
Early Decision Program	0	0	0	0
Baccalaureate/M.D.	n/a	n/a	n/a	n/a
M.D./Ph.D.	9	13	0	22
Matriculated	81	21	0	**102**

Applications accepted from International Applicants: Yes

Matriculant Demographics: 2008–2009 First Year Class

Men: 66   **Women:** 36

Matriculants' Self-Reported Race/Ethnicity

Mexican American	5	Korean	2
Cuban	0	Vietnamese	3
Puerto Rican	0	Other Asian	3
Other Hispanic	5	Total Asian	20
Total Hispanic	8	Native American	3
Chinese	3	Black	1
Asian Indian	4	Native Hawaiian	4
Pakistani	1	White	82
Filipino	4	Unduplicated Number	
Japanese	3	of Matriculants	102

Science and Math Majors: 61%
Matriculants with:
    Baccalaureate degree: 97%
    Graduate degree(s): 14%

Specialty Choice

2004, 2005, 2006 Graduates, Specialty Choice (As reported by program directors to GME Track™)

Anesthesiology	13%
Emergency Medicine	13%
Family Practice	11%
Internal Medicine	9%
Obstetrics/Gynecology	2%
Orthopaedic Surgery	4%
Pediatrics	13%
Psychiatry	2%
Radiology	4%
Surgery	5%

Financial Information

Source: 2007–2008 LCME I-B survey and 2008–2009 AAMC TSF questionnaire

	Residents	Non-residents
Total Cost of Attendance	$39,494	$58,400
Tuition and Fees	$21,934	$40,840
Other (includes living expenses)	$17,560	$17,560
Health Insurance (can be waived)	$0	$0

Average 2008 Graduate Indebtedness: $132,170
% of Enrolled Students Receiving Aid: 94%

Criminal Background Check

This medical school requires a criminal background check prior to matriculation.

University of Vermont College of Medicine

Burlington, Vermont

The University of Vermont College of Medicine
Office of Admissions, E215 Given Building
89 Beaumont Avenue
Burlington, Vermont 05405
T 802 656 2154   F 802 656 9663

Admissions www.med.uvm.edu/Admissions
Main www.med.uvm.edu
Financial www.uvm.edu/financialaid
E-mail medadmissions@uvm.edu

Public Institution

Dr. Frederick C. Morin III, Dean

Dr. Janice M. Gallant, Associate Dean for Admissions

Dr. Karen Richardson-Nassif, Associate Dean for Faculty and Staff Development and Diversity

Dr. G. Scott Waterman, Associate Dean for Student Affairs

Tiffany Delaney, Director of Admissions

General Information

The University of Vermont College of Medicine is located in Burlington, Vermont, (pop. 40,000). Established in 1822, it is the seventh oldest medical school in the U.S. The education of students remains the principal mission of the College, with teaching hospital partner Fletcher Allen Health Care, adjacent to the College in Burlington. A 100,000-square-foot Medical Education Center and Ambulatory Care Center opened in Fall 2005 to serve the College's 400 medical students, 275 residents, and support care for a population base of over 1 million people.

Mission Statement

The overarching goal of our educational program is to provide our students with a knowledge base that will allow them to practice the science and art of medicine in a framework that offers a foundation for lifelong learning.

Curricular Highlights

Community Service Requirement: Required.
Research/Thesis Requirement: Optional.

The Vermont Integrated Curriculum (VIC) progresses from the study of Foundations of Medicine, both clinical and basic science, to applications in Clinical Clerkship, to senior scholarship and supervised patient management in Advanced Integration. Areas of focus include progressive skill development, health care systems, preventive care, and a greater understanding of applied sciences, particularly genetics, ethics and epidemiology. VIC also places emphasis on professionalism, cultural competency, scholarly research, teaching skills, and community service.

USMLE

Step 1: Required. Students must record a passing score for graduation, but not promotion.
Step 2: Clinical Skills (CS): Required. Students must record a passing total score to graduate.
Step 2: Clinical Knowledge (CK): Required. Students must record a passing total score to graduate.

Selection Factors

The Committee on Admissions seeks a diverse student body. We look for evidence of excellence accompanied by genuine concern for the welfare of others. Effective interpersonal skills are important, and successful applicants often have a history of service to the community. Selection is based upon a past pattern of academic performance plus an assessment of the applicant's fitness for the study and practice of medicine in terms of aptitude, interests, experience, motivation, leadership abilities, and maturity. Letters of recommendation and a personal interview are required and form an important part of the application process. Students from groups underrepresented in medicine are encouraged to apply. The University of Vermont does not discriminate on the basis of race, color, sex, sexual orientation, religion, age, handicap, national origin, or Vietnam veteran status.

Financial Aid

Financial aid funds are distributed according to relative need for both in- and out-of-state students. Entering students are considered for awards on the same basis as those already enrolled. An applicant's financial status has no bearing on the admission determination.

Information about Diversity Programs

The College of Medicine strongly encourages applications from those who have the potential to increase the overall diversity of the class based on a variety of factors such as economic hardship, first generation college graduates, race, and cultural background.

Campus Information

Setting

Located in Burlington, recently named "the healthiest city in America", the University of Vermont College of Medicine, in partnership with Fletcher Allen Health Care, comprises the only academic medical center in the state. Burlington is a vibrant community located on the shores of Lake Champlain, between the Adirondack and Green Mountains. With year-round recreational opportunities, this progressive community has been frequently cited as one of the most livable cities in the U.S. Boston and New York are both within a half-day's drive, and Montreal is just 100 miles north of campus.

Enrollment

For 2008, total enrollment was: 402

Special Features

The University of Vermont College of Medicine is known for innovations in instructional technology and was honored in 2007 by Campus Technology magazine. All of the advances in technology aim to help our students bridge distance and time and to make learning more interactive, engaging, and effective.

Housing

While the college does offer limited campus housing options, the majority of medical students find rooms, apartments or houses in the surrounding area via a housing list maintained by the college. Many housing opportunities are within easy walking or bicycling distance from campus.

Satellite Campuses/Facilities

Students have the opportunity to serve clinical rotations at Fletcher Allen Health Care, our affiliated hospital in Burlington, as well as practice sites in Vermont.

Application Process and Requirements 2010–2011

Primary Application Service: AMCAS
Earliest filing date: June 1, 2009
Latest filing date: November 1, 2009

Secondary Application Required?: Yes
Sent to: All Applicants
Contact: Admissions Office,
(802) 656-2154, medadmissions@uvm.edu
Fee: Yes, $85
Fee waiver available: Yes
Earliest filing date: June 15, 2009
Latest filing date: December 30, 2009

MCAT® required?: Yes
Latest MCAT® considered: September 2009
Oldest MCAT® considered: December 2006

Early Decision Program: School does have EDP
Applicants notified: October 1, 2009
EDP available for: Both Residents
and Non-residents

Regular Acceptance Notice
Earliest date: October 16, 2009
Latest date: Until class is full
Applicant's Response to Acceptance
Offer – Maximum Time: Two weeks

Requests for Deferred
Entrance Considered: Yes

Deposit to Hold Place in Class: Yes
Deposit (Resident): $100
Deposit (Non-resident): $100
Deposit due: With response to acceptance offer
Applied to tuition: Yes
Deposit refundable: Yes
Refundable by: May 15, 2010

Estimated number of new entrants: 114
EDP: 5, special program: 4

Start Month/Year: August 2010

Interview Format: Campus interview with admissions committee member. Regional interviews are not available.

Other Programs

PREPARATORY PROGRAMS
Postbaccalaureate Program: Yes
http://learn.uvm.edu/?Page=postbac.html

COMBINED DEGREE PROGRAMS
Baccalaureate/M.D.: No
M.D./M.P.H.: No
M.D./M.B.A.: No
M.D./J.D.: No
M.D./Ph.D.: Yes, www.med.uvm.edu/mdphd

Premedical Coursework

Course	Req.	Rec.	Lab.	Hrs.
Inorganic Chemistry	•		•	8
Behavioral Sciences		•		
Biochemistry		•		4
Biology	•		•	8
Biology/Zoology				
Calculus				
College English		•		
College Mathematics		•		

Course	Req.	Rec.	Lab.	Hrs.
Computer Science				
Genetics		•		4
Humanities		•		
Organic Chemistry	•		•	8
Physics	•		•	8
Psychology				
Social Sciences		•		
Other				

Selection Factors: 2008 Accepted Applicants

Proportion of Accepted Applicants with Relevant Experience (Data Self-Reported to AMCAS)		
Community Service/Volunteer		77%
Medically-Related Work		88%
Research		82%

Shaded bar represents school's accepted scores ranging from the 10th percentile to the 90th percentile   School Median ○   National Median ○

Overall GPA 2.0 2.1 2.2 2.3 2.4 2.5 2.6 2.7 2.8 2.9 3.0 3.1 3.2 3.3 3.4 3.5 3.6 3.7 (3.8) 3.9 4.0
Science GPA 2.0 2.1 2.2 2.3 2.4 2.5 2.6 2.7 2.8 2.9 3.0 3.1 3.2 3.3 3.4 3.5 3.6 (3.7) 3.8 3.9 4.0

MCAT® Total Numeric Score 9 10 11 12 13 14 15 16 17 18 19 20 21 22 23 24 25 26 27 28 29 30 (31) 32 33 34 35 36 37 38 39 40 41 42 43

Writing Sample			J	K	L	M	N	O	P	(Q)	R	S	T
Verbal Reasoning	3	4	5	6	7	8	9	(10)	11	12	13	14	15
Biological Sciences	3	4	5	6	7	8	9	10	(11)	12	13	14	15
Physical Sciences	3	4	5	6	7	8	9	(10)	(11)	12	13	14	15

Acceptance & Matriculation Data for 2008–2009 First Year Class

	Resident	Non-resident	International	Total
Applications	91	5289	392	5772
Interviewed	63	556	28	647
Deferred	2	1	1	4
Matriculants				
Early Assurance Program	n/a	n/a	n/a	n/a
Early Decision Program	4	0	0	4
Baccalaureate/M.D.	n/a	n/a	n/a	n/a
M.D./Ph.D.	3	1	0	4
Matriculated	34	74	3	**111**

Applications accepted from International Applicants: No

Matriculant Demographics: 2008–2009 First Year Class

Men: 54   **Women:** 57

Matriculants' Self-Reported Race/Ethnicity

Mexican American	0	**Korean**	1
Cuban	0	**Vietnamese**	1
Puerto Rican	1	**Other Asian**	3
Other Hispanic	7	**Total Asian**	14
Total Hispanic	8	**Native American**	0
Chinese	5	**Black**	2
Asian Indian	2	**Native Hawaiian**	1
Pakistani	0	**White**	92
Filipino	2	**Unduplicated Number**	
Japanese	0	**of Matriculants**	111

Science and Math Majors: 60%
Matriculants with:
Baccalaureate degree: 100%
Graduate degree(s): 14%

Specialty Choice

2004, 2005, 2006 Graduates, Specialty Choice (As reported by program directors to GME Track™)	
Anesthesiology	6%
Emergency Medicine	9%
Family Practice	6%
Internal Medicine	19%
Obstetrics/Gynecology	7%
Orthopaedic Surgery	2%
Pediatrics	16%
Psychiatry	3%
Radiology	6%
Surgery	6%

Financial Information

Source: 2007–2008 LCME I-B survey and 2008–2009 AAMC TSF questionnaire

	Residents	Non-residents
Total Cost of Attendance	$47,597	$68,153
Tuition and Fees	$28,470	$48,490
Other (includes living expenses)	$19,127	$19,663
Health Insurance (can be waived)	$0	$0

Average 2008 Graduate Indebtedness: $140,553
% of Enrolled Students Receiving Aid: 88%

Criminal Background Check

This medical school requires a criminal background check prior to matriculation.

Eastern Virginia Medical School
Norfolk, Virginia

Office of Admissions
Eastern Virginia Medical School
700 W. Olney Road
Norfolk, Virginia 23507-1607
T 757 446 5812   **F** 757 446 5896

Admissions www.evms.edu/admissions
Main www.evms.edu
Financial www.evms.edu/students/
fin-aid/budgets/md.html
E-mail mclendm@evms.edu

Public Institution

Dr. Gerald J. Pepe, Dean and Provost

*Dr. Michael J. Solhaug,
Associate Dean for Admissions*

*Gail C. Williams, Assistant Dean for Student
Affairs and Director of Minority Affairs*

Michelle D. Byers, Director of Financial Aid

Susan L. Castora, Director of Admissions

General Information

Established in 1973 to enhance the quality and diversity of health care throughout the Hampton Roads region, the mission of EVMS is deeply rooted in the education and training of primary care physicians, arming them with the requisite scientific, academic, and humanistic skills most relevant to today's practice of medicine. EVMS provides health care for more than one quarter of Virginia's population as well as neighboring regions of North Carolina.

Mission Statement

EVMS is a public institution dedicated to medical and health education, biomedical research, and the enhancement of health care in the Commonwealth of Virginia.

Curricular Highlights

Community Service Requirement: Optional.
Research/Thesis Requirement: Optional.

The first two years focus on clinical medicine through two vehicles: the Theresa A. Thomas Professional Skills Teaching and Assessment Center and a Longitudinal Mentorship with a generalist physician in community practice. Careful coordination between basic sciences and generalist disciplines permits an integrated curriculum. Weekly small-group sessions introduce students to clinical problem-solving. This early introduction to clinical medicine teaches medical history-taking and physical examination along with the application of basic science knowledge to patient care. Third-year clinical clerkships focus on ambulatory care in community-based sites in balance with inpatient care experiences. In addition to the required clerkships are rotations in substance abuse, geriatrics, and surgical subspecialties.

For those interested in generalist medicine, electives are offered in special populations and rural health care, and an elective honors track in generalist medicine. Elective opportunities are available for those interested in research or subspecialty care. Students are graded as Honors, High Pass, Pass, or Fail.

USMLE

Step 1: Required. Students must record a passing score for promotion.
Step 2: Clinical Skills (CS): Required. Students must record a passing total score to graduate.
Step 2: Clinical Knowledge (CK): Required. Students must record a passing total score to graduate.

Selection Factors

EVMS does not discriminate on the basis of sex, race, creed, age, national origin, marital status, or handicap. A supplementary application packet is sent to those applicants receiving a favorable initial screening of their completed AMCAS application. The Admissions Committee considers the entire academic record, including science and overall GPA, MCAT scores, exposure to the medical field, maturity, character, and motivation. The application fee will be waived if a fee waiver is granted by AMCAS. Preference is given to legal residents of Virginia. EVMS seeks persons with personal and background traits that indicate a high potential for becoming a primary care physician. Applicants who have completed one or more years in a medical school accredited by the LCME can be considered for transfer into the second or third year only to fill vacancies that may arise with the withdrawal of previously enrolled students. All transfers must meet the requirements stated for general admission.

Financial Aid

Scholarships are limited. Loans constitute the majority of aid received. Students may fully meet the costs of medical school at EVMS, providing they meet all federal criteria, meet citizenship requirements, are creditworthy, and maintain satisfactory academic progress. Federal scholarships are available for those interested in primary care. The Tuition Assistance Grant Program provides annual grants for state residents. Applicants for financial assistance must file the FAFSA and other additional required forms.

Information about Diversity Programs

EVMS is committed to producing a diverse physician workforce to meet the health care needs of the region. Applicants from rural or other underserved regions and those who have been disadvantaged or underrepresented for economic, racial, or social reasons, and who possess the motivation and aptitude required for the study of medicine are strongly encouraged to apply.

Campus Information

Setting
The EVMS complex includes the Children's Hospital of the King's Daughters and Sentara Norfolk General Hospital. The campus is minutes from downtown shopping areas and cultural attractions.

Enrollment
For 2008, total enrollment was: 445

Special Features
EVMS has numerous Centers of Excellence including the world-renowned Jones Institute for Reproductive Medicine, the Strelitz Diabetes Institute, and the Glennan Center for Geriatric Medicine. The Theresa A. Thomas Professional Skills Teaching and Assessment Center is a leader in the use and training of standardized patients for assessing medical competencies of our students and residents, as well as those from institutes around the world.

Housing
EVMS's Hague Club Apartments offers one- and two-bedroom apartments. Additional housing is located in nearby neighborhoods.

Satellite Campuses/Facilities
EVMS partners with 33 local area hospitals, including Sentara Norfolk General Hospital, the Children's Hospital of the King's Daughters, the U.S. Naval Medical Center in Portsmouth, and the Veterans Affairs Hospital in Hampton.

Application Process and Requirements 2010–2011

Primary Application Service: AMCAS
Earliest filing date: June 1, 2009
Latest filing date: November 15, 2009

Secondary Application Required?: Yes
Sent to: Screened applicants
URL: www.evms.edu/admissions
Fee: Yes, $100
Fee waiver available: Yes
Earliest filing date: July 2009
Latest filing date: January 2010

MCAT® required?: Yes
Latest MCAT® considered: September 2009
Oldest MCAT® considered: 2006

Early Decision Program: School does have EDP
Applicants notified: October 1, 2009
EDP available for: Both Residents and Non-residents

Regular Acceptance Notice
Earliest date: October 15, 2009
Latest date: Until class is full
Applicant's Response to Acceptance
Offer – Maximum Time: Two weeks

Requests for Deferred
Entrance Considered: Yes

Deposit to Hold Place in Class: Yes
Deposit (Resident): $100
Deposit (Non-resident): $100
Deposit due: With response to acceptance offer
Applied to tuition: Yes
Deposit refundable: Yes
Refundable by: May 15, 2010

Estimated number of new entrants: 115
EDP: 2, special program: n/a

Start Month/Year: August 2010

Interview Format: Panel interviews. Regional interviews are not available.

Other Programs

PREPARATORY PROGRAMS
Postbaccalaureate Program: Yes,
www.evms.edu/hlthprof/ms-bio-medical/index.html
Summer Program: No

COMBINED DEGREE PROGRAMS
Baccalaureate/M.D.: Yes
M.D./M.P.H.: Yes,
www.evms.edu/education/joint-md-mph.html
M.D./M.B.A.: No
M.D./J.D.: No
M.D./Ph.D.: No

Premedical Coursework

Course	Req.	Rec.	Lab.	Sems.	Course	Req.	Rec.	Lab.	Sems.
Inorganic Chemistry	•		•	2	Computer Science				
Behavioral Sciences					Genetics				
Biochemistry					Humanities				
Biology	•		•	2	Organic Chemistry	•		•	2
Biology/Zoology					Physics	•		•	2
Calculus					Psychology				
College English					Social Sciences				
College Mathematics					Other				

Selection Factors: 2008 Accepted Applicants

Proportion of Accepted Applicants with Relevant Experience (Data Self-Reported to AMCAS®)		Community Service/Volunteer	72%
		Medically-Related Work	90%
		Research	75%

Shaded bar represents school's accepted scores ranging from the 10th percentile to the 90th percentile ● **School Median** ● **National Median**

Overall GPA 2.0 2.1 2.2 2.3 2.4 2.5 2.6 2.7 2.8 2.9 3.0 3.1 **3.2 3.3 3.4 3.5 (3.6) 3.7 3.8 3.9** 4.0
Science GPA 2.0 2.1 2.2 2.3 2.4 2.5 2.6 2.7 2.8 2.9 3.0 **3.1 3.2 3.3 3.4 (3.5) 3.6 3.7 3.8 3.9** 4.0

MCAT® Total Numeric Score 9 10 11 12 13 14 15 16 17 18 19 20 21 22 23 24 25 26 27 **28 29 30 (31) 32 33 34 35** 36 37 38 39 40 41 42 43

Writing Sample			J	K	L	M	N	O	P	(Q)	R	S	T
Verbal Reasoning	3	4	5	6	7	8	9	(10)	11	12	13	14	15
Biological Sciences	3	4	5	6	7	8	9	10	(11)	12	13	14	15
Physical Sciences	3	4	5	6	7	8	9	(10)	(11)	12	13	14	15

Acceptance & Matriculation Data for 2008–2009 First Year Class

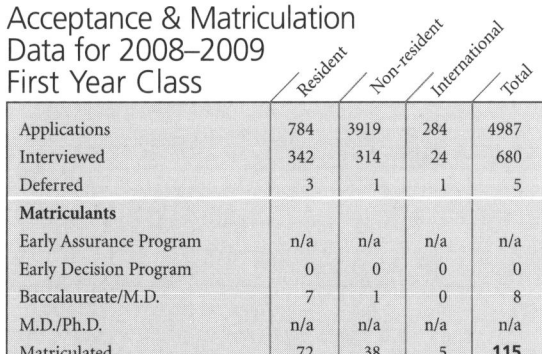

	Resident	Non-resident	International	Total
Applications	784	3919	284	4987
Interviewed	342	314	24	680
Deferred	3	1	1	5
Matriculants				
Early Assurance Program	n/a	n/a	n/a	n/a
Early Decision Program	0	0	0	0
Baccalaureate/M.D.	7	1	0	8
M.D./Ph.D.	n/a	n/a	n/a	n/a
Matriculated	72	38	5	**115**

Applications accepted from International Applicants: Yes

Specialty Choice

2004, 2005, 2006 Graduates, Specialty Choice (As reported by program directors to GME Track™)	
Anesthesiology	3%
Emergency Medicine	11%
Family Practice	10%
Internal Medicine	20%
Obstetrics/Gynecology	5%
Orthopaedic Surgery	2%
Pediatrics	16%
Psychiatry	3%
Radiology	5%
Surgery	6%

Matriculant Demographics: 2008–2009 First Year Class

Men: 65   **Women:** 50

Matriculants' Self-Reported Race/Ethnicity

Mexican American	2	**Korean**	2
Cuban	0	**Vietnamese**	3
Puerto Rican	1	**Other Asian**	5
Other Hispanic	1	**Total Asian**	22
Total Hispanic	4	**Native American**	1
Chinese	5	**Black**	3
Asian Indian	4	**Native Hawaiian**	0
Pakistani	2	**White**	78
Filipino	1	**Unduplicated Number**	
Japanese	0	**of Matriculants**	115

Science and Math Majors: 74%
Matriculants with:
   Baccalaureate degree: 99%
   Graduate degree(s): 24%

Financial Information

Source: 2007–2008 LCME I-B survey and 2008–2009 AAMC TSF questionnaire

	Residents	Non-residents
Total Cost of Attendance	$43,398	$63,746
Tuition and Fees	$25,196	$45,544
Other (includes living expenses)	$15,825	$15,825
Health Insurance (can be waived)	$2,377	$2,377

Average 2008 Graduate Indebtedness: $144,721
% of Enrolled Students Receiving Aid: 90%

Criminal Background Check

This medical school requires a criminal background check prior to matriculation.

University of Virginia School of Medicine

Charlottesville, Virginia

Medical School Admissions Office
PO Box 800725
University of Virginia School of Medicine
Charlottesville, Virginia 22908
T 434 924 5571   F 434 982 2586

Admissions www.healthsystem.virginia.edu/internet/admissions
Main www.healthsystem.virginia.edu/internet/som
Financial www.healthsystem.virginia.edu/internet/financial-aid
E-mail medsch-adm@virginia.edu

Public Institution

Dr. Steven T. DeKosky, Vice President and Dean, School of Medicine

Dr. R.J. Canterbury, Associate Dean for Admissions

Dr. Norman Oliver, Associate Dean for Diversity

Nancy Zimmer, Director of Financial Aid

Lesley L. Thomas, Director of Admissions

General Information

The University of Virginia School of Medicine was opened for instruction in 1825, making it one of the oldest medical schools in the South. Both the School of Medicine and the University of Virginia Hospital are located on the grounds of the University of Virginia in Charlottesville.

Mission Statement

The mission of the University of Virginia School of Medicine is: to educate students to fulfill the need for practitioners and scientists; to provide cost-effective, high-quality patient care at primary, secondary, and tertiary levels; to produce new knowledge required to advance health by conducting research; and, to provide public service as needed by citizens or by public jurisdictions.

Curricular Highlights

Community Service Requirement: Required. Community service learning activities in Year 1.
Research/Thesis Requirement: Optional. A thesis is required for Generalist Scholars only.

The University of Virginia curriculum integrates scientific knowledge, clinical care, and research throughout the entire four years of medical school. The cornerstone of the curriculum is clinical problem solving with the focus on the patient and the physician–patient relationship. Lectures (never more than half a day), self-study from course syllabi and computer-aided instruction provide the factual content necessary for problem solving. Students have three or four afternoons free each week in years 1 and 2 for productive self-study or elective activities. Small-group activities maximize interactions between students and faculty. Basic science concepts are presented in the context of clinical cases. The Practice of Medicine course in years 1 and 2 teaches professionalism, interviewing skills, physical diagnosis, and ethics in small groups. The elective program of the fourth year offers students the opportunity to pursue their own interests. An innovative clerkship model allows students to tailor their clinical experience to meet their particular interests and needs. Students may choose from a wide variety of electives, including clinical experience, graduate courses, and research activities.

USMLE

Step 1: Required. Students must record a passing score for promotion.
Step 2: Clinical Skills (CS): Required. Students must record a passing total score to graduate.
Step 2: Clinical Knowledge (CK): Required. Students must record a passing total score to graduate.

Selection Factors

All applicants must have completed at least 90 semester hours of course work in a U.S. or Canadian college or university. The Committee on Admissions does not discriminate on the basis of race, gender, sexual preference, creed, national origin, age, or disability. Grades, MCAT scores, work and volunteer experience, letters of recommendation, and the interview influence committee decisions.

Financial Aid

In addition to Federal Stafford Loans, the University of Virginia School of Medicine provides robust school-funded scholarships and loans to students who demonstrate need via the Free Application for Federal Student Aid (FAFSA). Parental financial information is required for all applicants who wish to receive aid from school funds. Student employment is not encouraged. Financial aid applications are available online on January 1 or immediately after acceptance.

Information about Diversity Programs

The University of Virginia encourages applications from qualified applicants from groups that are underrepresented in medicine. Systems in place to facilitate preparation and success of students include: (1) a six-week summer enrichment program; (2) extensive tutorial and other academic support programs upon admission; and (3) need-based and merit-based financial assistance. For more information, please contact Dr. Norm Oliver, Associate Dean for Diversity, at mno3p@virginia.edu.

Campus Information

Setting

The University of Virginia Health System is one of the nation's 100 Top Hospitals with state-of-the-art emergency, operating, and labor and delivery rooms. The medical center is located in the heart of Charlottesville, with significant historical sites located nearby, including Thomas Jefferson's Monticello.

Enrollment

For 2008, total enrollment was: 569

Special Features

The University of Virginia Health System includes the School of Medicine, the University Hospital, and other special centers of excellence, including the Heart Center, Kidney Center, Digestive Health Center, Cancer Center, Transplant Center, and Primary Care Center. As part of its Global Health Initiative, UVA has twenty-seven sites in developing countries around the world where students are encouraged to participate in direct patient care, public health services, health education and/or research activities.

Housing

Most medical students choose to live in the community close by the medical school and hospital. There are ample housing opportunities in the area, with rents ranging from $300 to $800 per month.

Satellite Campuses/Facilities

During the third-year clinical clerkships, students will spend approximately half their time at the University Health System. They also spend an average of 20 weeks at the Roanoke Memorial Hospital in Roanoke, VA, the Salem Veterans Affairs Hospital, and the Fairfax INOVA Hospital in Fairfax, VA. Housing and meals are provided at offsite clinical locations.

Application Process and Requirements 2010–2011

Primary Application Service: AMCAS
Earliest filing date: June 1, 2009
Latest filing date: November 1, 2009

Secondary Application Required?: Yes
Sent to: All applicants
Contact: Lesley L. Thomas, J.D., (434) 924-5571, llt6p@virginia.edu
Fee: Yes, $80
Fee waiver available: Yes
Earliest filing date: June 1, 2009
Latest filing date: January 4, 2010

MCAT® required?: Yes
Latest MCAT® considered: September 2009
Oldest MCAT® considered: April 2007

Early Decision Program: School does not have EDP
Applicants notified: n/a
EDP available for: n/a

Regular Acceptance Notice
Earliest date: October 16, 2009
Latest date: Until class is full
Applicant's Response to Acceptance Offer – Maximum Time: Three weeks

Requests for Deferred Entrance Considered: Yes

Deposit to Hold Place in Class: No
Deposit (Resident): n/a
Deposit (Non-resident): n/a
Deposit due: n/a
Applied to tuition: n/a
Deposit refundable: n/a
Refundable by: n/a

Estimated number of new entrants: 148
EDP: n/a, special program: n/a

Start Month/Year: August 2010

Interview Format: Two one-on-one, half-hour interviews. Regional interviews are not available.

Other Programs

PREPARATORY PROGRAMS
Postbaccalaureate Program: Yes, www.uvapostbacpremed.info postbacpremed@virginia.edu
Summer Program: Yes, www.healthsystem.virginia.edu/internet/academic-support/maap1-A.cfm

COMBINED DEGREE PROGRAMS
Baccalaureate/M.D.: No
M.D./M.P.H.: Yes, www.healthsystem.virginia.edu/internet/phs/mph/jointmdmph.cfm
M.D./M.B.A.: Yes
M.D./J.D.: No
M.D./Ph.D.: Yes, www.healthsystem.virginia.edu/internet/mstp/
Additional Program: Yes, www.healthsystem.virginia.edu/internet/bio-ethics/MABioethics.cfm

Premedical Coursework

Course	Req.	Rec.	Lab.	Sems.	Course	Req.	Rec.	Lab.	Sems.
Inorganic Chemistry	•		•	2	Computer Science				
Behavioral Sciences					Genetics				
Biochemistry		•			Humanities				
Biology	•		•	2	Organic Chemistry	•		•	2
Biology/Zoology					Physics	•		•	2
Calculus					Psychology				
College English					Social Sciences				
College Mathematics					Other				

Selection Factors: 2008 Accepted Applicants

Proportion of Accepted Applicants with Relevant Experience (Data Self-Reported to AMCAS)

Community Service/Volunteer	69%
Medically-Related Work	90%
Research	87%

Shaded bar represents school's accepted scores ranging from the 10th percentile to the 90th percentile. School Median ● National Median ●

Overall GPA 2.0 2.1 2.2 2.3 2.4 2.5 2.6 2.7 2.8 2.9 3.0 3.1 3.2 3.3 3.4 3.5 3.6 3.7 (3.8) 3.9 4.0
Science GPA 2.0 2.1 2.2 2.3 2.4 2.5 2.6 2.7 2.8 2.9 3.0 3.1 3.2 3.3 3.4 3.5 3.6 3.7 (3.8) 3.9 4.0

MCAT® Total Numeric Score 9 10 11 12 13 14 15 16 17 18 19 20 21 22 23 24 25 26 27 28 29 30 31 (32)(33)(34) 35 36 37 38 39 40 41 42 43

Writing Sample			J	K	L	M	N	O	P	(Q)	R	S	T
Verbal Reasoning	3	4	5	6	7	8	9	(10)	(11)	12	13	14	15
Biological Sciences	3	4	5	6	7	8	9	10	(11)	(12)	13	14	15
Physical Sciences	3	4	5	6	7	8	9	10	(11)	(12)	13	14	15

Acceptance & Matriculation Data for 2008–2009 First Year Class

	Resident	Non-resident	International	Total
Applications	736	3418	148	4302
Interviewed	186	337	25	548
Deferred	2	2	0	4
Matriculants				
Early Assurance Program	0	0	0	0
Early Decision Program	0	0	0	0
Baccalaureate/M.D.	n/a	n/a	n/a	n/a
M.D./Ph.D.	1	7	0	8
Matriculated	77	65	3	**145**

Applications accepted from International Applicants: Yes

Matriculant Demographics: 2008–2009 First Year Class

Men: 80   **Women:** 65

Matriculants' Self-Reported Race/Ethnicity

Mexican American	2	Korean	2
Cuban	3	Vietnamese	2
Puerto Rican	2	Other Asian	3
Other Hispanic	9	Total Asian	25
Total Hispanic	16	Native American	1
Chinese	8	Black	11
Asian Indian	8	Native Hawaiian	0
Pakistani	1	White	107
Filipino	2	Unduplicated Number	
Japanese	1	of Matriculants	145

Science and Math Majors: 66%
Matriculants with:
Baccalaureate degree: 100%
Graduate degree(s): 6%

Specialty Choice

2004, 2005, 2006 Graduates, Specialty Choice (As reported by program directors to GME Track™)

Anesthesiology	6%
Emergency Medicine	7%
Family Practice	8%
Internal Medicine	19%
Obstetrics/Gynecology	5%
Orthopaedic Surgery	4%
Pediatrics	12%
Psychiatry	4%
Radiology	6%
Surgery	5%

Financial Information

Source: 2007–2008 LCME I-B survey and 2008–2009 AAMC TSF questionnaire

	Residents	Non-residents
Total Cost of Attendance	$52,021	$62,021
Tuition and Fees	$32,650	$42,650
Other (includes living expenses)	$17,395	$17,395
Health Insurance (can be waived)	$1,976	$1,976

Average 2008 Graduate Indebtedness: $118,329
% of Enrolled Students Receiving Aid: 91%

Criminal Background Check

This medical school requires a criminal background check prior to matriculation.

Virginia Commonwealth University School of Medicine

Richmond, Virginia

Virginia Commonwealth University
School of Medicine
P.O. Box 980565
Richmond, Virginia 23298-0565
T 804 828 9629   **F** 804 828 1246

Admissions www.medschool.vcu.edu
Main www.medschool.vcu.edu
Financial www.medschool.vcu.edu/finaid/
financial.html
E-mail somume@vcu.edu

Public Institution

Dr. Jerome F. Strauss III, Dean

Dr. Michelle Whitehurst-Cook, Associate Dean for Admissions

Donna Jackson, Director of Student Outreach Programs

Dr. Glenda Palmer, Asst. Dean of Student Affairs/Dir. of Financial Aid

Agnes L. Mack, Director of Admissions

General Information

The School of Medicine, which has been in continuous operation since 1838, is the founding institution of Virginia Commonwealth University. The vitality of VCU's clinical, educational, and research programs is reflected in the caliber of its faculty, the success of its patient care programs, and the level of research funding.

Mission Statement

The mission of the School of Medicine is constant improvement of the quality of health care for citizens of Virginia, using innovative, scholarly activity to create new knowledge, to provide better systems of medical education, and to develop more effective health care methods. The primary aim of the School of Medicine is to provide a diverse academic environment appropriate for the education of its students and continuing education directed toward the needs of practicing physicians.

Curricular Highlights

Community Service Requirement: Optional.
Research/Thesis Requirement: Optional.

The first year is spent studying normal structure and function in a traditional discipline format. The second year emphasizes the pathogenesis of disease and its manifestations and is taught in an organ system manner. Pathogenesis, pathology, pharmacology, and the major manifestations and principles of management are discussed in each of the major body systems. In the longitudinal clinical experience for first- and second-year students, students spend two afternoons per month in a small group learning the fundamentals of clinical medicine. This is supplemented by a clinical experience in the office of a primary care physician two afternoons per month. The clinical experience is integrated with the basic sciences in a way that enhances and enriches students' learning. There is a computer lab with over 40 workstations and a full array of commercial and in-house, faculty-developed educational software. Third-year rotations are at the University and Veterans Affairs Hospitals, with ambulatory care rotations at non-university primary care sites. A select number of students will complete the third and fourth years at the Inova campus in Northern Virginia. The fourth year is primarily elective time with two required rotations.

USMLE

Step 1: Required. Students must record a passing score for promotion.
Step 2: Clinical Skills (CS): Required. Students must record a passing score in each section to graduate.
Step 2: Clinical Knowledge (CK): Required. Students must record a passing score in each section to graduate.

Selection Factors

Applicants are selected on the basis of their potential as prospective physicians as well as students of medicine. Attributes of character, personality factors, academic skills, and exposure to medicine are considered along with academic performance, GPA, MCAT scores, letters of recommendation, and personal interviews at the School of Medicine.

Financial Aid

Assistance to students in meeting the cost of their medical education is available in the form of loans and scholarship. Financial counseling is done through the School of Medicine Financial Aid Office. The FAFSA (Free Application for Federal Student Aid) is required of all students who want aid. For need-based scholarship and grant aid the NeedAccess online form should be completed. This information is used to award grants from the Department of Health and Human Services and institutional need-based aid. Completion of these forms will allow the Financial Aid Office to give students an accurate picture of what their eligibility for aid will be within 48 hours.

Information about Diversity Programs

The office of Student Outreach Programs endeavors to provide support for the school's diverse population. Student Outreach's objectives are to recruit and retain students from disadvantaged or non-traditional backgrounds to an environment conducive for exchange of ideas where students learn from faculty and peers. The main goal of the program is to provide medical school graduates that will best meet the healthcare needs of the state and nation.

Campus Information

Setting
The school is located in downtown Richmond near cultural, historical, and government centers. The medical education buildings are directly across the street from the main hospital.

Enrollment
For 2008, total enrollment was: 741

Special Features
The 779-bed VCU Health Systems Hospital, including our new critical care tower, has both the largest ER and neonatal intensive care units in the state and is one of the largest university-owned medical centers in the U.S. This facility and the full service Veterans and Inova Fairfax Hospitals afford students an unparalleled clinical experience.

Housing
Single student housing is available on campus. Off-campus housing is plentiful, varied in style, and reasonable in cost and ranges from inner city, suburban to rural.

Satellite Campuses/Facilities
There is a regional campus at Inova Hospital, Fairfax, VA, which is used for third- and fourth-year training.

Application Process and Requirements 2010–2011

Primary Application Service: AMCAS
Earliest filing date: June 1, 2009
Latest filing date: October 15, 2009

Secondary Application Required?: Yes
Sent to: Screened applicants
Contact: Shenia Tyler
(804) 828-9629, shenia.tyler@vcu.edu
Fee: Yes, $80
Fee waiver available: Yes
Earliest filing date: June 1, 2009
Latest filing date: January 26, 2010

MCAT® required?: Yes
Latest MCAT® considered: September 2009
Oldest MCAT® considered: August 2006

Early Decision Program: School does have EDP
Applicants notified: October 1, 2009
EDP available for: Both Residents
and Non-residents

Regular Acceptance Notice
Earliest date: October 16, 2009
Latest date: Until class is full
Applicant's Response to Acceptance
Offer – Maximum Time: Two weeks

Requests for Deferred
Entrance Considered: Yes

Deposit to Hold Place in Class: Yes
Deposit (Resident): $100
Deposit (Non-resident): $100
Deposit due: With response to acceptance offer
Applied to tuition: Yes
Deposit refundable: Yes
Refundable by: May 15, 2010

Estimated number of new entrants: 192
EDP: 5, special program: n/a

Start Month/Year: August 2010

Interview Format: Single, one-on-one interview
Regional interviews are not available.

Other Programs

PREPARATORY PROGRAMS
Postbaccalaureate Program: Yes,
www.medschool.vcu.edu/graduate/premed_cert/
index.html
Summer Program: No,
www.healthdisparities.vcu.edu/workforce/
pipeline.html

COMBINED DEGREE PROGRAMS
Baccalaureate/M.D.: Yes, www.honors.vcu.edu/
M.D./M.P.H.: Yes, www.medschool.vcu.edu/
admissions/mdmph.html
M.D./M.B.A.: No
M.D./J.D.: No
M.D./Ph.D.: Yes, www.vcu.edu/mdphd/
Additional Program: Yes, www.had.vcu.edu
Suzanne Havasy, (804) 828-0719, shavasy@hsc.vcu.edu

Premedical Coursework

Course	Req.	Rec.	Lab.	Sems.	Course	Req.	Rec.	Lab.	Sems.
Inorganic Chemistry	•		•	2	Computer Science				
Behavioral Sciences					Genetics				
Biochemistry					Humanities				
Biology	•		•	2	Organic Chemistry	•		•	2
Biology/Zoology					Physics	•		•	2
Calculus					Psychology				
College English	•			2	Social Sciences				
College Mathematics	•			2	Other				

Selection Factors: 2008 Accepted Applicants

Proportion of Accepted Applicants with Relevant Experience (Data Self-Reported to AMCAS®)		
Community Service/Volunteer	76%
Medically-Related Work	91%
Research	82%

Shaded bar represents school's accepted scores ranging from the 10th percentile to the 90th percentile   **School Median** ● **National Median** ●

Overall GPA	2.0	2.1	2.2	2.3	2.4	2.5	2.6	2.7	2.8	2.9	3.0	3.1	3.2	3.3	3.4	3.5	3.6	(3.7)	3.8	3.9	4.0
Science GPA	2.0	2.1	2.2	2.3	2.4	2.5	2.6	2.7	2.8	2.9	3.0	3.1	3.2	3.3	3.4	3.5	(3.6)	3.7	3.8	3.9	4.0

MCAT® Total Numeric Score 9 10 11 12 13 14 15 16 17 18 19 20 21 22 23 24 25 26 27 28 29 (30) 31 (32) 33 34 35 36 37 38 39 40 41 42 43

Writing Sample			J	K	L	M	N	O	P	(Q)	R	S	T
Verbal Reasoning	3	4	5	6	7	8	9	(10)	11	12	13	14	15
Biological Sciences	3	4	5	6	7	8	9	10	(11)	12	13	14	15
Physical Sciences	3	4	5	6	7	8	9	10	(11)	12	13	14	15

Acceptance & Matriculation Data for 2008–2009 First Year Class

	Resident	Non-resident	International	Total
Applications	824	5213	117	6154
Interviewed	408	448	0	856
Deferred	4	1	0	5
Matriculants				
Early Assurance Program	0	0	0	0
Early Decision Program	1	1	0	2
Baccalaureate/M.D.	8	3	0	11
M.D./Ph.D.	2	4	0	6
Matriculated	108	81	3	**192**

Applications accepted from International Applicants: Only Canadian

Specialty Choice

2004, 2005, 2006 Graduates, Specialty Choice (As reported by program directors to GME Track™)	
Anesthesiology	5%
Emergency Medicine	5%
Family Practice	9%
Internal Medicine	22%
Obstetrics/Gynecology	6%
Orthopaedic Surgery	2%
Pediatrics	12%
Psychiatry	3%
Radiology	7%
Surgery	6%

Matriculant Demographics: 2008–2009 First Year Class

Men: 104   **Women:** 88

Matriculants' Self-Reported Race/Ethnicity

Mexican American	0	**Korean**	7
Cuban	2	**Vietnamese**	7
Puerto Rican	1	**Other Asian**	6
Other Hispanic	0	**Total Asian**	56
Total Hispanic	3	**Native American**	1
Chinese	11	**Black**	8
Asian Indian	26	**Native Hawaiian**	2
Pakistani	1	**White**	122
Filipino	2	**Unduplicated Number**	
Japanese	0	**of Matriculants**	192

Science and Math Majors: 70%
Matriculants with:
Baccalaureate degree: 99%
Graduate degree(s): 18%

Financial Information

Source: 2007–2008 LCME I-B survey
and 2008–2009 AAMC TSF questionnaire

	Residents	Non-residents
Total Cost of Attendance	$54,775	$68,580
Tuition and Fees	$27,720	$41,525
Other (includes living expenses)	$25,050	$25,050
Health Insurance (can be waived)	$2,005	$2,005

Average 2008 Graduate Indebtedness: $153,147
% of Enrolled Students Receiving Aid: 89%

Criminal Background Check

This medical school requires a criminal background check prior to matriculation.

University of Washington School of Medicine

Seattle, Washington

Office of Admissions
Health Sciences Center A-300
Box 356340, University of Washington
Seattle, Washington 98195-6340
T 206 543 7212   F 206 616 3341

Admissions http://uwmedicine.washington.edu/
Education/MDProgram/Admissions
Main http://uwmedicine.washington.edu/
Financial http://uwmedicine.washington.edu/
Education/MDProgram/StudentAffairsAndServices/
FinancialAid
E-mail askuwsom@u.washington.edu

Public Institution

Dr. Paul G. Ramsey, Dean

Dr. Carol C. Teitz, Associate Dean for Admissions

Dr. David Acosta, Associate Dean for Multicultural Affairs

Diane Noecker, Financial Aid Officer

Patricia T. Fero, Director of Admissions

Dr. Peter Eveland, Associate Dean for Student Affairs

General Information

Ranked as the top medical school training primary care physicians for 15 years, and first among public medical schools in federal research funding, the UWSOM is dedicated to improving the health of the public by advancing medical knowledge, providing outstanding primary and specialty care to people of the region, and preparing tomorrow's physicians and scientists. The top-ranked programs in family medicine and rural health are enhanced by volunteer clinical faculty in the WWAMI region who provide community-based medical education in the states of Washington, Wyoming, Alaska, Montana, and Idaho. The UWSOM is committed to building and sustaining a diverse academic community and to assuring that access to education and training is open to all segments of society.

Mission Statement

The UWSOM has a dual mission: 1) meeting the health care needs of our region, especially by recognizing the importance of primary care and providing service to underserved populations, and 2) advancing knowledge and assuming leadership in the biomedical sciences and academic medicine.

Curricular Highlights

Community Service Requirement: Optional.
Research/Thesis Requirement: Required.
Independent Investigative Inquiry is required.

The curriculum in the first two years integrates basic sciences and clinical medicine in both discipline-based and organ-systems courses. Patient contact begins in the first year via com-

munity preceptorships and the Introduction to Clinical Medicine course, administered in a college system. The college groups consist of a faculty mentor who guides 24 students for 4 years in acquiring fundamental clinical skills including physical exam and diagnosis, case presentation and write-up, clinical reasoning, communication with patients and colleagues, and professionalism and ethics. Opportunities range from rural or underserved experiences to bench research. Problem-based learning, observed standardized clinical examinations (OSCE), and special capstone courses provide transitions from 2nd to 3rd year and from 4th year to residency. Required clerkships leave ample time for electives allowing students to identify and develop diverse career interests. Opportunities are provided for a longitudinal interdisciplinary clerkship and for clerkships in communities across the WWAMI region, as well as international electives. Certificate programs include the Indian Health, Global Health, Hispanic Health and Underserved Pathways.

USMLE

Step 1: Required. Students must record a passing score for promotion.
Step 2: Clinical Skills (CS): Required. Students must record a passing total score to graduate.
Step 2: Clinical Knowledge (CK): Required. Students must record a passing total score to graduate.

Selection Factors

Candidates are considered on the basis of motivation, maturity, integrity, and academic performance. Demonstrated humanitarian qualities, community service, ability to communicate with and relate to a diverse group of individuals, as well as knowledge of issues in health care, ability to think analytically, and intellectual curiosity are important considerations. At least 40 hours of M.D. shadowing is expected. Strong preference is given to residents of the WWAMI states; less than 5% of the class is from outside the WWAMI region. Applicants with a demonstrated interest in research may apply for the M.D./Ph.D. program (MSTP) regardless of residency. Only U.S. citizens or permanent residents are considered for either program. Competitive candidates are asked to send additional materials. Matriculation is contingent

on the outcome of a criminal background check initiated upon acceptance. Candidates may apply no more than 3 times. Prerequisites have changed for the entering class of 2010.

Financial Aid

Financial status has no bearing on admission. All applicants for aid must submit data for an analysis of need through FAFSA. Applications are available in January. The application deadline of February 28 must be met, regardless of admission status, in order to receive highest priority for aid; applicants should apply on line (*www.fafsa.ed.gov*) or mail the FAFSA form by mid-February. Most aid is in the form of loans.

Information about Diversity Programs

UWSOM is committed to creating an inclusive and diverse learning environment for all students and training culturally competent physicians to care for the region's increasingly diverse population. We welcome applicants from groups underrepresented in medicine and those committed to working with underserved groups. The Office of Multicultural Affairs supports student activities that promote inclusion, equity and diversity in all forms.

Campus Information

Setting

Classrooms and hospitals of the UWSOM are located across five states and run the gamut from primary to tertiary care settings including a level I trauma hospital, and renowned research facilities. Cultural and recreational opportunities abound.

Enrollment

For 2008, total enrollment was: 854

Special Features

A unique aspect of the UWSOM is the WWAMI program of decentralized medical education. Students take a portion of their clinical training at sites away from the UW-Seattle campus. Offers of admission are contingent upon agreement to participate in the WWAMI program.

Housing

On-campus housing is available, but the majority of students live off-campus. Average rent $800–$900/month.

Application Process and Requirements 2010–2011

Primary Application Service: AMCAS
Earliest filing date: June 1, 2009
Latest filing date: November 1, 2009

Secondary Application Required?: Yes
Sent to: Screened applicants
URL: http://depts.washington.edu/mdadmit/secondary/
Contact: Patricia Fero, (206) 543-7212, patf@u.washington.edu
Fee: Yes, $35
Fee waiver available: Yes
Earliest filing date: July 15, 2009
Latest filing date: January 15, 2010

MCAT® required?: Yes
Latest MCAT® considered: September 2009
Oldest MCAT® considered: September 2007

Early Decision Program: School does not have EDP
Applicants notified: n/a
EDP available for: n/a

Regular Acceptance Notice
Earliest date: November 1, 2009
Latest date: Until Class is Full
Applicant's Response to Acceptance Offer – Maximum Time: Two weeks before May 15, one week thereafter

Requests for Deferred Entrance Considered: Yes

Deposit to Hold Place in Class: No
Deposit (Resident): n/a
Deposit (Non-resident): n/a
Deposit due: n/a
Applied to tuition: n/a
Deposit refundable: n/a
Refundable by: n/a

Estimated number of new entrants: 216
EDP: n/a, special program: n/a

Start Month/Year: August 2010

Interview Format: A three-member panel interviews each applicant.

Other Programs

PREPARATORY PROGRAMS
Postbaccalaureate Program: No
Summer Program: Yes, (206) 685-2489
http://depts.washington.edu/omca/SMDEP/
Prematriculation Program: Yes,
http://depts.washington.edu/omca/PREMAT/
Mary Walls, (206) 616-3047,
mwalls@u.washington.edu

COMBINED DEGREE PROGRAMS
Baccalaureate/M.D. : No
M.D./M.P.H.: Yes, http://depts.washington.edu/epidem
Kate O'Brien, (206) 685-1762, epi@u.washington.edu
M.D./M.B.A.: No
M.D./J.D.: No
M.D./Ph.D.: Yes, www.mstp.washington.edu/
admissions, (206) 685-0762, Maureen Holstad,
mstp@u.washington.edu

Premedical Coursework

Course	Req.	Rec.	Lab.	Qtrs.
Inorganic Chemistry				
Behavioral Sciences				
Biochemistry		•		1-2
Biology	•			2-4
Biology/Zoology				
Calculus				
College English		•		1
College Mathematics				

Course	Req.	Rec.	Lab.	Qtrs.
Computer Science				
Genetics		•		
Humanities				2-4
Organic Chemistry				
Physics		•		2
Psychology				
Social Sciences		•		2-4
Inorgan./Organ. Chem		•		2-4

Selection Factors: 2008 Accepted Applicants

Proportion of Accepted Applicants with Relevant Experience (Data Self-Reported to AMCAS)		
Community Service/Volunteer		70%
Medically-Related Work		90%
Research		77%

Shaded bar represents school's accepted scores ranging from the 10th percentile to the 90th percentile ▬   School Median ● National Median ●

Overall GPA	2.0	2.1	2.2	2.3	2.4	2.5	2.6	2.7	2.8	2.9	3.0	3.1	3.2	3.3	3.4	3.5	3.6	(3.7)	3.8	3.9	4.0
Science GPA	2.0	2.1	2.2	2.3	2.4	2.5	2.6	2.7	2.8	2.9	3.0	3.1	3.2	3.3	3.4	3.5	3.6	(3.7)	3.8	3.9	4.0

MCAT® Total Numeric Score 9 10 11 12 13 14 15 16 17 18 19 20 21 22 23 24 25 26 27 28 29 30 (31) 32 33 34 35 36 37 38 39 40 41 42 43

Writing Sample			J	K	L	M	N	O	P	(Q)	R	S	T
Verbal Reasoning	3	4	5	6	7	8	9	(10)	11	12	13	14	15
Biological Sciences	3	4	5	6	7	8	9	10	(11)	12	13	14	15
Physical Sciences	3	4	5	6	7	8	9	(10)	(11)	12	13	14	15

Acceptance & Matriculation Data for 2008–2009 First Year Class

	Resident	Non-resident	International	Total
Applications	1137	3415	77	4629
Interviewed	761	156	0	917
Deferred	6	0	0	6
Matriculants				
Early Assurance Program	n/a	n/a	n/a	n/a
Early Decision Program	0	0	0	0
Baccalaureate/M.D.	n/a	n/a	n/a	n/a
M.D./Ph.D.	2	8	0	10
Matriculated	195	21	0	**216**

Applications accepted from International Applicants: No
*Resident includes: WA, WY, AK, MT, ID

Matriculant Demographics: 2008–2009 First Year Class

Men: 98   **Women:** 118

Matriculants' Self-Reported Race/Ethnicity

Mexican American	8	**Korean**	5
Cuban	0	**Vietnamese**	3
Puerto Rican	1	**Other Asian**	5
Other Hispanic	4	**Total Asian**	37
Total Hispanic	12	**Native American**	4
Chinese	9	**Black**	4
Asian Indian	8	**Native Hawaiian**	1
Pakistani	1	**White**	175
Filipino	3	**Unduplicated Number**	
Japanese	5	**of Matriculants**	216

Science and Math Majors: 62%
Matriculants with:
   Baccalaureate degree: 99%
   Graduate degree(s): 9%

Specialty Choice

2004, 2005, 2006 Graduates, Specialty Choice (As reported by program directors to GME Track™)	
Anesthesiology	8%
Emergency Medicine	8%
Family Practice	14%
Internal Medicine	19%
Obstetrics/Gynecology	6%
Orthopaedic Surgery	3%
Pediatrics	11%
Psychiatry	4%
Radiology	2%
Surgery	7%

Financial Information

Source: 2007–2008 LCME I-B survey and 2008–2009 AAMC TSF questionnaire

	Residents	Non-residents
Total Cost of Attendance	$38,158	$64,563
Tuition and Fees	$19,122	$45,527
Other (includes living expenses)	$19,036	$19,036
Health Insurance (can be waived)	$0	$0

Average 2008 Graduate Indebtedness: $112,530
% of Enrolled Students Receiving Aid: 91%

Criminal Background Check

This medical school requires a criminal background check prior to matriculation.

Marshall University
Joan C. Edwards School of Medicine
Huntington, West Virginia

Admissions Office, Marshall University
Joan C. Edwards School of Medicine
1600 Medical Center Drive
Huntington, West Virginia 25701-3655
T 800 544 8514   **F** 304 691 1744

Admissions http://musom.marshall.edu/admissions
Main http://musom.marshall.edu
Financial www.marshall.edu/sfa
E-mail warren@marshall.edu

Public Institution

Dr. Charles H. McKown Jr.,
Vice President and Dean

Cynthia A. Warren, Assistant Dean for
Admissions and Student Affairs

Nadine Hamrick, Associate Director of
Student Financial Aid

Dr. Aaron M. McGuffin, Senior Associate Dean
for Medical Education

Dr. Marie C. Veitia,
Associate Dean for Student Affairs

General Information
The Marshall University School of Medicine
was developed under the Veterans
Administration Medical Assistance and Health
Training Act passed by Congress in 1972. The
School of Medicine was granted full accreditation and graduated its first class in 1981. The
School of Medicine is a community-based program. The school's many affiliations provide
the opportunity to experience medical practice
in varied settings: a $32 million ambulatory
care center, the Veterans Affairs Medical
Center, successful rural clinics, highly specialized tertiary-care services in community hospitals, offices of private physicians, and others.
Students' educational opportunities are further
enhanced by three recently opened facilities:
the Edwards Comprehensive Cancer Center,
the Robert C. Byrd Biotechnology Science
Center and the Byrd Clinical Center.

Mission Statement
The Marshall University School of Medicine
has a special mission to respond to the health
care needs of West Virginians. We emphasize
training in the primary care specialties and
encourage graduates to practice in the state's
underserved rural areas. Marshall is now tied
for first place in the nation in the percentage of
graduates who choose to enter family medicine.

Curricular Highlights
Community Service Requirement: Optional.
Research/Thesis Requirement: Optional.

Students integrate basic science information
with clinical medicine the first two years. Year-

one consists of the traditional foundational
disciplines of medicine: Anatomy, Biochemistry,
Cell Biology, Histology and Physiology. Year-
two is an Integrated Systems Curriculum consisting of 10 blocks: Core Principles, Infectious
Agents & Antimicrobials, Neoplasia &
Hematology, Nervous System, Cardiovascular
System, Pulmonary System & ENT, Gastro-
intestinal System, Renal & Endocrine Systems,
Muscoskeletal, Genitourinary, Women's &
Men's Health, and Dermatology, Toxicology
and Eye. Throughout both years students have
direct patient contact through the Mentorship
Program giving them a natural framework to
integrate their growing knowledge of the traditional sciences basic to medicine. During both
years students learn the foundational principles of patient care including the skills of history taking and the physical exam. In addition,
topics such as preventive medicine, ethics, professionalism, and biostatistics and epidemiology are woven through the curriculum. During
the third and fourth years, students rotate
through clerkships at participating community
hospitals and other locations in the clinical
fields of medicine, surgery, pediatrics, psychiatry, family practice, obstetrics-gynecology, and
emergency medicine. Two months of rural
health care at approved sites are required of all
students. Twenty-three weeks are devoted to
electives in the senior year. A letter grading system (A, B, C, F) is utilized.

USMLE
Step 1: Required. Students must record a passing
score for promotion.
Step 2: Clinical Skills (CS): Required. Students
must record a passing total score to graduate.
Step 2: Clinical Knowledge (CK): Required.
Students must record a passing total score to
graduate.

Selection Factors
There is no discrimination because of race,
gender, religion, age, handicap, sexual orientation, or national origin. Qualified members of
groups who are underrepresented in medicine
are encouraged to apply. Applicants are evaluated on the basis of their academic records,
MCAT scores, recommendations from instructors, and personal qualifications as judged
through interviews. Interviews are arranged

only by invitation of the Admissions
Committee. As a state-assisted institution, the
School of Medicine gives preference in selection of students to West Virginia residents. A
limited number of positions will be available
to well-qualified non-residents from states
contiguous to West Virginia or to non-residents who have strong ties to West Virginia.
Other non-residents are not considered. Only
applicants who are U.S. citizens or who have
permanent resident visas are eligible for
admission. The School of Medicine considers
for transfer admission those applicants who
are currently in good standing at an allopathic
medical school. Positions are limited by attrition and are rarely available. The residency
policy for regular admissions also applies to
transfer admissions with the exception that
only U.S. citizens are considered.

Financial Aid
The financial needs of the applicant are not a
consideration in the admission process. There
are a variety of resources for financial assistance available to medical students. The supplemental application fee will be waived for
individuals who have been granted an AMCAS
fee waiver.

Campus Information
Enrollment
For 2008, total enrollment was: 281

Special Features
Distinguishing features for students at
Marshall include options and flexibility and an
emphasis on compassion, integrity, leadership,
and professionalism. Students determine their
own career goals after exploring primary care
and specialty rotations at Marshall and other
sites, as well as electives, which can include
wilderness medicine and international health
experiences. Over the past four years, Marshall
has become a leader in promoting childhood
obesity awareness and intervention through
their "Let's Get Moving" program.

Housing
The medical school maintains a list
of apartments.

Application Process and Requirements 2010–2011

Primary Application Service: AMCAS
Earliest filing date: June 1, 2009
Latest filing date: November 15, 2009

Secondary Application Required?: Yes
Sent to: State residents and those from states bordering West Virginia (NR fee: $100)
Contact: Cynthia A. Warren, (800) 544-8514, warren@marshall.edu
Fee: Yes, $50
Fee waiver available: Yes
Earliest filing date: July 15, 2009
Latest filing date: December 31, 2009

MCAT® required?: Yes
Latest MCAT® considered: September 2009
Oldest MCAT® considered: January 2007

Early Decision Program: School does not have EDP
Applicants notified: n/a
EDP available for: n/a

Regular Acceptance Notice
Earliest date: October 15, 2009
Latest date: Until class is full
Applicant's Response to Acceptance
Offer – Maximum Time: Two weeks

Requests for Deferred Entrance Considered: Yes

Deposit to Hold Place in Class: No
Deposit (Resident): n/a
Deposit (Non-resident): n/a
Deposit due: n/a
Applied to tuition: n/a
Deposit refundable: n/a
Refundable by: n/a

Estimated number of new entrants: 78
EDP: n/a, special program: n/a

Start Month/Year: August 2010

Interview Format: Two one-on-one interviews. Regional interviews are not available.

Other Programs

PREPARATORY PROGRAMS
Postbaccalaureate Program: No
Summer Program: No

COMBINED DEGREE PROGRAMS
Baccalaureate/M.D.: No
M.D./M.P.H.: No
M.D./M.B.A.: No
M.D./J.D.: No
M.D./Ph.D.: Yes, Richard Niles, Ph.D., (304) 696-7323, niles@marshall.edu

Premedical Coursework

Course	Req.	Rec.	Lab.	Hrs.	Course	Req.	Rec.	Lab.	Hrs.
Inorganic Chemistry	•		•	8	Computer Science				
Behavioral Sciences	•			6	Genetics				
Biochemistry		•			Humanities				
Biology					Organic Chemistry	•		•	8
Biology/Zoology	•		•	8	Physics	•		•	8
Calculus					Psychology				
College English	•			6	Social Sciences	•			6
College Mathematics					Other				

Selection Factors: 2008 Accepted Applicants

Proportion of Accepted Applicants with Relevant Experience (Data Self-Reported to AMCAS)		
Community Service/Volunteer		61%
Medically-Related Work		72%
Research		58%

Shaded bar represents school's accepted scores ranging from the 10th percentile to the 90th percentile   School Median ●   National Median ●

Overall GPA 2.0 2.1 2.2 2.3 2.4 2.5 2.6 2.7 2.8 2.9 3.0 3.1 3.2 3.3 3.4 3.5 ③.6 3.7 3.8 3.9 4.0
Science GPA 2.0 2.1 2.2 2.3 2.4 2.5 2.6 2.7 2.8 2.9 3.0 3.1 3.2 3.3 3.4 3.5 ③.6 3.7 3.8 3.9 4.0

MCAT® Total Numeric Score 9 10 11 12 13 14 15 16 17 18 19 20 21 22 23 24 25 ㉖ 27 28 29 30 31 ㉜ 33 34 35 36 37 38 39 40 41 42 43

Writing Sample			J	K	L	M	N	Ⓞ	P	Ⓠ	R	S	T
Verbal Reasoning	3	4	5	6	7	8	⑨	⑩	11	12	13	14	15
Biological Sciences	3	4	5	6	7	8	⑨	10	⑪	12	13	14	15
Physical Sciences	3	4	5	6	7	⑧	9	10	⑪	12	13	14	15

Acceptance & Matriculation Data for 2008–2009 First Year Class

	Resident	Non-resident	International	Total
Applications	209	1095	12	1316
Interviewed	156	90	0	246
Deferred	6	7	0	13
Matriculants				
Early Assurance Program	0	0	0	0
Early Decision Program	0	0	0	0
Baccalaureate/M.D.	n/a	n/a	n/a	n/a
M.D./Ph.D.	0	0	0	0
Matriculated	57	21	0	**78**

Applications accepted from International Applicants: No

Matriculant Demographics: 2008–2009 First Year Class

Men: 35   **Women:** 43

Matriculants' Self-Reported Race/Ethnicity

Mexican American	0	Korean	0
Cuban	0	Vietnamese	0
Puerto Rican	1	Other Asian	2
Other Hispanic	0	Total Asian	14
Total Hispanic	1	Native American	0
Chinese	0	Black	1
Asian Indian	11	Native Hawaiian	0
Pakistani	0	White	61
Filipino	1	Unduplicated Number	
Japanese	0	of Matriculants	78

Science and Math Majors: 72%
Matriculants with:
          Baccalaureate degree: 97%
          Graduate degree(s): 18%

Specialty Choice

2004, 2005, 2006 Graduates, Specialty Choice (As reported by program directors to GME Track™)

Anesthesiology	5%
Emergency Medicine	7%
Family Practice	16%
Internal Medicine	10%
Obstetrics/Gynecology	8%
Orthopaedic Surgery	2%
Pediatrics	20%
Psychiatry	3%
Radiology	6%
Surgery	5%

Financial Information

Source: 2007–2008 LCME I-B survey and 2008–2009 AAMC TSF questionnaire

	Residents	Non-residents
Total Cost of Attendance	$33,872	$59,462
Tuition and Fees	$16,588	$42,178
Other (includes living expenses)	$15,164	$15,164
Health Insurance (can be waived)	$2,120	$2,120

Average 2008 Graduate Indebtedness: $147,902
% of Enrolled Students Receiving Aid: 91%

Criminal Background Check

This medical school requires a criminal background check prior to matriculation.

West Virginia University School of Medicine

Morgantown, West Virginia

Office of Student Services
West Virginia University School of Medicine
Health Sciences Center, P.O. Box 9111
Morgantown, West Virginia 26506
T 304 293 2408   F 304 293 7814

Admissions www.hsc.wvu.edu/som/students/
aboutSoM/admissionProcess/index.asp
Main www.hsc.wvu.edu/som/
Financial www.hsc.wvu.edu/fin/medbud.htm
E-mail medadmissions@hsc.wvu.edu

Public Institution

Dr. James E. Brick, Interim Dean

Dr. Bruce Freeman, Chair,
Admissions Committee

Dr. G. Anne Cather, Associate Dean
for Student Services

Candace Frazier, Financial Aid Officer

Beth Ann McCormick, Admissions Associate

General Information

WVU has served for more than 100 years as a public institution of health professions education. The Robert C. Byrd Health Sciences Center has more than 1,900 students in Medicine, Dentistry, Pharmacy, Nursing and Allied Health. The Morgantown campus includes: the Physician Office Center, Ruby Memorial Hospital, Chestnut Ridge Psychiatric Hospital, HealthSouth Regional Rehabilitation Hospital, Mary Babb Randolph Cancer Center, and the WVU Eye Institute. New construction includes the Blanchette Rockefeller Neurosciences Institute, research labs and additions to the Cancer Center. There are three campuses: Morgantown, Charleston, and Eastern Division. Morgantown serves north and central WV with primary and tertiary care. Charleston is the oldest regional medical education campus in the U.S. and serves as a regional referral center for southern WV. Eastern provides a broad, community-based education emphasizing primary care and rural health in a longitudinal curriculum.

Mission Statement

The mission of the West Virginia University School of Medicine is to improve the health of West Virginians through the education of health professionals, through basic/clinical scientific research and research in rural health care delivery, through the provision of continuing professional education, and through participation in the provision of direct and supportive health care.

Curricular Highlights

Community Service Requirement: Required. 100 hours.

Research/Thesis Requirement: Optional.

WVU's education provides a strong foundation for any medical specialty. The basic medical sciences are covered in the MS1 and MS2 years in lecture and problem-based learning formats with computer-based testing. The Physical Diagnosis course begins in MS1 year and continues through MS2 year. Summer externships are available. The MS2 year has an integrated, organ-based approach. A traditional MS3 curriculum serves as a foundation in general medicine in the major clinical disciplines. The MS4 year is 50% required and 50% elective rotations. Three months of rural rotations are required. International travel scholarships are available.

USMLE

Step 1: Required. Students must record a passing score for promotion.
Step 2: Clinical Skills (CS): Required. Students must record a passing total score to graduate.
Step 2: Clinical Knowledge (CK): Required. Students must record a passing total score to graduate.

Selection Factors

WV residents are given preference for admission. There are available spaces for well-qualified non-residents, especially for those with strong state ties. Admission is based upon scholarship, MCAT scores, personal qualifications noted on interview, recommendations, community service, leadership, and medical experiences. The school does not discriminate on the basis of race, sex, creed, national origin, age, or disability. Approximately one third of the students are assigned to MS3 and MS4 years at the Charleston Division and a smaller number of students are assigned to the Eastern Division.

Financial Aid

A number of scholarship awards are available based on financial need and merit. Multiple loan funds are also available. Students' spouses with reasonable training and experience often find work near the medical school, at WVU, or in Morgantown. Medical students are discouraged from seeking outside employment while enrolled.

Information about Diversity Programs

The Health Careers Opportunity Program is available for disadvantaged students or those from groups underrepresented in medicine.

Campus Information

Setting

There are three clinical campuses. The Morgantown campus (*www.morgantown.com*) is a vibrant, active community and the medical, cultural, and commercial hub of the region. It has been named "#1 Dreamtown in America," and "Best Small City In The East." Clinical campuses are also located in the Charleston and Eastern Divisions. Charleston is the state capitol and serves as a hub for business and industry. The Charleston Area Medical Center is the largest in the state and serves as the regional referral center. The Eastern Division is located in the eastern panhandle of the state and serves a large nine-county area. It is associated with two hospitals, the VA system and several health centers.

Enrollment

For 2008, total enrollment was: 432

Special Features

WVU School of Medicine is highly respected for its clinical and rural education. It is a recent recipient of the AAMC Community Service Award, and the AAFP's Top 10 in students going into Family Medicine. Our computer laptop program provides electronic testing and prepares students well for the USMLE exams. Primary and tertiary care facilities are state-of-the-art. MPH and International Medicine tracks are available. Community service is required.

Housing

On-campus housing is not available. Affordable housing is available nearby, with average rents of $600–$800/month.

Satellite Campuses/Facilities

Two regional campuses are located at the Charleston (*www.hsc.wvu.edu/charleston*) and Eastern Divisions (*www.hsc.wvu.edu/eastern*) for MS3 and MS4 year clinical rotations.

Application Process and Requirements 2010–2011

Primary Application Service: AMCAS
Earliest filing date: June 1, 2009
Latest filing date: November 1, 2009

Secondary Application Required?: Yes
Sent to: Select applicants by secure e-mail
Contact: Beth Ann McCormick,
1-800-543-5650, medadmissions@hsc.wvu.edu
Fee: Yes, $100
Fee waiver available: Yes
Earliest filing date: July 15, 2009
Latest filing date: January 1, 2010

MCAT® required?: Yes
Latest MCAT® considered: September 2009
Oldest MCAT® considered: January 2008

Early Decision Program: School does have EDP
Applicants notified: October 1, 2009
EDP available for: Both Residents
and Non-residents

Regular Acceptance Notice
Earliest date: October 15, 2009
Latest date: Until class is full
Applicant's Response to Acceptance
Offer – Maximum Time: Two weeks

Requests for Deferred
Entrance Considered: Yes

Deposit to Hold Place in Class: Yes
Deposit (Resident): $100
Deposit (Non-resident): $100
Deposit due: With response to acceptance offer
Applied to tuition: Yes
Deposit refundable: Yes
Refundable by: May 15, 2010

Estimated number of new entrants: 110
EDP: 10, special program: 4

Start Month/Year: August 2010

Interview Format: Interview and tour,
Morgantown campus. Regional tours can
be arranged.

Other Programs

PREPARATORY PROGRAMS
Postbaccalaureate Program: No
Summer Program: No

COMBINED DEGREE PROGRAMS
Baccalaureate/M.D.: No
M.D./M.P.H.: Yes, www.hsc.wvu.edu/som/cmed/degree_programs/md_mph.asp
M.D./M.B.A.: No
M.D./J.D.: No
M.D./Ph.D.: Yes, www.hsc.wvu.edu/som/resoff/gradprograms/mdphd_main.asp
Additional Program: Yes, www.hsc.wvu.edu/som/students/aboutSoM/admissionProcess/medStepProgram.asp

Premedical Coursework

Course	Req.	Rec.	Lab.	Hrs.
Inorganic Chemistry	•		•	8
Behavioral Sciences	•			6
Biochemistry		•		4-8
Biology				
Biology/Zoology	•		•	8
Calculus				
College English	•			6
College Mathematics				

Course	Req.	Rec.	Lab.	Hrs.
Computer Science				
Genetics				
Humanities				
Organic Chemistry	•		•	8
Physics	•		•	8
Psychology				
Social Sciences	•			6
Adv. Cell & Molecular Biology		•		4-8

Selection Factors: 2008 Accepted Applicants

Proportion of Accepted Applicants with Relevant Experience (Data Self-Reported to AMCAS)		
Community Service/Volunteer		77%
Medically-Related Work		84%
Research		69%

Shaded bar represents school's accepted scores ranging from the 10th percentile to the 90th percentile. School Median ● National Median ●

Overall GPA	2.0	2.1	2.2	2.3	2.4	2.5	2.6	2.7	2.8	2.9	3.0	3.1	3.2	3.3	3.4	3.5	3.6	3.7	(3.8)	3.9	4.0
Science GPA	2.0	2.1	2.2	2.3	2.4	2.5	2.6	2.7	2.8	2.9	3.0	3.1	3.2	3.3	3.4	3.5	3.6	(3.7)	3.8	3.9	4.0

MCAT® Total Numeric Score 9 10 11 12 13 14 15 16 17 18 19 20 21 22 23 24 25 26 27 28 29 (30) 31 (32) 33 34 35 36 37 38 39 40 41 42 43

Writing Sample			J	K	L	M	N	O	(P)	(Q)	R	S	T
Verbal Reasoning	3	4	5	6	7	8	(9)	(10)	11	12	13	14	15
Biological Sciences	3	4	5	6	7	8	9	(10)	(11)	12	13	14	15
Physical Sciences	3	4	5	6	7	8	9	(10)	(11)	12	13	14	15

Acceptance & Matriculation Data for 2008–2009 First Year Class

	Resident	Non-resident	International	Total
Applications	218	2669	92	2979
Interviewed	140	270	0	410
Deferred	1	0	0	1
Matriculants				
Early Assurance Program	0	0	0	0
Early Decision Program	9	0	0	9
Baccalaureate/M.D.	n/a	n/a	n/a	n/a
M.D./Ph.D.	1	2	0	3
Matriculated	64	44	1	**109**

Applications accepted from International Applicants: No

Matriculant Demographics: 2008–2009 First Year Class

Men: 64   **Women:** 45

Matriculants' Self-Reported Race/Ethnicity

Mexican American	0	**Korean**	1
Cuban	0	**Vietnamese**	2
Puerto Rican	0	**Other Asian**	2
Other Hispanic	0	**Total Asian**	16
Total Hispanic	0	**Native American**	0
Chinese	7	**Black**	0
Asian Indian	2	**Native Hawaiian**	0
Pakistani	2	**White**	93
Filipino	1	**Unduplicated Number**	
Japanese	1	**of Matriculants**	109

Science and Math Majors: 75%
Matriculants with:
    Baccalaureate degree: 99%
    Graduate degree(s): 3%

Specialty Choice

2004, 2005, 2006 Graduates, Specialty Choice (As reported by program directors to GME Track™)	
Anesthesiology	4%
Emergency Medicine	3%
Family Practice	9%
Internal Medicine	18%
Obstetrics/Gynecology	6%
Orthopaedic Surgery	3%
Pediatrics	11%
Psychiatry	6%
Radiology	5%
Surgery	6%

Financial Information

Source: 2007–2008 LCME I-B survey
and 2008–2009 AAMC TSF questionnaire

	Residents	Non-residents
Total Cost of Attendance	$36,176	$59,972
Tuition and Fees	$20,164	$43,960
Other (includes living expenses)	$16,012	$16,012
Health Insurance (not applicable)	$0	$0

Average 2008 Graduate Indebtedness: $135,008
% of Enrolled Students Receiving Aid: 91%

Criminal Background Check

This medical school requires a criminal background check prior to matriculation.

Medical College of Wisconsin
Milwaukee, Wisconsin

Office of Admissions
Medical College of Wisconsin
8701 Watertown Plank Road
Milwaukee, Wisconsin 53226
T 414 456 8246   **F** 414 955 0121

Admissions www.mcw.edu/medicalschool
Main www.mcw.edu
Financial www.mcw.edu/acad/finaid
E-mail medschool@mcw.edu

Private Institution

Dr. Johnathan Ravdin, Dean and Executive Vice President

Michael T. Istwan, Director of Admissions

Dr. Dawn Bragg, Assistant Dean for Student Affairs – Diversity

Linda L. Paschal, Director of Student Financial Services

General Information

The Medical College of Wisconsin became a private, free-standing school of medicine in 1967. Located on the Milwaukee Regional Medical Campus, it maintains strong relationships and educational programs with institutions statewide. Major affiliated teaching hospitals include Froedtert Hospital, the VA Medical Center, and Children's Hospital of Wisconsin. Affiliations also include area hospitals and a number of healthcare facilities.

Mission Statement

The Medical College of Wisconsin is a private, academic institution dedicated to leadership and excellence in advancing the prevention, diagnosis and treatment of disease and injury through: Education: Preparing the physicians and scientists of tomorrow while enhancing the skills of today's health professionals. Discovery: Creating new knowledge in basic, translational and patient-based research to improve human health. Patient Care: Providing effective, compassionate, expert care for patients. Community Engagement: Partnering with public and private organizations to enhance learning, research, patient care and the health of the community.

Curricular Highlights

Community Service Requirement: Optional.
Research/Thesis Requirement: Optional.
The curriculum provides a foundation for a career in any discipline of medicine. In the first two years, students learn the basic sciences and experience the clinical environment through a mentor course and clinically related course work in the Clinical Continuum. Clinical topics covered include medical interviewing, human behavior, information management,

ethics, palliative care, physical exam, and health policy. In the third year, students rotate through required clinical clerkships and an optional elective experience to gain exposure to major clinical disciplines. In the fourth year, four one-month rotations are required including two subinternships, one each in a medically and surgically-oriented specialty, a Medicine rotation, and an Integrated Selective. Five one-month electives are available to senior students. Joint degree programs or an Honors in Research program are available to students with specific research interests. A five-year extended curriculum is available to students who wish to extend their studies over a longer period.

USMLE

Step 1: Required. Students must record a passing score for promotion.
Step 2: Clinical Skills (CS): Required. Students must only record a score.
Step 2: Clinical Knowledge (CK): Required. Students must record a passing total score to graduate.

Selection Factors

Student selection is based on a careful analysis of the suitability for the medical profession. Academic achievement and MCAT scores are carefully evaluated. Subjective factors include the personal statement, experiences, recommendations and interviews. Interviews are integral, done only at the college and required before acceptance. Applications are reviewed on a rolling basis by date of completion. Interviews are conducted and offers are also made on a rolling basis until the class is filled. Candidates are encouraged to complete the application in a timely fashion. The Medical College of Wisconsin does not discriminate on the basis of race, gender, creed, disability, age, national origin or sexual orientation.

Financial Aid

Most financial assistance, including federal and institutional scholarships and loans, is awarded on basis of need. Financial aid award letters are developed using the Federal Methodology formula. Applicants are encouraged to begin the application process as soon as they are interviewed. To matriculate, a student must provide a current clean credit report as defined in the

College's credit report policy. A student must be a U.S. citizen or eligible non-citizen to receive aid from federal administered programs. International applicants must file proof of financial support before acceptance.

Information about Diversity Programs

The college encourages applications from students of diverse backgrounds. In addition to academic credentials, letters of recommendation, and personal interviews, a student's motivation and educational background are carefully considered. The Office of Academic Affairs/Diversity offers various programs to assist students, demonstrating the college's commitment to their recruitment, retention and graduation.

Campus Information

Setting
Located on the Milwaukee Regional Medical Center Campus, in a suburb seven miles west of downtown Milwaukee, the College offers a safe comfortable environment to live and study, with easy access to the city and its advantages.

Enrollment
For 2008, total enrollment was: 820

Special Features
Froedtert Hospital and Children's Hospital of Wisconsin are nationally ranked, Level One trauma centers. Children's has been selected as one of the ten best Children's Hospital in the country. With over $125 million in grant funds, the College conducted 3,000 studies and had 1,500 clinical trials in progress during the past year.

Housing
Student housing is not provided. A list of available housing is maintained and students live within easy driving or walking distance of campus.

Satellite Campuses/Facilities
The Milwaukee Regional Medical Campus provides students with the opportunity to complete their clinical requirements at this location.

Application Process and Requirements 2010–2011

Primary Application Service: AMCAS
Earliest filing date: June 1, 2009
Latest filing date: November 1, 2009

Secondary Application Required?: Yes
Sent to: All applicants
Contact: Michael Istwan, (414) 456-8246, mistwan@mcw.edu
Fee: Yes, $70
Fee waiver available: Yes
Earliest filing date: July 1, 2009
Latest filing date: January 31, 2010

MCAT® required?: Yes
Latest MCAT® considered: September 2009
Oldest MCAT® considered: 2007

Early Decision Program: School does have EDP
Applicants notified: October 1, 2009
EDP available for: Both Residents and Non-residents

Regular Acceptance Notice
Earliest date: October 15, 2009
Latest date: Until class is full
Applicant's Response to Acceptance Offer – Maximum Time: One month

Requests for Deferred Entrance Considered: Yes

Deposit to Hold Place in Class: Yes
Deposit (Resident): $100
Deposit (Non-resident): $100
Deposit due: One month after acceptance
Applied to tuition: Yes
Deposit refundable: Yes
Refundable by: May 15, 2010

Estimated number of new entrants: 204
EDP: 10, special program: n/a

Start Month/Year: August 2010

Interview Format: Two, thirty-minute interviews. Regional interviews are not available.

Other Programs

PREPARATORY PROGRAMS
Postbaccalaureate Program: No
Summer Program: No

COMBINED DEGREE PROGRAMS
Baccalaureate/M.D.: No
M.D./M.P.H.: No
M.D./M.B.A.: No
M.D./J.D.: No
M.D./Ph.D.: Yes, www.mcw.edu/mstp

Premedical Coursework

Course	Req.	Rec.	Lab.	Hrs.
Inorganic Chemistry	•		•	8
Behavioral Sciences				
Biochemistry		•		
Biology	•		•	8
Biology/Zoology				
Calculus		•		
College English	•			6
College Mathematics	•			4

Course	Req.	Rec.	Lab.	Hrs.
Computer Science				
Genetics				
Humanities				
Organic Chemistry	•		•	8
Physics	•			8
Psychology				
Social Sciences				
Other				

Selection Factors: 2008 Accepted Applicants

Proportion of Accepted Applicants with Relevant Experience (Data Self-Reported to AMCAS®)		
Community Service/Volunteer		71%
Medically-Related Work		91%
Research		82%

Shaded bar represents school's accepted scores ranging from the 10th percentile to the 90th percentile   School Median ● National Median ●

Overall GPA 2.0 2.1 2.2 2.3 2.4 2.5 2.6 2.7 2.8 2.9 3.0 3.1 3.2 3.3 3.4 **3.5 3.6 3.7** (3.8) 3.9 4.0
Science GPA 2.0 2.1 2.2 2.3 2.4 2.5 2.6 2.7 2.8 2.9 3.0 3.1 3.2 3.3 **3.4 3.5 3.6** (3.7) 3.8 3.9 4.0

MCAT® Total Numeric Score 9 10 11 12 13 14 15 16 17 18 19 20 21 22 23 24 25 26 **27 28 29 30** (31) 32 **33 34 35** 36 37 38 39 40 41 42 43

Writing Sample			J	K	L	M	N	O	(P)	(Q)	R	S	T
Verbal Reasoning	3	4	5	6	7	8	9	(10)	11	12	13	14	15
Biological Sciences	3	4	5	6	7	8	9	10	(11)	12	13	14	15
Physical Sciences	3	4	5	6	7	8	9	(10)	(11)	12	13	14	15

Acceptance & Matriculation Data for 2008–2009 First Year Class

	Resident	Non-resident	International	Total
Applications	643	5549	237	6429
Interviewed	203	475	2	680
Deferred	17	11	0	28
Matriculants				
Early Assurance Program	n/a	n/a	n/a	n/a
Early Decision Program	6	3	0	9
Baccalaureate/M.D.	n/a	n/a	n/a	n/a
M.D./Ph.D.	1	5	0	6
Matriculated	74	137	1	**212**

Applications accepted from International Applicants: Yes

Matriculant Demographics: 2008–2009 First Year Class

Men: 116   **Women:** 96

Matriculants' Self-Reported Race/Ethnicity

Mexican American	9	Korean	4
Cuban	0	Vietnamese	3
Puerto Rican	1	Other Asian	2
Other Hispanic	0	Total Asian	44
Total Hispanic	10	Native American	3
Chinese	18	Black	10
Asian Indian	14	Native Hawaiian	1
Pakistani	1	White	153
Filipino	0	Unduplicated Number	
Japanese	3	of Matriculants	212

Science and Math Majors: 74%
Matriculants with:
    Baccalaureate degree: 100%
    Graduate degree(s): 7%

Specialty Choice

2004, 2005, 2006 Graduates, Specialty Choice (As reported by program directors to GME Track™)	
Anesthesiology	8%
Emergency Medicine	10%
Family Practice	12%
Internal Medicine	14%
Obstetrics/Gynecology	5%
Orthopaedic Surgery	4%
Pediatrics	9%
Psychiatry	4%
Radiology	6%
Surgery	8%

Financial Information

Source: 2007–2008 LCME I-B survey and 2008–2009 AAMC TSF questionnaire

	Residents	Non-residents
Total Cost of Attendance	$48,010	$53,630
Tuition and Fees	$33,385	$39,005
Other (includes living expenses)	$12,130	$12,130
Health Insurance (cannot be waived)	$2,495	$2,495

Average 2008 Graduate Indebtedness: $155,534
% of Enrolled Students Receiving Aid: 95%

Criminal Background Check

This medical school requires a criminal background check prior to matriculation.

University of Wisconsin
School of Medicine and Public Health

Madison, Wisconsin

Admissions Committee
2130 Health Sciences Learning Center
University of Wisconsin School of Medicine
and Public Health
750 Highland Avenue
Madison, Wisconsin 53705-2221
T 608 263 4925   F 608 262 4226

Admissions www.med.wisc.edu/education/
admissions
Main www.med.wisc.edu
Financial www.finaid.wisc.edu/index.php
E-mail medadmissions@mailplus.wisc.edu

Public Institution

Dr. Robert N. Golden, Dean

Lucy J. Wall, Assistant Dean for Admissions

*Dr. Gloria V. Hawkins, Assistant Dean
for Multicultural Affairs*

*Amy J. Schrader, Senior Advisor Student
Financial Services*

General Information

The University of Wisconsin School of
Medicine and Public Health has had a four-
year program in medicine since 1924 and has
the largest research commitment of any school
or college on campus, receiving more than
$215 million in extramural research support in
fiscal 2006. National surveys consistently rank
UW Hospital and Clinics among the finest
academic medical centers in the United States.

Mission Statement

The University of Wisconsin School of
Medicine and Public Health is committed to
meeting the health needs of Wisconsin and
beyond through excellence in education,
research, patient care, and service. The UW
School of Medicine and Public Health seeks to
be one of the preeminent medical schools by
excelling in the creation, integration, and
transfer of knowledge through a combination
of basic, translational, and clinical research, a
greater emphasis on active learning, and consistently outstanding patient care.

Curricular Highlights

Community Service Requirement: Optional.
Research/Thesis Requirement: Optional.

The curriculum introduces students to the
generalist practice of medicine by exposing
them to community-based settings in the first
and second years. There is a focus on active
learning; case-based problem-solving; interdisciplinary teaching by basic science and clinical
faculty throughout the first and second years; a
four-year curriculum that prepares students
for either a primary care or specialty career;
diverse clinical clerkship experiences around
the state, including inner-city and rural sites;
and a six-week one-on-one preceptorship with
an experienced clinician in Year 4. The senior

year provides elective opportunities for study
at other institutions and abroad. Opportunities
for research are available to medical students
in individually arranged programs.

USMLE

Step 1: Required. Students must record a passing
score for promotion.
Step 2: Clinical Skills (CS): Required. Students
must only record a score.
Step 2: Clinical Knowledge (CK): Required.
Students must only record a score.

Selection Factors

The Admissions Committee seeks students
with diverse backgrounds and interests.
Breadth of academic and nonacademic interests and experiences, ability to communicate
with others, motivation for medicine, personal
characteristics, and intellectual ability are some
of the factors considered. Preference is given to
residents of Wisconsin. Non-resident applicants compete for relatively few places.
Secondary applications and interview invitations are sent to selected applicants.

Financial Aid

All financial aid allocated by the University of
Wisconsin School of Medicine and Public
Health is awarded on the basis of proven need.
Need is calculated as the necessary expenses
incurred while attending medical school minus
the resources provided to the student by outside agencies, personal resources. Priority for
financial aid, especially grant awards, will be
given to students with the greatest need. The
major proportion of total financial aid is available in the form of loans.

Information about Diversity Programs

The University of Wisconsin School of Medicine
and Public Health is committed to increasing
the number of physicians from groups underrepresented in medicine and those showing
evidence of socioeconomically and education-
ally-disadvantaged backgrounds. Applications
are encouraged from persons with socioeconomic disadvantages and from members of
groups underrepresented in medicine.

Campus Information

Setting

The University of Wisconsin School of
Medicine and Public Health and the Ebling
Health Sciences Library are located in the new
Health Sciences Learning Center. It is connected to the University of Wisconsin Hospital and
Clinics and the School of Pharmacy on the
west side of campus. The Learning Center features sophisticated instructional technologies,
including advanced digital capabilities
throughout its lecture halls, classrooms, clinical training and assessment areas, computing
facilities, and distance education centers. The
building was designed to enhance individual
and small-group learning.

Enrollment

For 2008, total enrollment was: 649

Special Features

The UW medical degree program includes
opportunities for global health experiences, a
research honors track, rural and urban medicine tracks, the M.P.H. dual degree, service in
the community including free medical clinics.
There is a balance between strong primary care
and strong cuttng-edge research.

Housing

Housing information is available at
www.housing.wisc.edu. Additional private housing is widely available within the city of
Madison.

Satellite Campuses/Facilities

The typical UW medical student spends at
least 16 weeks at clinical sites outside Madison
and throughout the state of Wisconsin. Other
locations are LaCrosse, Marshfield, Green Bay,
and Milwaukee teaching hospitals, and community clinics in other cities.

Application Process and Requirements 2010–2011

Primary Application Service: AMCAS
Earliest filing date: June 1, 2009
Latest filing date: November 1, 2009

Secondary Application Required?: Yes
Sent to: Selected applicants
URL: Invitation only
Fee: Yes, $56
Fee waiver available: Yes
Earliest filing date: July 15, 2009
Latest filing date: December 1, 2009

MCAT® required?: Yes
Latest MCAT® considered: September 2009
Oldest MCAT® considered: April 2006

Early Decision Program: School does have EDP
Applicants notified: October 1, 2009
EDP available for: Residents only

Regular Acceptance Notice
Earliest date: October 16, 2009
Latest date: Until class is full
Applicant's Response to Acceptance
Offer – Maximum Time: Two weeks

Requests for Deferred
Entrance Considered: Yes

Deposit to Hold Place in Class: No
Deposit (Resident): n/a
Deposit (Non-resident): n/a
Deposit due: n/a
Applied to tuition: n/a
Deposit refundable: n/a
Refundable by: n/a

Estimated number of new entrants: 148
EDP: 2, special program: 15

Start Month/Year: Mid-August 2010

Interview Format: Selected applicants are invited to interview. Regional interviews are not available.

Other Programs

PREPARATORY PROGRAMS
Postbaccalaureate Program: No
Summer Program: No

COMBINED DEGREE PROGRAMS
Baccalaureate/M.D.: No
M.D./M.P.H.: Yes, www.pophealth.wisc.edu/MPH/
M.D./M.B.A.: No
M.D./J.D.: No
M.D./Ph.D.: Yes, http://mstp.med.wisc.edu/

Premedical Coursework

Course	Req.	Rec.	Lab.	Sems.
Inorganic Chemistry	•		•	2
Behavioral Sciences		•		
Biochemistry	•			1
Biology				
Biology/Zoology	•		•	1
Calculus		•		
College English		•		
College Mathematics	•			1

Course	Req.	Rec.	Lab.	Sems.
Computer Science				
Genetics				
Humanities		•		
Organic Chemistry	•			1
Physics	•		•	2
Psychology		•		
Social Sciences		•		
Statistics	•			1
Advanced level biology	•		•	1

Selection Factors: 2008 Accepted Applicants

Proportion of Accepted Applicants with Relevant Experience (Data Self-Reported to AMCAS)		
Community Service/Volunteer	71%
Medically-Related Work	89%
Research	85%

Shaded bar represents school's accepted scores ranging from the 10th percentile to the 90th percentile.   School Median ●   National Median ●

Overall GPA	2.0	2.1	2.2	2.3	2.4	2.5	2.6	2.7	2.8	2.9	3.0	3.1	3.2	3.3	3.4	3.5	3.6	3.7	(3.8)	3.9	4.0
Science GPA	2.0	2.1	2.2	2.3	2.4	2.5	2.6	2.7	2.8	2.9	3.0	3.1	3.2	3.3	3.4	3.5	3.6	(3.7)	3.8	3.9	4.0

MCAT® Total Numeric Score 9 10 11 12 13 14 15 16 17 18 19 20 21 22 23 24 25 26 27 28 29 30 3[(32)]33 34 35 36 37 38 39 40 41 42 43

Writing Sample				J	K	L	M	N	O	P	(Q)	R	S	T
Verbal Reasoning	3	4	5	6	7	8	9	(10)	11	12	13	14	15
Biological Sciences	3	4	5	6	7	8	9	10	(11)	12	13	14	15
Physical Sciences	3	4	5	6	7	8	9	10	(11)	12	13	14	15

Acceptance & Matriculation Data for 2008–2009 First Year Class

	Resident	Non-resident	International	Total
Applications	648	2611	5	3264
Interviewed	309	146	0	455
Deferred	10	2	0	12
Matriculants				
Early Assurance Program	n/a	n/a	n/a	n/a
Early Decision Program	4	0	0	4
Baccalaureate/M.D.	0	0	0	0
M.D./Ph.D.	0	8	0	8
Matriculated	119	44	0	**163**

Applications accepted from International Applicants: No

Matriculant Demographics: 2008–2009 First Year Class

Men: 76   **Women:** 87

Matriculants' Self-Reported Race/Ethnicity

Mexican American	5	Korean	2
Cuban	0	Vietnamese	3
Puerto Rican	1	Other Asian	4
Other Hispanic	5	Total Asian	30
Total Hispanic	11	Native American	0
Chinese	9	Black	8
Asian Indian	11	Native Hawaiian	0
Pakistani	0	White	129
Filipino	1	Unduplicated Number	
Japanese	0	of Matriculants	163

Science and Math Majors: 69%
Matriculants with:
Baccalaureate degree: 99%
Graduate degree(s): 15%

Specialty Choice

2004, 2005, 2006 Graduates, Specialty Choice (As reported by program directors to GME Track™)	
Anesthesiology	9%
Emergency Medicine	8%
Family Practice	12%
Internal Medicine	11%
Obstetrics/Gynecology	5%
Orthopaedic Surgery	2%
Pediatrics	16%
Psychiatry	4%
Radiology	5%
Surgery	5%

Financial Information

Source: 2007–2008 LCME I-B survey and 2008–2009 AAMC TSF questionnaire

	Residents	Non-residents
Total Cost of Attendance	$41,492	$52,616
Tuition and Fees	$23,102	$34,226
Other (includes living expenses)	$16,395	$16,395
Health Insurance (can be waived)	$1,995	$1,995

Average 2008 Graduate Indebtedness: $134,271
% of Enrolled Students Receiving Aid: 87%

Criminal Background Check

This medical school requires a criminal background check prior to matriculation.

Information About Canadian Medical Schools
Accredited by the LCME and by the CACMS

The 17 medical schools in Canada are members of the Association of Faculties of Medicine of Canada (*www.afmc.ca*) and affiliate members of the AAMC. They participate in the activities of both associations. Canadian medical schools are accredited jointly by the Liaison Committee on Medical Education (*www.lcme.org*, LCME) and the Committee on Accreditation of Canadian Medical Schools (*www.afmc.ca/education-cacms-e.php*, CACMS). All are M.D. degree-granting schools with high-quality educational programs.

Admission policies and procedures of Canadian schools are similar in many respects to those followed in U.S. schools; thus, many of the suggestions for applicants in chapters 1 through 9 will also apply. Schools vary with respect to the emphasis placed on selection factors, and applicants are encouraged to refer to the individual school entries for additional details.

Fifteen Canadian medical schools offer four-year educational programs; two, McMaster and Calgary, are three-year programs. Some students at the Université de Montréal are admitted into a one-year preparatory program prior to beginning the M.D. curriculum. McGill University's five-year M.D. program includes an initial year that must be completed by graduates of the province of Quebec's Collège d'enseignement général et professionnel (CÉGEP).

Selection Criteria

As reflected in the individual school entries in this chapter, Canadian medical schools vary with respect to the number of years of undergraduate instruction required of applicants. Medical schools also vary with respect to recommended content during premedical undergraduate education. Table 13-A shows that physics, inorganic and organic chemistry, biology,

biochemistry, humanities, and English are the most common subjects required in undergraduate education by the Canadian medical schools.

Language of Instruction

Three Canadian medical schools — Laval, Montréal and Sherbrooke, all located in the province of Quebec — require students to be fluent in French as all instruction is in that language. Instruction in the other 14 schools is in English, and the University of Ottawa offers the M.D. curriculum in both French and English.

Residency Requirements

In Canada, universities fall under provincial jurisdiction and the majority of places in each faculty of medicine are allocated to permanent residents of the province in which the university is located.

TABLE 13-A

Subjects Required by Two or More Canadian Medical Schools, 2010–2011 Entering Class

Required Subject	No. of Schools (n=17)
Biochemistry	6
Biology	7
Calculus	2
College English	4
College Mathematics	3
Humanities	3
Inorganic Chemistry	7
Organic Chemistry	8
Physics	6
Social Sciences	2

NOTE: Figures based on data provided fall 2009. Three of the 17 medical schools (Northern Ontario, McMaster and Western Ontario) did not indicate specific course requirements and are not included in the tabulations.

Not all faculties of medicine accept applications from international students. Conversely, some faculties of medicine may reserve positions for international students, possibly as part of agreements with foreign governments and institutions. Statistics compiled by the Association of Faculties of Medicine of Canada (www.afmc.ca) show that most medical schools admit international students. In 2006–07, 233 U.S. students applied to Canadian medical schools and recorded a 9.9% success rate. In the same year, 426 non-U.S. international students applied to Canadian medical schools and recorded a 5.6% success rate. The success rate for Canadian applicants was 26.2%. Additional information about Canadian medical schools can be found in the Association of Faculties of Medicine of Canada publication, Admission Requirements of Canadian Faculties of Medicine (2009) (www.afmc.ca/ publications-admission-2009-e.php).

Positions filled by international students in Canadian medical schools are not necessarily subsidized by provincial/territorial governments. As such, international students, including U.S. students, may pay higher tuition and fees compared to those of Canadian residents.

Academic Record/Suitability

Although an excellent academic record is a very important factor in gaining admission to a Canadian medical school, great deal of effort is expended in assessing applicants' suitability for a medical career based on other factors. Personal suitability is assessed in a variety of ways by the schools; applicants who can demonstrate that they possess the qualities considered important in the practice of medicine may sometimes be admitted even if their academic record is not outstanding. Alternately, applicants with outstanding records who do not possess these qualities may not gain a place in medical school.

Most applicants to Canadian medical schools are interviewed prior to accept-

ance, so the interview information in Chapter 7 will be useful.

Medical College Admission Test (MCAT®)

Eleven Canadian medical schools require applicants to take the MCAT: Alberta, British Columbia, Calgary, Dalhousie, Manitoba, McGill, Memorial, Queen's, Saskatchewan, Toronto, and Western Ontario.

Other Considerations

Canadian faculties of medicine do not discriminate on the basis of race, religion, or gender in admitting new students. The admission of Aboriginal students (First Nations, Inuit, Métis) is encouraged at several Canadian medical schools, including Laval, Sherbrook, Montréal, McGill, Ottawa, Queen's, Western Ontario, Northern Ontario School of Medicine, Saskatchewan, Alberta and British Columbia.

The number of female applicants has risen dramatically in recent years, with correspondingly larger proportions of women in schools' entering classes. Women comprised 57 percent of the

2006–2007 applicant pool, and the success rate for women was slightly higher than that for men. The 2006 entering classes at the 17 Canadian medical schools reporting data about male and female matriculants included 58 percent women and 42 percent men. Overall, 25 percent of applicants received at least one offer of admission.

Expenses/Financial Aid

Tuition and student fees for Canadian and non-Canadian students in the 2008 entering class are provided in Table 13-B and in individual school entries. Expenses vary from school to school and from student to student. Tuition at several Canadian schools is slightly higher for the first year than for successive years. Tuition and fees at all Canadian universities are expected to increase substantially in the next several years. Some financial aid information is provided in the individual school entries. Eligible Canadian students may apply for a Canadian Student Loan, or they may apply to the Department of Education in their province for a provincial student loan.

TABLE 13-B

Tuition and Student Fees for 2008–2009 First-Year Students at Canadian Medical Schools (In Canadian Dollars)

Categories of Students	Range	Average
In-Province	$3,577–$18,921	$12,212*
Canada, Out-of-Province	$7,267–$18,921	$13,861*
Visa	$20,944–$91,862	$39,719*

NOTE: Figures based on data provided fall 2008

* Average In-Province data were derived from all 17 Canadian schools. Average Out-of-Province data were derived from all 17 Canadian schools reporting. Average visa data were derived from 10 schools which accept foreign students.

Source: Association of Faculties of Medicine of Canada

Ontario Medical School Application Service (OMSAS)

The Ontario Medical School Application Service (OMSAS) is a non-profit, centralized application service for applicants to the six medical schools in Ontario. OMSAS provides only the application processing service; each medical school is autonomous in reaching its admission decisions. All applications to the Ontario medical schools must be made through OMSAS.

The online application, COMPASS. OMSAS, is available in early July. Completed applications must be received at OMSAS by October 1. Official transcripts and references must be received at OMSAS by October 1. Applicants are advised to submit their application and supporting documents prior to the deadline. For the instruction booklet containing information about application procedures and admission requirements, visit *www.ouac.on.ca/omsas/*.

Information Sources

Additional information about admission requirements, the curricula of Canadian medical schools, and medical education in Canada is provided in catalogs available from each school, and can be downloaded free of charge from the AFMC Web site (*www.afmc.ca*). A printed version of Admission Requirements of Canadian Faculties of Medicine can also be ordered from:

The Association of Faculties of Medicine of Canada
265 Carling Avenue, Suite 800
Ottawa, ON K1S 2E1
Canada
(613) 730-0687
Information is also available at *www.afmc.ca*.

University of Alberta
Faculty of Medicine and Dentistry
Edmonton, Alberta

2-45 Medical Sciences Building
University of Alberta
Faculty of Medicine and Dentistry
Edmonton, Alberta
Canada, T6G 2H7
T 780 492 6350   **F** 780 492 9531

Admissions www.med.ualberta.ca/education/ugme/
Main www.med.ualberta.ca
Financial www.registrar.ualberta.ca/ro.cfm?id=287
E-mail admission@med.ualberta.ca

Public Institution

Dr. Thomas Marrie, Dean

M. Healey, Admissions Officer

Dr. Marc Moreau, Assistant Dean

General Information
The Faculty of Medicine at the University of Alberta was founded in 1913. The Medical Sciences Building, the Clinical Sciences Building, the Walter C. Mackenzie Health Sciences Centre, and the University of Alberta Hospitals are located on the university campus. Clinical instruction is also given at the Royal Alexandra Hospital, Edmonton General Hospital, Misericordia Hospital, Alberta Hospital, Glenrose Hospital, Cross Cancer Institute, and Grey Nuns Hospital. Counseling services and student health services are available to all University of Alberta students.

Mission Statement
Dedicated to the optimizations of health through scholarship and leadership in our education programs, in fundamental and applied research, and in the prevention and treatment of illness in conjunction with the Capital Health Authority and other partners. Vision: To be nationally and internationally recognized leaders investing in education, research and service, making important contributions to health.

Curricular Highlights
Community Service Requirement: Required. Rural Family Medicine training.
Research/Thesis Requirement: Optional.

The Faculty of Medicine conducts a fully accredited, four-year program leading to the degree of doctor of medicine. Each of the first two years consists of 33 weeks of instruction, from early September until mid-May. The final two years are conducted as a continuum, during which each student has a four-week holiday period. The first two years of the curriculum are an integrated systems-based program covering the basic and clinical sciences. It is primarily case-based and uses a mixture of lectures and small-group sessions with some problem-based learning. The last two years are

composed of a student internship of at least 56 weeks, during which the student is assigned to hospitals affiliated with the faculty for clinical study and experience, a selective program in medicine and surgery, and an elective program that allows students to develop their own curriculum and spend a minimum of 12 weeks in one or more subject areas of their choice. Throughout the program, emphasis is on self-education; much instruction is on a small-group basis. A graduate training program leading to eligibility for specialist qualifications by the Royal College of Physicians and Surgeons of Canada is offered in most clinical specialties.

USMLE
Step 1: Optional.
Step 2: Clinical Skills (CS): Optional.
Step 2: Clinical Knowledge (CK): Optional.

Selection Factors
The Admissions Committee selects applicants without discrimination to gender, race, religion, or age, and attempts to apply five criteria: undergraduate academic achievement, employment history, extracurricular activities, letters of recommendation, and the MCAT. Final applicants will be required to attend an interview at the University of Alberta at their own expense. Preference is given to Alberta residents. The University of Alberta does not accept applications from international students. Rejected applicants are given the opportunity to reapply for admission. Applicants who have been asked to withdraw or who have been suspended or expelled from any medical school will not usually be considered. There are five positions over the regular quota of 133 for the M.D. program to Aboriginal applicants.

Financial Aid
Loans are available under the Canada Student Loan Plan or the Province of Alberta Loan Plan to Canadian citizens or permanent residents who have been in Canada and in Alberta for 12 months prior to the beginning of the academic term.

Information about Diversity Programs
Five positions for aboriginal and eight for rural applicants.

Campus Information

Setting
The University of Alberta is in a dynamic city with all amenities of big city living. Edmonton is home to the most expansive urban park in North America. Providing the city with 22 parks, the river valley boasts 1,500 km of trails used for walking, biking, and cross-country skiing. The city boasts sports franchises, one of North America's finest concert halls (the Winspear Centre), a symphony orchestra, a vibrant theatre scene, and a summer packed with major arts and cultural events.

Enrollment
For 2008, total enrollment was: 563

Special Features
Students train in one of Canada's leading clinical, research, and teaching hospitals. The UAH treats more than 700,000 patients annually and is recognized as a national leader in organ and tissue transplant, both in success rates and in transplant volumes. Other major facilities are the Stollery Children's Hospital, Alberta Diabetes Institute and the future Mazankowski Alberta Heart Institute and Lois Hole Women's Pavilion.

Housing
The University of Alberta offers residence service. The two main facilities on campus, the Lister Centre and HUB Centre, have been updated and have new additions. Information on housing can be found on the University of Alberta, Office of the Registrar and Student Awards, Web site at *www.registrar.ualberta.ca.*

Application Process and Requirements 2010–2011

Primary Application Service: School-specific
Fee: $115
Earliest filing date: July 2, 2009
Latest filing date: November 1, 2009

Secondary Application Required?: Yes
Sent to: All applicants
URL: n/a
Fee: n/a
Fee waiver available: No
Earliest filing date: July 2, 2009
Latest filing date: November 1, 2009

MCAT® required?: Yes
Latest MCAT® considered: September 2009
Oldest MCAT® considered: 1991

Early Decision Program: School does have EDP
Applicants notified: May 15, 2010
EDP available for: Both residents and non-residents

Regular Acceptance Notice
Earliest date: May 15, 2010
Latest date: Until class is full
Applicant's Response to Acceptance
Offer – Maximum Time: 10 business days

Requests for Deferred
Entrance Considered: Yes

Deposit to Hold Place in Class: Yes
Deposit (Resident): $1,000
Deposit (Non-resident): $1,000
Deposit due: With response to acceptance offer
Applied to tuition: Yes
Deposit refundable: No
Refundable by: n/a

Estimated number of new entrant: 155
EDP: 0, special program: n/a

Start Month/Year: August 2010

Interview Format: Multiple Mini Interview (MMI).

Other Programs

PREPARATORY PROGRAMS
Postbaccalaureate Program: No
Summer Program: No

COMBINED DEGREE PROGRAMS
Baccalaureate/M.D.: No
M.D./M.P.H.: No
M.D./M.B.A.: No
M.D./J.D.: No
M.D./Ph.D.: Yes, www.med.ualberta.ca/research/mdphd.cfm

Premedical Coursework

Course	Req.	Rec.	Lab.	Sems.	Course	Req.	Rec.	Lab.	Sems.
Inorganic Chemistry	•			6	Computer Science				
Behavioral Sciences					Genetics				
Biochemistry	•			3	Humanities				
Biology	•			6	Organic Chemistry	•			6
Biology/Zoology					Physics	•			6
Calculus					Psychology				
College English	•			6	Social Sciences				
College Mathematics					Statistics	•			3

Selection Factors: 2008 Accepted Applicants

Proportion of Accepted Applicants with Relevant Experience (Data Self-Reported to AMCAS®)	Community Service/Volunteer Medically-Related Work Research	DATA NOT COLLECTED

Shaded bar represents school's accepted scores ranging from the 10th percentile to the 90th percentile ▬   School Median ● National Median ●

Overall GPA	2.0	2.1	2.2	2.3	2.4	2.5	2.6	2.7	2.8	2.9	3.0	3.1	3.2	3.3	3.4	3.5	3.6	3.7	(3.8)	3.9	4.0
Science GPA	2.0	2.1	2.2	2.3	2.4	2.5	2.6	2.7	2.8	2.9	3.0	3.1	3.2	3.3	3.4	3.5	3.6	3.7	(3.8)	3.9	4.0

MCAT® Total Numeric Score 9 10 11 12 13 14 15 16 17 18 19 20 21 22 23 24 25 26 27 28 29 30 31 32 33 34 35 36 37 38 39 40 41 42 43

Writing Sample			J	K	L	M	N	O	P	(Q)	R	S	T
Verbal Reasoning	3	4	5	6	7	8	9	(10)	11	12	13	14	15
Biological Sciences	3	4	5	6	7	8	9	10	11	(12)	13	14	15
Physical Sciences	3	4	5	6	7	8	9	10	(11)	12	13	14	15

Acceptance & Matriculation Data for 2008–2009 First Year Class

	Resident	Non-resident	International	Total
Applications	612	537	n/a	1149
Interviewed	309	68	n/a	377
Deferred	0	0	0	0
Matriculants	0	0	0	0
Early Assurance Program	0	0	0	0
Early Decision Program	n/a	n/a	n/a	n/a
Baccalaureate/M.D.	n/a	n/a	n/a	n/a
M.D./Ph.D.	0	0	0	0
Matriculated	142	13	n/a	**155**

Applications accepted from International Applicants: No

Matriculant Demographics: 2008–2009 First Year Class

Men: 85   **Women:** 70

Matriculants' Self-Reported Race/Ethnicity

Mexican American   Korean
Cuban   Vietnamese
Puerto Rican   Other Asian
Other Hispani
Total Hispanic   **DATA NOT COLLECTED**
Chinese
Asian Indian
Pakistani   Total Asian
Filipino   **Unduplicated Number**
Japanese   **of Matriculants**

Science and Math Majors: 85%
Matriculants with:
Baccalaureate degree: 112
Graduate degree(s): 6

Specialty Choice

2004, 2005, 2006 Graduates, Specialty Choice

Anesthesiology
Emergency Medicine
Family Practice

DATA NOT COLLECTED

Psychiatry
Radiology
Surgery

Financial Information

	Residents	Non-residents
Total Cost of Attendance	$13,944	$13,944
Tuition and Fees	$11,791	$11,791
Other (includes living expenses)	n/r	n/r
Health Insurance (can be waived)	n/r	n/r

Average 2008 Graduate Indebtedness: n/r
% of Enrolled Students Receiving Aid: n/r

Criminal Background Check

This medical school requires a criminal background check prior to matriculation.

University of Calgary Faculty of Medicine

Calgary, Alberta

Office of Admissions
University of Calgary, Faculty of Medicine
3330 Hospital Drive, N.W.
Calgary, Alberta
Canada, T2N 4N1
T 403 220 4262 **F** 403 210 8148

Admissions www.medicine.ucalgary.ca
Main www.medicine.ucalgary.ca
Financial www.ucalgary.ca/UofC/students/awards
E-mail ucmedapp@ucalgary.ca

Public Institution

Dr. Thomas Feasby, Dean of Medicine

Adele Meyers, Admissions Officer

Claudia Barrett, Interim Director, Awards and Financial Aid

General Information
The Faculty of Medicine at the University of Calgary accepted its first students in September 1970. In 1972, the Faculty of Medicine moved into its permanent facilities in the Calgary Health Sciences Centre. The centre has been designed to complement the objectives of the faculty's integrated teaching program.

Mission Statement
We wish to be a medical school which is: responsive to community and societal needs; determined to shape the future of society; rooted in basic research and discovery; committed to excellence and pursuit of excellence and to continuous improvement in all endeavors; and committed to innovation and creativity.

Curricular Highlights
Community Service Requirement: Optional. Strongly recommended.
Research/Thesis Requirement: Optional.

The curriculum is based on clinical presentations of the way patients present to physicians. One hundred twenty clinical presentations have been defined, ranging from simple to complex, and they are grouped by body system and human development. The clinical presentation curriculum teaches the basic science and clinical knowledge pertinent to each clinical presentation and provides an approach to the solution of the clinical problems. The Introductory Clinical Skills of Communication and Physical Examination commence in the first weeks of the curriculum. The curriculum maintains an active learning environment with more than 25 percent of scheduled instructional activities spent in small-group, case-based learning sessions. Students have the opportunity to reinforce in a clinical setting what they have learned in the body systems as they progress through each of the systems. The curriculum also focuses on the relevance of the

family and the community in health and disease. The school employs a pass/fail grading system. Each academic year lasts about 11 months. At the end of the three years, students will be granted the M.D. degree. The school's philosophy is to produce generalist physicians who can proceed to further training in specialty, family medicine, or research.

USMLE
Step 1: Optional.
Step 2: Clinical Skills (CS): Optional.
Step 2: Clinical Knowledge (CK): Optional.

Selection Factors
The Admissions Committee selects applicants without discrimination to gender, race, religion, or age, and attempts to apply six criteria: undergraduate academic achievement, employment history, extracurricular activities, an essay, letters of recommendation, and the MCAT. Final applicants will be required to attend an interview at the University of Calgary at their own expense. Final applicants will also be required to write an on-site essay on a topic assigned by the Admissions Committee. Preference is given to Alberta residents. The University of Calgary does not accept applications from individual international students. Presently, seats for international students are limited to those students who come from institutions/countries with whom the Faculty of Medicine has a formal, contractual agreement. Rejected applicants are given the opportunity to reapply for admission. Applicants who have been asked to withdraw or who have been suspended or expelled from any medical school will not usually be considered.

Financial Aid
The majority of students obtain financial aid through student loans and lines of credit. Because students attend school 11 months each year, summer employment is unlikely, and, therefore, financial support must be sufficient to meet their requirements over the subsequent three years. The student awards officer will provide information about student loans, bursaries, and awards. The financial status of the applicant does not affect acceptance into the program. Students receive a total stipend of $3,420 for the third (final) year.

Campus Information

Setting
The school is located on a hospital site one kilometer from the main university campus.

Enrollment
For 2008, total enrollment was: 444

Special Features
The Health Sciences Centre offers students state-of-the-art facilities. Students are encouraged to pursue electives in developing countries.

Housing
There are residences on the main campus, as well as apartment buildings and condominiums within walking distance. The average cost per month of a one-bedroom apartment near the hospital is $850.

Satellite Campuses/Facilities
Students have clinical experiences on-site at the Foothills Medical Centre, as well as at two other general hospitals and the children's hospital in Calgary. During the final year, they may rotate through hospitals in smaller centers in the province, in addition to doing electives outside of Alberta.

Application Process and Requirements 2010–2011

Primary Application Service: School-specific
Earliest filing date: July 1, 2009
Latest filing date: October 15, 2009

Secondary Application Required?: No
Sent to: n/a
URL: n/a
Fee: n/a
Fee waiver available: n/a
Earliest filing date: n/a
Latest filing date: n/a

MCAT® required?: Yes
Latest MCAT® considered: September 2009
Oldest MCAT® considered: April 1999

Early Decision Program: School does not have EDP
Applicants notified: n/a
EDP available for: n/a

Regular Acceptance Notice
Earliest date: May 15, 2010
Latest date: Varies
Applicant's Response to Acceptance Offer – Maximum Time: Two weeks. Less for offers to applicants on the waitlist.

Requests for Deferred Entrance Considered: Yes

Deposit to Hold Place in Class: Yes
Deposit (Resident): $500
Deposit (Non-resident): $500
Deposit due: With response to acceptance offer
Applied to tuition: Yes
Deposit refundable: No
Refundable by: n/a

Estimated number of new entrants: 150
EDP: 0, special program: n/a

Start Month/Year: August 2010

Interview Format: A series of short standardized interviews.

Other Programs

PREPARATORY PROGRAMS
Postbaccalaureate Program: No
Summer Program: No

COMBINED DEGREE PROGRAMS
Baccalaureate/M.D.: No
M.D./M.P.H.: Yes
M.D./M.B.A.: Yes
M.D./J.D.: No
M.D./Ph.D.: Yes, http://gse.myweb.med.ucalgary.ca/x.pro/ModShow/ShowPage/1022
Additional Program: Yes, MD/MSc

Premedical Coursework

Course	Req.	Rec.	Lab.	Sems.	Course	Req.	Rec.	Lab.	Sems.
Inorganic Chemistry		•		2	Computer Science				
Behavioral Sciences					Genetics				
Biochemistry		•		2	Humanities				
Biology		•		2	Organic Chemistry		•		2
Biology/Zoology					Physics		•		2
Calculus		•		1	Psychology		•		1
College English		•		2	Social Sciences		•		1
College Mathematics					Statistics		•		1

Selection Factors: 2008 Accepted Applicants

Proportion of Accepted Applicants with Relevant Experience (Data Self-Reported to AMCAS®)		
Community Service/Volunteer		99%
Medically-Related Work		95%
Research		35%

Shaded bar represents school's accepted scores ranging from the 10th percentile to the 90th percentile ▪   School Median ●   National Median ●

Overall GPA	2.0	2.1	2.2	2.3	2.4	2.5	2.6	2.7	2.8	2.9	3.0	3.1	3.2	3.3	3.4	3.5	3.6	(3.7)	3.8	3.9	4.0
Science GPA	2.0	2.1	2.2	2.3	2.4	2.5	2.6	2.7	2.8	2.9	3.0	3.1	3.2	3.3	3.4	3.5	3.6	3.7	3.8	3.9	4.0

MCAT® Total Numeric Score				**DATA NOT COLLECTED**							

Writing Sample			J	K	L	M	N	O	P	(Q)	R	S	T
Verbal Reasoning	3	4	5	6	7	8	9	(10)	11	12	13	14	15
Biological Sciences	3	4	5	6	7	8	9	10	(11)	12	13	14	15
Physical Sciences	3	4	5	6	7	8	9	10	(11)	12	13	14	15

Acceptance & Matriculation Data for 2008–2009 First Year Class

	Resident	Non-resident	International	Total
Applications	715	690	0	1405
Interviewed	324	108	0	432
Deferred	4	1	0	5
Matriculants				
Early Assurance Program	0	0	0	0
Early Decision Program	n/a	n/a	n/a	n/a
Baccalaureate/M.D.	n/a	n/a	n/a	n/a
M.D./Ph.D.	9	0	0	9
Matriculated	128	22	0	**150**

Applications accepted from International Applicants: No

Specialty Choice

2004, 2005, 2006 Graduates, Specialty Choice	
Anesthesiology	4
Emergency Medicine	2
Family Practice	32
Internal Medicine	18
Obstetrics/Gynecology	5
Orthopaedic Surgery	6
Pediatrics	5
Psychiatry	11
Radiology	3
Surgery	13

Matriculant Demographics: 2008–2009 First Year Class

Men: 74   **Women:** 76

Matriculants' Self-Reported Race/Ethnicity

Mexican American	Korean
Cuban	Vietnamese
Puerto Rican	Other Asian
Other Hi...	
Total Hi...	
Chinese	
Asian In...	Total Asian
Pakistani	Unduplicated Number
Filipino	of Matriculants
Japanese	

DATA NOT COLLECTED

Science and Math Majors: 80%
Matriculants with:
    Baccalaureate degree: 89%
    Graduate degree(s): 21%

Financial Information

	Residents	Non-residents
Total Cost of Attendance	$35,000	$86,000
Tuition and Fees	$14,000	$65,000
Other (includes living expenses)	$21,000	$21,000
Health Insurance (can be waived)	$193	$193

Average 2008 Graduate Indebtedness: $100,000
% of Enrolled Students Receiving Aid: 90%

Criminal Background Check

This medical school does not require a criminal background check prior to matriculation.

University of British Columbia Faculty of Medicine

Vancouver, British Columbia

MD Undergraduate Program
Faculty of Medicine, Dean's Office
University of British Columbia
317-2194 Health Sciences Mall
Vancouver, British Columbia
Canada, V6T 1Z3
T 604 822 4482   F 604 822 6061

Admissions www.med.ubc.ca/admissionsmd
Main www.med.ubc.ca/home.htm
Financial www.med.ubc.ca/education/md_ugrad/
financial_assistance.htm
E-mail admissions.md@ubc.ca

Public Institution

Dr. Gavin C.E. Stuart, Dean, Facility of Medicine

Dr. Michael Clifford Fabian, Associate Dean, Admissions

Lori Charvat, Associate Dean, Equity

Jennifer Fong, Student Financial Assistant Officer

Denis Hughes, Director, Admissions

Shelley Small, Joan Munro, Christine Wood, and Jennifer Young, Admissions Coordinator

General Information

The expansion and distribution of the UBC Faculty of Medicine undergraduate program began on March 15, 2002, creating a partnership in medical education with the University of Northern British Columbia, the University of Victoria, and the regional Health Authorities. The expansion provides an education model for other Canadian jurisdictions, contributes to meeting federal health care recommendations, and advances BC's economic and educational capacity. The photograph above was provided by Bunting Coady Architects.

Mission Statement

The M.D. Undergraduate Program recruits, admits, educates, and supports students who will graduate with defined and demonstrated personal qualities, competencies, knowledge, and behaviors rooted in the vision, missions, and values of UBC and its Faculty of Medicine, and in an ethical context of social responsibility for the health needs of British Columbians.

Curricular Highlights

Community Service Requirement: Required.
Research/Thesis Requirement: Optional.

The program is built on principles of student self-directed learning, integration of biomedical and social sciences, early clinical contact, information management, professional development, and social responsibility. See the UBC Web site for information at *www.med.ubc.ca/ education/md_ugrad/Schedule_Courses.htm.*

USMLE

Step 1: Optional.
Step 2: Clinical Skills (CS): Optional.
Step 2: Clinical Knowledge (CK): Optional.

Selection Factors

The selection of candidates for admission to UBC's medical school is governed by guidelines established by the Senate of UBC, and is the responsibility of the Faculty of Medicine Admissions Selection Committee. See the Web site for selection criteria at *www.med.ubc.ca/ education/md_ugrad/MD_Undergraduate_ Admissions/Selection.htm.* The UBC Faculty of Medicine's Associate Dean of Admissions oversees the selection process to ensure that all applicants are given careful consideration without regard to age, gender, sexual orientation, race, ancestry, color, place of origin, family status, physical or mental disability, political belief, religion, or marital or economic status.

Financial Aid

UBC and the Faculty of Medicine are committed to ensuring that financial circumstances are not a barrier to qualified domestic students. Graduates who practice in rural areas are eligible for a number of financial incentives. For information regarding financial aid and awards, please contact the Student Financial Assistance Officer Faculty of Medicine, M.D. Undergraduate Program by telephone at (604) 875-5834, or toll free at (1-877) 875-7800. E-mail may be sent to studentfinances@ medd.med.ubc.ca. Additional information is available at *www.med.ubc.ca/education/ md_ugrad/financial_assistance.htm.*

Information about Diversity Programs

The UBC Faculty of Medicine is committed to increasing opportunities for Aboriginal (Status or Non-Status Indians, Treaty, First Nations, Metis, or Inuit) applicants through the Aboriginal Admissions Subcommittee. Contact James Andrew, Aboriginal Programs Coordinator, for more information at james.andrew@ubc.ca or 604-822-3236. Applicants with disabilities are considered in accordance with UBC's policy on Academic Accommodation for Students with Disabilities. The Northern Medical Program provides an opportunity to complete undergraduate train-ing in a northern regional centre and may be of particular interest to those applicants who come from, or are interested in, rural, remote, or northern communities.

Campus Information

Setting

The UBC Faculty of Medicine launched an innovative, distributed medical education program in collaboration with the Government of British Columbia, the University of Northern British Columbia, the University of Victoria, and provincial regional Health Authorities. The first of its kind in Canada, the program creates opportunities for medical education across BC, doubling undergraduate class sizes at sites in the North, on Vancouver Island, in the Fraser Valley, in the BC interior, and in Vancouver.

Enrollment

For 2008, total enrollment was: 256

Special Features

The 40,000 square meter UBC Life Sciences Centre is located on the University of British Columbia campus. It houses basic science departments and teaching and research laboratories. The Northern Health Sciences Centre (UNBC) and the Medical Sciences Building (UVic) use state-of-the-art technology in the delivery of medical education. The buildings contain labs, lecture halls, classrooms, small seminar rooms, and student common areas.

Housing

For detailed information regarding housing, please contact the appropriate program site. For the Island Medical Program, go to *http://imp.uvic.ca/current/affairs/impoffice.php.* For the Northern Medical Program, go to *www.unbc. ca/nmp/nmp.html.* For the Vancouver Fraser Medical Program, go to *www.med.ubc.ca/ education/md_ugrad/student_affairs.htm.*

Satellite Campuses/Facilities

The Island Medical Program (IMP) at the University of Victoria, the Northern Medical Program (NMP) at the University of Northern British Columbia, and the UBC-based Vancouver Fraser Medical Program (VFMP).

Application Process and Requirements 2010–2011

Primary Application Service: School-specific
Earliest filing date: Early June 2009
Latest filing date: Early September 2009

Secondary Application Required?: Yes
Sent to: Applicable applicants
Contact: Admissions Officer, (604) 822-4482, admissions.md@ubc.ca
Fee: $105 – $185
Fee waiver available: No
Earliest filing date: Early January 2010
Latest filing date: Mid-January 2010

MCAT® required?: Yes
Latest MCAT® considered: September 2009
Oldest MCAT® considered: July 2004

Early Decision Program: School does not have EDP
Applicants notified: n/a
EDP available for: n/a

Regular Acceptance Notice
Earliest date: Mid-May 2010
Latest date: Until Class is Full
Applicant's Response to Acceptance Offer – Maximum Time: Varies

Requests for Deferred Entrance Considered: Yes

Deposit to Hold Place in Class: Yes
Deposit (Resident): $500
Deposit (Non-resident): $500
Deposit due: With response to acceptance offer
Applied to tuition: Yes
Deposit refundable: No
Refundable by: n/a

Estimated number of new entrants: 256
EDP: n/a, special program: n/a

Start Month/Year: August 2010

Interview Format: Multiple Mini-Interview. Regional interviews are not available.

Other Programs

PREPARATORY PROGRAMS
Postbaccalaureate Program: Yes, www.med.ubc.ca/education/md_postgrad.htm
Summer Program: No

COMBINED DEGREE PROGRAMS
Baccalaureate/M.D.: No
M.D./M.P.H.: No
M.D./M.B.A.: No
M.D./J.D.: No
M.D./Ph.D.: Yes, www.med.ubc.ca/education/md_ugrad/mdphd.htm

Premedical Coursework

Course	Req.	Rec.	Lab.	Sems.	Course	Req.	Rec.	Lab.	Sems.
Inorganic Chemistry	•			2	Computer Science				
Behavioral Sciences		•			Genetics		•		
Biochemistry	•			2	Humanities				
Biology	•			2	Organic Chemistry	•			2
Biology/Zoology					Physics		•		
Calculus					Psychology				
College English	•			2	Social Sciences				
College Mathematics					Other		•		

Selection Factors: 2008 Accepted Applicants

Proportion of Accepted Applicants with Relevant Experience (Data Self-Reported to AMCAS®)		
Community Service/Volunteer		100%
Medically-Related Work		50%
Research		50%

Shaded bar represents school's accepted scores ranging from the 10th percentile to the 90th percentile ▨   School Median ● National Median ●

Overall GPA	2.0	2.1	2.2	2.3	2.4	2.5	2.6	2.7	2.8	2.9	3.0	3.1	3.2	3.3	3.4	3.5	3.6	(3.7)	3.8	3.9	4.0
Science GPA	2.0	2.1	2.2	2.3	2.4	2.5	2.6	2.7	2.8	2.9	3.0	3.1	3.2	3.3	3.4	3.5	(3.6)	3.7	3.8	3.9	4.0

MCAT® Total Numeric Score 9 10 11 12 13 14 15 16 17 18 19 20 21 22 23 24 25 26 27 28 29 30 31 32 33 34 35 36 37 38 39 40 41 42 43

Writing Sample			J	K	L	M	N	O	(P)	Q	R	S	T
Verbal Reasoning	3	4	5	6	7	8	(9)	10	11	12	13	14	15
Biological Sciences	3	4	5	6	7	8	9	10	(11)	12	13	14	15
Physical Sciences	3	4	5	6	7	8	9	(10)	11	12	13	14	15

Acceptance & Matriculation Data for 2008–2009 First Year Class

	Resident	Non-resident	International	Total
Applications	986	820	0	1806
Interviewed	607	41	0	648
Deferred	2	0	0	2
Matriculants				
Early Assurance Program	n/a	n/a	n/a	n/a
Early Decision Program	n/a	n/a	n/a	n/a
Baccalaureate/M.D.	n/a	n/a	n/a	n/a
M.D./Ph.D.	3	0	0	3
Matriculated	244	12	0	**256**

Applications accepted from International Applicants: No

Matriculant Demographics: 2008–2009 First Year Class

Men: 108   **Women:** 148

Matriculants' Self-Reported Race/Ethnicity

Mexican American	Korean
Cuban	Vietnamese
Puerto Rican	Other Asian
Other H	
Total Hi	
Chinese	**DATA NOT COLLECTED**
Asian In	
Pakistani	Total Asian
Filipino	**Unduplicated Number**
Japanese	**of Matriculants**

Science and Math Majors: 83%
Matriculants with:
  Baccalaureate degree: 196
  Graduate degree(s): 42

Specialty Choice

2004, 2005, 2006 Graduates, Specialty Choice

Anesthesiology
Emergency Medicine
Family Practice

DATA NOT COLLECTED

Psychiatry
Radiology
Surgery

Financial Information

	Residents	Non-residents
Total Cost of Attendance	n/c	n/c
Tuition and Fees	$14,857	$14,857
Other (includes living expenses)	$12,000	$12,000
Health Insurance	n/c	n/c

Average 2008 Graduate Indebtedness: n/c
% of Enrolled Students Receiving Aid: n/c

Criminal Background Check

This medical school requires a criminal background check prior to matriculation.

University of Manitoba
Faculty of Medicine
Winnipeg, Manitoba

Chair, Admissions Committee
Faculty of Medicine
University of Manitoba
260-727 McDermot Avenue
Winnipeg, Manitoba
Canada, R3E 3P5
T 204 789 3499   **F** 204 789 3929

Admissions www.umanitoba.ca/medicine/admissions
Main www.umanitoba.ca/medicine
Financial http://umanitoba.ca/admin/financial_services
E-mail registrar_med@umanitoba.ca

Public Institution

Dr. D. Sandham, Dean

Dr. F. Aoki and B.A. MacKalski, Assistant Deans, Admissions

Ms. Beth Jennings, Administrator, Admissions and Enrolment Services

General Information
Medical education in Manitoba is designed to provide students with the knowledge and experience they need to practice medicine in a profession where new developments in science and public health policy create an ever-changing environment. In the first two years of the program, the subject matter is divided into blocks which cover core concepts in health and medicine, human development, and body systems. Clinical Skills, Problem-Solving, Medical Humanities, Law, Laboratory and Investigative Medicine, Health Equity and Survival Tactics are integrated into the six blocks. The final two years, called the "clerkship," are spent in direct contact with patients and doctors in a clinical setting in which students gain experience with increasing responsibility for patient care and management. General teaching facilities are located in the medical buildings, and facilities for clinical instruction are provided in the teaching hospitals affiliated with the University of Manitoba and in related institutions. The varied settings in which medicine is practiced in Winnipeg and in rural and northern Manitoba also provide students with the opportunity to study community medicine outside the major teaching institutions. For more information on the institution, please visit the Web site.

Mission Statement
The mission of the Faculty of Medicine is to: develop, deliver, and evaluate high quality educational programs for undergraduate and postgraduate students of medicine and medical rehabilitation, for graduate students and postdoctoral fellows in basic medical sciences and for physicians to practice; to conduct research and other scholarly enquiry into the basic and applied medical sciences; and to provide advice, disseminate information to health professions and plan for the development and delivery of

health care services; and to help improve health status and service delivery to the Province of Manitoba and the wider community.

Curricular Highlights
Community Service Requirement: Optional.
Research/Thesis Requirement: Optional.

For information regarding curriculum, scheduling, and enrichment programs, please refer to the links posted at: *www.umanitoba.ca/faculties/medicine/education/undergraduate.html.*

USMLE
Step 1: Optional.
Step 2: Clinical Skills (CS): Optional.
Step 2: Clinical Knowledge (CK): Optional.

Selection Factors
Selection by the Admissions Committee is made on the basis of (1) adjusted grade-point (GPA is calculated on a 4.5 scale); (2) MCAT; and (3) personal assessment score (PAS). All students must be Canadian citizens or permanent residents of Canada. Preference is given to residents of Manitoba and Aboriginal applicants, although a limited number of Out of Province applicants are accepted. For more information, see the Applicant Information Bulletin: *www.umanitoba.ca/faculties/medicine/admissions.*

Financial Aid
Under the Canadian Students Loan Act, Canadians can obtain interest-free loans during their undergraduate course in medicine. Bursaries from the University, the Manitoba Medical College Foundation, and the provincial government are available to deserving students. Applications for these bursaries are available when classes commence. Students may also obtain assistance from the W. K. Kellogg Student Loan Program. Several entrance scholarships are also offered annually.

Information about Diversity Programs
The Health Careers Access Program: University of Manitoba's Access program provides support to persons who have traditionally not had the opportunity for advanced education because of social, economic, or cultural reasons or lack of formal education. This program is exclusive to Aboriginal (Metis, Status, Non-

Status, Inuit) residents of Manitoba with a strong interest in becoming a health professional. Sponsorship includes academic and personal support and may include some financial assistance. These programs are funded by Manitoba Education and Training, Advanced Education and Skills Training Division.

Campus Information
Setting
The Faculty of Medicine is located at the Bannatyne Campus. Facilities for instruction are provided there, including the Clinical Learning and Simulation Facility. In addition to the affiliated teaching hospitals students also have access to the Institutes and Centres of Cell Biology, Health Policy, Child Health, CancerCare Manitoba, Cardiovascular Sciences, Spinal Cord Reseach; St. Boniface General Hospital Research Centre; the National Microbiology Laboratory; and the Institute for Biodiagnostics (NRC).

Enrollment
For 2008, total enrollment was: 387

Housing
On-campus housing is not available at the Bannatyne Campus. However affordable apartments are available nearby. See: *http://umanitoba.ca/student/housing.*

Application Process and Requirements 2010–2011

Primary Application Service: School-specific
Earliest filing date: August 15, 2009
Latest filing date: October 9, 2009

Secondary Application Required?: Yes
Sent to: All applicants
URL: www.umanitoba.ca/medicine/admissions
Fee: Yes, $95
Fee waiver available: No
Earliest filing date: Same as primary application.
Latest filing date: October 9, 2009

MCAT® required?: Yes
Latest MCAT® considered: September 2009
Oldest MCAT® considered: April 2006

Early Decision Program: School does not have EDP
Applicants notified: n/a
EDP available for: n/a

Regular Acceptance Notice
Earliest date: May 15, 2010
Latest date: Until class is full
Applicant's Response to Acceptance
Offer – Maximum Time: Two weeks or as specified in the offer.

Requests for Deferred
Entrance Considered: Yes

Deposit to Hold Place in Class: Yes
Deposit (Resident): $500
Deposit (Non-resident): $500
Deposit due: With response to acceptance offer
Applied to tuition: Yes
Deposit refundable: No
Refundable by: n/a

Estimated number of new entrants: 110
EDP: n/a, special program: n/a

Start Month/Year: August 28, 2010

Interview Format: Multi-Mini Interview (MMI).

Other Programs

PREPARATORY PROGRAMS
Postbaccalaureate Program: No
Summer Program: Yes, www.umanitoba.ca/medicine/media/EarlyExposureExperienceInfo Sheet.pdf

Combined Degree Programs
Baccalaureate/M.D.: Yes, http://umanitoba.ca/medicine/education/undergraduate/preclerkship/bsc_med.html
M.D./M.P.H.: No
M.D./M.B.A.: No
M.D./J.D.: No
M.D./Ph.D.: Yes, Dr. D. Eisenstat, eisensta@cc.umanitoba.ca

Premedical Coursework

Course	Req.	Rec.	Lab.	Hrs.	Course	Req.	Rec.	Lab.	Hrs.
Inorganic Chemistry					Computer Science				
Behavioral Sciences					Genetics		•		
Biochemistry	•			6	Humanities		•		
Biology		•			Organic Chemistry		•		
Biology/Zoology		•			Physics		•		
Calculus					Psychology				
College English					Social Sciences		•		
College Mathematics					Other				

Selection Factors: 2008 Accepted Applicants

Proportion of Accepted Applicants with Relevant Experience (Data Self-Reported to AMCAS)	DATA NOT COLLECTED

Shaded bar represents school's accepted scores ranging from the 10th percentile to the 90th percentile   School Median ● National Median ●

Overall GPA	2.0	2.1	2.2	2.3	2.4	2.5	2.6	2.7	2.8	2.9	3.0	3.1	3.2	3.3	3.4	3.5	3.6	3.7	3.8	3.9	(4.0)
Science GPA	2.0	2.1	2.2	2.3	2.4	2.5	2.6	2.7	2.8	2.9	3.0	3.1	3.2	3.3	3.4	3.5	3.6	3.7	3.8	3.9	4.0

MCAT® Total Numeric Score	DATA NOT COLLECTED

			J	K	L	M	N	O	P	Q	R	S	T
Writing Sample			J	K	L	M	N	O	P	(Q)	R	S	T
Verbal Reasoning	3	4	5	6	7	8	9	(10)	11	12	13	14	15
Biological Sciences	3	4	5	6	7	8	9	10	(11)	12	13	14	15
Physical Sciences	3	4	5	6	7	8	9	10	(11)	12	13	14	15

Acceptance & Matriculation Data for 2008–2009 First Year Class

	Resident	Non-resident	International	Total
Applications	282	666	0	948
Interviewed	243	75	0	318
Deferred	4	0	0	4
Matriculants				
Early Assurance Program	0	0	0	0
Early Decision Program	n/a	n/a	n/a	n/a
Baccalaureate/M.D.	n/a	n/a	n/a	n/a
M.D./Ph.D.	0	0	0	0
Matriculated	99	11	0	**110**

Applications accepted from International Applicants: No

Specialty Choice

2004, 2005, 2006 Graduates, Specialty Choice
Anesthesiology
Emergency Medicine
Family Practice
DATA NOT COLLECTED
Psychiatry
Radiology
Surgery

Matriculant Demographics: 2008–2009 First Year Class

Men: 60   **Women:** 50

Matriculants' Self-Reported Race/Ethnicity

Mexican American   Korean
Cuban   Vietnamese
Puerto Rican   Other Asian
Other

DATA NOT COLLECTED

Total
Chinese
Asian Indian   White
Pakistani   Total Asian
Filipino   Unduplicated Number
Japanese   of Matriculants

Science and Math Majors: Data not collected
Matriculants with:
   Baccalaureate degree: 100%
   Graduate degree(s): 12%

Financial Information

	Residents	Non-residents
Total Cost of Attendance	n/r	n/r
Tuition and Fees	$7,595	$7,595
Other (includes living expenses)	n/r	n/r
Health Insurance (can be waived)	n/r	n/r

Average 2008 Graduate Indebtedness: n/r
% of Enrolled Students Receiving Aid: n/r

Criminal Background Check

This medical school does not require a criminal background check prior to matriculation.

Memorial University of Newfoundland
Faculty of Medicine
St. John's, Newfoundland

Memorial University of Newfoundland
Faculty of Medicine
St. John's, Newfoundland/Labrador
Canada, A1B 3V6
T 709 777 6615   **F** 709 777 8422

Admissions www.med.mun.ca/admissions
Main www.med.mun.ca/med
Financial www.edu.gov.nf.ca/studentaid
E-mail munmed@mun.ca

Public Institution

Dr. J. Rourke, Dean of Medicine

Janet McHugh, Admissions Officer

Dr. W. Parsons, Assistant Dean for Admissions

General Information
Memorial is the only university in the province of Newfoundland. The university was established as Memorial College in 1925 and incorporated as a university in 1949. In 1959, campus buildings were erected on a 1,000-acre site. There are some 12,000 undergraduates and a faculty of about 1,000 (including visiting professors) working on the campus, which is situated on the periphery of St. John's. The medical school is fully accredited by the Committee on Accreditation of Canadian Medical Schools (CACMS) of the Association of Canadian Medical Colleges and the Canadian Medical Association and the Liaison Committee on Medical Education (LCME) of the Association of American Medical Colleges and the American Medical Association. Thus, the medical school is equivalent in every respect to other medical schools in Canada and the United States. Approved teaching programs for interns and residents are under the direction of the medical school. Research work is being conducted both in the hospitals and in the Health Sciences Centre.

Mission Statement
Our purpose is to enhance the health of people by educating physicians and health scientists, by conducting research in clinical and basic medical sciences and applied health sciences, and by promoting the skills and attitudes of lifelong learning.

Curricular Highlights
Community Service Requirement: Optional.
Research/Thesis Requirement: Optional.

The curriculum, the physical structure, and the administrative organization of the school were planned to allow for maximum cooperation among the various basic science and clinical disciplines. The M.D. degree is granted upon completion of the fourth year. Canadian students take the LMCC (Medical Council of Canada) Examinations and U.S. students take the USMLE (United States Medical Licensing Examination) Step 1 and Step 2. During the first year of the medical program, students take introductory courses in cell structure and functions, biochemistry, physiology, molecular genetics, pharmacology, microbiology, anatomy, behavioral science, ethics, interviewing skills, and community medicine. In the second half of the first year and the second year, teaching has a systems approach; material from anatomy, physiology, pathology, and clinical medicine is presented in an integrated manner. The third year is a structured clinical clerkship that includes eight weeks of electives, and the fourth year is made up of electives and selectives. Rotations for Rural Medicine take place in the first, third, and fourth years. A pass/fail system is used for grading. Medical students may apply through the Offices of Undergraduate Medical Education and Research/Graduate Studies for the M.D./Ph.D. program.

USMLE
Step 1: Must only record a score.
Step 2: Clinical Skills (CS): Must only record a score.
Step 2: Clinical Knowledge (CK): Optional.

Selection Factors
The school admits students on the basis of residency priority as follows: bona fide residents of Newfoundland and Labrador, of New Brunswick, of Prince Edward Island, of other Canadian provinces, and non-Canadians. In every case, a high academic standard is required. Age by itself is not used as a basis for selection or rejection. However, both age and length of time away from full-time academic studies may be taken into consideration. Normally, the medical school does not accept transfer students from other medical schools. In rare circumstances, a transfer applicant may be considered if there is space available.

Financial Aid
Financial assistance is available to medical students through government student loan programs. Information can be obtained by contacting the Student Affairs Office at: Student Affairs Office, Faculty of Medicine, Memorial University of Newfoundland, St. John's, NL, A1B 3VC; by telephone: (709) 777-6690; or by e-mail: mdray@mun.ca.

Information about Diversity Programs
Although there is no formal affirmative action process at this medical school, the Admissions Committee does take into consideration the background of applicants in making its decisions.

Campus Information
Setting
The Faculty of Medicine is housed with the Health Sciences Centre, Janeway Children's Hospital, H.Bliss Murphy Cancer Centre, Telemedicine Centre, Centre for Offshore and Remote Medicine, and Nursing and Pharmacy Schools.

Enrollment
For 2008, total enrollment was: 244

Special Features
Health services are open to all students on campus.

Housing
On-campus housing for single and married students is provided. In addition, the university maintains a list of approved off-campus accommodations.

Application Process and Requirements 2010–2011

Primary Application Service: School-specific
Earliest filing date: July 1, 2009
Latest filing date: October 15, 2009

Secondary Application Required?: No
Sent to: n/a
URL: n/a
Fee: n/a
Fee waiver available: n/a
Earliest filing date: n/a
Latest filing date: n/a

MCAT® required?: Yes
Latest MCAT® considered: September 2009
Oldest MCAT® considered: 2004

Early Decision Program: School does not have EDP
Applicants notified: n/a
EDP available for: n/a

Regular Acceptance Notice
Earliest date: March 1, 2010
Latest date: Until class is full
Applicant's Response to Acceptance
Offer – Maximum Time: Two weeks

Requests for Deferred
Entrance Considered: Yes

Deposit to Hold Place in Class: Yes
Deposit (Resident): $200
Deposit (Non-resident): $200
Deposit due: With response to acceptance offer
Applied to tuition: Yes
Deposit refundable: No
Refundable by: n/a

Estimated number of new entrants: 64
EDP: n/a, special program: n/a

Start Month/Year: September 2010

Interview Format: One hour interview with two interviewers. Regional interviews are not available.

Other Programs

PREPARATORY PROGRAMS
Postbaccalaureate Program: No
Summer Program: Yes,
MedQuest, 709-777-6029, mdray@mun.ca

COMBINED DEGREE PROGRAMS
Baccalaureate/M.D.: No
M.D./M.P.H.: No
M.D./M.B.A.: No
M.D./J.D.: No
M.D./Ph.D.: Yes, www.med.mun.ca/admissions

Premedical Coursework

Course	Req.	Rec.	Lab.	Sems.	Course	Req.	Rec.	Lab.	Sems.
Inorganic Chemistry		•			Computer Science				
Behavioral Sciences		•			Genetics				
Biochemistry		•			Humanities				
Biology		•			Organic Chemistry			•	
Biology/Zoology					Physics			•	
Calculus		•			Psychology				
College English	•			2	Social Sciences				
College Mathematics		•			Other				

Selection Factors: 2008 Accepted Applicants

Proportion of Accepted Applicants with Relevant Experience (Data Self-Reported to AMCAS®)		
Community Service/Volunteer	100%
Medically-Related Work	75%
Research	50%

Shaded bar represents school's accepted scores ranging from the 10th percentile to the 90th percentile   School Median ●   National Median ●

Overall GPA	2.0	2.1	2.2	2.3	2.4	2.5	2.6	2.7	2.8	2.9	3.0	3.1	3.2	3.3	3.4	3.5	3.6	3.7	(3.8)	3.9	4.0
Science GPA	2.0	2.1	2.2	2.3	2.4	2.5	2.6	2.7	2.8	2.9	3.0	3.1	3.2	3.3	3.4	3.5	3.6	3.7	3.8	3.9	4.0

MCAT® Total Numeric Score			**DATA NOT COLLECTED**					

Writing Sample			J	K	L	M	N	O	P	(Q)	R	S	T
Verbal Reasoning	3	4	5	6	7	8	9	(10)	11	12	13	14	15
Biological Sciences	3	4	5	6	7	8	9	(10)	11	12	13	14	15
Physical Sciences	3	4	5	6	7	8	9	(10)	11	12	13	14	15

Acceptance & Matriculation Data for 2008-2009 First Year Class

	Resident	Non-resident	International	Total
Applications	155	531	14	700
Interviewed	115	105	7	227
Deferred	1	0	0	1
Matriculants				
Early Assurance Program	0	0	0	0
Early Decision Program	n/a	n/a	n/a	n/a
Baccalaureate/M.D.	n/a	n/a	n/a	n/a
M.D./Ph.D.	n/a	n/a	n/a	n/a
Matriculated	47	16	1	**64**

Applications accepted from International Applicants: Yes

Specialty Choice

2004, 2005, 2006 Graduates, Specialty Choice	
Anesthesiology	4%
Emergency Medicine	3%
Family Practice	36%
Internal Medicine	9%
Obstetrics/Gynecology	5%
Orthopedic Surgery	3%
Pediatrics	11%
Psychiatry	10%
Radiology	10%
Surgery	8%

Matriculant Demographics: 2008–2009 First Year Class

Men: 24   **Women:** 40

Matriculants' Self-Reported Race/Ethnicity

Mexican American   Korean
Cuban   Vietnamese
Puerto Rican   Other Asian
Other Hispa   Native A
Total Hispan
Chinese   **DATA NOT COLLECTED**
Asian Indian
Pakistani
Filipino   **Unduplicated Number**
Japanese   **of Matriculants**

Science and Math Majors: 90%
Matriculants with:
Baccalaureate degree: 100%
Graduate degree(s): 19%

Financial Information

	Residents	Non-residents
Total Cost of Attendance	$27,400	$51,400
Tuition and Fees	$6,250	$30,000
Other (includes living expenses)	$20,988	$20,790
Health Insurance (can be waived)	$162	$610

Average 2008 Graduate Indebtedness: $100,000
% of Enrolled Students Receiving Aid: 80%

Criminal Background Check

This medical school does not require a criminal background check prior to matriculation.

Dalhousie University Faculty of Medicine

Halifax, Nova Scotia

Admissions and Student Affairs
Room C-124, Lower Level
Clinical Research Centre, Dalhousie University
Halifax, Nova Scotia
Canada, B3H 4H7
T 902 494 1874   F 902 494 6369

Admissions http://admissions.medicine.dal.ca
Main www.medicine.dal.ca
Financial http://as01.ucis.dal.ca/staccts/
2006-2007/MD.pdf
E-mail medicine.admissions@dal.ca

Public Institution

Dr. Harold Cook, Dean

Dr. Evelyn Sutton, Assistant Dean, Admissions and Student Affairs

General Information

Dalhousie University, a privately endowed institution founded in 1838, established the Faculty of Medicine in 1868. The main responsibility of the Faculty of Medicine is to the three Maritime Provinces of Canada (Nova Scotia, New Brunswick, and Prince Edward Island), which have a population of 1.7 million. The teaching hospitals located in the immediate vicinity of the medical school have a total of 2,300 beds covering inpatient and outpatient services in all branches of medicine.

Mission Statement

The Faculty of Medicine, Dalhousie University, strives to benefit society through equal commitment to exemplary patient care, education and the discovery and advancement of knowledge. We aim to create and maintain a learning and research environment of national and international stature, enabling our graduates and us to serve the health needs of the Maritime Provinces and Canada.

Curricular Highlights

Community Service Requirement: Optional.
Research/Thesis Requirement: Optional.

Dalhousie aims to provide a basic education that would permit a graduate to enter any branch of postgraduate training. Medicine One and Two begin in early September and extend through May. Medicine Three begins in late August/early September and ends the following September. Medicine Four begins in late September and extends until the following May. In the first year, students have extensive patient contact hours, with great emphasis on the development of clinical skills. During the first two years, students work in small groups with a tutor. The curriculum is organized around clinical problems to provide an integrated context for students to learn both basic and clinical science, and to begin the development of clinical reasoning skills. The third and fourth years are predominantly clinical, with

third year comprised of 12-week units in the major disciplines. The fourth year is arranged with initial blocks of elective time. Students finish with a unit in Continuing and Preventive Care. Dalhousie offers postgraduate medical trainees university-arranged and university-supervised clinical training which meets national accreditation standards. In all provinces with the exception of Quebec, the basis for licensure for the majority of trainees in a postgraduate training program affiliated with a CACMS/LCME medical school is successful completion of the two-part Medical Council of Canada Qualifying Examination (MCCQE), plus certification by either the College of Family Physicians of Canada or the Royal College of Physicians and Surgeons of Canada. The family medicine program at Dalhousie is a two-year integrated training experience following the M.D., leading to certification by the College of Family Physicians of Canada. Specialty training is conducted in affiliated teaching hospitals in both Halifax and Saint John. Dalhousie University currently holds Royal College approval for 41 specialty training programs. The Faculty of Medicine maintains an active program of continuing medical education for practicing physicians in the Maritime Provinces. Research and graduate education take place in all the basic science departments and in most of the clinical departments.

USMLE

Step 1: Optional.
Step 2: Clinical Skills (CS): Optional.
Step 2: Clinical Knowledge (CK): Optional.

Selection Factors

Sources of information and factors considered by the Admissions Committee include academic requirements, ability as judged on university records and on the MCAT, confidential assessments received from referees of the applicant's choice and from any others the committee may wish to consult, interviews (selected applicants only), and place of residence. Detailed comments and explanations on these selection factors may be obtained in the Faculty of Medicine Calendar. Dalhousie does not discriminate on the basis of race, sex, creed, national origin, age, or handicap.

Financial Aid

A few entrance scholarships and entrance bursaries are awarded to students in the first year who are residents of the Maritime Provinces. The Dalhousie Medical Alumni Association Entrance Scholarship, the Dr. E. James Gordon Scholarship, and the Halifax Medical Society Entrance Scholarship are available to anyone regardless of residency. A number of bursaries and prizes are available in each year.

Information about Diversity Programs

Students from groups underrepresented in medicine will be considered on their individual merits. Dalhousie University is an affirmative action and equal opportunity educational institution.

Campus Information

Setting

Dalhousie Medical School plays a direct and vital role in patient care in the Maritimes. Our students and residents experience "distributed learning" in over 100 teaching sites, including tertiary and community hospitals, continuing care facilities and rural physician offices throughout the Maritimes.

Enrollment

For 2008, total enrollment was: 397

Housing

University housing and a comprehensive Student Health Service are available.

Application Process and Requirements 2010–2011

Primary Application Service: School-specific
Earliest filing date: September 1, 2009
Latest filing date: November 2, 2009

Secondary Application Required?: No
Sent to: n/a
URL: http://admissions.medicine.dal.ca/application.htm
Fee: n/a
Fee waiver available: n/a
Earliest filing date: n/a
Latest filing date: n/a

MCAT® required?: Yes
Latest MCAT® considered: 2009
Oldest MCAT® considered: 2004

Early Decision Program: School does not have EDP
Applicants notified: n/a
EDP available for: n/a

Regular Acceptance Notice
Earliest date: May 15, 2010
Latest date: Varies
Applicant's Response to Acceptance Offer – Maximum Time: Three weeks

Requests for Deferred Entrance Considered: No

Deposit to Hold Place in Class: Yes
Deposit (Resident): $200
Deposit (Non-resident): $200
Deposit due: With response to acceptance offer
Applied to tuition: Yes
Deposit refundable: No
Refundable by: n/a

Estimated number of new entrants: 98
EDP: n/a, special program: n/a

Start Month/Year: September 2010

Interview Format: Interview format is Multiple Mini Interview. Regional interviews are not available.

Other Programs

PREPARATORY PROGRAMS
Postbaccalaureate Program: No
Summer Program: No

COMBINED DEGREE PROGRAMS
Baccalaureate/M.D.: No
M.D./M.P.H.: No
M.D./M.B.A.: No
M.D./J.D.: No
M.D./Ph.D.: No

Premedical Coursework

Course	Req.	Rec.	Lab.	Hrs.
Inorganic Chemistry		•		
Behavioral Sciences				
Biochemistry				
Biology		•		
Biology/Zoology				
Calculus				
College English				
College Mathematics				

Course	Req.	Rec.	Lab.	Hrs.
Computer Science				
Genetics				
Humanities		•		
Organic Chemistry		•		
Physics		•		
Psychology				
Social Sciences		•		
Other				

Selection Factors: 2007 Accepted Applicants

Proportion of Accepted Applicants with Relevant Experience (Data Self-Reported to AMCAS®)	**DATA NOT COLLECTED**

Shaded bar represents school's accepted scores ranging from the 10th percentile to the 90th percentile   School Median ● National Median ●

Overall GPA	DATA NOT REPORTED
Science GPA	

MCAT® Total Numeric Score 9 10 11 12 13 14 15 16 17 18 19 20 21 22 23 24 25 26 27 28 29 30 31 32 33 34 35 36 37 38 39 40 41 42 43

Verbal Reasoning	
Physical Sciences	DATA NOT REPORTED
Biological Sciences	
Writing Sample	

Acceptance & Matriculation Data for 2008–2009 First Year Class

	Resident	Non-resident	International	Total
Applications	308	270	0	578
Interviewed	250	50	0	300
Deferred				
Matriculants				
Early Assurance Program	n/a	n/a	n/a	n/a
Early Decision Program	n/a	n/a	n/a	n/a
Baccalaureate/M.D.	n/a	n/a	n/a	n/a
M.D./Ph.D.	n/a	n/a	n/a	n/a
Matriculated				**92**

Applications accepted from International Applicants: Yes

Matriculant Demographics: 2008–2009 First Year Class

Men: 54   **Women:** 48

Matriculants' Self-Reported Race/Ethnicity

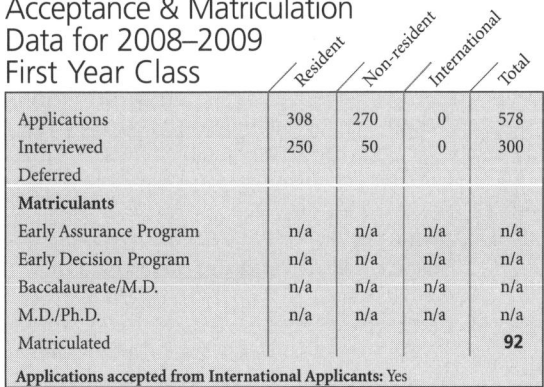

Mexican American	Korean
Cuban	Vietnamese
Puerto Rican	Other Asian
Other	
Total	**DATA NOT COLLECTED**
Chinese	
Asian	
Pakistani	Total Asian
Filipino	**Unduplicated Number**
Japanese	**of Matriculants**

Science and Math Majors: n/r
Matriculants with:
   Baccalaureate degree: n/r
   Graduate degree(s): n/r

Specialty Choice

2004, 2005, 2006 Graduates, Specialty Choice
Anesthesiology
Emergency Medicine
Family Practice
DATA NOT COLLECTED
Psychiatry
Radiology
Surgery

Financial Information

	Residents	Non-residents
Total Cost of Attendance	n/r	n/r
Tuition and Fees	n/r	n/r
Other (includes living expenses)	n/r	n/r
Health Insurance (not applicable)	n/r	n/r

Average 2008 Graduate Indebtedness: n/r
% of Enrolled Students Receiving Aid: n/r

Criminal Background Check

This school does not require a criminal background check prior to matriculation.

McMaster University, Michael G. DeGroote School of Medicine

Hamilton, Ontario

Michael G. DeGroote School of Medicine
McMaster University
MD Admissions, MDCL 3115
1200 Main Street West
Hamilton, Ontario
Canada, L8N 3Z5
T 905 525 9140 x22235   **F** 905 546 0349

Admissions www.fhs.mcmaster.ca/mdprog/
admissions/admissions.htm
Main www.fhs.mcmaster.ca/mdprog
Financial www.sfas.mcmaster.ca
E-mail mdadmit@mcmaster.ca

Public Institution

Dr. John Kelton, Dean and Vice President, Health Sciences

Dr. Harold Reiter, Chair, M.D. Admissions

Dr. Alan Neville, Assistant Dean, M.D. Program

Cathy Oudshoorn, M.D. Program Administrator

General Information

The Faculty of Health Sciences at McMaster University offers programs in health sciences education, including undergraduate and post-graduate medical education. The clinical programs use the teaching hospital and extensive ambulatory facilities of the McMaster Division of the Hamilton Health Sciences Corporation, but they also involve clinical teaching units at the major Hamilton hospitals and surrounding community health care centers.

Mission Statement

"Together, Advancing Health Through Learning and Discovery."

Curricular Highlights

Community Service Requirement: Optional.
Research/Thesis Requirement: Optional.

The three-year M.D. program at McMaster uses an approach to learning that will apply throughout a physician's career. The components have been organized in a logical manner, with early exposure to patients. Flexibility is ensured to allow for the variety of backgrounds and career goals. Graduates of McMaster's Medical Program will have developed the knowledge, ability, and attitudes necessary to qualify for further education in any medical career. The goals for students include the following: the development of competency in problem-based learning and problem-solving, the development of personal characteristics and attitudes compatible with effective health care, the development of clinical and communication skills, and the development of the skills to be a lifelong, self-directed learner and self-reflective practitioner. To achieve these objectives, students are introduced to patients within the first Medical Foundation block of the curriculum. They are presented with a

series of tutorial cases and questions requiring the understanding of principles and data collection. Much of the students' learning occurs within the small-group tutorial. Faculty members serve as tutors or sources of expert knowledge. The medical program is arranged as a preclerkship sequence of five Medical Foundations followed by clerkship. A Professional Competencies curriculum runs horizontally across the Foundations and into the clerkship. There are elective opportunities, both in block periods and horizontal electives taken concurrently. The clerkship emphasizes the clinical application of concepts learned in the earlier Foundations and consists of experience in inpatient and ambulatory settings. These include internal medicine, family medicine, emergency medicine, surgery, psychiatry, obstetrics-gynecology, anesthesia, and pediatrics. Students will have the opportunity to work in both teaching hospital and community hospital environments.

USMLE

Step 1: Optional.
Step 2: Clinical Skills (CS): Optional.
Step 2: Clinical Knowledge (CK): Optional.

Selection Factors

Students and members of the community and faculty are involved in the assessment of applicants. The aim is to select students who not only have the necessary academic standards, but who also display characteristics that are deemed to be important for the study and practice of medicine. These include characteristics that suggest sensitivity to the needs of the community; sensitivity to the emotional, psychological, and physical aspects of patients; the ability to detect and solve problems; the ability to learn independently; the ability to function as a member of a small group; and the ability to plan one's career in a way that reflects the needs of the community. Applicants rating highest in academic achievement and in noncognitive qualities will be invited to the interview. From these applicants, 182 students will be selected for three campuses.

Financial Aid

The M.D. Program and the University Financial Aid Program offer a large bursary

program to assist students in financial need. The M.D. Program administers a small loans program for students in further need.

Campus Information

Setting

Beginning in 2008, McMaster consists of three campuses – the Hamilton campus sits on the main McMaster University campus in Hamilton Ontario; the Waterloo Regional campus, which opened in 2007, is situated in Kitchener, Ontario and the Niagara Regional Campus, which opened in 2008, is located in St. Catharines Ontario.

Enrollment

For 2008, total enrollment was: 494

Special Features

McMaster's undergraduate medical program has become internationally known for its small-group, problem-based learning approach to medical education. Most recently, the school has been renamed in honor of the landmark and generous donation from philanthropist Michael G. DeGroote.

Housing

The McMaster Housing Office maintains a list of affordable housing in the area for students.

Satellite Campuses/Facilities

Tutorial and clinical training opportunities exist at McMaster University and in community hospitals throughout Central West Ontario. Satellite campuses are now open in the Waterloo region (21 students admitted/year) and Niagara region (15 students admitted/year).

Application Process and Requirements 2010–2011

Primary Application Service: OMSAS
Earliest filing date: July 1, 2009
Latest filing date: September 15, 2009

Secondary Application Required?: Yes
Sent to: OMSAS
URL: www.ouac.on.ca/omsas
Fee: Yes, $210
Fee waiver available: No
Earliest filing date: July 1, 2009
Latest filing date: September 15, 2009

MCAT® required?: Yes
Latest MCAT® considered: September 2009
Oldest MCAT® considered: September 2004

Early Decision Program
School does not have EDP
Applicants notified: n/a
EDP available for: n/a

Regular Acceptance Notice
Earliest date: May 15, 2010
Latest date: Until class is full

Applicant's Response to Acceptance
Offer – Maximum Time: Two weeks

Requests for Deferred
Entrance Considered: Yes

Deposit to Hold Place in Class: Yes
Deposit (Resident): $1,000
Deposit (Non-resident): $1,000
Deposit due: With acceptance of offer
Applied to tuition: Yes
Deposit refundable: No
Refundable by: n/a

Estimated number of new entrants: 182
EDP: 0, special program: 0

Start Month/Year: Late August 2010

Interview Format: Multiple mini-interviews. Regional interviews are not available.

Other Programs

PREPARATORY PROGRAMS
Postbaccalaureate Program: No
Summer Program: No

COMBINED DEGREE PROGRAMS
Baccalaureate/M.D.: No
M.D./M.P.H.: No
M.D./M.B.A.: No
M.D./J.D.: No
M.D./Ph.D.: Yes, https://gradapplication.mcmaster.ca/account/instructions.asp

Premedical Coursework

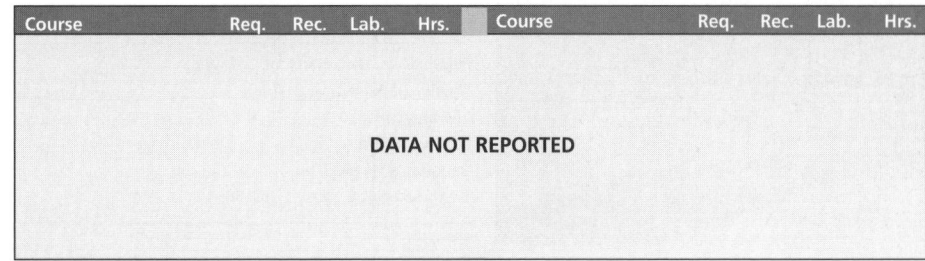

Course	Req.	Rec.	Lab.	Hrs.	Course	Req.	Rec.	Lab.	Hrs.
				DATA NOT REPORTED					

Selection Factors: 2008 Accepted Applicants

Proportion of Accepted Applicants with Relevant Experience (Data Self-Reported to AMCAS®)			Community Service/Volunteer Medically-Related Work Research	DATA NOT COLLECTED

Shaded bar represents school's accepted scores ranging from the 10th percentile to the 90th percentile   School Median ● National Median ●

	Overall GPA																																		
	Science GPA									DATA NOT COLLECTED																									

MCAT® Total Numeric Score	9	10	11	12	13	14	15	16	17	18	19	20	21	22	23	24	25	26	27	28	29	30	31	32	33	34	35	36	37	38	39	40	41	42	43
Writing Sample							J	K	L		M	N	O	P	Q															R		S			T
Verbal Reasoning	3	4									DATA NOT COLLECTED																						14		15
Biological Sciences	3	4																															14		15
Physical Sciences	3	4	5	6	7		8		9		10		11		12		13		14		15														

Acceptance & Matriculation Data for 2008–2009 First Year Class

	Resident	Non-resident	International	Total
Applications	3680	991	67	4738
Interviewed	491	54	1	546
Deferred	1	0	0	1
Matriculants				
Early Assurance Program	0	0	0	0
Early Decision Program	n/a	n/a	n/a	n/a
Baccalaureate/M.D.	n/a	n/a	n/a	n/a
M.D./Ph.D.	n/a	n/a	n/a	n/a
Matriculated	167	16	0	**183**

Applications accepted from International Applicants: Yes

Specialty Choice

2004, 2005, 2006 Graduates, Specialty Choice
Anesthesiology
Emergency Medicine
Family Practice
DATA NOT COLLECTED
Psychiatry
Radiology
Surgery

Matriculant Demographics: 2008–2009 First Year Class

Men: 66   **Women:** 117

Matriculants' Self-Reported Race/Ethnicity

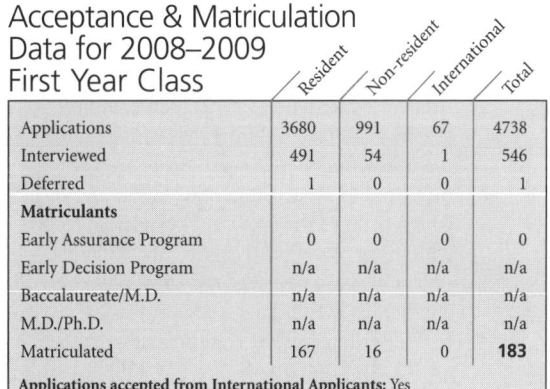

Mexican American   Korean
Cuban   Vietnamese
Puerto Rican   Other Asian
Other H...   ...rican
Total His...   **DATA NOT COLLECTED**   ...aiian
Chinese
Asian In...
Pakistan...   ...otal Asian
Filipino   **Unduplicated Number**
Japanese   **of Matriculants**

Science and Math Majors: 79%
Matriculants with:
Baccalaureate degree: 90%
Graduate degree(s): 14%

Financial Information

	Residents	Non-residents
Total Cost of Attendance	$21,921	$ 94,862
Tuition and Fees	$18,921	$91,862
Other (includes living expenses)	n/c	n/c
Health Insurance (can be waived)	n/c	n/c

Average 2008 Graduate Indebtedness: $120,000
% of Enrolled Students Receiving Aid: 70%

Criminal Background Check

This medical school requires a criminal background check prior to matriculation.

University of Ottawa Faculty of Medicine

Ottawa, Ontario

Admissions, University of Ottawa
Faculty of Medicine
451 Smyth Road
Ottawa, Ontario
Canada, K1H 8M5
T 613 562 5409   F 613 562 5651

Admissions www.uottawa.ca/whychoose
Main www.medicine.uottawa.ca/eng
Financial www.uottawa.ca/student/englishguide/
1section/finance
E-mail admissmd@uottawa.ca

Public Institution

Dr. Jacques Bradwejn, Dean

Chantal Renaud, Admissions Officer

*Dr. Richard L. Hebert,
Assistant Dean, Admissions*

*Dr. Arlington Dungy, Associate Dean,
Alumni and Student Affairs*

General Information

The University of Ottawa received its charter from the province of Ontario in 1866. It was founded by the Missionary Oblates of Mary Immaculate, who were its administrators until 1965, when important structural reforms were introduced through an act of the legislative assembly of the province of Ontario. The management, discipline, and control of the university are free from the restrictions and control of any outside body, whether lay or religious. The Faculty of Medicine was established in 1945.

Mission Statement

We explore, we learn, we care. We develop society's leaders who improve the health of Canadians and communities worldwide. We do this through the integration of education, research, patient care, and technology in an inclusive environment, in both official languages.

Curricular Highlights

Community Service Requirement: Optional.
Research/Thesis Requirement: Optional.

Students acquire the knowledge, skills, and attitudes necessary to recognize, understand, and apply effective, efficient strategies for the prevention and treatment of common and important health problems. Emphasis is placed on self-learning principles, and facts are assimilated in a multidisciplinary fashion, within the context of clinical problems. Lectures and seminars are used to discuss basic concepts. Training occurs in ambulatory, primary, secondary, distributed and tertiary settings. The program emphasizes health promotion and disease prevention and is responsive to individual needs and the health care system. The

program fosters the qualities of trust and compassion, communication skills, ethical professional conduct, and patient advocacy. The program is scheduled over four calendar years and is divided into two stages. The preclerkship includes 70 weeks of study of essential biomedical principles and consists of multidisciplinary units. Students learn communication and clinical skills in an integrated fashion with the study of body systems. The clerkship, of two years duration, is devoted to clinical rotations; an extended period is available for elective study.

USMLE

Step 1: Optional.
Step 2: Clinical Skills (CS): Optional.
Step 2: Clinical Knowledge (CK): Optional.

Selection Factors

Academic excellence, the detailed autobiographical sketch, and interview rating are the main selection factors used. Academics are measured by an assessment of marks and by a comparison of the applicant's academic record with those of the other applicants. No preference is given to one academic program over another. In selecting its students, the University of Ottawa reserves the right to assess, in the applicant's program, the level of difficulty of the courses and/or their pertinence for future medical studies and the performance achieved by the candidate. The selection is not made by quota. No candidate will be admitted without an interview. It is highly desirable that the candidate who has a broad exposure to biology and physical sciences also have a broad exposure to the arts, humanities, and social sciences. In view of the limited number of places available, a candidate whose GPA is below 3.5 has considerably less chance of being admitted. Sex, race, age, religion, and socioeconomic status play no part in the selection process.

Financial Aid

Students may apply to the Student Financial Aid Office of the university and to their respective provincial governments for loan assistance. The Ontario Medical Association Bursaries and Loan Fund, the Kellogg Foundation Loan Fund, and a special bursaries

fund are administered by the Awards Committee of the Faculty. The Association of Professors of the University also provides bursaries. Most of these awards are made on the basis of demonstrable financial need and good academic standing.

Information about Diversity Programs

In 2005, the Faculty established a dedicated admissions program for candidates of Aboriginal ancestry as part of its mission to improve access to better health care for Aboriginal peoples and to better serve society's needs.

Campus Information

Setting

The Faculty of Medicine is located in a building which also houses the Faculty of Health Sciences. The building is located off the main campus within a health sciences complex where a few of the affiliated teaching hospitals are also located. Medical students have access to the many student services on main campus (downtown) through the services of a shuttle.

Enrollment

For 2008, total enrollment was: 613

Special Features

Medical students benefit from a diverse learning environment with a laptop-supported Web-based curriculum and case-based learning (CBL) approach combined with traditional learning methods.

Housing

A good number of medical students live in groups of 2 or 3 and share costs in affordable townhouses in a residential area within close proximity (5 to 10 minutes walking distance) of the campus. The Admissions Office also puts together a housing file of availabilities for newly admitted students' perusal. Housing information (off-campus and residencies) is available at: *www.uottawa.ca/students/housing/*.

Application Process and Requirements 2010–2011

Primary Application Service: OMSAS
Earliest filing date: July 2009
Latest filing date: September 15, 2009

Secondary Application Required?: No
Sent to: n/a
URL: n/a
Fee: n/a
Fee waiver available: No
Earliest filing date: n/a
Latest filing date: n/a

MCAT® required?: No
Latest MCAT® considered: n/a
Oldest MCAT® considered: n/a

Early Decision Program
School does not have EDP
Applicants notified: n/a
EDP available for: n/a

Regular Acceptance Notice
Earliest date: May 15, 2010
Latest date: Until class is full

Applicant's Response to Acceptance
Offer – Maximum Time: Two weeks

Requests for Deferred
Entrance Considered: Yes

Deposit to Hold Place in Class: Yes
Deposit (Resident): $1,000
Deposit (Non-resident): n/a
Deposit due: with acceptance
Applied to tuition: Yes
Deposit refundable: No
Refundable by: n/a

Estimated number of new entrants: 143
EDP: n/a, special program: n/a

Start Month/Year: September 2010

Interview Format: Semi-structured, 45-minute interviews. Regional interviews are not available.

Other Programs

PREPARATORY PROGRAMS
Postbaccalaureate Program: No
Summer Program: No

COMBINED DEGREE PROGRAMS
Baccalaureate/M.D.: No
M.D./M.P.H.: No
M.D./M.B.A.: No
M.D./J.D.: No
M.D./Ph.D.: No

Premedical Coursework

Course	Req.	Rec.	Lab.	Sems.
Inorganic Chemistry	•		•	2
Behavioral Sciences				
Biochemistry	•			2
Biology				
Biology/Zoology	•		•	2
Calculus				
College English				
College Mathematics				

Course	Req.	Rec.	Lab.	Sems.
Computer Science				
Genetics				
Humanities	•			2
Organic Chemistry	•		•	2
Physics				
Psychology				
Social Sciences				
Other				

Selection Factors: 2008 Accepted Applicants

Proportion of Accepted Applicants with Relevant Experience (Data Self-Reported to AMCAS®)	DATA NOT COLLECTED

Shaded bar represents school's accepted scores ranging from the 10th percentile to the 90th percentile ● School Median ● National Median

	2.0	2.1	2.2	2.3	2.4	2.5	2.6	2.7	2.8	2.9	3.0	3.1	3.2	3.3	3.4	3.5	3.6	3.7	3.8	3.9	4.0
Overall GPA																					
Science GPA																					

MCAT® Total Numeric

DATA NOT COLLECTED

Writing Sample
Verbal Reasoning
Biological Sciences
Physical Sciences

Acceptance & Matriculation Data for 2008–2009 First Year Class

	Resident	Non-resident	International	Total
Applications	2436	833	n/a	3269
Interviewed	532	n/r	n/r	532
Deferred	2	n/r	n/r	2
Matriculants				
Early Assurance Program	n/a	n/a	n/a	n/a
Early Decision Program	n/a	n/a	n/a	n/a
Baccalaureate/M.D.	n/a	n/a	n/a	n/a
M.D./Ph.D.	n/a	n/a	n/a	n/a
Matriculated	131	12	0	**143**

Applications accepted from International Applicants: No

Specialty Choice

2004, 2005, 2006 Graduates, Specialty Choice
Anesthesiology
Emergency Medicine
Family Practice
DATA NOT COLLECTED
Psychiatry
Radiology
Surgery

Matriculant Demographics: 2008–2009 First Year Class

Men: 54   **Women:** 89

Matriculants' Self-Reported Race/Ethnicity

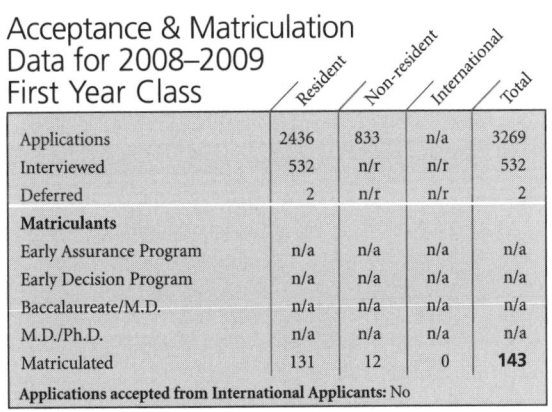

Mexican American
Cuban
Puerto Rican
Other
Total H
Chines
Asian
Pakista...
Filipino
Japanese

Korean
Vietnamese
Other Asian

DATA NOT COLLECTED

Unduplicated Number of Matriculants

Science and Math Majors: 66%
Matriculants with:
    Baccalaureate degree: 76%
    Graduate degree(s): 27%

Financial Information

	Residents	Non-residents
Total Cost of Attendance	n/a	n/a
Tuition and Fees	$15,976	n/a
Incidental fees	$581	n/a
Health Insurance (Voluntary)	$180	n/a

Average 2008 Graduate Indebtedness: n/a
% of Enrolled Students Receiving Aid: n/a

Criminal Background Check

This medical school requires a criminal background check prior to matriculation.

Queen's University Faculty of Health Sciences School of Medicine

Kingston, Ontario

Admissions Office, Queen's University
School of Medicine
68 Barrie Street
Kingston, Ontario
Canada, K7L 3N6
T 613 533 3307   **F** 613 533 3190

Admissions http://meds.queensu.ca/
undergraduate/prospective_students
Main http://meds.queensu.ca/home
Financial http://meds.queensu.ca/undergrad/
student_information/financial_awards_or_loans
E-mail queensmd@queensu.ca

Public Institution

*Dr. David Walker, Dean, Faculty of
Health Science*

Jennifer Saunders, Admissions Officer

Dr. Anthony J. Sanfilippo, Associate Dean

General Information

The School of Medicine is an integral part of
Queen's University. With a legacy of over 150
years of quality teaching and research, the
environment and the flexibility of the curriculum complement innovative programs that
provide the breadth of training required for
practice throughout Canada.

Mission Statement

The mission of Queen's Medicine is to advance
our tradition of preparing excellent physicians
and leaders in health care. We embrace a spirit
of inquiry and innovation in education and
research.

Curricular Highlights
Community Service Requirement: Optional.
Research/Thesis Requirement: Optional.

The four-year Undergraduate Medical Program
is structured in three sequential phases allowing
students to progress from foundational knowledge through specific specialty applications and
finally through clinical engagement during an
eighteen-month clerkship. Our medical program is well known for the opportunities it provides for close personal interaction between students and faculty members, and for students
obtaining relevant extensive hands-on clinical
experiences under supervision, particularly in
an ambulatory setting. Our medical culture
offers opportunities for students to engage in
the administration, development and evaluation
of our medical curriculum and our governance
structures. Our graduates are highly successful
in obtaining postgraduate training positions
and are known to be committed and enthusiastic professionals within their communities.

USMLE
Step 1: Optional.
Step 2: Clinical Skills (CS): Optional.
Step 2: Clinical Knowledge (CK): Optional.

Selection Factors

Students are selected on the basis of a strong
academic record and assessment of personal
characteristics considered to be most appropriate for the study of medicine at Queen's
University and for the subsequent practice of
medicine. Candidates to be invited for an
interview are determined based on converted
GPA and MCAT results. Candidates who do
not make the academic cut based on their
undergraduate grade point average, but who
have completed graduate work are considered
separately. Candidates meeting the academic
requirements are then assessed based on confidential letters of reference, the autobiographic
sketch, and the personal interview. These candidates will be ranked for offers and placement
on the waiting list. The Admissions Committee
does not give preference to applicants who
have studied in any particular university program nor any particular level of training. Place
of residence and location of the university
where studies have been undertaken are not
criteria in selection. Age, gender, race, and religion are not factors considered in the selection
process.

Financial Aid

Student financial assistance at Queen's
University is offered through merit-based
(scholarships) and need-based (bursaries,
awards, and work-study) funding. The Student
Awards Web site is located at:
www.queensu.ca/registrar/awards.

Information about Diversity Programs

The Admissions Committee recognizes the
critical shortage of aboriginal physicians in
Canada and the need to educate more aboriginal physicians to serve as role models and to
address the health care needs of Canada's aboriginal people. The committee has developed an
alternate process for assessment of aboriginal
candidates. Up to a maximum of four qualified
aboriginal students per year may be admitted
to the M.D. program by the alternate process.
Aboriginal candidates may also choose to apply
through the regular admission process.

Campus Information

Setting
The campus is located in Kingston, Ontario, a
true university town with the benefits of a
small community such as affordable cost-of-
living, a peaceful waterfront, and minimal traffic and the cultural richness of an urban centre, including acclaimed restaurants, pubs, theatre and music. Kingston is ideally situated
between Toronto, Montreal, and Ottawa.

Enrollment
For 2008, total enrollment was: 400

Special Features
Queen's University School of Medicine produces physicians equipped to handle the complex, ever-changing world of 21st-century
health care. Small class sizes, frequent interaction with professors, and a strong mentorship
program make for a close-knit community at
the school. A regional education model allows
students to experience a broad range of healthcare settings, while exposure to advanced
health sciences research nurtures innovation
and critical thinking. Early and extensive
hands-on clinical experience is another distinctive feature of the program. Queen's offers all
the advantages of one of Canada's leading
medical schools — including an international
reputation for exceptional graduates — in an
intimate, supportive learning environment.

Housing
Information on Queen's housing and residence
is available at *www.queensu.ca/dsao/housing/
ah1.htm* and *https://housing.queensu.ca/
residence.* Most medical students prefer to find
their own accommodations, generally living
within a 15-minute walk from campus.

Satellite Campuses/Facilities
Clinical rotations occur in Kingston teaching
hospitals and in affiliated regional sites in
Southeastern Ontario.

Application Process and Requirements 2010–2011

Primary Application Service: OMSAS
Earliest filing date: July 2009
Latest filing date: October 1, 2009

Secondary Application Required?: No
Sent to: n/a
URL: n/a
Fee: n/a
Fee waiver available: n/a
Earliest filing date: n/a
Latest filing date: n/a

MCAT® required?: Yes
Latest MCAT® considered: September 2009
Oldest MCAT® considered: September 2004

Early Decision Program
School does not have EDP
Applicants notified: n/a
EDP available for: n/a

Regular Acceptance Notice
Earliest date: May 15, 2010
Latest date: Until class is full

Applicant's Response to Acceptance
Offer – Maximum Time: Two weeks

Requests for Deferred
Entrance Considered: Yes

Deposit to Hold Place in Class: Yes
Deposit (Resident): $1,000
Deposit (Non-resident): $1,000
Deposit due: With response to firm acceptance
Applied to tuition: Yes
Deposit refundable: No
Refundable by: n/a

Estimated number of new entrants: 100
EDP: n/a, special program: n/a

Start Month/Year: September 2010

Interview Format: Panel interviews. Regional interviews are not available.

Other Programs

PREPARATORY PROGRAMS
Postbaccalaureate Program: No
Summer Program: No

COMBINED DEGREE PROGRAMS
Baccalaureate/M.D.: No
M.D./M.P.H.: No
M.D./M.B.A.: No
M.D./J.D.: No
M.D./Ph.D.: No

Premedical Coursework

Course	Req.	Rec.	Lab.	Sems.
Inorganic Chemistry				
Behavioral Sciences				
Biochemistry				
Biology				
Biology/Zoology				
Calculus				
College English				
College Mathematics				

Course	Req.	Rec.	Lab.	Sems.
Computer Science				
Humanities	•			2
Organic Chemistry				
Physics				
Psychology				
Social Sciences	•			2
Physical Science	•			2
Biological Science	•			2

Selection Factors: 2008 Accepted Applicants

Proportion of Accepted Applicants with Relevant Experience (Data Self-Reported to AMCAS®)	Community Service/Volunteer Medically-Related Work Research	**DATA NOT COLLECTED**

Shaded bar represents school's accepted scores ranging from the 10th percentile to the 90th percentile. School Median ● National Median ●

Overall GPA	2.0 2.1 2.2 2.3 2.4 2.5 2.6 2.7 2.8 2.9 3.0 3.1 3.2 3.3 3.4 3.5 3.6 3.7 3.8	3.9 4.0
Science GPA	2.0 2.1	.9 4.0
MCAT® Total Numeric		41 42 43
Writing Sample	**DATA NOT COLLECTED**	T
Verbal Reasoning		15
Biological Sciences		15
Physical Sciences		15

Acceptance & Matriculation Data for 2008–2009 First Year Class

	Resident	Non-resident	International	Total
Applications	1851	n/a	n/a	1851
Interviewed	490	n/a	n/a	489
Deferred	5	n/a	n/a	5
Matriculants				
Early Assurance Program	0	0	0	0
Early Decision Program	n/a	n/a	n/a	n/a
Baccalaureate/M.D.	n/a	n/a	n/a	n/a
M.D./Ph.D.	n/a	n/a	n/a	n/a
Matriculated	100	n/a	n/a	**100**

Applications accepted from International Applicants: No

Specialty Choice

2004, 2005, 2006 Graduates, Specialty Choice
Anesthesiology
Emergency Medicine
Family Practice
DATA NOT COLLECTED
Psychiatry
Radiology
Surgery

Matriculant Demographics: 2008–2009 First Year Class

Men: 48　　　　**Women:** 52

Matriculants' Self-Reported Race/Ethnicity

Mexican American
Cuban
Puerto Rican
Other
Total H
Chines
Asian I
Pakistan
Filipino
Japanese

Korean
Vietnamese
Other Asian

DATA NOT COLLECTED

Total Asian
Unduplicated Number of Matriculants

Science and Math Majors: 0%
Matriculants with:
　　　　Baccalaureate degree: 0%
　　　　Graduate degree(s): 0%

Financial Information

	Residents	Non-residents
Total Cost of Attendance	n/r	n/r
Tuition and Fees	$16,345	$16,345
Other (includes living expenses)	$0	$0
Health Insurance (not applicable)	n/a	n/a

Average 2008 Graduate Indebtedness: n/r
% of Enrolled Students Receiving Aid: n/r

Criminal Background Check

This medical school requires a criminal background check prior to matriculation.

University of Toronto Faculty of Medicine

Toronto, Ontario

University of Toronto, Faculty of Medicine
Medical Sciences Building, Room 2135
1 King's College Circle
Toronto, Ontario
Canada, M5S 1A8
T 416 978 7928 F 416 971 2163

Admissions www.facmed.utoronto.ca/programs/md/admissions/0910.htm
Main www.facmed.utoronto.ca
Financial www.facmed.utoronto.ca/programs/md/admissions/finance.htm
E-mail medicine.admiss@utoronto.ca

Public Institution

Catharine Whiteside, Dean

Dr. M. Shandling, Associate Dean, Admissions and Student Financial Services

Dr. David McKnight, Associate Dean, Equity and Professionalism

Bill Gregg, Associate Registrar, Student Financial Services

Deborah L. Coombs, Coordinator, Admissions and Awards

Leslie Taylor, Admissions Officer

General Information

Founded in 1843 as a school of medicine, the University of Toronto's Faculty of Medicine is an integral component of one of North America's largest health science complexes. Through the University of Toronto, the Faculty is affiliated with a network of teaching hospitals and community-based health units that offer the Faculty's students a broad spectrum of educational experiences. Placements, including core clerkship placements, are not limited to the major teaching hospitals and will extend into the surrounding regions.

Mission Statement

We prepare future health leaders, contribute to our communities, and improve the health of individuals and populations through the discovery, application and communication of knowledge.

Curricular Highlights

Community Service Requirement: Required. Community placement during a longitudinal course.

Research/Thesis Requirement: Optional.

The four-year curriculum is focused on student-centered learning. The preclerkship phase (approximately 82 weeks) consists of six multidisciplinary courses, each of which is built upon a series of patient-based cases. Selected lectures, seminars, and laboratory exercises will complement small-group, problem-based learning sessions. Following the preclerkship, students spend approximately 78 weeks as clinical clerks. This phase of medical education enables the student to participate in the study and care of patients as a member of a clinical team working in different hospital services. Each rotation includes community experiences as well as elements of problem-based learning and basic science. As part of the clerkship, students spend a total of 17 weeks in elective rotations to allow them to explore areas of medicine of particular interest. During the clerkship, students apply to the Canadian Resident Matching Service to select the program with which they wish to do their postgraduate training. Applications must be submitted in the fall, and students are notified in March as to the program to which they have been matched.

USMLE

Step 1: Optional.
Step 2: Clinical Skills (CS): Optional.
Step 2: Clinical Knowledge (CK): Optional.

Selection Factors

Applicants are judged initially upon their academic and nonacademic records. All applicants are required to take the MCAT. Selected applicants are invited to appear for an interview in Toronto. Definite preference is given to Canadian residents. A maximum of seven places will be offered to applicants with student visas. Sex, race, and religion are not considered in determining those applicants to whom places are offered. Successful candidates must be deemed by the Admissions Committee to be acceptable in all aspects of the admissions process. This may include cumulative grade-point average, MCAT scores, reference letters, nonacademic factors, English proficiency, performance on interview, and any other criteria put forward by the faculty.

Financial Aid

Financial aid is available under the Province of Ontario Student Assistance Program, the Canada Student Loan Program, and the University of Toronto Faculty of Medicine Bursary and Loan Programs. Applicants are referred to the University of Toronto, Faculty of Medicine Web site for details and regulations governing these awards. Applicants are advised not to plan to earn money in time-consuming work that may jeopardize their standing during the academic year.

Information about Diversity Programs

The Faculty of Medicine supports mentorship and role-modeling for students from under-represented groups through a number of programs. These include summer mentorship programs organized by the Faculty in collaboration with the Association for the Advancement of Blacks in Health Sciences. These programs include both black and Aboriginal students.

Campus Information

Setting

The Faculty of Medicine provides the only M.D. training program in the Greater Toronto area, with a catchment population of five million people. The main campus is located in the center of Toronto, one of the world's most culturally diverse cities. Toronto is the largest city in Canada, the fifth largest in North America, and is home to five professional sports franchises, major film and jazz festivals, the third largest live theatre centre in the English-speaking world and thousands of ethnic restaurants.

Enrollment

For 2008, total enrollment was: 886

Special Features

The University of Toronto's Faculty of Medicine is an integral component of one of North America's largest health science complexes. The Faculty of Medicine provides the only M.D. training program in the Greater Toronto area, providing an extraordinary environment for clinical care, research, and education.

Housing

Limited on-campus housing is available, and affordable housing is available within a short radius. Rents average $500–$1000 per month.

Satellite Campuses/Facilities

Student rotations are divided among ten fully affiliated and fifteen partially affiliated teaching hospitals, as well as a large number of community health practices. Placements, including core clerkship placements, are not limited to the major teaching hospitals and will extend into the surrounding regions.

Application Process and Requirements 2010–2011

Primary Application Service: OMSAS
Earliest filing date: July 6, 2009
Latest filing date: September 15, 2009

Secondary Application Required?: No
Sent to: n/a
URL: n/a
Fee: n/a
Fee waiver available: n/a
Earliest filing date: n/a
Latest filing date: n/a

MCAT® required?: Yes
Latest MCAT® Considered: September 2009
Oldest MCAT® Considered: September 2004

Early Decision Program
School does not have EDP
Applicants notified: n/a
EDP available for: n/a

Regular Acceptance Notice
Earliest date: May 15, 2010
Latest date: Until class is full

Applicant's Response to Acceptance
Offer – Maximum Time: Normally two weeks from date of offer.

Requests for Deferred
Entrance Considered: No

Deposit to Hold Place in Class: Yes
Deposit (Resident): $1,000
Deposit (Non-resident): $1,000
Deposit due: With response to acceptance of offer
Applied to tuition: Yes
Deposit refundable: No
Refundable by: n/a

Estimated number of new entrants: 224
EDP: 0, special program: n/a

Start Month/Year: August 23, 2010

Interview Format: Forty-five minute interview with faculty and student. Regional interviews are not available.

Other Programs

PREPARATORY PROGRAMS
Postbaccalaureate Program: No
Summer Program: No

COMBINED DEGREE PROGRAMS
Baccalaureate/M.D.: No
M.D./M.P.H.: No
M.D./M.B.A.: No
M.D./J.D.: No
M.D./Ph.D.: Yes, www.utoronto.ca/mdphd

Premedical Coursework

Course	Req.	Rec.	Lab.	Sems.
Inorganic Chemistry				
Behavioral Sciences				
Biochemistry				
Biology				
Biology/Zoology				
Calculus				
College English				
College Mathematics				

Course	Req.	Rec.	Lab.	Sems.
Computer Science				
Humanities	•			2
Organic Chemistry				
Physics				
Psychology				
Social Sciences	•			2
Life Science	•			4
Language	•			2
Statistics		•		1

Selection Factors: 2008 Accepted Applicants

Proportion of Accepted Applicants with Relevant Experience (Data Self-Reported to AMCAS)	Community Service/Volunteer Medically-Related Work Research	DATA NOT COLLECTED

Shaded bar represents school's accepted scores ranging from the 10th percentile to the 90th percentile   School Median ●   National Median ●

Overall GPA	2.0	2.1	2.2	2.3	2.4	2.5	2.6	2.7	2.8	2.9	3.0	3.1	3.2	3.3	3.4	3.5	3.6	3.7	3.8	(3.9)	4.0
Science GPA	2.0	2.1	2.2	2.3	2.4	2.5	2.6	2.7	2.8	2.9	3.0	3.1	3.2	3.3	3.4	3.5	3.6	3.7	3.8	3.9	4.0

MCAT® Total Numeric Score	DATA NOT COLLECTED

Writing Sample			J	K	L	M	N	O	P	(Q)	R	S	T
Verbal Reasoning	3	4	5	6	7	8	9	(10)	11	12	13	14	15
Biological Sciences	3	4	5	6	7	8	9	10	11	(12)	13	14	15
Physical Sciences	3	4	5	6	7	8	9	10	(11)	12	13	14	15

Acceptance & Matriculation Data for 2008–2009 First Year Class

	Resident	Non-resident	International	Total
Applications	2709	n/a	25	2734
Interviewed	517	n/a	1	518
Deferred	0	n/a	n/a	0
Matriculants				
Early Assurance Program	n/a	n/a	n/a	n/a
Early Decision Program	n/a	n/a	n/a	n/a
Baccalaureate/M.D.	n/a	n/a	n/a	n/a
M.D./Ph.D.	5	n/a	0	5
Matriculated	224	n/a	0	**224**

Applications accepted from International Applicants: Yes

Matriculant Demographics: 2008–2009 First Year Class

Men: 111   **Women:** 113

Matriculants' Self-Reported Race/Ethnicity

Mexican American   Korean
Cuban   Vietnamese
Puerto Rican   Other Asian
Other H
Total H   DATA NOT COLLECTED
Chines
Asian I
Pakistan   Total Asian
Filipino   **Unduplicated Number**
Japanese   **of Matriculants**

Science and Math Majors: 95%
Matriculants with:
Baccalaureate degree: 69
Graduate degree(s): 27

Specialty Choice

2004, 2005, 2006 Graduates, Specialty Choice

Anesthesiology	7%
Emergency Medicine	1%
Family Practice	23%
Internal Medicine	21%
Obstetrics/Gynecology	3%
Orthopedic Surgery	5%
Pediatrics	4%
Psychiatry	6%
Radiology	8%
Surgery	4%

Financial Information

	Residents	Non-residents
Total Cost of Attendance	$37,354	$65,155
Tuition and Fees	$18,504	$46,305
Other (includes living expenses)	$18,850	$18,850
Health Insurance (not applicable)	n/a	n/a

Average 2008 Graduate Indebtedness: $95,311
% of Enrolled Students Receiving Aid: 82%

Criminal Background Check

This medical school requires a criminal background check prior to matriculation.

Northern Ontario School of Medicine
Ontario, Canada

West Campus	East Campus	
955 Oliver Rd	935 Ramsey Lake Rd	**Admissions** www.nosm.ca/education/ume/ general.aspx?id=384
Thunder Bay, ON, P7B 5E1	Sudbury, ON, P3E 2C6	**Main** www.normed.ca
T 807 766 7300	**T** 705 675 4883	**Financial** www.nosm.ca/educatioon/ume/ general.aspx?id=384
F 807 766 7370	**F** 705 675 4858	**E-mail** nosmadmit@normed.ca

Public Institution

Dr. Roger Strasser, Founding Dean

Tracy Al-idrissi, Director, Admissions

Dr. Joel Lanphear, Associate Dean, Undergraduate Medical Education

Dr. Blair Schoales, Assistant Dean, Admissions

General Information
The Northern Ontario School of Medicine is the first new medical school in Canada in the 21st century. It is the Faculty of Medicine of Laurentian University, Sudbury, and of Lakehead University, Thunder Bay. With main campuses in Thunder Bay and Sudbury, the school has multiple teaching and research sites distributed across Northern Ontario, including large and small communities.

Mission Statement
The Northern Ontario School of Medicine is a pioneering faculty of medicine working to the highest international standards. Its overall mission is to educate skilled physicians and undertake health research suited to community needs. In fulfilling this mission NOSM will become a cornerstone of community health care in Northern Ontario.

Curricular Highlights
Community Service Requirement: Optional.
Research/Thesis Requirement: Optional.

Grounded in Northern Ontario, our four-year M.D. program provides students with a unique mix of learning opportunities in a diverse range of sites, including Aboriginal and Francophone communities. Patient-Centered Medicine (PCM) was chosen as the major underlying concept of health and medicine in the development of the M.D. program. PCM is a comprehensive clinical method with six interactive components supported by substantial and growing research evidence. PCM links well to Learner-Centered Education (LCE), which was chosen as the underlying concept of education for the medical school. Throughout the four-year program, the curriculum is organized around five themes: 1. Northern and

Rural Health, 2. Personal and Professional Aspects of Medical Practice, 3. Social and Population Health, 4. The Foundations of Medicine, and 5. Clinical Skills in Healthcare. The focus of the Northern Ontario School of Medicine program is on graduating skilled physicians who are ready and able to pursue further training and clinical practice anywhere, but who will have a special affinity for, and comfort in, Northern Ontario. The curriculum is highly integrated, with students undertaking most learning in small-group, patient-centered Case-Based Learning. The cases present complex real-life scenarios, which present people in their home/family/community context. In addition to small-group learning, students participate in hands-on practical classes, self-directed learning, and clinical education in a range of different health service and community settings. Through the mix of themes and different learning modalities, the program covers core curricula, ensuring that students gain a strong grounding in the basic medical sciences, the humanities, social and behavioral sciences, and clinical medicine. Clinical education starts at the beginning of the program and occurs in a diverse range of settings.

USMLE
Step 1: Optional
Step 2: Clinical Skills (CS): Optional
Step 2: Clinical Knowledge (CK): Optional

Selection Factors
Applications that meet the minimum requirement are assigned a score based on the grade point average, the autobiographic sketch and school submission questions, and context. Context is primarily based on place(s) of residence of one year or more. Advantage is given to those applicants from within Northern Ontario, rural and remote areas in the rest of Canada, and Aboriginal and Francophone applicants. Based on the total application score, the top-ranked candidates are invited to participate in the admission interviews. The final selection for admission is based on a combination of the total application and interview scores. Check our Web site for current information.

Financial Aid
Financial assistance is available to medical students through provincial and federal student loan programs. The Northern Ontario School of Medicine also has bursaries and other awards available for students enrolled in the medical program.

Information about Diversity Programs
Aboriginal applicants are given modest advantage. Aboriginal applicants can select either the General or Aboriginal Admission Stream. A minimum of 2 program seats are designated for Aboriginal students.

Campus Information
Setting
The Northern Ontario School of Medicine is the Faculty of Medicine of both Lakehead University in Thunder Bay, Ontario and Laurentian University in Sudbury, Ontario. Two new buildings, one on each campus, house the medical school.

Enrollment
For 2008, total enrollment was: 58

Housing
On campus housing is available through our host universities, Lakehead and Laurentian University.

Satellite Campuses/Facilities
While the majority of the first two years will be spent in either Thunder Bay or Sudbury, students will spend a month during the first year in an Aboriginal community. In the second year, there will be two placements of six weeks in rural and remote communities throughout Northern Ontario. The majority of third year will be spent in the small urban and large rural communities of Northern Ontario. The Clinical Clerkship in the 4th year is primarily in hospitals of Thunder Bay, Sudbury, and other large urban northern centers.

Application Process and Requirements 2010–2011

Primary Application Service: OMSAS
Earliest filing date: July 2009
Latest filing date: October 1, 2009

Secondary Application Required?: No
Sent to: n/a
URL: n/a
Fee: No
Fee waiver available: n/a
Earliest filing date: n/a
Latest filing date: n/a

MCAT® required?: No
Latest MCAT® considered: n/a
Oldest MCAT® considered: n/a

Early Decision Program
School does not have EDP
Applicants notified: n/a
EDP available for: n/a

Regular Acceptance Notice
Earliest date: May 2010
Latest date: Until class is full

Applicant's Response to Acceptance Offer – Maximum Time: Two weeks

Requests for Deferred Entrance Considered: Yes

Deposit to Hold Place in Class: Yes
Deposit (Resident): $1,000
Deposit (Non-resident): $1,000
Deposit due: n/r
Applied to tuition: Yes
Deposit refundable: No
Refundable by: n/a

Estimated number of new entrants: 56
EDP: n/a, special program: n/a

Start Month/Year: August 2010

Interview Format: Multiple mini-interviews. Regional interviews are not available.

Other Programs

PREPARATORY PROGRAMS
Postbaccalaureate Program: No
Summer Program: No

COMBINED DEGREE PROGRAMS
Baccalaureate/M.D.: No
M.D./M.P.H.: No
M.D./M.B.A.: No
M.D./J.D.: No
M.D./Ph.D.: No

Premedical Coursework

Course	Req.	Rec.	Lab.	Hrs.	Course	Req.	Rec.	Lab.	Hrs.
Inorganic Chemistry					Computer Science				
Behavioral Sciences									
Biochemistry									
Biology		DATA NOT COLLECTED							
Biology/Zoology									
Calculus									
College English					Social Sciences				
College Mathematics					Other				

Selection Factors: 2008 Accepted Applicants

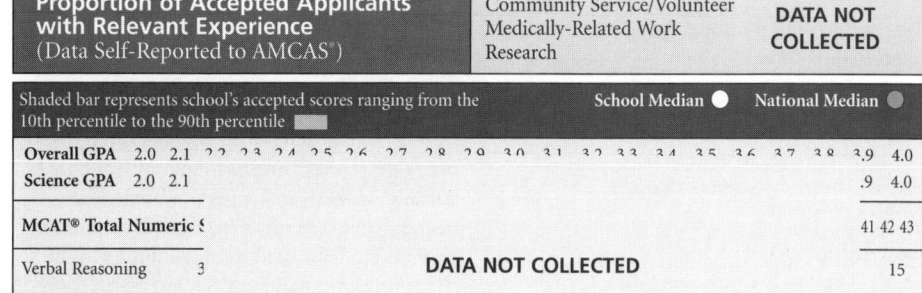

Proportion of Accepted Applicants with Relevant Experience (Data Self-Reported to AMCAS®)										Community Service/Volunteer Medically-Related Work Research									**DATA NOT COLLECTED**			

Shaded bar represents school's accepted scores ranging from the 10th percentile to the 90th percentile. School Median ● National Median ●

Overall GPA	2.0	2.1	2.2	2.3	2.4	2.5	2.6	2.7	2.8	2.9	3.0	3.1	3.2	3.3	3.4	3.5	3.6	3.7	3.8	3.9	4.0
Science GPA	2.0	2.1																		.9	4.0
MCAT® Total Numeric Score							DATA NOT COLLECTED													41	42	43
Verbal Reasoning	3																				15
Physical Sciences	3																				15
Biological Sciences	3																				15
Writing Sample				J	K	L	M	N	O	P	Q	R	S								T

Acceptance & Matriculation Data for 2008–2009 First Year Class

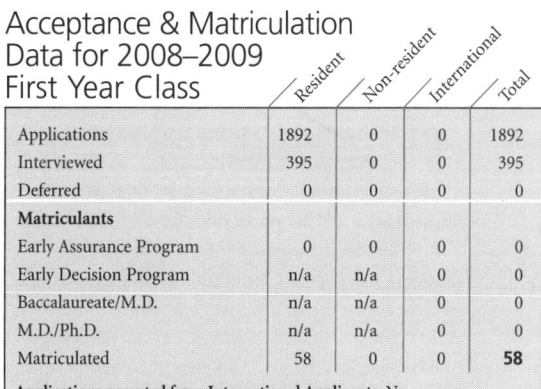

	Resident	Non-resident	International	Total
Applications	1892	0	0	1892
Interviewed	395	0	0	395
Deferred	0	0	0	0
Matriculants				
Early Assurance Program	0	0	0	0
Early Decision Program	n/a	n/a	0	0
Baccalaureate/M.D.	n/a	n/a	0	0
M.D./Ph.D.	n/a	n/a	0	0
Matriculated	58	0	0	**58**

Applications accepted from International Applicants: No

Matriculant Demographics: 2008–2009 First Year Class

Men: 15   **Women:** 43

Matriculants' Self-Reported Race/Ethnicity

Mexican American   Korean
Cuban   Vietnamese
Puerto Rican   Other Asian
Other   Native American
Total
Chinese   **DATA NOT COLLECTED**
Asian
Pakistani
Filipino   **Unduplicated Number**
Japanese   **of Matriculants**

Science and Math Majors: n/a
Matriculants with:
   Baccalaureate degree: 58
   Graduate degree(s): 14

Specialty Choice

2004, 2005, 2006 Graduates, Specialty Choice
Anesthesiology
Emergency Medicine
Family Practice
DATA NOT COLLECTED
Psychiatry
Radiology
Surgery

Financial Information

	Residents	Non-residents
Total Cost of Attendance	n/r	n/r
Tuition and Fees	$17,920	n/r
Other (includes living expenses)	n/r	n/r
Health Insurance	n/a	n/a

Average 2008 Graduate Indebtedness: n/c
% of Enrolled Students Receiving Aid: n/c

Criminal Background Check

This medical school requires a criminal background check prior to matriculation.

The University of Western Ontario, Schulich School of Medicine & Dentistry

London, Ontario

Admissions & Student Affairs
Schulich School of Medicine & Dentistry
The University of Western Ontario
London, Ontario
Canada, N6A 5C1
T 519 661 3744   F 519 850 2958

Admissions www.schulich.uwo.ca/education/
admissions/medicine
Main www.schulich.uwo.ca
Financial n/a
E-mail admissions.medicine@schulich.uwo.ca

Public Institution

Dr. Carol P. Herbert, Dean

Dr. Francis Chan, Associate Dean, Admissions & Student Affairs

Dr. Barbara Lent, Associate Dean for Equity/Gender Issues and Faculty Health

Dr. Tom Scott, Associate Dean, Windsor Program

Pamela Bere, Manager, Admissions & Student Affairs and Equity/Gender Issues and Faculty Health

General Information

The Schulich School of Medicine & Dentistry at The University of Western Ontario (Western) has a long tradition of excellence, beginning with the founding of the medical school in 1881. The School is home to more than 1,800 faculty and 2,700 students in medicine, dentistry, medical sciences, graduate and postgraduate training. Western is one of Canada's oldest post-secondary institutions and is committed to providing the best student experience among Canada's leading research-intensive universities.

Mission Statement

The Schulich School of Medicine & Dentistry provides outstanding education within a research-intensive environment where tomorrow's physicians, dentists, and health researchers learn to be socially responsible leaders in the advancement of human health.

Curricular Highlights

Community Service Requirement: Required.
Research/Thesis Requirement: Optional.

Programs of Study: As of Fall 2008, the Doctor of Medicine program was offered from two home sites – London, Ontario and Windsor, Ontario. Twenty-four students each year will complete all of their academic studies on the campus of the University of Windsor and graduate from The University of Western Ontario. The new Windsor initiative is a partnership between Western, the University of Windsor and London and Windsor hospitals. Curriculum and clinical training will be equiva-

lent at both sites. The undergraduate curriculum is patient-centered in content and student-centered in delivery. It is designed to provide students with an opportunity to acquire the knowledge, skills, and attitudes required to advance to postgraduate training leading to clinical practice, research, or other medical careers. The format is a blend of lectures, laboratory experience, small-group problem-based learning sessions, and supervised clinical experiences. The curriculum in first and second year provides students with solid grounding in the basic and clinical sciences. System-based courses include: Introduction to Medicine, Blood & Oncology, Digestive System & Nutrition, Emergency Care, Endocrine & Metabolism, Heart & Circulation, Infection & Immunity, Musculoskeletal System, Respiration & Airways, Neurosciences, Eye, & Ear, Psychiatry & Behavioral Sciences, Reproduction, and Urinary System. Students are also introduced to Community Health and have numerous opportunities for community involvement. The Clinical Methods courses span two years. During the first year, students participate in patient contact emphasizing a patient-centered approach. During third-year Clerkships, students become active members of clinical care teams in family medicine, medicine, obstetrics and gynecology, pediatrics, psychiatry, and surgery. Under faculty and senior resident supervision, clerks are given graded responsibility in the diagnosis, investigation, and management of patients in hospital, clinic, and outpatient settings. All third-year students are required to complete a community Clinical Clerkship in a region outside London or Windsor for a minimum of four weeks through Schulich's Southwestern Ontario Medical Education Network, to ensure students at all levels gain an understanding and experience of the practice of medicine from both a rural/regional and a tertiary care/urban perspective. Fourth-year Clinical Electives are arranged entirely by the student in any area of medicine. After completion of the Clinical Electives, students return in February for the Transition Period, to complete advanced learning opportunities in basic and clinical sciences. This permits students to further integrate the basic and clinical aspects of medicine in light of their clinical experience.

USMLE

Step 1: Optional.
Step 2: Clinical Skills (CS): Optional.
Step 2: Clinical Knowledge (CK): Optional.

Selection Factors

Admission consideration is based on academic achievement, MCAT scores, and a personal interview score. Only those applicants deemed competitive will be selected for an interview.

Financial Aid

The Schulich School of Medicine & Dentistry makes financial assistance for students in need a top priority.

Information about Diversity Programs

Schulich Medicine has designated three seats in each entering class for First Nations, Metis, and Inuit students who provide proof of Indigenous status or ancestral Indigenous origin.

Campus Information

Setting

Western is located in London, Ontario (approximately halfway between Toronto, Ontario and Detroit, Michigan). The Windsor-based portion of the M.D. program operates from the campus of the University of Windsor, just across the border from Detroit.

Enrollment

For 2008, total enrollment was: 569

Special Features

The Schulich School of Medicine & Dentistry is one of Canada's top centers for medical research and education, with more than $140 million annually in research funding and 49 accredited postgraduate specialty programs.

Housing

For housing information, see: *www.has.uwo.ca/housing/offcampus/index.htm.*

Regional/Satellite Campuses/Facilities:

The Windsor-based portion of the M.D. Program is situated on the campus of the University of Windsor.

Application Process and Requirements 2010–2011

Primary Application Service: OMSAS
Earliest filing date: July 2009
Latest filing date: September 2009

Secondary Application Required?: No
Sent to: n/a
URL: n/a
Fee: No
Fee waiver available: No
Earliest filing date: n/a
Latest filing date: n/a

MCAT® required?: Yes
Latest MCAT® considered: September 2009
Oldest MCAT® considered: September 2004

Early Decision Program
School does not have EDP
Applicants notified: n/a
EDP available for: n/a

Regular Acceptance Notice
Earliest date: May 2010
Latest date: Until class is full

Applicant's Response to Acceptance
Offer – Maximum Time: Two weeks

Requests for Deferred
Entrance Considered: No

Deposit to Hold Place in Class: Yes
Deposit (Resident): $1,000
Deposit (Non-resident): $1,000
Deposit due: With response form
Applied to tuition: Yes
Deposit refundable: No
Refundable by: n/a

Estimated number of new entrants: 147
EDP: 0, special program: n/a

Start Month/Year: September 2010

Interview Format: One physician, one community person, one senior medical student. Regional interviews are not available.

Other Programs

PREPARATORY PROGRAMS
Postbaccalaureate Program: No
Summer Program: No

COMBINED DEGREE PROGRAMS
Baccalaureate/M.D.: No
M.D./M.P.H.: No
M.D./M.B.A.: No
M.D./J.D.: No
M.D./Ph.D.: Yes,
www.schulich.uwo.ca/medicine/md_phd/index.php
ADDITIONAL PROGRAM
www.eng.uwo.ca/undergraduate/
ProgramInformation/program_information.htm

Premedical Coursework

Course	Req.	Rec.	Lab.	Sems.
Inorganic Chemistry				
Behavioral Sciences				
Biochemistry				
Biology				
Biology/Zoology				
Calculus				
College English				

Course	Req.	Rec.	Lab.	Sems.
College Mathematics				
Genetics				
Humanities				
Organic Chemistry				
Physics				
Psychology				
Social Sciences				

Selection Factors: 2008 Accepted Applicants

Proportion of Accepted Applicants with Relevant Experience (Data Self-Reported to AMCAS)	
Community Service/Volunteer	100%
Medically-Related Work	70%
Research	25%

Shaded bar represents school's accepted scores ranging from the 10th percentile to the 90th percentile   School Median ●   National Median ●

Overall GPA	2.0	2.1	2.2	2.3	2.4	2.5	2.6	2.7	2.8	2.9	3.0	3.1	3.2	3.3	3.4	3.5	3.6	(3.7)	3.8	3.9	4.0
Science GPA	2.0	2.1	2.2	2.3	2.4	2.5	2.6	2.7	2.8	2.9	3.0	3.1	3.2	3.3	3.4	3.5	3.6	(3.7)	3.8	3.9	4.0

MCAT® Total Numeric Score	DATA NOT COLLECTED

Writing Sample			J	K	L	M	N	O	P	(Q)	R	S	T
Verbal Reasoning	3	4	5	6	7	8	9	(10)	11	12	13	14	15
Biological Sciences	3	4	5	6	7	8	9	10	(11)	12	13	14	15
Physical Sciences	3	4	5	6	7	8	(9)	10	11	12	13	14	15

Acceptance & Matriculation Data for 2008–2009 First Year Class

	Resident	Non-resident	International	Total
Applications	1803	n/r	n/a	1803
Interviewed	473	n/r	n/a	473
Deferred	n/r	n/r	0	0
Matriculants				
Early Assurance Program	0	0	0	0
Early Decision Program	n/a	n/a	n/a	n/a
Baccalaureate/M.D.	n/a	n/a	n/a	n/a
M.D./Ph.D.	18	n/r	n/a	18
Matriculated	n/r	n/r	n/r	**147**

Applications accepted from International Applicants: No

Specialty Choice

2004, 2005, 2006 Graduates, Specialty Choice	
Anesthesiology	8
Emergency Medicine	13
Family Practice	47
Internal Medicine	18
Obstetrics/Gynecology	5
Orthopaedic Surgery	5
Pediatrics	4
Psychiatry	4
Radiology	4
Surgery	7

Matriculant Demographics: 2008–2009 First Year Class

Men: 79   **Women:** 68

Matriculants' Self-Reported Race/Ethnicity

Mexican American	Korean
Cuban	Vietnamese
Puerto Rican	Other Asian
Other Hispa	
Total Hispan	
Chinese	DATA NOT COLLECTED
Asian Indian	
Pakistani	Total Asian
Filipino	Unduplicated Number
Japanese	of Matriculants

Science and Math Majors: 86%
Matriculants with:
    Baccalaureate degree: 100%
    Graduate degree(s): 15%

Financial Information

	Residents	Non-residents
Total Cost of Attendance	n/r	n/r
Tuition and Fees	$17,224	$17,224
Other (includes living expenses)	$16,050	$16,050
Health Insurance	n/a	n/a

Average 2008 Graduate Indebtedness: $120,000
% of Enrolled Students Receiving Aid: 50%

Criminal Background Check

This medical school requires a criminal background check prior to matriculation.

Université Laval
Faculty of Medicine
Quebec, Quebec

Admissions Committee
Universite Laval Faculty of Medicine
Quebec, Quebec
Canada, G1K 7P4
T 418 656 2131 x2492   **F** 418 656 2733

Admissions www.reg.ulaval.ca/p4.html
Main www.fmed.ulaval.ca
Financial www.bbaf.ulaval.ca/bbaf/entree.htm
E-mail admission@fmed.ulaval.ca

Public Institution

Dr. Pierre J. Durand, Dean

Dr. Evens Villeneuve, Admission Committee Chairman

Guy Labrecque Sr., Admission Committee

General Information
Universite Laval was established by a Royal Charter in 1852 granted by Queen Victoria. It was named after Monseigneur de Laval, first bishop of Quebec. For more than 150 years, the medical school has been dedicated to the formation of health professionals through high standard teaching programs and research activities. Research opportunities are provided in all the basic sciences and in many fields of clinical investigation. The clinical teaching is provided through a network of affiliated health institutions. Residence accommodations are provided for many students. There is a University Health Service for students, as well as vocational guidance, and counseling services.

Mission Statement
The overall goal of the program is to assure a theoretical and clinical formation which prepares students for practicing medicine competently in a contemporary health system, with emphasis on an approach which is scientific, ethical, global, and humanistic. In addition, the program strives to prepare students for a lifetime of continued learning.

Curricular Highlights
Community Service Requirement: Optional.
Research/Thesis Requirement: Optional.

The curriculum aims to prepare students to undertake any career in medicine. During the first two years, the program provides early introduction to clinical problems and interdepartmental teaching by both basic science and clinical faculty. This part of the curriculum is designed to be flexible and can be spread over three calendar years. The basic clinical clerkships are given in the third and fourth years and provide a basic exposure to each major clinical discipline, including family medicine. Both faculty and students monitor the curriculum.

USMLE
Step 1: Optional.
Step 2: Clinical Skills (CS): Optional.
Step 2: Clinical Knowledge (CK): Optional.

Selection Factors
Preference is given to applicants from the province of Quebec. Admission requirements for application from Quebec colleges (CEGEP) and universities include a standardized autobiographical note and Multiple Mini Interviews which is a subjective structured admission tool with 10 short-interview stations. This test evaluates different personal characteristics of the candidates. A few outstanding French-speaking candidates are admitted from other Canadian provinces and the United States. These candidates are selected on the basis of different parameters: scholastic achievement, interview, and curriculum vitae. Sex, race, religion, age, and socioeconomic status are not considered in the selection process.

Financial Aid
Financial aid is available to Quebec residents through the Bursaries Division of the Provincial Ministry of Education. Summer scholarships of $4,200 to $5,000 are also available to students who wish to devote their vacation period to research. There is no financial assistance for foreign applicants.

Information about Diversity Programs
Laval University School of Medicine, associated with other Quebec medical schools, has a program focused on integrating more aboriginal students with four dedicated seats each year.

Campus Information

Setting
The medical school is located in Quebec, a city famous for its walled old city center. Public transportation is widely available and makes travel very easy. Quebec is a lively French city with abundant cultural activities. There are several public parks, cultural institutions, cinemas, shopping areas, and natural areas. The city is surrounded by lakes, rivers, and mountains and enjoys four distinct seasons. Water and snow activities are easily accessible.

Enrollment
For 2008, total enrollment was: 218

Special Features
The medical school has a international exchange program for talented students. Laval has reciprocity agreements with several countries, including Cuba, Peru, Nicaragua, India, Mali, Senegal, and China. The program has two stages: first, five to six weeks of observation and second, three months of medical training.

Housing
Universite Laval boasts four residences with 2,400 Internet-equipped, comfortable rooms. Three of the residences are equipped with modern communal kitchens. For more information, see *www.ulaval.ca/sres* or call the Residence Office at (418) 656-2921 or e-mail sres@sres.ulaval.ca.

Regional/Satellite Campuses/Facilities:
Students rotate among several general and specialized hospitals and affiliated ambulatory care centers. Locations are spread throughout the city and in several towns in the eastern part of the province of Quebec.

Application Process and Requirements 2010–2011

Primary Application Service: School-specific
Earliest filing date: November 15, 2009
Latest filing date: March 1, 2010 (Quebec colleges), February 1, 2010 (all others)

Secondary Application Required?: No
Sent to: Bureau du Régistraire, Pavillon J-Charles Bonefant local 2440 Université Laval, G1K 7P4 Québec Qc
URL: n/a
Fee: n/a
Fee waiver available: No
Earliest filing date: n/a
Latest filing date: Same as primary application

MCAT® required?: No
Latest MCAT® considered: n/a
Oldest MCAT® considered: n/a

Early Decision Program
School does not have EDP
Applicants notified: n/a
EDP available for: n/a

Regular Acceptance Notice
Earliest date: May 4, 2010
Latest date: Until class is full

Applicant's Response to Acceptance
Offer – Maximum Time: 10 days after the offer

Requests for Deferred
Entrance Considered: No

Deposit to Hold Place in Class: No
Deposit (Resident): n/a
Deposit (Non-resident): n/a
Deposit due: n/a
Applied to tuition: n/a
Deposit refundable: n/a
Refundable by: n/a

Estimated number of new entrants: 218
EDP: n/a, special program: n/a

Start Month/Year: September 2010

Interview Format: Multiple Mini Interview (MMI). Ten OSCE-style stations.

Other Programs

PREPARATORY PROGRAMS
Postbaccalaureate Program: Yes, www.fmed.ulaval.ca
Summer Program: No
Additional: Three Month International Study Abroad, Guy Labrecque, (418) 656-2131 #2492, guy.labrecque@fmed.ulaval.ca

COMBINED DEGREE PROGRAMS
Baccalaureate/M.D.: Yes, Dr. Joan Glenn (418) 656-2131 #2492, joan.glenn@fmed.ulaval.ca
M.D./M.P.H.: No
M.D./M.B.A.: No
M.D./J.D.: No
M.D./Ph.D.: Yes, Dr. Lucie Rochefort (418) 656-2131 #5709 lucie.rochefort@fmed.ulaval.ca

Premedical Coursework

Course	Req.	Rec.	Lab.	Hrs.
Inorganic Chemistry	•		•	1
Behavioral Sciences				
Biochemistry	•			1
Biology	•		•	2
Biology/Zoology			•	
Calculus				
College English				
College Mathematics	•			2

Course	Req.	Rec.	Lab.	Sems.
Computer Science				
Genetics				
Humanities				
Organic Chemistry	•		•	1
Physics	•		•	3
Psychology				
Social Sciences				
Other				

Selection Factors: 2008 Accepted Applicants

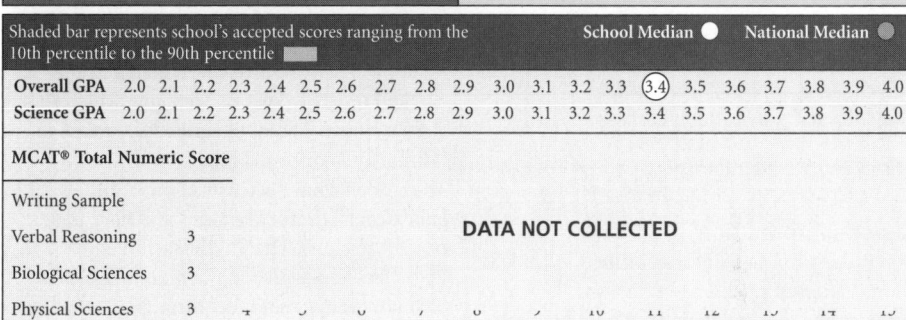

Proportion of Accepted Applicants with Relevant Experience (Data Self-Reported to AMCAS®)	**DATA NOT COLLECTED**

Shaded bar represents school's accepted scores ranging from the 10th percentile to the 90th percentile ▮   School Median ● National Median ●

Overall GPA	2.0	2.1	2.2	2.3	2.4	2.5	2.6	2.7	2.8	2.9	3.0	3.1	3.2	3.3	(3.4)	3.5	3.6	3.7	3.8	3.9	4.0
Science GPA	2.0	2.1	2.2	2.3	2.4	2.5	2.6	2.7	2.8	2.9	3.0	3.1	3.2	3.3	3.4	3.5	3.6	3.7	3.8	3.9	4.0

MCAT® Total Numeric Score

Writing Sample		
Verbal Reasoning	3	**DATA NOT COLLECTED**
Biological Sciences	3	
Physical Sciences	3	

Acceptance & Matriculation Data for 2008–2009 First Year Class

	Resident	Non-resident	International	Total
Applications	1816	61	106	1983
Interviewed	n/r	n/r	n/r	n/r
Deferred	n/r	n/r	n/r	n/r
Matriculants				
Early Assurance Program	0	0	0	0
Early Decision Program	n/a	n/a	n/a	n/a
Baccalaureate/M.D.	n/a	n/a	n/a	n/a
M.D./Ph.D.	n/a	n/a	n/a	n/a
Matriculated	214	3	1	**218**

Applications accepted from International Applicants: Yes

Matriculant Demographics: 2008–2009 First Year Class

Men: 67   **Women:** 151

Matriculants' Self-Reported Race/Ethnicity

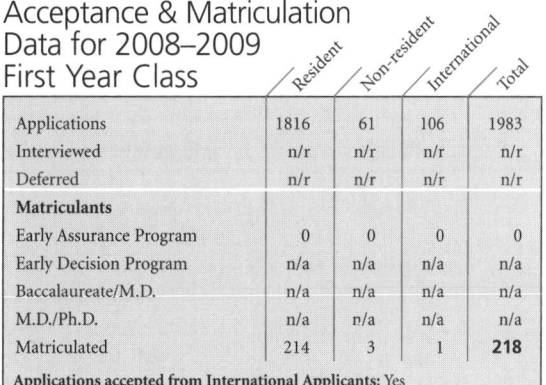

Mexican American	Korean
Cuban	Vietnamese
Puerto Rican	Other Asian
Other Hispanic	African American
Total Hispanic	Native American
Chinese	Canadian
Asian Indian	
Pakistani	Total Asian
Filipino	Unduplicated Number of Matriculants
Japanese	

DATA NOT COLLECTED

Science and Math Majors: 80%
Matriculants with:
Baccalaureate degree: 60%
Graduate degree(s): 4%

Specialty Choice

2004, 2005, 2006 Graduates, Specialty Choice
Anesthesiology
Emergency Medicine
Family Practice
DATA NOT COLLECTED
Psychiatry
Radiology
Surgery

Financial Information

	Residents	Non-residents
Total Cost of Attendance	$5,000	$16,000
Tuition and Fees	$1,800	$12,000
Other (includes living expenses)	$15,000	$15,000
Health Insurance (can be waived)	n/r	$700

Average 2008 Graduate Indebtedness: n/r
% of Enrolled Students Receiving Aid: 33%

Criminal Background Check

This medical school does not require a criminal background check prior to matriculation.

McGill University Faculty of Medicine
Montréal, Quebec

Admissions Office
McGill University Faculty of Medicine
3655 Promenade Sir William Osler
Montréal, Quebec
Canada, H3G 1Y6
T 514 398 3517   **F** 514 398 4631

Admissions www.mcgill.ca/medicine/admissions/
Main www.mcgill.ca/medicine/
Financial www.mcgill.ca/studentaid/
E-mail admissions.med@mcgill.ca

Public Institution

Dr. Richard I. Levin, Dean

Dr. Joyce Pickering, Associate Dean, Medical Education & Student Affairs

France Drolet, Director of Admissions

Judy Stymest, Director, Scholarships, Student Aid & International Services

Michel Dansereau, Admissions Officer

General Information
The Faculty of Medicine, established in 1829, is a foundation of medicine in Canada. Clinical facilities include four major teaching hospitals, several affiliated hospitals, specialized centers, and research units. In the Québec health care system, all patients are available for medical student teaching, giving McGill graduates extensive clinical exposure. McGill's Faculty of Medicine is accredited by the LCME, allowing American students to return to the U.S. for residency.

Mission Statement
The advancement of learning through teaching, scholarship, and service to society by offering to outstanding undergraduate and graduate students the best education available; by carrying out scholarly activities judged to be excellent when measured against the highest international standards; and by providing service to society in well-suited ways by virtue of academic strengths. Within this context, the mission of the Faculty of Medicine is to pursue internationally significant scholarship and to provide undergraduate, graduate, and professional programs of the highest academic quality in order to contribute to the well-being of mankind.

Curricular Highlights
Community Service Requirement: Optional.
Research/Thesis Requirement: Optional.

The objectives of the curriculum correspond to the mission statement of the Faculty of Medicine and aim to equip the student to meet the most stringent standards of medical practice and professionalism to ensure career-long excellence in whole-person care. The graduate will be able to function responsibly, in a supervised clinical setting, at the level of an "undifferentiated" physician. The program emphasizes the fundamental sciences and scientific methodology as pillars of medical knowledge. It provides traditional lectures and small group teaching, as well as laboratory and computer teaching. There are five components to the curriculum: The Basis of Medicine which provides a system-based, integrated approach to normal and abnormal functions of the body. The students have extensive opportunities for hands-on laboratory sessions and have patient contact sessions. The Physicianship and Physician Apprenticeship component consists of small groups that meet throughout the four years of the program. The focus is on the roles of the physician as a professional and healer; to the knowledge, skills, attitudes and behaviors required of professionalism and healer. The Introduction to Clinical Medicine provides a clinical experience, using both in-patient and ambulatory settings and utilizes our Medical Simulation Centre. The Core and Senior Clerkships are the last two components which involve many rotations in both urban and rural environments, along with plenty of opportunity for electives. All students must successfully complete the Medical Council of Canada exam (MCC-QE-I), USMLE Step 2 CK, or a McGill Exit exam to graduate.

USMLE
Step 1: Optional. Students must only record a score.
Step 2: Clinical Skills (CS): Required. Students must record a passing total score to graduate.
Step 2: Clinical Knowledge (CK): Required. Students must record a passing total score to graduate.

Selection Factors
Pre-selection is based upon academic achievement (GPA, MCAT, Science GPA), personal characteristics and accomplishments evidenced through an autobiographical sketch, C.V. and references. All candidates are reviewed without regard to ethnic, religious, linguistic, or sociocultural background or gender. There are no strict cut-offs for applicants, though successful applicants tend to have an overall undergraduate degree GPA of 3.5+ and an MCAT total of 30+. Only pre-selected applicants get interviews in the multiple-mini interview (MMI) format. Admission decisions are final and are not subject to appeal.

Financial Aid
The McGill Student Aid Office assists students with the financial resources necessary to help cover the cost of school. The Web site gives information about government aid programs, McGill loans and bursaries, scholarship funding, debt management, individualized budget counseling, and the Work-Study program.

Information about Diversity Programs
A few reserved places are available for qualified First Nations or Inuit candidates.

Campus Information
Setting
The campus spans 80 acres of downtown Montréal, home to countless cultures and festivities. It is within walking distance of major hospitals, advanced teaching facilities, shops, housing, and Mount-Royal, the city's central park and natural forest.

Enrollment
For 2008, total enrollment was: 675

Special Features
The Sir Mortimer B. Davis-Jewish General, Douglas Mental Health University Institute, and the St. Mary's Hospital Centre, along with the McGill University Health Centre (Montreal Children's, Montreal General, Montreal Neurological, Royal Victoria Hospitals, and Montreal Chest Institute) make up the teaching hospital network not to mention affiliated urban and rural hospitals. The McGill Medical Simulation Centre is also included in teaching facilities.

Housing
Three styles of housing are available, along with wonderful off-campus housing. For more information, see: *www.mcgill.ca/residences/* or */offcampus/*.

Application Process and Requirements 2010–2011

Primary Application Service: School-specific
Earliest filing date: September 1, 2009
Latest filing date: November 15, 2009 - non-residents; January 15, 2010 - residents

Secondary Application Required?: No
Sent to: n/a
URL: www.mcgill.ca/medicine/admissions/
Fee: Yes, $85
Fee waiver available: No
Earliest filing date: n/a
Latest filing date: n/a

MCAT® required?: Yes
Latest MCAT® considered: October 2009
Oldest MCAT® considered: November 2006

Early Decision Program
School does not have EDP
Applicants notified: n/a
EDP available for: n/a

Regular Acceptance Notice
Earliest date: Early March 2010
Latest date: Until Class is Full

Applicant's Response to Acceptance
Offer – Maximum Time: Two weeks

Requests for Deferred
Entrance Considered: Yes

Deposit to Hold Place in Class: Yes
Deposit (Resident): $500
Deposit (Non-resident): $500
Deposit due: With response to acceptance offer
Applied to tuition: Yes
Deposit refundable: Yes
Refundable by: May 15, 2010 - non-residents; June 15, 2010 - residents

Estimated number of new entrants: 175
EDP: n/a, special program: 7

Start Month/Year: Mid-August 2010

Interview Format: Multiple mini-interview (MMI) format with personal interview. Regional interviews are not available.

Other Programs

PREPARATORY PROGRAMS
Postbaccalaureate Program: No
Summer Program: No

COMBINED DEGREE PROGRAMS
Baccalaureate/M.D.: No
M.D./M.P.H.: No
M.D./M.B.A.: Yes, www.mcgill.ca/medicine/admissions/programs/md-mba/
M.D./J.D.: No
M.D./Ph.D.: Yes, www.mcgill.ca/medicine/admissions/programs/md-phd/

Premedical Coursework

Course	Req.	Rec.	Lab.	Hrs.
Inorganic Chemistry	•		•	6
Behavioral Sciences				
Biochemistry		•		
Biology	•		•	6
Biology/Zoology				
Calculus				
College English				
College Mathematics				

Course	Req.	Rec.	Lab.	Hrs.
Computer Science				
Genetics				
Humanities				
Organic Chemistry	•		•	3
Physics	•		•	6
Psychology				
Social Sciences				
Cell/Molecular Biology		•		
Statistics		•		

Selection Factors: 2008 Accepted Applicants

Proportion of Accepted Applicants with Relevant Experience (Data Self-Reported to AMCAS®)	DATA NOT COLLECTED

Shaded bar represents school's accepted scores ranging from the 10th percentile to the 90th percentile   School Median ●   National Median ●

Overall GPA	2.0	2.1	2.2	2.3	2.4	2.5	2.6	2.7	2.8	2.9	3.0	3.1	3.2	3.3	3.4	3.5	3.6	3.7	(3.8)	3.9	4.0
Science GPA	2.0	2.1	2.2	2.3	2.4	2.5	2.6	2.7	2.8	2.9	3.0	3.1	3.2	3.3	3.4	3.5	3.6	3.7	(3.8)	3.9	4.0

MCAT® Total Numeric Score 9 10 11 12 13 14 15 16 17 18 19 20 21 22 23 24 25 26 27 28 29 30 31 32 (33) 34 35 36 37 38 39 40 41 42 43

Writing Sample				J	K	L	M	N	O	P	(Q)	R	S	T
Verbal Reasoning	3	4	5	6	7	8	9	(10)	11	12	13	14	15
Biological Sciences	3	4	5	6	7	8	9	10	11	(12)	13	14	15
Physical Sciences	3	4	5	6	7	8	9	10	11	(12)	13	14	15

Acceptance & Matriculation Data for 2008–2009 First Year Class

	Resident	Non-resident	International	Total
Applications	730	566	104	1400
Interviewed	317	52	48	417
Deferred	0	0	0	0
Matriculants				
Early Assurance Program	n/a	n/a	n/a	n/a
Early Decision Program	0	0	0	0
Baccalaureate/M.D.	n/a	n/a	n/a	n/a
M.D./Ph.D.	2	1	0	3
Matriculated	159	9	7	**175**

Applications accepted from International Applicants: Yes

Matriculant Demographics: 2008–2009 First Year Class

Men: 77   **Women:** 98

Matriculants' Self-Reported Race/Ethnicity

Mexican American   Korean
Cuban   Vietnamese
Puerto Rican   Other Asian
Other
Total
Chines
Asian
Pakist
Filipino   **Unduplicated Number**
Japanese   **of Matriculants**

DATA NOT COLLECTED

Science and Math Majors: 82%
Matriculants with:
     Baccalaureate degree: 54%
     Graduate degree(s): 10%

Specialty Choice

2004, 2005, 2006 Graduates, Specialty Choice	
Anesthesiology	1
Emergency Medicine	2
Family Practice	22
Internal Medicine	19
Obstetrics/Gynecology	4
Orthopaedic Surgery	2
Pediatrics	9
Psychiatry	2
Radiology	2
Surgery	5

Financial Information

	Residents	Non-residents
Total Cost of Attendance	$20,769	$49,105
Tuition and Fees	$4,893	$24,822
Other (includes living expenses)	$16,021	$23,589
Health Insurance (can be waived)	$0	$693

Average 2008 Graduate Indebtedness: n/c
% of Enrolled Students Receiving Aid: n/c

Criminal Background Check

This school does not require a criminal background check prior to matriculation.

Université de Montréal School of Medicine

Montréal, Quebec

Admissions Committee
Université de Montréal School of Medicine
P.O. Box 6128, Station Centre-Ville
Montréal Quebec H3C 3J7
T 514 343 6265   **F** 514 343 6629

Admissions www.med.umontreal.ca/etudes/
programme_formation/doctorate_medicine/
admission.html
Main www.med.umontreal.ca
Financial n/a
E-mail admmed@ere.umontreal.ca

Public Institution

Dr. Jean-Lucien Rouleau,
Dean of Faculty of Medicine

Dr. Christian Bourdy, President
of Admissions Committee

Dr. Christian Bourdy, Vice Dean,
Undergraduate Studies

General Information

The Faculty of Medicine of the Université de Montréal can be traced back to a school first established in Montréal in 1843 and incorporated in 1845 under the name of École de Médecine et de Chirurgie de Montréal. In 1891 the school merged with the Faculté de Médecine of the Montréal Branch of Laval University, which had been founded in 1877. In 1920, by an act of the Quebec legislature, the Montréal branch of Laval University was granted its independence, and the school of medicine became known by its present name. All instruction is in French, and clinical instruction is carried out at 15 affiliated teaching hospitals and research centers.

Mission Statement

The Faculty of Medicine of the Université de Montréal seeks through its undergraduate medical program to provide medical knowledge, clinical skills and professional attitudes so that students will be able to enter postgraduate training in family medicine or medical specialization, or fields related to research, teaching, or health care management.

Curricular Highlights

Community Service Requirement: Optional.
Research/Thesis Requirement: Optional.

In September 1993, a new four-year curriculum came into effect. It consists of two years (70 weeks) of problem-based learning during which students are exposed to biomedical and psychosocial sciences basic to medicine. Courses are interdisciplinary and system-based. Early introduction to clinical skills takes place in a continuous fashion throughout those two preclinical years. Clinical exposure begins with Year 1. Forty-five hours of electives are mandatory during each of the first two

years. The third and fourth years consist of an 80-week clerkship. In the new curriculum, formal lecturing is reduced to a minimum and replaced by active methods, especially problem-based learning and small-group discussion. A premedical year devoted to basic biological and behavioral sciences is restricted to students having just graduated from the provincial colleges of general and professional education (CEGEP). Students who have completed one to three years at the university level in others than biomedical fields are also eligible for the premedical year. Residency training in the teaching hospitals is under the responsibility of the Faculty of Medicine. Various courses and symposia are organized by the continuing medical education division.

USMLE

Step 1: Optional.
Step 2: Clinical Skills (CS): Optional.
Step 2: Clinical Knowledge (CK): Optional.

Selection Factors

Candidates accepted must be either Canadian citizens or landed immigrants, but due consideration is given to French-speaking applicants from other provinces of Canada. Selection of candidates is competitive and based on a global score derived from scholastic records and interviews. Interviews (Multiple Mini-Interviews), conducted on the site of the medical school, are granted to about one-third of the applicants on the basis of their scholastic records. This interview can be eliminatory. For candidates holding a Ph.D. degree, performance in research may constitute an important selection factor. No consideration is given to race, sex, creed, or age.

Financial Aid

Financial aid is available to students through the Bursaries Division of the Department of Education, the Kellogg Foundation Loan Fund, the Scholarships and Loan Committee of the university, and the Jean Frappier Fund. Summer scholarships are also available.

Information about Diversity Programs

Since 2008, a yearly total of four positions are

reserved for Quebec aboriginal students (First Nations and Inuit) in the Faculties of Medicine in Quebec.

Campus Information

Setting

The medical school is located in the main campus of the Université de Montréal in downtown Montréal, which can be reached by buses and subways. University and community-based hospitals associated with the University are spread in the downtown area and suburbs.

Enrollment

For 2008, total enrollment was: 1,242

Housing

On-campus housing is available.

Satellite Campuses/Facilities

Since 2004, there is a regional campus in the city of Trois-Rivières, located 125 kilometers east of Montréal. Each year, thirty-two students start medical school on Trois-Rivières campus, most of them at the pre-medical level. The currula at the Montréal campus and Trois-Rivières campus are identical. Clinical training is completed at community hospitals in the Mauricie region.

Application Process and Requirements 2010–2011

Primary Application Service: School-specific
Earliest filing date: December 1, 2009
Latest filing date: January 15, 2010

Secondary Application Required?: No
Sent to:
URL: n/a
Fee: No
Fee waiver available: No
Earliest filing date: n/a
Latest filing date: n/a

MCAT® required?: No
Latest MCAT® considered: n/a
Oldest MCAT® considered: n/a

Early Decision Program
School does not have EDP
Applicants notified: n/a
EDP available for: n/a

Regular Acceptance Notice
Earliest date: May 15, 2010
Latest date: Until class is full

Applicant's Response to Acceptance
Offer – Maximum Time: Two weeks

Requests for Deferred
Entrance Considered: No

Deposit to Hold Place in Class: Yes
Deposit (Resident): $200
Deposit (Non-resident): $200
Deposit due: With response to acceptance offer
Applied to tuition: Yes
Deposit refundable: No
Refundable by: n/a

Estimated number of new entrants: 279
EDP: n/a, special program: 1

Start Month/Year: August 2010

Interview Format: Multiple Mini-Interviews (MMI). Regional interviews are not available.

Other Programs

PREPARATORY PROGRAMS
Postbaccalaureate Program: No
Summer Program: No

COMBINED DEGREE PROGRAMS
Baccalaureate/M.D.: No
M.D./M.P.H.: No
M.D./M.B.A.: No
M.D./J.D.: No
M.D./Ph.D.: No

Premedical Coursework

Course	Req.	Rec.	Lab.	Sems.
Inorganic Chemistry	•			2
Behavioral Sciences				
Biochemistry				
Biology	•			2
Biology/Zoology				
Calculus	•			2
College English				
College Mathematics	•			

Course	Req.	Rec.	Lab.	Sems.
Computer Science				
Genetics				
Humanities				
Organic Chemistry	•			1
Physics	•			3
Psychology				
Social Sciences				

Selection Factors: 2008 Accepted Applicants

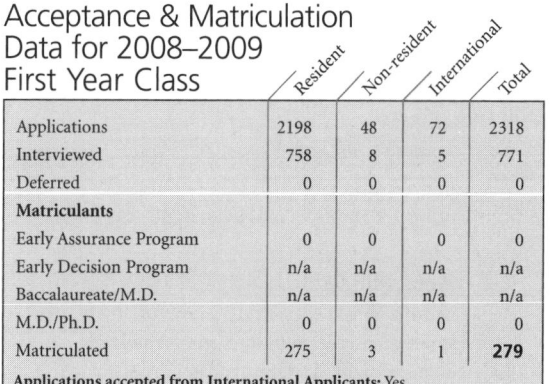

Proportion of Accepted Applicants with Relevant Experience (Data Self-Reported to AMCAS®)	Community Service/Volunteer Medically-Related Work Research	DATA NOT COLLECTED

Shaded bar represents school's accepted scores ranging from the 10th percentile to the 90th percentile.   School Median ●   National Median ●

	2.0	2.1	2.2	2.3	2.4	2.5	2.6	2.7	2.8	2.9	3.0	3.1	3.2	3.3	3.4	3.5	3.6	(3.7)	3.8	3.9	4.0
Overall GPA																		(3.7)			
Science GPA																		(3.7)			

MCAT® Total Numeric Score

Writing Sample	
Verbal Reasoning	3
Biological Sciences	3
Physical Sciences	3

DATA NOT COLLECTED

Acceptance & Matriculation Data for 2008–2009 First Year Class

	Resident	Non-resident	International	Total
Applications	2198	48	72	2318
Interviewed	758	8	5	771
Deferred	0	0	0	0
Matriculants				
Early Assurance Program	0	0	0	0
Early Decision Program	n/a	n/a	n/a	n/a
Baccalaureate/M.D.	n/a	n/a	n/a	n/a
M.D./Ph.D.	0	0	0	0
Matriculated	275	3	1	**279**

Applications accepted from International Applicants: Yes

Specialty Choice

2004, 2005, 2006 Graduates, Specialty Choice
Anesthesiology
Emergency Medicine
Family Practice
DATA NOT COLLECTED
Psychiatry
Radiology
Surgery

Matriculant Demographics: 2008–2009 First Year Class

Men: 81   **Women:** 198

Matriculants' Self-Reported Race/Ethnicity

Mexican American
Cuban
Puerto Rican
Other
Total
Chine
Asian
Pakist
Filipino
Japanese

Korean
Vietnamese
Other Asian

DATA NOT COLLECTED

Unduplicated Number of Matriculants

Science and Math Majors: 65%
Matriculants with:
Baccalaureate degree: 35
Graduate degree(s): 3

Financial Information

	Residents	Non-residents
Total Cost of Attendance	n/r	n/r
Tuition and Fees	$4,000	$23,000
Other (includes living expenses)	$2,000	$2,000
Health Insurance (can be waived)	n/r	n/r

Average 2008 Graduate Indebtedness: $35,000
% of Enrolled Students Receiving Aid: 60%

Criminal Background Check

This school does not require a criminal background check prior to matriculation.

University of Sherbrooke
Faculty of Medicine

Sherbrooke, Quebec

Admission Office, University of Sherbrooke
Faculty of Medicine and Health Sciences
3001, 12e Avenue Nord
Sherbrooke, Quebec
Canada, J1H 5N4
T 819 564 5208   F 819 820 6809

Admissions www.usherbrooke.ca/
doctorat_medecine
Main www.usherbrooke.ca
Financial www.usherbrooke.ca
E-mail admission-med@usherbrooke.ca

Public Institution

Dr. Rejean Hebert, Dean

Dr. Daniel J.Cote, Chair, Admissions Committee

Dr. Jocelyne Faucher, Vice Dean, Student Affairs

Dr. Paul Grand'Maison, Vice Dean, Undergraduate Medical Education

Dr. Guy Waddell, M.D. Program Director

General Information

Officially founded in February 1961, the Faculty of Medicine at the University of Sherbrooke is a French-speaking institution. It admitted its first students in September 1966. The Faculty opened two outside campuses in September 2006 and offers its whole M.D. program in a distributed approach. The first is located in Saguenay, the central city of Quebec peripheral region. The second one is located in Moncton, the central French-speaking city in the province of New Brunswick. Students complete the program either in the central campus in Sherbrooke (144–148 admitted students,) or in Moncton (24 students,) or in Saguenay (24 students).

Mission Statement

Improved health and well-being of people and populations through education, research, clinical services, and knowledge transfer.

Curricular Highlights

Community Service Requirement: Optional.
Research/Thesis Requirement: Optional.

The M.D. degree is granted after successful completion of the four-year course. Teaching is given through small-group problem-based learning in an integrated and system-based curriculum. Audiovisual facilities, seminars, small-group discussions, panels, field work, and case studies are used extensively. Teaching of clinical skills starts during the first month of the program and is offered through a continuous and integrated program throughout the preclinical years. The program is offered in three different sites: Moncton (New Brunswick), Saguenay and Sherbrooke (Quebec). Community-based education is a

major characteristic of the clerkship. The clerkship is 18 months long. Clinical training starts with the winter trimester of the third year. Clerkship rotations are offered in a network of primary to tertiary health care institutions located in urban, suburban, peripheral, rural and remote areas in the Province of Québec and New Brunswick which offer complementary experience to the students. Each student must spend at least 1/3 of their clerkship in community-based settings. Postgraduate programs are available in most clinical disciplines including community health. A joint M.D./M.Sc. program is offered to students who are enrolled in the M.D. program with outstanding academic records. Its objective is to form physicians who will have achieved a scientific approach of medicine and who will also be able to pursue scientific activities among a team.

USMLE

Step 1: Optional.
Step 2: Clinical Skills (CS): Optional.
Step 2: Clinical Knowledge (CK): Optional.

Selection Factors

Admission to the Faculty of Medicine is primarily based on ability and premedical achievement, as demonstrated by students academic records. Learning skills tests (MMI and/or TAAMUS) are included in the selection. Candidates from the province of Quebec are required to participate in the Multiple Mini Interviews (MMI) in addition to the Test d'aptitudes à l'apprentissage de la médecine à l'Université de Sherbrooke (TAAMUS). One-hundred and seventy (170) places are reserved for applicants from the province of Quebec (3 of these positions may be filled by French-speaking students coming from Western Canadian provinces and Territories). In addition, twenty-four (24) places are reserved for applicants from New Brunswick, one (1) place is available for an applicant from Prince Edward Island, one (1) place is available for an applicant from Newfoundland and three (3) places are available for applicants from Nova Scotia. One (1) to six (6) places are available for Canadian Forces candidates. One (1) to four (4) places are available for applicants from

First Nations and Inuits from Quebec and one (1) place is available for a qualified foreign applicant with a student visa. In 2008, two-hundred and one (201) students entered into the program. Approximately the same number should enter the program next year (2009–2010). Applicants must be fluent in both written and spoken French language.

Financial Aid

Financial aid is available to resident students through the Bursaries Division of the Provincial Ministry of Education, the Scholarships and Loans Committee of the university, and a few private foundations.

Campus Information

Setting

The Faculty's main campus is located on the Health Sciences Campus of the University in a joint building with the 682-bed University Hospital and major Research Center.

Enrollment

For 2008, total enrollment was: 749

Satellite Campuses/Facilities

Our Saguenay satellite campus is located at the Université du Québec à Chicoutimi and at the Chicoutimi regional Hospital. Our Moncton satellite campus is located at the Université de Moncton and partners with Hospital Georges L. Dumont, the French-speaking regional hospital in Moncton.

Application Process and Requirements 2010–2011

Primary Application Service: School-specific
Earliest filing date: November 1, 2009
Latest filing date: All candidates must return their admission form before January 15, 2010, except for Quebec College students with no (0) university credit who can return their admission form until March 1, 2010.

Secondary Application Required?: No
Sent to: Bureau de la registraire - Université de Sherbrooke
URL: n/a
Fee: Yes, $70
Fee waiver available: No
Earliest filing date: n/a
Latest filing date: n/a

MCAT® required?: No
Latest MCAT® considered: n/a
Oldest MCAT® considered: n/a

Early Decision Program
School does not have EDP
Applicants notified: n/a
EDP available for: n/a

Regular Acceptance Notice
Earliest date: May 2010
Latest date: Varies

Applicant's Response to Acceptance
Offer – Maximum Time: Varies. 1–15 days, depending on when the acceptance notice is sent.

Requests for Deferred
Entrance Considered: No

Deposit to Hold Place in Class: Yes
Deposit (Resident): $200
Deposit (Non-resident): $200
Deposit due: With response to acceptance offer
Applied to tuition: Yes
Deposit refundable: No
Refundable by: n/a

Estimated number of new entrants: 204
EDP: n/a, special program: n/a

Start Month/Year: August 2010

Interview Format: The process includes learning skills tests (MMI and/or TAAMUS). Regional interviews are not available.

Other Programs

PREPARATORY PROGRAMS
Postbaccalaureate Program: No
Summer Program: No

COMBINED DEGREE PROGRAMS
Baccalaureate/M.D.: No
M.D./M.P.H.: No
M.D./M.B.A.: No
M.D./J.D.: No
M.D./Ph.D.: Yes, Dr. Claude Asselin, www.usherbrooke.ca/doctorat_medecine (819) 564-5276, Claude.Asselin@USherbrooke.ca
MD-M.Sc. master degrees: Yes, www.usherbrooke.ca/doctorat_medecine Dr. Claude Asselin, (819) 564-5276, Claude.Asselin@USherbrooke.ca

Premedical Coursework

Course	Req.	Rec.	Lab.	Sems.	Course	Req.	Rec.	Lab.	Sems.
Inorganic Chemistry					Computer Science				
Behavioral Sciences					Genetics				
Biochemistry					Humanities				
Biology	•		•	2	Organic Chemistry	•		•	3
Biology/Zoology					Physics	•		•	3
Calculus					Psychology				
College English					Social Sciences				
College Mathematics	•		•	2	Other				

Selection Factors: 2008 Accepted Applicants

Proportion of Accepted Applicants with Relevant Experience (Data Self-Reported to AMCAS®)		
Community Service/Volunteer	0
Medically-Related Work	0
Research	0

Shaded bar represents school's accepted scores ranging from the 10th percentile to the 90th percentile ▪   School Median ●   National Median ●

Overall GPA	2.0	2.1	2.2	2.3	2.4	2.5	2.6	2.7	2.8	2.9	3.0	3.1	3.2	3.3	3.4	3.5	3.6	3.7	3.8	3.9	4.0
Science GPA	2.0	2.1																		.9	4.0
MCAT® Total Numeric S																				41 42 43
Verbal Reasoning	3					**DATA NOT COLLECTED**														15
Physical Sciences	3																				15
Biological Sciences	3																				15
Writing Sample						J	K	L	M	N	O	P	Q	R	S						T

Acceptance & Matriculation Data for 2008–2009 First Year Class

	Resident	Non-resident	International	Total
Applications	1668	109	72	1849
Interviewed	693	81	1	775
Deferred	0	0	0	0
Matriculants				
Early Assurance Program	0	0	0	0
Early Decision Program	0	0	0	0
Baccalaureate/M.D.	0	0	0	0
M.D./Ph.D.	0	0	0	0
Matriculated	167	33	1	**201**

Applications accepted from International Applicants: Yes

Matriculant Demographics: 2008–2009 First Year Class

Men: 80   **Women:** 121

Matriculants' Self-Reported Race/Ethnicity

Mexican American	Korean
Cuban	Vietnamese
Puerto Rican	Other Asian
Other H	
Total Hi	**DATA NOT COLLECTED**
Chinese	
Asian In	
Pakistan	Total Asian
Filipino	**Unduplicated Number**
Japanese	**of Matriculants**

Science and Math Majors: n/a
Matriculants with:
     Baccalaureate degree: 14%
     Graduate degree(s): 1%

Specialty Choice

2004, 2005, 2006 Graduates, Specialty Choice
Anesthesiology
Emergency Medicine
Family Practice
DATA NOT COLLECTED
Psychiatry
Radiology
Surgery

Financial Information

	Residents	Non-residents
Total Cost of Attendance	$10,330	$17,600-31,000
Tuition and Fees	$4,330	$11,600-25,000
Other (includes living expenses)	$600/month	600/month
Health Insurance (waived)	n/a	n/a

Average 2008 Graduate Indebtedness: $26,000
% of Enrolled Students Receiving Aid: 52%

Criminal Background Check

This medical school does not require a criminal background check prior to matriculation.

University of Saskatchewan College of Medicine
Saskatoon, Saskatchewan

Admissions
University of Saskatchewan College of Medicine
A204 Health Sciences Bld, 107 Wiggins Rd
Saskatoon, Saskatchewan
Canada, S7N 5E5
T 306 966 8554   **F** 306 966 2601

Admissions www.medicine.usask.ca/admissions
Main www.medicine.usask.ca
Financial www.usask.ca/calendar/scholarships
E-mail med.admissions@usask.ca

Public Institution

Dr. William L. Albritton, Dean

Dr. Barry Ziola, Director, Admissions & Student Affairs

Heather Mandeville, Administrative Coordinator, Admissions & Student Affairs

General Information
The University of Saskatchewan began teaching medical students in a two-year medical sciences program in 1926. The present college was introduced in 1953, with a four-year curriculum leading to the M.D. degree. In 1968, the curriculum changed to five years with a one-year premedical university requirement. The curriculum reverted to a four-year program in 1988 with a minimum two-year premedical requirement. Clinical teaching is based at the Royal University, St. Paul's, and Saskatoon City Hospitals in Saskatoon, and the Plains Health Centre and General Hospital in Regina. Students also complete rotations in Saskatchewan Health Regions. The class size is 84 students with future possible expansions to 100 students.

Mission Statement
The College of Medicine is a departmentalized collegial unit of the University of Saskatchewan. The mission is to improve health through excellence in education, research, and clinical care.

Curricular Highlights
Community Service Requirement: Optional.
Research/Thesis Requirement: Optional.

The College of Medicine provides a curriculum leading to the general professional education of the physician; graduates may select careers in family medicine, specialty practice, or research. The current curriculum was launched in the fall of 1997. Phase A (31 weeks) provides students with an overview of the basic science disciplines appropriate to the study of medicine, as well as an introduction to professional skills (including primary clinical skills) within the context of developing the patient-doctor relationship. This phase includes a two-week clinical experience done

in one of the Saskatchewan Health Districts. Phase B (33 weeks) enables students to acquire specific knowledge in those subjects bridging the basic and clinical sciences and to enhance basic clinical skills. Phase C (15 weeks), enables learning of the principles and methods in core clinical knowledge and linking courses. Phase D (64 weeks) of clinical clerkships provides an opportunity to apply the knowledge, skills, and attitudes students have acquired to the management of patients. Provision is made for clinical electives. Learning in the basic and clinical sciences has been organized by body systems with a problem-solving emphasis.

USMLE
Step 1: n/a
Step 2: Clinical Skills (CS): n/a
Step 2: Clinical Knowledge (CK): n/a

Selection Factors
The Admissions Committee considers academic ability and personal qualities assessed through scholastic records, letters of recommendation, and results of an interview. All eligible candidates are interviewed during a weekend in March.

Financial Aid
Various loan funds and scholarships are available. A limited number of bursaries enable students to engage in research between the end of one academic year and the beginning of another.

Information about Diversity Programs
There is an Aboriginal Access Program for Canadian residents of Aboriginal ancestry. For more information, contact the Admissions office.

Campus Information

Setting
Our medical school is situated on 755 hectares of land, in the heart of the city of Saskatoon on the scenic bank of the South Saskatchewan River. Much of the original architecture remains from the University's opening in 1909, and greystone buildings ornamented with garrets and turrets are a monument of fine craftsmanship. The University of Saskatchewan has

the largest collection of health sciences in Canada.

Enrollment
For 2008, total enrollment was: 272

Housing
As a student at the University of Saskatchewan, you have several options for finding appropriate, affordable housing. Students may choose from both on- and off-campus accommodations. Living in residence offers the opportunity to meet people from all colleges and cultures and you will become more familiar with the opportunities offered at university, both social and academic. To find out more about housing and residence at the University of Saskatchewan, please visit *http://explore.usask.ca/about/housing/*.

Satellite Campuses/Facilities
The University of Saskatchewan College of Medicine has a distributive learning environment in which a number of clinical educational experiences take place in a number of Saskatchewan Health Regions and teaching hospitals. Students will be assigned to a core set of rotations centered either in the Saskatoon Health Region or in the Regina/Qu'Appelle Health Region.

Application Process and Requirements 2010–2011

Primary Application Service: School-specific
Earliest filing date: July 1, 2009
Latest filing date: October 30, 2009

Secondary Application Required?: No
Sent to: n/a
URL: www.medicine.usask.ca/admissions
Fee: n/a
Fee waiver available: n/a
Earliest filing date: n/a
Latest filing date: n/a

MCAT® required?: Yes
Latest MCAT® considered: September 2009
Oldest MCAT® considered: April 2004

Early Decision Program
School does not have EDP
Applicants notified: May 15, 2010
EDP available for: n/a

Regular Acceptance Notice
Earliest date: May 15, 2010
Latest date: Until Class is Full

Applicant's Response to Acceptance
Offer – Maximum Time: Two weeks

Requests for Deferred
Entrance Considered: Yes

Deposit to Hold Place in Class: Yes
Deposit (Resident): $500
Deposit (Non-resident): $500
Deposit due: With response to acceptance offer
Applied to tuition: Yes
Deposit refundable: No
Refundable by: n/a

Estimated number of new entrant: 84
EDP: 0, special program: n/a

Start Month/Year: August 2010

Interview Format: Multiple Mini Interview. Regional Interviews are not available.

Other Programs

PREPARATORY PROGRAMS
Postbaccalaureate Program: No
Summer Program: No

COMBINED DEGREE PROGRAMS
Baccalaureate/M.D.: No
M.D./M.P.H.: No
M.D./M.B.A.: No
M.D./J.D.: No
M.D./Ph.D.: Yes, www.medicine.usask.ca/research/clinical_programs

Premedical Coursework

Course	Req.	Rec.	Lab.	Hrs.
Inorganic Chemistry	•		•	3
Behavioral Sciences				
Biochemistry	•			6
Biology	•		•	6
Biology/Zoology				
Calculus				
College English	•			6
College Mathematics				

Course	Req.	Rec.	Lab.	Hrs.
Computer Science				
Genetics				
Humanities	•			
Organic Chemistry	•		•	3
Physics	•		•	6
Psychology				
Social Sciences	•			6
Other				

Selection Factors: 2008 Accepted Applicants

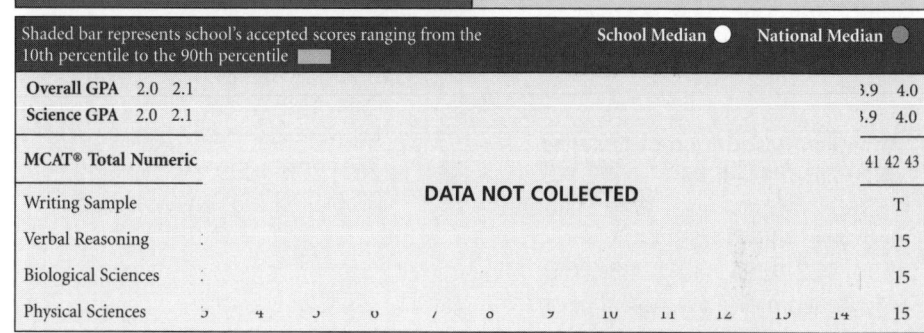

Proportion of Accepted Applicants with Relevant Experience (Data Self-Reported to AMCAS®)		**DATA NOT COLLECTED**	

Shaded bar represents school's accepted scores ranging from the 10th percentile to the 90th percentile. School Median ● National Median ●

Overall GPA	2.0 2.1	3.9 4.0
Science GPA	2.0 2.1	3.9 4.0
MCAT® Total Numeric		41 42 43
Writing Sample	**DATA NOT COLLECTED**	T
Verbal Reasoning		15
Biological Sciences		15
Physical Sciences	3 4 5 6 7 8 9 10 11 12 13 14	15

Acceptance & Matriculation Data for 2008–2009 First Year Class

	Resident	Non-resident	International	Total
Applications	223	368	n/a	591
Interviewed	202	50	n/a	252
Deferred	2	0	n/a	2
Matriculants				
Early Assurance Program	n/a	n/a	n/a	n/a
Early Decision Program	n/a	n/a	n/a	n/a
Baccalaureate/M.D.	n/a	n/a	n/a	n/a
M.D./Ph.D.	n/a	n/a	n/a	n/a
Matriculated	84	n/a	n/a	**84**

Applications accepted from International Applicants: No

Specialty Choice

2004, 2005, 2006 Graduates, Specialty Choice
Anesthesiology
Emergency Medicine
Family Practice
Internal Medicine
DATA NOT COLLECTED
Psychiatry
Radiology
Surgery

Matriculant Demographics: 2008–2009 First Year Class

Men: 33   **Women:** 51

Matriculants' Self-Reported Race/Ethnicity

Mexican American	n/a	**Korean**	n/a
Cuban	n/a	**Vietnamese**	n/a
Puerto Rican	n/a	**Other Asian**	n/a
Other			/a
Total			/a
Chine	**DATA NOT COLLECTED**		/a
Asian			/a
Pakist			/a
Filipin			
Japanese	n/a	of Matriculants	60

Science and Math Majors: n/a
Matriculants with:
 Baccalaureate degree: 39%
 Graduate degree(s): 2%

Financial Information

	Residents	Non-residents
Total Cost of Attendance	n/r	n/r
Tuition and Fees	$11,460	n/r
Other (includes living expenses)	n/r	n/r
Health Insurance (can be waived)	n/a	n/a

Average 2008 Graduate Indebtedness: n/r
% of Enrolled Students Receiving Aid: n/r

Criminal Background Check

This medical school does not require a criminal background check prior to matriculation.

Resources for
Other Health Careers

1. **American Association of Colleges
   of Osteopathic Medicine**
   5550 Friendship Boulevard, Suite 310
   Chevy Chase, MD 20815-7231
   (301) 968-4100; *www.aacom.org*

2. **American Association of Colleges
   of Pharmacy**
   1727 King Street
   Alexandria, VA 22314-2815
   (703) 739-2330; *www.aacp.org*

3. **American Association of Colleges
   of Podiatric Medicine**
   15850 Crabbs Branch Way, Suite 320
   Rockville, MD 20855-4307
   (800) 922-9266; (301) 948-9760
   info@aacpm.org; *www.aacpm.org*

4. **American Association
   of Dental Schools**
   1400 K Street, N.W., Suite 1100
   Washington, D.C. 20005
   (202) 289-7201; *www.adea.org*

5. **Association of American
   Veterinary Medical Colleges**
   1101 Vermont Avenue, N.W., Suite 301
   Washington, D.C. 20005-3521
   (202) 371-9195; *www.aavmc.org*

6. **Association of Schools
   and Colleges of Optometry**
   6110 Executive Boulevard, Suite 420
   Rockville, MD 20852
   (301) 231-5944
   admini@opted.org; *www.opted.org*

7. **Association of Schools
   of Public Health**
   1101 15th Street, N.W., Suite 910
   Washington, D.C., 20005
   (202) 296-1099
   info@asph.org; *www.asph.org*

Publications for the Health Professions

1. 300 Ways to Put Your Talent to Work in the Health Field

Single copy, $15 member,
$18.00 non-member
National Health Council
1730 M Street, N.W., Suite 500
Washington, D.C. 20036
(202) 785-3910;
*www.nationalhealthcouncil.org/
pubs/pubs_index.htm*

2. Autsin, L., What's Holding You Back? 8 Critical Choices for Women's Success

$14.00
Basic Books, 2000
*www.perseusbooksgroup.com/basic/
home.jsp*

3. Bickel, J., Women in Medicine: Getting In, Growing & Advancing

$38.95
Sage, 2000
(805) 499-9774; *www.sagepub.com*

4. Educational Survival Skills Study Guide

Free
Office of Statewide Health
Planning and Development
Health Professions Career
Opportunity Program
1600 Ninth Street, Room 441
Sacramento, CA 95814
*www.oshpd.ca.gov/HWDD/pdfs/
StudySkills.pdf*

5. Financial Advice and Health Careers Resources Directory for Students

Free
Office of Statewide Health
Planning and Development
Health Professions Careers
Opportunity Program
1600 Ninth Street, Room 441
Sacramento, CA 95814
*www.oshpd.ca.gov/HWDD/pdfs/
FinancialAdvice.pdf*

6. The Journal for Minority Medical Students

$5.00, published quarterly
Spectrum Unlimited
630 Goldpoint Trace
Woodstock, GA 30189
(800) 661-3319, (504) 433-5040

7. Kaltreider, Nancy B., Dilemmas of a Double Life, Women Balancing Careers and Relationship

$44.95
Jason Aronson, Inc., 1997
(800) 462-6420;
www.rowmanlittlefield.com/Catalog/

8. Minorities in Medicine: A Guide for Premedical Students

Free
Office of Statewide Health Planning
and Development
Health Professions Career
Opportunity Program
1600 Ninth Street, Room 441
Sacramento, CA 95814
*www.oshpd.ca.gov/HWDD/pdfs/
MinoritiesMedicine.pdf*

9. Minority Student Opportunities in United States Medical Schools

$15.00, published bi-annually
Association of American
Medical Colleges
2450 N Street, N.W.
Washington, D.C. 20037
(202) 828-0416;
www.aamc.org/publications

10. More, E.S., Restoring the Balance: Women Physicians and the Profession of Medicine, 1850–1995.

$62.50 hardcover, $31.00 paperback
Harvard University Press, 2000
www.hup.harvard.edu

11. Need a Lift? College Financial Aid Handbook

$3.00, plus shipping
The American Legion
P.O. Box 1050
Indianapolis, IN 46206
888-453-4466;
www.emblem.legion.org

12. The Student Guide

U.S. Department of Education Federal
Student Aid Information Center
P.O. Box 84
Washington, D.C. 20044-0084
(800) 4-FED-AID, (800) 433-3243
*http://studentaid.ed.gov/students/
attachments/siteresources/Funding
EduBeyondHighSchool_0809.pdf*

13. Time Management for Students

Free
Office of Statewide Health
Planning and Development
Health Professions Career
Opportunity Program
1600 Ninth Street, Room 441
Sacramento, CA 95814
*www.oshpd.ca.gov/HWDD/pdfs/
TimeManagement.pdf*

14. Wear, D. (Ed), Women in Medical Education: An Anthology of Experience

$22.50 hardcover, $21.95 paperback
SUNY Press, 1996
*www.sunypress.edu/details.
asp?id=53512*

15. The Young Scientist: A Career Guide for Underrepresented Science Graduates

$5.00, published annually
Spectrum Unlimited
630 Goldpoint Trace
Woodstock, GA 30189
(504) 433-5040

You can change the face of medicine.

From left: Romeu Azevedo, M.D., Candelaria Martin, M.D., Kahlil Johnson, M.D., Claudine Morcos, M.D.

If you really want to make a difference in people's lives, consider a career in medicine. Too many African Americans, Latinos/as, and Native Americans don't get the care they need. Help us change this reality. Log on to **AspiringDocs.org™**, a new resource from the Association of American Medical Colleges, to learn more.

Tomorrow's Doctors, Tomorrow's Cures®

© 2009 AAMC

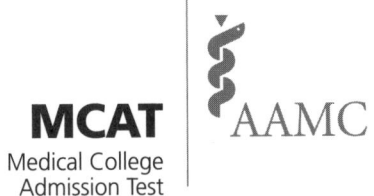

Available Now . . .
"The Official Guide to the MCAT Exam"

Inside You Will Find....

- Passages and questions from actual MCAT exams

- Detailed analyses of both the correct and incorrect answers

- Tips to help you come up with the right solutions

- An analysis of the types of questions you'll find on the exam

- Sample essays and scoring analyses

- The "difficulty levels" of questions, revealing what percentages of examinees answered correctly in the real-life test

- Data that show you how your scores compare to those who apply to medical school

- Data to help determine how likely you are to increase or decrease your scores upon a retake, and by how many points

- A look at how MCAT scores factor into the admissions decision, with insights from a former associate dean of admissions

- Data that show what percentage of applicants were admitted to medical school, based on MCAT scores and GPAs combined

- *and much more!*

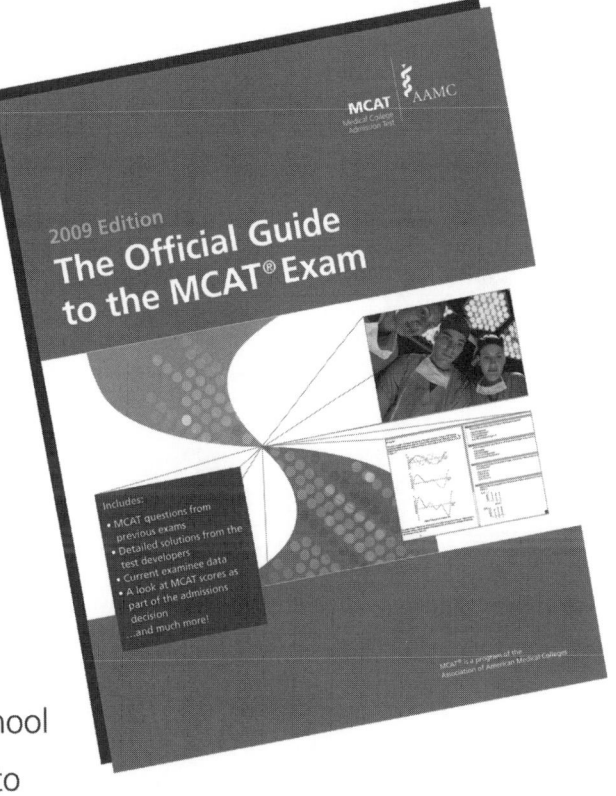

For pricing and ordering information, please visit www.aamc.org/officialmcatguide

MCAT® is a program of the
Association of American Medical Colleges

Created by the AAMC, FIRST *for Medical Education* offers a full range of **F**inancial **I**nformation, **R**esources, **S**ervices, and **T**ools for applicants, medical school students, residents, advisors, and financial aid officers. Our goal is to help medical school borrowers expand their financial literacy, make smart decisions about student loans, and manage their student debt wisely.

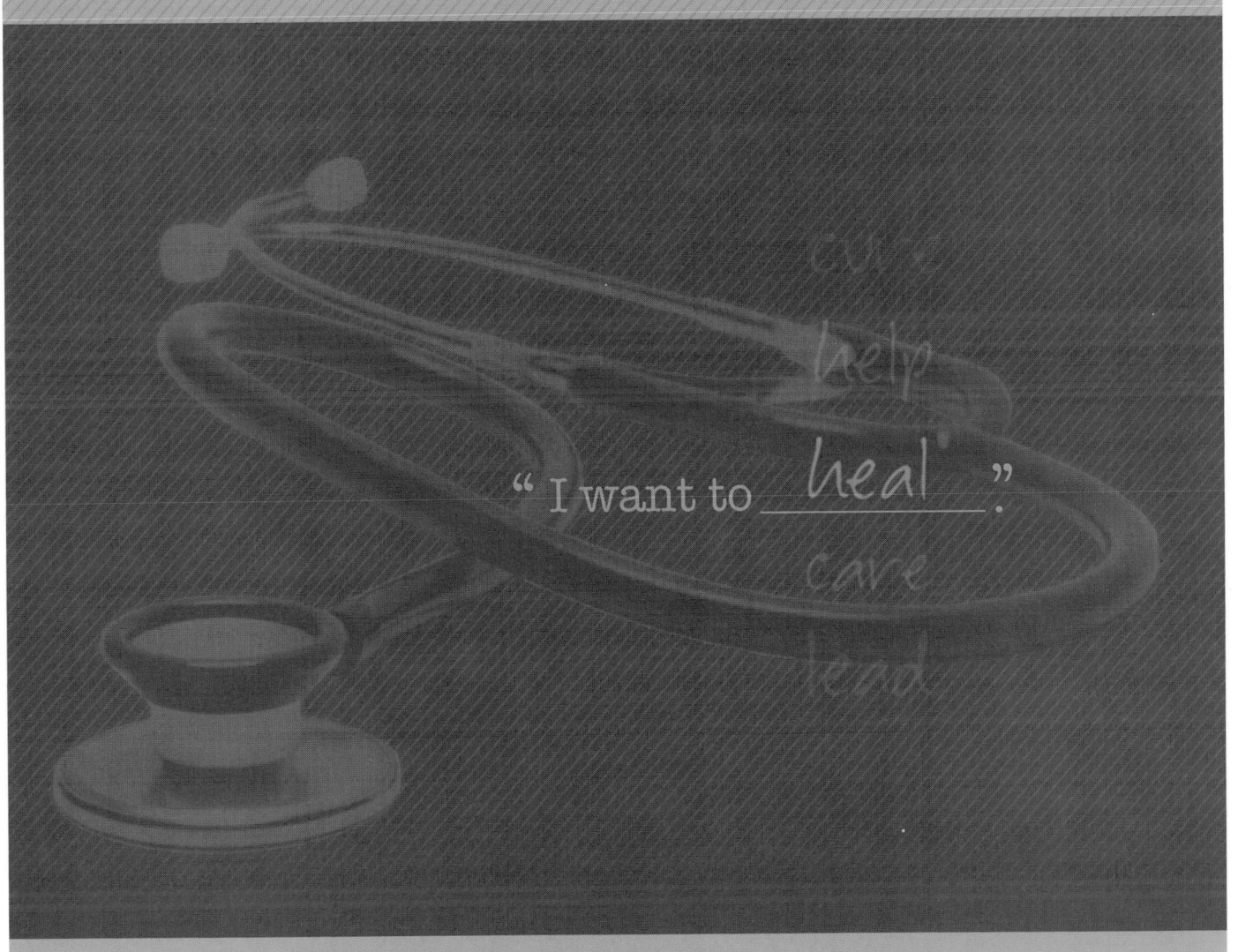

Take control of your debt! Log on to
www.aamc.org/first